Distal Radius Fractures

Evidence-Based Management

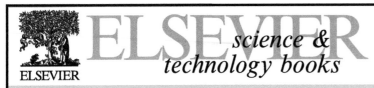

Companion Web Site: 9780323907583

https://www.elsevier.com/books-and-journals/book-companion/9780323757645

Distal Radius Fractures

Jesse Jupiter, Michel Chammas, Geert Alexander Buijze, Editors

ELSEVIER

Distal Radius Fractures

Evidence-Based Management

EDITED BY

JESSE JUPITER

Harvard Medical School, Department Of Orthopedic Surgery, Massachusetts General Hospital, Past President, American Shoulder and Elbow Surgeons, Past President, American Association of Hand Surgery

MICHEL CHAMMAS

Associate Dean, Montpellier-Nîmes Medical University, Montpellier, France

Professor of Orthopaedic Surgery, Hand and Upper Extremity Surgery Unit, Lapeyronie Hospital, Montpellier, France

Montpellier University Medical Center, Montpellier, France

EDITOR-IN-CHIEF

GEERT ALEXANDER BUIJZE

Hand and Upper Limb Surgery Unit, Clinique Générale, Annecy, France

Hand and Upper Extremity Surgery Unit, Lapeyronie Hospital, Montpellier University Medical Center, Montpellier, France

Department of Orthopaedic Surgery, Amsterdam University Medical Center, Amsterdam, Netherlands

ELSEVIER

Elsevier
Radarweg 29, PO Box 211, 1000 AE Amsterdam, Netherlands
The Boulevard, Langford Lane, Kidlington, Oxford OX5 1GB, United Kingdom
50 Hampshire Street, 5th Floor, Cambridge, MA 02139, United States

Notices

Knowledge and best practice in this field are constantly changing. As new research and experience broaden our
understanding, changes in research methods, professional practices, or medical treatment may become
necessary.

Practitioners and researchers must always rely on their own experience and knowledge in evaluating and using
any information, methods, compounds, or experiments described herein. In using such information or methods
they should be mindful of their own safety and the safety of others, including parties for whom they have a
professional responsibility.

To the fullest extent of the law, neither the Publisher nor the authors, contributors, or editors, assume any liability
for any injury and/or damage to persons or property as a matter of products liability, negligence or otherwise, or
from any use or operation of any methods, products, instructions, or ideas contained in the material herein.

Library of Congress Cataloging-in-Publication Data
A catalog record for this book is available from the Library of Congress

British Library Cataloguing-in-Publication Data
A catalogue record for this book is available from the British Library

ISBN: **978-0-323-75764-5**

For information on all Elsevier publications
visit our website at https://www.elsevier.com/books-and-journals

Publisher: Cathleen Sether
Acquisitions Editor: Belinda Kuhn
Editorial Project Manager: Megan Ashdown
Production Project Manager: Kiruthika Govindaraju
Cover Designer: Alan Studholme

Typeset by SPi Global, India

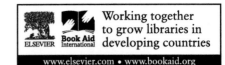

Working together
to grow libraries in
developing countries

www.elsevier.com • www.bookaid.org

This book is dedicated to all devoted healthcare workers on the COVID-19 frontline and their families whom we are humbly indebted for their immense sacrifices.

Contents

Section Editors

Laurent Obert
Orthopaedics, Traumatology, Plastic and Reconstructive Surgery Unit, Hand Surgery Unit, University Hospital J. Minjoz, Besançon, France

Robert J. Medoff
John A Burns School of Medicine, University of Hawaii, Kailua, HI, United States

Jong Pil Kim
Department of Orthopedic Surgery, Dankook University College of Medicine, Cheonan, South Korea

Yukichi Zenke
Department of Orthopaedics, University of Occupational and Environmental Health School of Medicine, Fukuoka, Japan

Andrew D. Duckworth
Edinburgh Orthopaedic Trauma and the University of Edinburgh, Royal Infirmary of Edinburgh, Edinburgh, United Kingdom

Niels W.L. Schep
Department of Trauma Surgery, Maasstad Hospital, Rotterdam, Netherlands

Michael Bouyer
Hand and Upper Limb Surgery Unit, Clinique Générale, Annecy, France

Thibault Lafosse
Hand and Upper Limb Surgery Unit, Clinique Générale, Annecy, France

Tommy R. Lindau
Pulvertaft Hand Centre, University Hospitals Derby and Burton; University of Derby, Derby, United Kingdom

Ruby Grewal
Roth | McFarlane Hand and Upper Limb Center, St Joseph's Health Care, London, ON, Canada

Job N. Doornberg
Department of Orthopaedic Surgery, Amsterdam University Medical Centre, University of Amsterdam, Amsterdam, The Netherlands; Flinders Medical Centre, Department of Orthopaedic Surgery, Flinders University, Adelaide, SA; Department of Orthopaedics and Trauma, Flinders Medical Centre, Adelaide, Australia

A. Lee Osterman
Philadelphia Hand to Shoulder Center, King of Prussia, PA, United States

Joost W. Colaris
Orthopedics, Erasmus MC; Resident Orthopedic Surgein, Orthopedic Surgery, ETZ, Tilburg, Rotterdam, Netherlands

Tamara Rozental
Department of Orthopaedics at Beth Israel Hospital, Harvard Medical School, Boston, MA, United States

Alexander Y. Shin
Department of Orthopedic Surgery, Mayo Clinic, Rochester, MN, United States

Joseph Dias
University Hospitals of Leicester, Leicester, United Kingdom

Peter Axelsson
Department of Hand Surgery, Institute of Clinical Sciences, Sahlgrenska Academy, University of Gothenburg; Department of Hand Surgery, Sahlgrenska University Hospital, Gothenburg, Sweden

Contributing Authors

Yukio Abe
Department of Orthopaedic Surgery, Saiseikai Shimonoseki General Hospital, Shimonoseki City, Yamaguchi, Japan

Márcio Aurélio Aita
Faculdade de Medicina do ABC, Centro Hospitalar Municipal de Santo André (University ABC Hospital), São Bernardo do Campo, São Paulo, Brazil

Jose Manuel Perez Alba
Orthopedic Surgery and Traumatology Service, Hospital Universitario del Vinalopo, Elche, Alicante, Spain

Daniel Axelrod
Division of Orthopaedic Surgery, McMaster University, Center for Evidence Based Orthopaedics, Hamilton, ON, Canada

Peter Axelsson
Department of Hand Surgery, Institute of Clinical Sciences, Sahlgrenska Academy, University of Gothenburg; Department of Hand Surgery, Sahlgrenska University Hospital, Gothenburg, Sweden

Thomas Bauer
Orthopedic and Traumatology Department,Hôpital Ambroise Pare, Paris University Hospitals, Boulogne-Billancourt, France

Katrina R. Bell
Edinburgh Orthopaedic, Royal Infirmary of Edinburgh, Edinburgh, United Kingdom; University of Edinburgh, Edinburgh, United Kingdom

J.H.J.M. Bessems
Orthopedics, Erasmus MC, Rotterdam, Netherlands

Mohit Bhandari
Division of Orthopaedic Surgery, McMaster University, Center for Evidence Based Orthopaedics, Hamilton, ON, Canada

Julia Blackburn
Pulvertaft Hand Centre, University Hospitals Derby and Burton, Derby, United Kingdom

Taco J. Blokhuis
Department of Trauma Surgery, Maastricht University Medical Centre, Maastricht, Netherlands

Michel E.H. Boeckstyns
Department of Orthopedic Surgery, Section of Hand Surgery, Herlev-Gentofte Hospital; Capio Private Hospital, Hellerup, Denmark

Michael Bouyer
Hand and Upper Limb Surgery Unit, Clinique Générale, Annecy, France

Vicente Carratalá Baixauli
Hand and Upper Limb Surgery Unit, Quirónsalud Valencia Hospital, Valencia, Spain

Maurizio Calcagni
Department of Plastic Surgery and Hand Surgery, University Hospital Zurich, Zurich, Switzerland

Andrea Chan
University of Toronto—Toronto Western Hospital, Toronto, ON, Canada

Christophe Chantelot
Orthopedic and Traumatology Department, Hôpital Roger Salengro, Lille University Hospital, Lille, France

Léo Chiche
Hand and Upper Extremity Surgery Unit, Lapeyronie Hospital, Montpellier University Medical Center, Montpellier, France

Kevin C. Chung
Department of Surgery, Michigan Medicine, Ann Arbor, MI, United States

Joost W. Colaris
Department of Orthopedics, Erasmus MC, Rotterdam, Netherlands

Fernando Corella Montoya
Hand Surgery Unit, Infanta Leonor Hospital;
Quirónsalud Madrid Hospital, Madrid, Spain

Elissa S. Davis
Department of Surgery, Michigan Medicine, Ann Arbor,
MI, United States

Francisco del Piñal
Institute for Hand and Plastic Surgery in Madrid and
Santander, Spain

Joseph Dias
University Hospitals of Leicester, Leicester, United
Kingdom

Job N. Doornberg
Department of Orthopaedic Surgery, Flinders Medical
Centre and Flinders University, Adelaide, SA,Australia;
Department of Orthopaedic Surgery, Amsterdam
University Medical Centre, Amsterdam; Department
of Orthopaedic Surgery, University Medical Centre
Groningen and Groningen University, Groningen,
The Netherlands

C.C. Drijfhout van Hooff
Department of Trauma Surgery, Maasstad Hospital,
Rotterdam, Netherlands

Andrew D. Duckworth
Edinburgh Orthopaedics, Royal Infirmary of Edinburgh,
Edinburgh, United Kingdom; University of Edinburgh,
Edinburgh, United Kingdom

Matthieu Ehlinger
Orthopedic and Traumatology Department, Hôpital de
Hautepierre, Strasbourg University Hospital,
Strasbourg, France

K.R. Esposito
Columbia University, Department of Orthopedic
Surgery, New York, NY, United States

Sybille Facca
Department of Hand Surgery, SOS Hand, University
Hospital of Strasbourg, FMTS, University of Strasbourg,
Strasbourg, France

Simon Farnebo
Department of Hand Surgery and Plastic Surgery, and
Burns; Department of Biomedical and Clinical Sciences,
Linköping, Linköping University, Linköping, Sweden

Per Fredrikson
Department of Hand Surgery, Institute of Clinical
Sciences, Sahlgrenska Academy, University of
Gothenburg, Gothenburg, Sweden

C.E. Freibott
Columbia University, Department of Orthopedic
Surgery, New York, NY, United States

Ignacio Miranda Gómez
Orthopedic Surgery and Traumatology Department,
Arnau de Vilanova Hospital, Valencia, Spain

Stéphanie Gouzou
Department of Hand Surgery, SOS Hand, University
Hospital of Strasbourg, FMTS, University of Strasbourg,
Strasbourg, France

Ruby Grewal
Roth | McFarlane Hand and Upper Limb Center,
St Joseph's Health Care, Western University, London,
ON, Canada

Marco Guidi
Department of Plastic Surgery and Hand Surgery,
University Hospital Zurich, Zurich, Switzerland

Pascal F.W. Hannemann
Department of Trauma Surgery, Maastricht University
Medical Centre, Maastricht, Netherlands

Carl M. Harper
Department of Orthopaedic Surgery, Harvard Medical
School, Beth Israel Deaconess Medical Center,
Boston, MA, United States

Sara F. Haynes
John Peter Smith Hospital, Department of Orthopaedic
Surgery, Fort Worth, TX, United States

R.L. Jaarsma
Department of Orthopaedic Surgery, Flinders Medical
Centre and Flinders University, Adelaide, SA, Australia

Herman Johal
Division of Orthopaedic Surgery, McMaster University, Center for Evidence Based Orthopaedics, Hamilton, ON, Canada

Nick Johnson
Pulvertaft Hand Centre, University Hospitals Derby and Burton, Derby; University Hospitals of Leicester, Leicester, United Kingdom

Hyoung-Seok Jung
Department of Orthopedic Surgery, Hospital of Chung-Ang University of Medicine, Seoul, Republic of Korea

Assaf Kadar
Roth|McFarlane Hand and Upper Limb Centre, St. Joseph's Health Care London; Department of Surgery, Division of Orthopaedic Surgery, Schulich School of Medicine & Dentistry, Western University, London, ON, Canada

Jong Pil Kim
Department of Orthopedic Surgery, Dankook University College of Medicine, Cheonan, South Korea

Steven M. Koehler
Department of Orthopaedic Surgery, SUNY Downstate Medical Center, Brooklyn, NY, United States

C.L.E. Laane
Trauma Research Unit, Department of Surgery, Erasmus MC, University Medical Center Rotterdam, Rotterdam, The Netherlands

Thibault Lafosse
Hand and Upper Limb Surgery Unit, Clinique Générale, Annecy, France

Hyun Il Lee
Department of Orthopedic Surgery, Ilsan Paik Hospital, Inje University, Goyang, South Korea

Jae-Sung Lee
Department of Orthopedic Surgery, Hospital of Chung-Ang University of Medicine, Seoul, Republic of Korea

Tommy R. Lindau
Pulvertaft Hand Centre, University Hospitals Derby and Burton; University of Derby, Derby, United Kingdom

Sandra Lindqvist
Department of Hand Surgery, Institute of Clinical Sciences, Sahlgrenska Academy, University of Gothenburg, Gothenburg, Sweden

Philippe Liverneaux
Department of Hand Surgery, SOS Hand, University Hospital of Strasbourg, FMTS, University of Strasbourg, Strasbourg, France

François Loisel
Orthopaedics, Traumatology, Plastic and Reconstructive Surgery Unit, Hand Surgery Unit, University Hospital J. Minjoz, Besançon, France

Francisco J. Lucas García
Hand and Upper Limb Surgery Unit, Quirónsalud Valencia Hospital, Valencia, Spain

Riccardo Luchetti
Rimini Hand and Upper Limb Surgery and Rehabilitation Center, Rimini, Italy

Jesse D. Meaike
Division of Plastic Surgery, Mayo Clinic, Rochester, MN, United States

Joshua J. Meaike
Department of Orthopedic Surgery, Mayo Clinic, Rochester, MN, United States

Robert J. Medoff
John A Burns School of Medicine, University of Hawaii, Kailua, HI, United States

Maartje Michielsen
Orthopedic Department, AZ Monica Hospital, Antwerp; Orthopedic Department, Antwerp University Hospital, Edegem, Belgium

Andrew Miller
Philadelphia Hand to Shoulder Center, Thomas Jefferson University Hospital, Philadelphia, PA, United States

Samuel G. Molyneux
Edinburgh Orthopaedics, Royal Infirmary of Edinburgh, Edinburgh, United Kingdom

Laurent Obert
Orthopaedics, Traumatology, Plastic and Reconstructive Surgery Unit, Hand Surgery Unit, University Hospital J. Minjoz, Besançon, France

A. Lee Osterman
Philadelphia Hand to Shoulder Center, King of Prussia, PA, United States

Ryan Paul
University of Toronto—Toronto Western Hospital, Toronto, ON, Canada

William F. Pientka, II
John Peter Smith Hospital, Department of Orthopaedic Surgery, Fort Worth, TX, United States

J.J.W. Ploegmakers
Department of Orthopedics, UMCG, Groningen, The Netherlands

Sasa Pocnetz
Pulvertaft Hand Centre, University Hospitals Derby and Burton, Derby, United Kingdom

A.R. Poublon
Department of Orthopedics, ETZ; Orthopedics, Elisabeth-TweeSteden Hospital, Tilburg, Netherlands

D. Ring
Department of Psychiatry and Perioperative Care, Dell Medical School, University of Texas at Austin, Austin, TX, United States

Tamara Rozental
Department of Orthopaedics at Beth Israel Hospital, Harvard Medical School, Boston, MA, United States

Marc Saab
Orthopedic and Traumatology Department, Hôpital Roger Salengro, Lille University Hospital, Lille, France

Natsumi Saka
Department of Orthopaedics, Teikyo University School of Medicine, Tokyo, Japan

Michael J. Sandow
Wakefield Orthopaedic Clinic, Adelaide, SA, Australia

Niels W.L. Schep
Department of Trauma Surgery, Maasstad Hospital, Rotterdam, Netherlands

B.J.A. Schoolmeesters
Department of Orthopaedic Surgery, Flinders Medical Centre and Flinders University, Adelaide, SA, Australia; Department of Orthopaedic Surgery, Amsterdam University Medical Centre, Amsterdam; Department of Orthopaedic Surgery, Amphia Hospital, Breda, The Netherlands

Alexander Y. Shin
Department of Orthopedic Surgery, Mayo Clinic, Rochester, MN, United States

S.C. Shoap
Columbia University, Department of Orthopedic Surgery, New York, NY, United States

Laura Sims
University of Saskatchewan, Saskatoon Orthopedic and Sports Medicine Center, Saskatoon, SK, Canada

R.J. Strauch
Columbia University, Department of Orthopedic Surgery, New York, NY, United States

Jason A. Strelzow
University of Chicago, Department of Orthopaedic Surgery and Rehabilitation Medicine, University of Chicago Medicine, Chicago, IL, United States

Nina Suh
Roth|McFarlane Hand and Upper Limb Centre, St. Joseph's Health Care London; Department of Surgery, Division of Orthopaedic Surgery, Schulich School of Medicine & Dentistry, Western University, London, ON, Canada

Youhei Takahashi
Department of Orthopaedic Surgery, Saiseikai Shimonoseki General Hospital, Shimonoseki City, Yamaguchi, Japan

Jin Bo Tang
Department of Hand Surgery, Affiliated Hospital of Nantong University, Nantong, Jiangsu, China

Jan A. Ten Bosch
Department of Trauma Surgery, Maastricht University Medical Centre, Maastricht, Netherlands

B. The
Department of Orthopaedic Surgery, Amphia Hospital, Breda, The Netherlands

Rick Tosti
Philadelphia Hand to Shoulder Center; Orthopaedic Surgery, Thomas Jefferson University Hospital, Philadelphia, PA, United States

A.E. van der Windt
Department of Orthopedics, Erasmus MC, Rotterdam, Netherlands

Matthias Vanhees
Orthopedic Department, AZ Monica Hospital, Antwerp; Orthopedic Department, Antwerp University Hospital, Edegem, Belgium

Paul Vernet
Department of Hand Surgery, SOS Hand, University Hospital of Strasbourg, FMTS, University of Strasbourg, Strasbourg, France

Frederik Verstreken
Orthopedic Department, AZ Monica Hospital, Antwerp; Orthopedic Department, Antwerp University Hospital, Edegem, Belgium

Timothy O. White
Edinburgh Orthopaedics, Royal Infirmary of Edinburgh, Edinburgh, United Kingdom

M.M.E. Wijffels
Trauma Research Unit, Department of Surgery, Erasmus MC, University Medical Center Rotterdam, Rotterdam, The Netherlands

Taylor Woolnough
Division of Orthopaedic Surgery, McMaster University, Center for Evidence Based Orthopaedics, Hamilton, ON, Canada

Grace Xiong
Harvard Combined Orthopaedic Surgery Residency, Harvard Medical School, Boston, MA, United States

Yukichi Zenke
Department of Orthopaedics, University of Occupational and Environmental Health School of Medicine, Fukuoka, Japan

Yiyang Zhang
Roth | McFarlane Hand and Upper Limb Center, St Joseph's Health Care, Western University, London, ON, Canada

Preface

The foundation of our hands merits judicious restoration. The most common fracture of all is the one involving the distal end of the radius. And with an increasing world-wide incidence, this topic merits frequent knowledge updates as well as the necessity to keep reevaluating the best evidence regarding its management. The philosophy of this evidence-based medicine range of books couldn't be better described than in the first (scaphoid fracture) edition by my inspiring mentor Professor David Ring: "As comfortable as habit can be, the one constant in life is change." Ergo, even though it may feel intuitive to pursue the lessons of our apprenticeship; advance means perpetually evolving our practice in line with the best available evidence.

This book is intended for anyone dealing with distal radius fractures (DRFs): all who are eager to keep up-to-date with the newest evidence on both diagnosis and treatment of simple "Colles" fractures as well as those seeking creative state-of-the-art solutions for managing more complex cases and sequalae—the whole spectrum is covered.

As most great innovations in DRF management now seem well behind and the previous decade was marked by a plethora of technique modifications, this new decade could be one of refinement by critical appraisal, where *Evidence-Based Management (EBM)* plays a major role shifting global paradigms toward universal cost-effective best practice. And at this time of the COVID-19 pandemic-related economic impact on global health care, there is an unprecedented need for improving evidence-based cost-effective treatment strategies.

The purpose of this book is to enhance your practice by bringing you the best of both worlds: *Evidence-Based Management & Expert-Based Opinion* combined. The innovative resultant format is what we like to label as *Best Practice*. While each chapter's core content is evidence-based management, it is encompassed by panels with practical expert-based content: case scenarios introducing key dilemmas engaging the reader to seek for the best solution as well as expert-based practice algorithms, step-by-step illustrated techniques, pearls and pitfalls from pioneers in the field.

The principles of this range of specialized EBM books are inspired by the pioneering work of Professor Mohit Bhandari and elucidated in Chapter 1. In brief, how does it work? Say you have a challenging psychiatric homeless patient who jumped from a height and among other severe injuries shattered her distal radius, as depicted on the cover of this book. Even though you may have been taught to "always ex-fix" these, a quick browse through Chapter 12 will give an evidence-based answer to your key question: what is the most effective treatment for this highly comminuted articular fracture? In fact, you may see that a bridging wrist spanning plate kept for 3 months is a safe and effective alternative with a predictable satisfactory result as in this case. Whereas in a complex articular fracture with good bone quality, you may want to consider dual plating and find the *Best Practice* along with Tips & Tricks in Chapter 11.

I wish to thank my former fellowship mentors, dear friends and co-editors Professors Jesse Jupiter and Michel Chammas for their precious and critical guidance as well as invaluable support in accomplishing this work. We are most grateful to all 17 Section Editors and 92 Contributing Authors from 17 countries around the world for investing their valuable spare time seeking the best available evidence and providing us with their highly valued experience to maximize the book's potential for the clinician. We are also indebted to Dr. David Slutsky for igniting this sequel of his inspiring cutting edge work. Moreover, this book could not have been realized without the excellent work and always optimistic support of editorial manager Mrs. Megan Ashdown. Finally and foremost, I wish to thank Erika, the love of my life and mother of our children, for supporting me throughout the "endless nights" needed to craft this book.

Now, feel free to pick any challenging topic and browse this book to help guide you toward *Evidence-Based Management* and enhance your *Best Practice* of the entire spectrum of DRFs and its sequalae.

Geert Alexander Buijze, Editor-in-Chief
Jesse Jupiter, Editor
Michel Chammas, Editor

CHAPTER 1

Principles of Evidence-Based Management of Distal Radius Fractures

TAYLOR WOOLNOUGH • DANIEL AXELROD • HERMAN JOHAL • MOHIT BHANDARI
Division of Orthopaedic Surgery, McMaster University, Center for Evidence Based Orthopaedics, Hamilton, ON, Canada

KEY POINTS

- Evidence-based management requires combination of the best evidence with patient values and provider preferences to make treatment decisions.
- The practice of evidence-based management involves question formulation, acquisition of related literature, appraisal of study quality, and the appropriate application of research findings to individual patients.
- Evidence-based management does not strictly depend on the results of randomized controlled trials, but more accurately involves the informed and effective use of all types of evidence.

Panel 1: Case Scenarios

CASE 1

A 75 year-old female trips and fall, landing on her outstretch right hand. She complains of right wrist pain when presenting to fracture clinic a few days later. Initial radiographs show a minimally displaced distal radius fracture (Fig.1A–C).

CASE 2

A 22 year-old male patient presents to the emergency room complaining of wrist pain after falling off a motorcycle,

Initial radiographs show a displaced radial styloid fracture (Fig. 2A–C).

How can you come to an evidence-based decision in the management of each of these patients' injuries?

What is the role of patients and provider preferences, practice environment and current literature in the end treatment chosen?

Continued

Distal Radius Fractures. https://doi.org/10.1016/B978-0-323-75764-5.00008-1

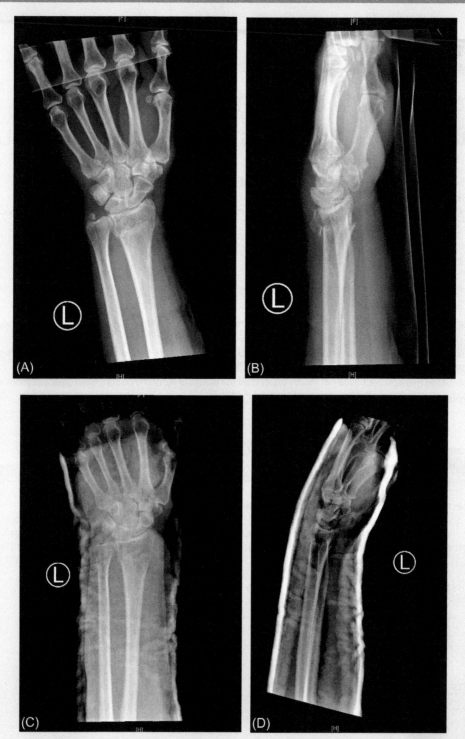

FIG. 1 (A, B) Initial radiographs showing a minimally displaced distal radius fracture. (C, D) Radiographs following initial reduction and immobilization in the emergency department.

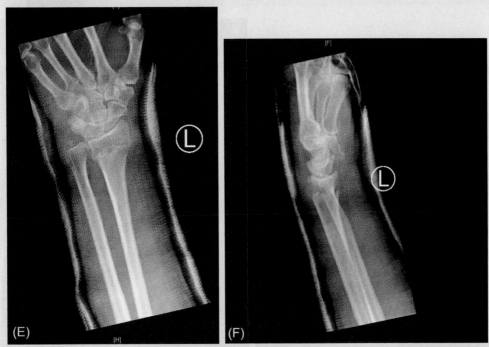

FIG. 1, CONT'D (E, F) Radiographs at two weeks demonstrating conversion to fiberglass casting material and mild shortening of the fracture with maintained sagital alignment.

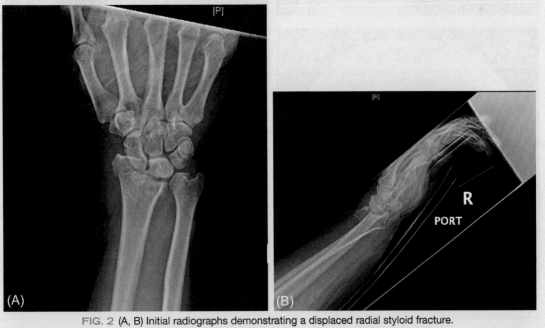

FIG. 2 (A, B) Initial radiographs demonstrating a displaced radial styloid fracture.

Continued

Panel 1: Case Scenarios—cont'd

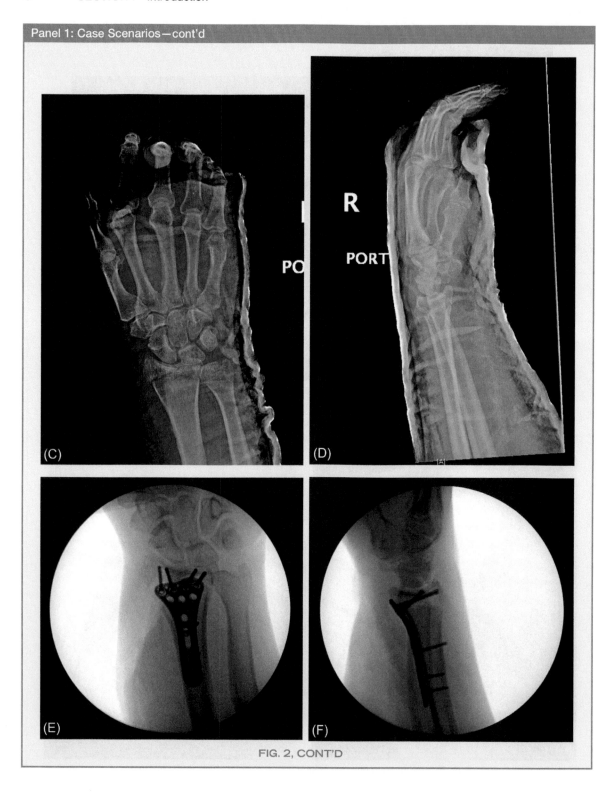

FIG. 2, CONT'D

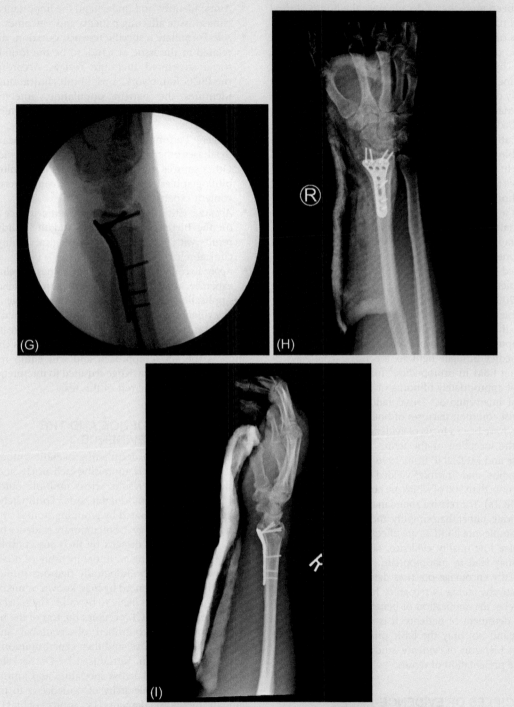

FIG. 2, CONT'D   (C, D) Radiographs following reduction and splint immobilization. (E–G) Intraoperative fluoroscopic images following open reduction and internal fixation with a volar locking plate. (H, I) Radiographs 2 weeks following fixation demonstrating maintained hardware position and fracture alignment.

It has been more than a decade since the *British Medical Journal* named the emergence of evidence-based medicine as one of the 15 greatest medical milestones since the inception of journal in 1840. First described in 1991 by Dr. Gordon Guyatt,[1] "evidence-based medicine" (EBM) describes a group of related principles initially developed by Dr. David Sackett and colleagues at McMaster University.[2] Evidence-based medicine is described in Dr. Sackett's seminal paper as, "integrating individual clinical expertise with the best available external clinical evidence from systematic research."[2] Gathering the best-available evidence requires a clear, clinically important question, followed by a thorough, systematic review of the literature, and finally a critical assessment of validity (i.e., relevance and quality) in light of the original question.[3] Dividing the paradigm of evidence-based medicine into three key components, practitioners are required to apply (1) gathered evidence in light of (2) clinical expertise and (3) patient values.[2, 3]

In 2000, less than 5 years after the seminal paper by Dr. Sackett, the Journal of Bone & Joint Surgery first published the term "evidenced-based orthopedics."[4] The development and popularization of evidence-based orthopedics brought light to the novel challenge of applying EBM in orthopedics,[5] for example, the difficulty of appropriately blinding or objectively assessing surgical interventions.[6] Distal radius fractures, among the most common fractures of both the young and the elderly, have been a focus of evidence-based orthopedics since the inception of the term.[7] A cursory search of Embase and MEDLINE from 1996 onwards for "distal" and "radius" and "fracture" yielded over 13,000 publications, more than 500 of which are randomized controlled trials (RCTs). The relative abundance of publications can complicate, rather than simplify, the application of EBM. For example, not all RCTs are of equal quality; failing to recognize low quality evidence, randomized or otherwise, may lead to inappropriate conclusions and can potentially encourage practices detrimental to patients. Alternatively, failing to recognize high quality evidence may delay the application of beneficial practices, again to the detriment of patients. It is vital for surgeons to understand not only the basic principles of EBM, but also the hierarchy of evidence, study design and quality, and the presentation of results.

PRINCIPLES OF EVIDENCE-BASED MANAGEMENT

The *Evidence Pathway* effectively organizes the key principles of evidence-based management into a simple algorithm:

- *Assess*: Identify, and understand the importance of, a clinical issue affecting patients and outcomes.
- *Ask*: Formulate a specific research question, directly related to the issue at hand, to be the foundation for a structured literature review. According to the PICO framework, a well-built clinical question identifies the patient population, intervention or exposure, comparator, and outcomes of interest.[8]
- *Acquire*: Perform an objective, systematic search of databases other sources to obtain relevant evidence. Other sources may include (but are not limited to) bibliographies, research conference abstracts, and content experts.
- *Appraise*: Critically evaluate acquired evidence based on the hierarchy of evidence and the validity of results with respect to methodological quality and clinical relevance.
- *Apply*: In conjunction with patient values and clinician expertise, apply the collected, evaluated evidence.

Application of this framework allows surgeons to make evidence-based decisions, particularly when faced with the sprawling literature base informing treatment of distal radius fractures. The remainder of this chapter unpacks the above approach and will equip readers with the practical knowledge required to interpret, summarize, and apply the rest of this text.

QUALITY OF EVIDENCE AND THE HIERARCHY OF EVIDENCE

For the busy clinician, deciphering an endless mountain of literature, personally appraising each article, and synthesizing numerous results across multiple outcomes may appear an insurmountable task.[9] Fortunately, this process can be accelerated by grouping studies by similarities in methodology. Contemporary evidence hierarchies separate study designs by their susceptibility to bias, thereby providing an initial measure of quality.[10] The findings of methodologically rigorous studies are less likely to be influenced by bias, known or unknown, and as such, are more likely to be valid. The most rigorous of designs, the RCT, occupies the top of the hierarchy, followed by controlled observational studies, uncontrolled case series, and then expert opinion. This broad grading system, introduced by Dr. Sackett, has been widely adopted across specialties and journals.[11] To understand the hierarchy of evidence is to understand the merits and demerits (i.e., sources of bias) associated with each study design.

Randomized controlled trials exist at the top of the hierarchy due to their unique ability to mitigate multiple sources of bias. Although relatively rare across the vista of surgical literature, the use of RCTs is increasing worldwide.[12] By randomly allocating patients to either an intervention (new treatment) or control arm (standard or no treatment), RCTs minimize the influence of selection bias by evenly distributing both known and unknown factors—potential confounding variables. Unfortunately, randomization alone does not mitigate other types of bias that can compromise study validity and necessitate demotion from Level I (highest quality) evidence to Level II. In addition to randomization, key methodological features of RCTs include allocation concealment, blinding, avoidance of expertise bias, minimization of attrition, and intention-to treat analysis.[13]

Allocation Concealment—The investigators enrolling patients are unable to determine which treatment arm the next patient will be assigned to. Acceptable methods include central (internet or telephone based) allocation, or the use of sequentially numbered, sealed, opaque envelopes. Allocation methodology susceptible to bias includes use of patient chart numbers, odd/even dates, or unsealed envelopes.

Blinding—Involved individuals are unaware of which treatment arm the patient has been allocated to. Groups that can be blinded include patients, clinicians, outcome collectors, outcome adjudicators, data analysts and manuscript writers. The more groups that are blinded, the less likelihood there is of performance or detection bias due to knowledge of treatment allocation.

Expertise Bias—The differential ability of a clinician to apply the intervention or procedure, due to skill or prior beliefs. This may occur when a surgeon is asked to perform a procedure that they lack proficiency in or that they believe to be ineffective, compared to the alternative treatment arm.

Attrition—Loss of patients to follow-up to the point where the final cohort may no longer represent the original cohort. Traditional thresholds have required at least 80% of patients to be included at final follow-up. Bias may occur if those who drop out of a trial systematically differ from those who remain.

Intention to Treat Principle—The analysis of patient outcomes by the treatment group to which they were allocated to, regardless of the treatment ultimately received during the trial. This form of analysis preserves the power imparted by randomization to balance the distribution of known and unknown factors among the treatment groups.

Despite RCTs representing the highest level of evidence, they may not be feasible or appropriate for the assessment of particular interventions. Particularly, for the investigation of potentially harmful exposures, rare outcomes, or outcomes that develop over a long period

of time, RCTs may be prohibitive based on ethical grounds or due to resource requirements. For example, using an RCT to explore the risk of flexor tendon rupture (a rare complication) after volar plating[14] may be inappropriate since meaningful comparison of infrequent events requires sample sizes that may prove impractically large for surgical trials.[15] Similarly, using an RCT to examine posttraumatic arthritis following intraarticular DRF[16] treatment may require many years, even decades, of follow-up that can be more reliably achieved through alternative study designs. Finally, conducting an RCT to examine the effect of a risk factor, take for example the effect of smoking on complication risk after distal radius fracture fixation, would require randomization of a harmful intervention (i.e., smoking).[17] In these and many other circumstances, observational study designs allow patient or provider preferences to determine which treatment (or exposure) group the patient is in. While the risk of selection bias pushes these nonrandomized studies down the evidence hierarchy, they are an invaluable tool to provide answers that RCTs cannot.

Within observational trial designs, differences in study design are often substantial and influence the risk of bias and thus level of evidence. Cohort studies involve the comparison of patients who are exposed to a risk factor (or treatment) to unexposed patients, who are then followed to determine the rate of occurrence of an outcome of interest.[13] Cohort studies may be prospective in nature, constituting a higher level evidence relative to retrospective cohort studies. A prospective design facilitates more rigorous data collection and patient follow-up but, like RCTs, feasibility challenges arise when attempting to follow large numbers of patients over long time intervals.[13] Like all observational studies, retrospective cohort studies involve the identification of exposed and unexposed patients. Previously reported outcomes are then gathered, typically through review of patient charts or databases, and analyzed. Retrospective cohort studies are considerably less time and resource intensive but are prone to additional sources of bias, such as recall bias.[13] Prospective designs allow investigators to study any outcome of interest while outcome choice in retrospective investigation is limited to outcomes that have been previously reported.

Prospective trial designs begin at a specified point when patients are either exposed or unexposed. These patients are then followed forward in time, to evaluate the impact of the exposure(s) on the outcomes of interest. Retrospective trial designs involves looking backwards from the present, into past records to identify patient outcomes and exposures.

Case-control studies invovle a retrospective observational design where a group of patients who have previously developed an outcome of interest (cases) are matched to a similar group of patients who do not have the outcome of interest (controls). These groups are then assessed for differences in previous risk factor exposures hypothesized to be associated with the outcome.[13] This is a particularly efficient design when assessing risk factors, rare outcomes, or outcomes that develop over a prolonged period of time, such as the effect of vitamin D insufficiency on distal radius fracture risk.[18] However, these studies still suffer from the limitations of retrospective enrollment and data collection, as outlined above.

> Recall bias is the differential likelihood of patients or providers to report an exposure in the setting of an adverse event or poor outcome

Case reports and case series are descriptive studies that involve detailed profiles of one or several patients. Without a control (i.e., unexposed) group for comparison, conclusions on causal associations between exposure and outcome cannot be made. Additionally, case series and case reports tend to describe the experience of a single surgeon or center, and therefore may have limited generalizability to other practice settings or populations. Largely for these reasons, case studies sit near the bottom of the evidence hierarchy. Nevertheless, case studies remain valuable for reporting rare events or new techniques, or for setting the groundwork preceding higher quality study designs.

> Generalizability refers to the ability to apply the findings of a study to a larger group of similar individuals.

Finally, systematic reviews and metaanalyses are summary studies that employ an organized, reproducible, and objective approach to the collection and synthesis of data from multiple primary studies. Metaanalyses synthesize results across relevant studies to increase the effective sample size, and provide a single pooled estimate of treatment effect. Metaanalyses are considered a higher level of evidence than RCTs; however, it is important to remember their quality is immediately dependent on the quality of included studies. Therefore, a metaanalysis of Level I RCTs represents the pinnacle of the hierarchy, whereas those including low-quality RCTs or observational studies may be classified lower than a single, high-quality RCT. Confidence in the effect estimate from a metaanalysis is dependent on homogeneity between the included trials; high heterogeneity between studies will produce a wide confidence interval that may be of little clinical value. Alternatively, results that are consistent and precise across trials increase confidence in the pooled effect estimate. Metaanalyses of this nature can be invaluable for well-informed, evidence-based decision making. While conventional metaanalyses include two interventions with head-to-head (direct) comparisons, multiple treatment options often exist (e.g., volar plate, percutaneous K-wires, external fixation) with or without direct evidence supporting one treatment over another.[19] The recent emergence of network-meta analyses addresses this discrepancy by using both direct and indirect comparisons to quantify the relative effectiveness of more than two treatment options simultaneously.[20, 21] While these studies are more complex in their pooling and analysis methodology, similar principles can be applied to their interpretation and application. Generally, network metaanalyses are performed from data obtained through randomized controlled trials; however, there has been a recent emergence to utilize all comparative studies to strengthen measures of association. Unlike standard pairwise metaanalyses that produce either odds ratios or relative risks, with associated confidence intervals and P values, network metaanalyses have the added advantage of generating ranking outputs which suggest which treatment is most likely to be the best intervention for a given outcome. This is done using Surface Under the Cumulative Ranking Curve (SUCRA) values that, in addition to direct and indirect pair-wise comparisons, represent the standard technique to report findings of network metaanalyses.

PRESENTATION OF RESEARCH FINDINGS

At this stage of the evidence pathway, all relevant studies have been gathered and assessed for both appropriateness of study design and likelihood of bias. It is now necessary to interpret the study findings as they relate to the clinical question. Authors may choose to present their findings using a variety of different outcome measures, the choice of which depends on the type of data being reported (e.g., continuous versus dichotomous). Complications associated with treatment are commonly reported as a dichotomous outcome using measures such as relative risk (RR) or odds ratio (OR); alternatively, functional scores and radiographic findings are commonly reported as continuous outcomes using mean difference (MD). Regardless of the type of data and measure, it is important to consider that point values are simply estimates of the effect direction and magnitude and, like all estimates, are universally associated with some degree of uncertainty. Confidence interval (CI) or standard deviation (SD) are common expressions of uncertainty.

Mean difference describes the absolute difference in means between treatment groups. So long as outcome measurements are the same across studies, MD may also be used in metaanalysis. Alternatively, standardized mean difference (SMD) may be used in a metaanalysis to express the effect size in each study relative to the outcome variability (i.e., standard deviation) in that study. Standardized mean difference is useful when the effect scale differs between studies; however, clinical interpretation of SMD is more difficult as the units are standard deviations.[22]

In a metaanalysis by Chaudry et al.[23] comparing volar locking plates to percutaneous K-wires, functional status was reported using the MD for Disabilities of the Arm, Shoulder, and Hand (DASH) scores at 6 and 12 months after postoperation.[24] The MD was 3.78, indicating patients treated with volar plating scored 3.78 points lower (i.e., less disability). The 95% CI of 1.23 to 6.32 indicates that the true mean difference lies within that range of values with 95% certainty. If the 95% CI of MD does not cross zero (i.e., no effect), it is likely that the treatment has an effect; accordingly, this finding is statistically significant according to the a priori threshold described by the authors.

This example illustrates another important consideration—the difference between statistically significant and clinically significant (i.e., relevant). The minimum threshold at which a change is likely to prove meaningful to informed patients and would therefore cause a patient or clinician to consider a change in management has been termed the minimally important difference (MID).[25, 26] Regarding DASH scores, previous study has found that patients are unable to perceive differences of less than 10 points.[27] Returning to the data from Chaudry et al.,[23] a DASH score reduction of 3.78 (95% CI 1.23 to 6.32) in the volar plating group falls below an MID of 10 points; thus, this difference is statistically significant but may lack clinical significance. This concept can have a large impact on how the findings of a study are interpreted by authors.[19]

Authors frequently present dichotomous data, such as number of patients experiencing a complication, using odds ratios (OR), relative risk (RR), and absolute risk ratio (ARR). In the metaanalysis by Zong et al.,[28] the authors compared complications of volar plating and percutaneous fixation with K-wires. In the pooled

sample, the absolute risk is 19.4% (85 events in 438 exposed patients) in the plating group and 50.8% in the K-wire group (222 events in 437 patients). The most straightforward way to interpret the difference in risk between these two groups is using risk difference (i.e., absolute risk reduction, ARR). In this example, the risk difference is 31.4%. Number needed to treat (NNT), the inverse of ARR, is often used to facilitate interpretation. In this example, the NNT is 3.2 (1/0.314), implying that for every three patients treated with plating instead of percutaneous fixation, one complication will be avoided.

More commonly in metaanalyses, relative statistics are used, namely relative risk and odds ratio. For both measures, a value of one—or a 95% CI including one—indicates the effect of two treatments is the same. Risk ratio, the more easily interpreted relative measure, describes risk in the treatment group relative to risk in the control group. Returning to the data set by Zong et al.,[28] risk ratio can be calculated as the risk in the plating group, 0.194, relative to the risk in the percutaneous fixation group, 0.508. Therefore, relative risk of postoperative complications is 0.382 favoring plating. Interpreting this value, patients treated with volar plates are 38.2% less likely to experience a postoperative complication than patients treated with percutaneous fixation with K-wires. Alternatively, relative risk reduction (RRR) can be calculated as $(RR - 1) \times 100\%$. After calculating RRR for this example, it can be seen that treating patients with volar plating reduces the risk of postoperative complications by 61.8% relative to percutaneous fixation with K-wires.

Relative measures are often preferred in metaanalyses, partly because they are more generalizable across multiple groups with different baseline risk.[29] When interpreting absolute and relative measures in the context of clinical significance, it is important to consider the event frequency: a 2% absolute risk reduction in an event that occurs 50% of the time is likely insignificant. Conversely, a 2% absolute risk reduction when baseline risk is 4% represents a relative risk reduction of 50%. A relative difference of that magnitude may be meaningful, particularly when considering serious complications such as malunion requiring reoperation.

Odds ratios, perhaps the most difficult relative measure for clinicians to interpret, are calculated by dividing the odds of an outcome occurring in the treatment group by the odds of the same outcome occurring in the control group. Risk ratio and OR are similar and equally valid but are not identical. When an intervention increases event probability, particularly with very common events, OR will be larger than RR, thereby overestimating the treatment effect.[30] The inverse also holds true, as demonstrated in the study by Zong et al.[28] The reported OR for postoperative complications (a frequent event) is 0.25 while the RR is 0.38; in this instance, odds ratio overestimates the beneficial treatment effect of volar plating.

If the confidence interval of an absolute measure does not cross zero, the difference between groups is considered statistically significant; the same is true if the CI of a relative measure does not cross one. It is important to recognize that CIs represent an estimate of the range of plausible truths made by sampling a subset of the population of interest.[30] The size of these intervals is influenced by individual and pooled sample sizes, measurement variability (i.e., standard deviation for continuous outcomes), and event frequency (i.e., absolute risk for dichotomous outcomes).[31] Narrow confidence intervals represent a more precise estimate of the true value. Due to the chance nature of sampling, the fragility of significant findings may be called into question. Fragility describes the minimum number of patients that would have to go from experiencing an event to not experiencing the event, or the inverse, for a finding to go from statistically significant to insignificant.[32] Emphasizing the importance of this concept, several analyses of orthopedic literature have found that a change of just two events would make findings nonsignificant.[33, 34]

This section on presentation of outcomes would be incomplete without an explanation of subgroup analysis. Authors often analyze subsets of participants (e.g., smokers versus nonsmokers, simple versus comminuted fractures) in an effort to draw additional conclusions from RCTs. Subgroup analyses may be planned prospectively or decided upon retrospectively; in both situations, these analyses are essentially observational (i.e., nonrandomized) comparisons and should be regarded accordingly. Subgroup findings are considered more reliable when differences between the subgroup and the overall study population are quantitative—being of the same direction of effect while differing in magnitude.[35] Subgroup findings are also more likely to be trustworthy when the effect is consistent across subgroups of independent studies. Alternatively, subgroup differences that are qualitative—differing in direction of treatment effect—are unlikely and should prompt skepticism.[35] Retrospective and/or multiple subgroups further degrade the quality of evidence. Ultimately, subgroup analyses should not be viewed as equivalent to RCT evidence and should seldom be the deciding factor in clinical decision-making.

MAKING RECOMMENDATIONS

Recommending a treatment for the majority of patients is not always a difficult decision, particularly when numerous, high quality (i.e., low risk of bias) RCTs demonstrate consistent benefit to patients with a highly favorable risk-benefit profile. For example, clinicians need not hesitate to offer arthroplasty over internal fixation for elderly patients with displaced femoral neck fractures.[36] However, considering distal radius fractures specifically, most interventions are only supported by observational data or RCTs with few patients at high risk of bias. In these instances, making a recommendation can be difficult and thus it is the job of the clinician to help patients weigh potential benefits of a treatment in the context of appreciable harms.

Many systems exist to structure and qualify treatment recommendations.[37] The Grading of Recommendations Assessment, Development and Evaluation (GRADE) classification has become the most widely used, endorsed by more than 100 organizations worldwide. Advantages of GRADE include clear implications of strong compared to weak recommendations, robust criteria for increasing or decreasing ratings of evidence quality, integration of patient values, and a transparent relationship between quality of evidence and associated recommendations.[38] This system describes both the strength of a recommendation and the quality of evidence supporting a recommendation. Evidence is graded as High, Moderate, Low, or Very Low quality.

Occupying the top of the evidence hierarchy, RCT evidence begins as "high quality evidence," while observational studies, the foundation of the evidence hierarchy, begin as "low quality evidence." The quality assessment of a pool of evidence is subsequently increased or decreased based on study methodological quality, sample size, effect size, precision, and other factors described previously in this chapter. After weighing the quality of evidence, the balance of wanted and unwanted effects (e.g., complications), patient values and preferences, and resource utilization, a strong or weak recommendation is made.[39] Strong recommendations indicate the advantages of a treatment clearly outweigh any undesirable effects, or the opposite, when harm is more probable than benefit. Weak recommendations indicate either a lack of evidence or an uncertain risk-benefit profile. In the case of a weak recommendation, patient values and provider expertise are often more influential in decision making.

The GRADE approach provides a pragmatic approach to evidence-based orthopedics. When used by surgeons, evidence grade and recommendation strength—both of which are brief, transparent summaries—can effectively streamline evidence-based decision-making. This is particularly true when navigating the expansive literature informing treatment of distal radius fractures, as will be seen throughout the following chapters. Panel 2 provides an example of evidence-based management for a patient with a distal radius fractures.

CONCLUSION

Nearly 30 years since the development of evidence-based medicine, the practice shift has faced numerous challenges. Critics draw attention to the emphasis on statistical benefits over clinically meaningful benefits, to rigid guidelines that ignore patient factors, and to an overall unmanageable quantity of evidence.[40] Throughout this introductory section, readers were presented with an objective, straightforward approach to applying evidence-based methodology. With an understanding of the hierarchy of evidence, clinicians will appreciate the value of observational data, particularly when randomized data are impractical to obtain. Further, with knowledge of the sources of bias and the benefits and drawbacks of various effect measures, it becomes clear that formation of recommendations is more patient-focused rather than less. The remainder of this text breaks the large evidence base into thorough yet manageable lessons that will leave readers with a practical approach to the evidence-based management of distal radius fractures.

REFERENCES

1. Guyatt G. Evidence-based medicine (editorial). *ACP J Club Arch.* 1991;https://doi.org/10.7326/ACPJC-1991-114-2-A16.
2. Sackett DL, Rosenberg J, Gray M, Haynes B, Richardson S. Evidence based practice: what it is and what it isn't. *Br Med J.* 1996;312:71. https://doi.org/10.1136/bmj.312.7023.71.
3. Bhandari M, Giannoudis PV. Evidence-based medicine: what it is and what it is not. *Injury.* 2006;37(4):302–306. https://doi.org/10.1016/j.injury.2006.01.034.
4. Wright JG, Swiontkowski MF. Introducing a new journal section: evidence-based orthopaedics. *J Bone Joint Surg.* 2000;82(6):759.
5. Schünemann HJ, Bone L. Evidence-based orthopaedics: a primer. In: *Clinical Orthopaedics and Related Research.* Lippincott Williams and Wilkins; 2003:117–132. https://doi.org/10.1097/01.blo.0000080541.81794.26.
6. Devereaux PJ, McKee MD, Yusuf S. Methodologic issues in randomized controlled trials of surgical interventions. In: *Clinical Orthopaedics and Related Research.* Lippincott Williams and Wilkins; 2003:25–32. https://doi.org/10.1097/01.blo.0000080539.81794.54.
7. Bhandari M, Guyatt GH, Swiontkowski MF. User's guide to the orthopaedic literature: how to use an article about a surgical therapy. *J Bone Joint Surg.* 2001;83(6):916–926. https://doi.org/10.2106/00004623-200106000-00015.
8. Oxman AD. Users' guides to the medical literature. I. How to get started. The evidence-based medicine working group. *JAMA J Am Med Assoc.* 1993;270(17):2093–2095. https://doi.org/10.1001/jama.270.17.2093.
9. Atkins D, Best D, Briss PA, et al. GRADE Working Group. Grading quality of evidence and strength of recommendations. *BMJ.* 2004;328:1490. https://doi.org/10.1136/bmj.328.7454.1490.
10. Wright JG, Swiontkowski MF, Heckman JD. Introducing levels of evidence to the journal. *J Bone Joint Surg.* 2003; https://doi.org/10.2106/00004623-200301000-00001.
11. Sackett DL. Rules of evidence and clinical recommendations on the use of antithrombotic agents. *Chest.* 1989;95(2 Suppl):2S–4S. https://doi.org/10.1378/chest.95.2_supplement.2s.
12. Ahmed Ali U, Van Der Sluis PC, Issa Y, et al. Trends in worldwide volume and methodological quality of surgical randomized controlled trials. *Ann Surg.* 2013;258(2):199–207. https://doi.org/10.1097/SLA.0b013e31829c7795.
13. Brighton B, Bhandari M, Tornetta P, Felson DT. Hierarchy of evidence: from case reports to randomized controlled trials. *Clin Orthop Relat Res.* 2003;413:19–24. https://doi.org/10.1097/01.blo.0000079323.41006.12.
14. Thorninger R, Madsen ML, Wæver D, Borris LC, Rölfing JHD. Complications of volar locking plating of distal radius fractures in 576 patients with 3.2 years follow-up. *Injury.* 2017;48(6):1104–1109. https://doi.org/10.1016/j.injury.2017.03.008.
15. Wittes J. Sample size calculations for randomized controlled trials. *Epidemiol Rev.* 2002;24(1):39–53. https://doi.org/10.1093/epirev/24.1.39.
16. Forward DP, Davis TRC, Sithole JS. Do young patients with malunited fractures of the distal radius inevitably develop symptomatic post-traumatic osteoarthritis? *J Bone Joint Surg (Br).* 2008;90-B(5):629–637. https://doi.org/10.1302/0301-620X.90B5.19448.
17. Hess DE, Carstensen SE, Moore S, Dacus AR. Smoking increases postoperative complications after distal radius fracture fixation: a review of 417 patients from a level 1 trauma center. *Hand.* 2018;https://doi.org/10.1177/1558944718810882.
18. Øyen J, Apalset EM, Gjesdal CG, Brudvik C, Lie SA, Hove LM. Vitamin D inadequacy is associated with low-energy distal radius fractures: a case-control study. *Bone.* 2011;48(5):1140–1145. https://doi.org/10.1016/j.bone.2011.01.021.
19. Woolnough T, Axelrod D, Bozzo A, et al. What is the relative effectiveness of the various surgical treatment options for distal radius fractures? A systematic review

and network meta-analysis of randomized controlled trials. *Clin Orthop Relat Res.*. 2020;5:10–97. https://doi.org/10.1097/CORR.0000000000001524 In press.

20. Chaudhry H, Foote CJ, Guyatt G, et al. Network meta-analysis: users' guide for surgeons: part II—certainty. *Clin Orthop Relat Res.* 2015;473(7):2172–2178. https://doi.org/10.1007/s11999-015-4287-9.

21. Foote CJ, Chaudhry H, Bhandari M, et al. Network meta-analysis: users' guide for surgeons: part I—credibility. *Clin Orthop Relat Res.* 2015;473(7):2166–2171. https://doi.org/10.1007/s11999-015-4286-x.

22. Egger M, Smith GD, Altman DG. *Systematic Reviews in Health Care: Meta-Analysis in Context.* 2nd ed. https://doi.org/10.1002/9780470693926.

23. Chaudhry H, Kleinlugtenbelt YV, Mundi R, Ristevski B, Goslings JC, Bhandari M. Are volar locking plates superior to percutaneous K-wires for distal radius fractures? A meta-analysis. *Clin Orthop Relat Res.* 2015;473(9):3017–3027. https://doi.org/10.1007/s11999-015-4347-1.

24. Westphal T, Piatek S, Schubert S, Schuschke T, Winckler S. Reliability and validity of the upper limb DASH questionnaire in patients with distal radius fractures. *Z Orthop Ihre Grenzgeb.* 2002;140(4):447–451. https://doi.org/10.1055/s-2002-33396.

25. Jaeschke R, Singer J, Guyatt GH. Measurement of health status. Ascertaining the minimal clinically important difference. *Control Clin Trials.* 1989;10(4):407–415. https://doi.org/10.1016/0197-2456(89)90005-6.

26. Johnston BC, Thorlund K, Schünemann HJ, et al. Improving the interpretation of quality of life evidence in meta-analyses: the application of minimal important difference units. *Health Qual Life Outcomes.* 2010;8(1):116. https://doi.org/10.1186/1477-7525-8-116.

27. Franchignoni F, Vercelli S, Giordano A, Sartorio F, Bravini E, Ferriero G. Minimal clinically important difference of the disabilities of the arm, shoulder and hand outcome measure (DASH) and its shortened version (quickDASH). *J Orthop Sports Phys Ther.* 2014;44(1):30–39. https://doi.org/10.2519/jospt.2014.4893.

28. Le Zong S, Kan SL, Su LX, Wang B. Meta-analysis for dorsally displaced distal radius fracture fixation: volar locking plate versus percutaneous Kirschner wires. *J Orthop Surg Res.* 2015;10(1):108. https://doi.org/10.1186/s13018-015-0252-2.

29. Engels EA, Schmid CH, Terrin N, Olkin I, Joseph L. Heterogeneity and statistical significance in meta-analysis: an empirical study of 125 meta-analyses. *Stat Med.* 2000;19(13):1707–1728. https://doi.org/10.1002/1097-0258(20000715)19:13<1707::AID-SIM491>3.0.CO;2-P.

30. Sinclair JC, Bracken MB. Clinically useful measures of effect in binary analyses of randomized trials. *J Clin Epidemiol.* 1994;47(8):881–889. https://doi.org/10.1016/0895-4356(94)90191-0.

31. Gardner MJ, Altman DG. Confidence intervals rather than P values: estimation rather than hypothesis testing. *Br Med J (Clin Res Ed).* 1986;292(6522):746–750. https://doi.org/10.1136/bmj.292.6522.746.

32. Walsh M, Srinathan SK, McAuley DF, et al. The statistical significance of randomized controlled trial results is frequently fragile: a case for a fragility index. *J Clin Epidemiol.* 2014;67(6):622–628. https://doi.org/10.1016/j.jclinepi.2013.10.019.

33. Khan M, Evaniew N, Gichuru M, et al. The fragility of statistically significant findings from randomized trials in sports surgery: a systematic survey. *Am J Sports Med.* 2017;45(9):2164–2170. https://doi.org/10.1177/0363546516674469.

34. Evaniew N, Files C, Smith C, et al. The fragility of statistically significant findings from randomized trials in spine surgery: a systematic survey. *Spine J.* 2015;15(10):2188–2197. https://doi.org/10.1016/j.spinee.2015.06.004.

35. Yusuf S, Wittes J, Probstfield J, Tyroler HA. Analysis and interpretation of treatment effects in subgroups of patients in randomized clinical trials. *JAMA J Am Med Assoc.* 1991;266(1):93–98. https://doi.org/10.1001/jama.1991.03470010097038.

36. Roberts KC, Brox WT, Jevsevar DS, Sevarino K. Management of hip Fractures in the elderly. *J Am Acad Orthop Surg.* 2015;23(2):131–137. https://doi.org/10.5435/JAAOS-D-14-00432.

37. Atkins D, Eccles M, Flottorp S, et al. Systems for grading the quality of evidence and the strength of recommendations I: critical appraisal of existing approaches. *BMC Health Serv Res.* 2004;4https://doi.org/10.1186/1472-6963-4-38.

38. Guyatt GH, Oxman AD, Vist GE, et al. GRADE: an emerging consensus on rating quality of evidence and strength of recommendations. *BMJ.* 2008;https://doi.org/10.1136/bmj.39489.470347.ad.

39. Guyatt G, Oxman AD, Akl EA, et al. GRADE guidelines: 1. Introduction—GRADE evidence profiles and summary of findings tables. *J Clin Epidemiol.* 2011;64(4):383–394. https://doi.org/10.1016/j.jclinepi.2010.04.026.

40. Greenhalgh T, Howick J, Maskrey N, et al. Evidence based medicine: a movement in crisis? *BMJ.* 2014;348https://doi.org/10.1136/bmj.g3725.

CHAPTER 2

Epidemiology of Distal Radius Fractures

ELISSA S. DAVIS • KEVIN C. CHUNG
Department of Surgery, Michigan Medicine, Ann Arbor, MI, United States

---

KEY POINTS

- Distal radius fractures primarily affect children, young adults, and the elderly.
- The incidence of distal radius fractures is increasing worldwide.
- Understanding the epidemiology of distal radius fractures helps guide treatment.

PANEL 1: CASE SCENARIO

A 65-year-old, right hand dominant female visited the emergency room with a swollen and deformed right wrist after a fall on an outstretched hand when she slipped on a wet floor at home. Radiographs reveal an intraarticular distal radius fracture with 30 degrees of dorsal angulation. How does the description and treatment of this fracture change if the patient is 10 or 25 years old?

IMPORTANCE OF THE PROBLEM

Upper extremity fractures are one of the most common injuries around the globe, with an estimated frequency of 67.6 fractures per 10,000 persons in the United States.[1–9] Distal radius and ulna fractures are the most common upper extremity fractures, occurring in 16.2/10,000 persons.[10] Although the incidence of distal radius fractures (DRFs) is increasing across all age groups, they are most common in the pediatric and elderly populations.[11–14] Research indicates that the first peak in the rate of DRFs occurs in the adolescent years. The second increase starts among adults greater than 50 years of age and peaks in the seventh to eighth decade of life (Fig. 1).[15] DRFs comprise about 25% and 18% of all fractures in the pediatric and elderly populations, respectively.[10]

Gender and racial differences also exist among DRF patients. Fig. 2 shows the gender distribution of DRFs by age.[15] Males have a higher incidence of fractures in the 0–19-year age group and females have a higher incidence in the 40–64-year age group. DRFs are also more common in woman than men with age > 65, especially among Caucasians.

An understanding of the heterogeneity of the DRF population helps surgeons provide better treatments that are tailored to unique patient characteristics. Assessing the epidemiology of DRFs is also critical in efforts to prevent these costly and debilitating injuries.

MAIN QUESTION

How does the epidemiology of distal radius fractures help guide treatment?

CURRENT OPINION

Pediatric DRFs rarely require anatomic reduction because children have remaining growth potential. On the other hand, young adult intraarticular DRFs often develop posttraumatic arthritis whether treated operatively or nonoperatively. Controversy also exists regarding operative versus nonoperative management of DRFs in the elderly population.

FINDING THE EVIDENCE

We identified articles that were published in the last 10 years. English, French, and German language studies were included.

The search results in PubMed are as follows:
"epidemiology of distal radius fracture" = 0

Distal Radius Fractures. https://doi.org/10.1016/B978-0-323-75764-5.00034-2

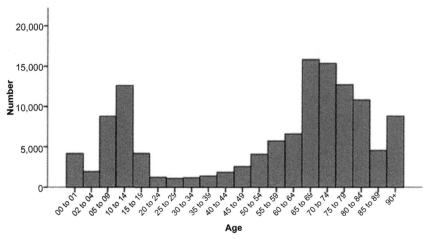

FIG. 1 Distal radius fracture distribution by age group.

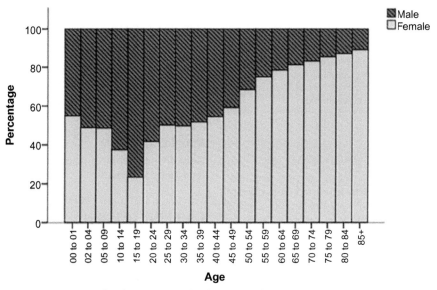

FIG. 2 Gender distribution in distal radius fractures by age group.

epidemiology of distal radius fracture = 387

"Radius Fractures/epidemiology"[Mesh] AND distal = 131

epidemiol* AND distal AND (radius OR radial) AND fracture* = 401

Total after removing duplicates = 412

The search results in Web of Science are as follows:

"epidemiology of distal radius fracture" = 1

epidemiology of distal radius fracture = 283

Total after removing duplicates = 283

No relevant articles were identified in the Cochrane database

QUALITY OF THE EVIDENCE

There is no level I or level II evidence available since epidemiology is mainly descriptive, looking at the incidence and distribution of health conditions; in this case, distal radius fractures.

Importance of the Problem:
Level III:
Systematic reviews of case series, case control, and retrospective comparative studies: 15
Pediatric Findings:
Level III:
Systematic reviews of case series, case control, and retrospective comparative studies: 18
Level V:
Expert opinion and summary of current concepts: 2
Young Adult Findings:
Level III:
Systematic reviews of case series, case control, and retrospective comparative studies: 5
Level V:
Expert opinion and summary of current concepts: 1
Elderly Findings:
Level III:
Systematic reviews of case series, case control, and retrospective comparative studies: 14
Level V:
Expert opinion and summary of current concepts: 2

FINDINGS

The Pediatric Population

The incidence of distal radius fractures in children and adolescents varies across studies but may be as high as 25%–33% of all fractures in this population.[16–19] Beattie et al. reported a fracture rate of 20.2/1000 children. Females and males accounted for 39% and 61% of their patient population, respectively, and 33% of fractures involved the distal radius/ulna. Randsborg et al. found a similar incidence of 18.0 fractures/1000 children less than 16 years of age. DRFs accounted for 31% of all fractures in their study.[19] Additional articles also reported a higher incidence of DRFs in male versus female children.[12, 13, 17, 20, 21]

The increasing overall incidence of DRFs in the pediatric population is well-documented.[12, 13, 17, 20, 22, 23] Landin, in a large study of pediatric fractures, suggested that increased sports participation contributed to an increase in fracture rate between 1950 and 1970.[17] De Putter et al. corroborated this in their study of Dutch children between 1997 and 2009. The authors found an increase in sports-related activities, soccer, and inline skating in particular, correlated with an increase in DRFs.[12] In addition to sports-related causes, trauma and falling onto an outstretched hand are hypothesized mechanisms of injury.[20, 22, 24] It is also possible that the increasing incidence of fractures is a result of better fracture detection methods and improved access to care.[23]

The literature indicates that the maximum fracture rate occurs at the age of puberty. In the 1960s, Alffram and Bauer found the peak age for forearm fractures to be 10–14 years of age.[25] For DRFs specifically, Bailey et al. identified peak ages of 11.5–12.5 and 13.5–14.5 for girls and boys, respectively.[21] Chung and Spilson identified a peak around 10 years of age.[1] Furthermore, Beattie et al. reported a bimodal distribution of DRFs with peaks at ages 6–7 and 13–14.[18] The higher occurrence of DRFs during puberty is likely related to bone mineral density at the distal radius during the growth spurt.[24, 26–29] Faulkner et al. demonstrated that the incidence of DRF coincides with a decline in size corrected bone mineral density and that gains in bone area precede the gain in bone mineral content.[29] The imbalance between bone strength and linear growth may explain why minor falls from standing height cause fractures in this age group.[20]

Skeletally immature individuals have remaining growth and remodeling potential. Therefore, anatomic reduction of the distal radius is rarely indicated. Casting alone is typically effective. Two studies with level III evidence of patients with malunited fractures both demonstrate that DRFs led to fewer complication than more proximal fractures.[30, 31] Although they are rare, complications from DRFs in children include re-fracture and synostosis. Re-fracture can occur if immobilization is removed too quickly and is associated with worse motion and deformity in observational studies.[30, 32] Synostosis is usually associated with high energy trauma.[33]

The Young Adult Population

Although DRFs are less frequent outside of the pediatric and elderly populations (Fig. 1), they are still a relatively common injury across all age groups. Recent US data showed that DRFs are the third most common fracture in the 18- to 34-year-old population following metacarpal and phalangeal fractures. In the 35- to 49-year-old group, DRFs were second in frequency only to phalangeal fractures.[10, 34] Sports injuries and car accidents are the most common causes of DRFs in young adults less than 50 years of age.

Although gender differences exist in the pediatric and elderly DRF populations, men and women in the 19- to 49-year age group have identical fracture rates. However, analyzing the 19- to 65-year age group reveals a two-times higher DRF rate among woman than men. This is presumably a result of greater osteoporotic fracture incidence in women over 50.[15] With respect to race, a majority (83%) of young adult DRFs occur in Caucasian individuals. However, this data point must be interpreted with caution. Differences in the likelihood of

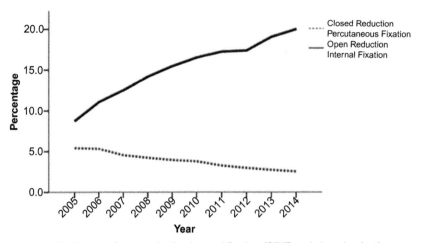

FIG. 3 Annual trend in the use of open reduction internal fixation (ORIF) and closed reduction percutaneous fixation (percentage).

reporting to emergency departments influence the results.[1, 35, 36]

The goal of DRF treatment is the same regardless of age: restore alignment using evidence-based treatments. In the young adult patient, the parameters for acceptable reduction are clear but the optimal method of fixation is inconclusive. Closed reduction and casting, percutaneous fixation, external fixation and open reduction and internal fixation (ORIF) are all treatment options for young adults with DRFs. Currently, there is a trend toward more operative interventions, as shown in Fig. 3.[15] In the young adult patient, the parameters for acceptable reduction are clear but the optimal method of fixation is inconclusive. Randomized, controlled trials are needed to determine the criteria for various treatments and evaluate the expected outcomes in this age group.

The Elderly Population

DRFs are the second most common fracture in the elderly population behind hip fractures. As previously noted, higher rates are seen in women than men with an up to sixfold increase in fractures in the elderly female compared to the elderly male. Unlike injuries in the younger population, DRFs in the elderly population are usually the result of low energy trauma, such as falling on an outstretched arm.[37–39] Furthermore, Caucasian women have the highest incidence of DRFs. These findings point to osteoporosis and osteopenia as common underlying conditions attributing to the fracture.

Numerous studies explored the association between decreased bone mineral density and DRF rates. For example, a recent study from China noted that elderly postmenopausal patients who experienced DRFs had significantly lower T-scores than a control group that did not experience DRFs. T-scores are a measure of bone mineral density compared to healthy 30-year olds. In a comparison between stable and unstable DRFs, the same researchers reported more unstable fractures in the group with the lower T-values.[40] Low bone mineral density has been well documented in other reports of women who suffer a DRF.[41–44] Researchers have also explored how DRFs and osteoporosis are associated with subsequent bone fractures in the elderly. A study from Mayo Clinic reported a 5-fold increase in risk for vertebral fractures among women and a 11-fold increase among men following their first distal forearm fracture.[45]

Decreased activity, hormonal changes, and Vitamin D deficiency all contribute to osteoporosis. DRF patients also have an increased level of bone turnover markers of formation and resorption. These markers are potentially useful in predicting future fragility fractures in the elderly. A study reported that individuals on hormonal therapy, particularly estrogen and progesterone, for 10 years had a 33% reduction in the risk of DRF. Individuals who took hormones for more than 15 years had a 63% reduction in risk.[46] Estrogen has protective effects on bone by inhibiting bone resorption. Furthermore, a recent epidemiologic report surveyed women with and without fractures to identify risk factors for DRFs. BMI was higher and calcium intake was lower in the fracture group. Bone mineral density was also significantly lower in the fracture group (T-2.74) than the control group

(T-1.69). In logistic regression analyses, only BMI and a fall within the past year were independent predictors of DRF.[40]

Premature mortality following hip and vertebral fragility fractures is well documented. However, there is conflicting evidence on mortality rates following DRFs. A recent study of 256 men and 1052 women over the age of 50 reported a 5% mortality rate at 1-year post-injury. Although men were on average 8 years younger than women at the time of fracture, they had a 2.2 times higher mortality rate. This difference was noticeable starting at 6 months' follow-up. The authors also examined classification systems as predictors of mortality. They found that extra articular fractures, such as AO type A and Frykman I, are predictors of mortality following DRF.[47]

The best treatment modality for elderly patients with DRF remains unresolved.[48–50] The distal radius practice guideline approved by the American Academy of Orthopaedic Surgeons in 2009 outlined the following recommendations with moderate strength in recommending surgical fixation over cast fixation:

Post reduction radial shortening >3 mm

Dorsal tilt >10 degrees

Intra articular displacement or step off >2 mm

These guidelines and the addition of appropriate use scoring system did not provide clear recommendations. Fixation devices have also evolved in recent years, but their influence on DRF outcomes is unclear.

Some DRF treatments are more popular than others, despite the lack of guidelines indicating their benefits. The authors of one study assessed trends in DRF treatment across 1 million patients in the United States between 2005 and 2014. Closed reduction and casting were the most frequent treatment modalities overall. However, the popularity of closed reduction declined steadily over the 10-year period, from 86% in 2005 to 77% in 2015. The use of closed reduction and percutaneous fixation also declined from 5% in 2005 to 3% in 2014. Meanwhile, internal fixation became more common, particularly among the elderly population, increasing from 8% in 2004 to 20% in 2014 (Fig. 3). Operative repair with ORIF is becoming more common outside of the United States as well.[51, 52]

The prior study also reported an 8% overall complication rate following DRF treatment. Complications occurred in 5% and 9% of nonsurgical and surgical patients, respectively. The latter group demonstrated significantly higher rates of nonunion, tendon rupture, contracture, mechanical symptoms, and complex regional pain syndrome. Only the rate of malunion was higher in the nonoperative group.[15]

The increase in surgical rates and internal fixation devices in particular has significant ramifications from a cost perspective. This will undoubtedly be a source of scrutiny as the era of episode-based bundle payments becomes a reality in the United States.[53]

RECOMMENDATION

In patients with an intraarticular displaced distal radius fracture, evidence suggests:

Recommendation	Overall Quality
Pediatric Populations	⊕⊕⊕⊕
• Treatment paradigm remains mainly nonoperative in the pediatric population	HIGH
Young Adult Population	⊕⊕⊕◯
• Achieve AAOS guidelines (Radial shortening <3 mm, Dorsal tilt <10 degrees, and intraarticular displacement or step off <2 mm) when considering methods of treatment	MODERATE
Elderly Population	⊕⊕⊕◯
• Workup for osteoporosis when indicated with low impact trauma	MODERATE

CONCLUSION

The rates of DRFs are increasing across all populations. High energy mechanisms of injury predominate in younger age groups, especially among males. In the elderly, females who experienced low energy causes of fracture are more common, and an osteoporosis workup should be considered. Treatment options vary by age group. Alignment as well as functional demand of the patient should be considered.

PANEL 2: PEARLS AND PITFALLS

Pearls:

• When deciding how best to treat a distal radius fracture, consider not only fracture characteristics and alignment but also the age and functional demand of the patient.

Pitfalls:

• Remember to consider an osteoporosis workup for elderly patients with low energy distal radius fractures. Risk factors include postmenopausal status, age over 50, low body weight, Caucasian/Asian race, and smoking history.

REFERENCES

1. Chung KC, Spilson SV. The frequency and epidemiology of hand and forearm fractures in the United States. *J Hand Surg [Am]*. 2001;26:908–915.
2. Jerrhag D, Englund M, Karlsson MK, Rosengren BE. Epidemiology and time trends of distal forearm fractures in adults—a study of 11.2 million person-years in Sweden. *BMC Musculoskelet Disord*. 2017;18:240.
3. Hevonkorpi TP, Launonen AP, Huttunen TT, Kannus P, Niemi S, Mattila VM. Incidence of distal radius fracture surgery in Finns aged 50 years or more between 1998 and 2016—too many patients are yet operated on? *BMC Musculoskelet Disord*. 2018;19:70.
4. Solvang HW, Nordheggen RA, Clementsen S, Hammer OL, Randsborg PH. Epidemiology of distal radius fracture in Akershus, Norway, in 2010-2011. *J Orthop Surg Res*. 2018;13:199.
5. Armstrong KA, von Schroeder HP, Baxter NN, Zhong T, Huang A, McCabe SJ. Stable rates of operative treatment of distal radius fractures in Ontario, Canada: a population-based retrospective cohort study (2004–2013). *Can J Surg*. 2019;62:386–392.
6. Stirling ERB, Johnson NA, Dias JJ. Epidemiology of distal radius fractures in a geographically defined adult population. *J Hand Surg Eur Vol*. 2018;43:974–982.
7. Jo YH, Lee BG, Kim HS, Kim JH, Lee CH, Kim SJ, et al. Incidence and seasonal variation of distal radius fractures in Korea: a population-based study. *J Korean Med Sci*. 2018;33(7):e48.
8. Jennison T, Brinsden M. Fracture admission trends in England over a ten-year period. *Ann R Coll Surg Engl*. 2019;101:208–214.
9. Nellans KW, Kowalski E, Chung KC. The epidemiology of distal radius fractures. *Hand Clin*. 2012;28:113–125.
10. Karl JW, Olson PR, Rosenwasser MP. The epidemiology of upper extremity fractures in the United States, 2009. *J Orthop Trauma*. 2015;29:e242–e244.
11. Melton 3rd LJ, Amadio PC, Crowson CS, O'Fallon WM. Long-term trends in the incidence of distal forearm fractures. *Osteoporos Int*. 1998;8:341–348.
12. de Putter CE, van Beeck EF, Looman CW, Toet H, Hovius SE, Selles RW. Trends in wrist fractures in children and adolescents, 1997–2009. *J Hand Surg [Am]*. 2011;36:1810–1815 e2.
13. Hagino H, Yamamoto K, Ohshiro H, Nose T. Increasing incidence of distal radius fractures in Japanese children and adolescents. *J Orthop Sci*. 2000;5:356–360.
14. Thompson PW, Taylor J, Dawson A. The annual incidence and seasonal variation of fractures of the distal radius in men and women over 25 years in Dorset, UK. *Injury*. 2004;35:462–466.
15. Azad A, Kang HP, Alluri RK, Vakhshori V, Kay HF, Ghiassi A. Epidemiological and treatment trends of distal radius fractures across multiple age groups. *J Wrist Surg*. 2019;8:305–311.
16. Cooper C, Dennison EM, Leufkens HG, Bishop N, van Staa TP. Epidemiology of childhood fractures in Britain: a study using the general practice research database. *J Bone Miner Res*. 2004;19:1976–1981.
17. Landin LA. Fracture patterns in children. Analysis of 8,682 fractures with special reference to incidence, etiology and secular changes in a Swedish urban population 1950–1979. *Acta Orthop Scand Suppl*. 1983;202:1–109.
18. Rennie L, Court-Brown CM, Mok JY, Beattie TF. The epidemiology of fractures in children. *Injury*. 2007;38:913–922.
19. Randsborg PH, Gulbrandsen P, Saltyte Benth J, et al. Fractures in children: epidemiology and activity-specific fracture rates. *J Bone Joint Surg Am*. 2013;95:e42.
20. Ryan LM, Teach SJ, Searcy K, et al. Epidemiology of pediatric forearm fractures in Washington, DC. *J Trauma*. 2010;69:S200–S205.
21. Bailey DA, Wedge JH, McCulloch RG, Martin AD, Bernhardson SC. Epidemiology of fractures of the distal end of the radius in children as associated with growth. *J Bone Joint Surg Am*. 1989;71:1225–1231.
22. Khosla S, Melton 3rd LJ, Dekutoski MB, Achenbach SJ, Oberg AL, Riggs BL. Incidence of childhood distal forearm fractures over 30 years: a population-based study. *JAMA*. 2003;290:1479–1485.
23. Mathison DJ, Agrawal D. An update on the epidemiology of pediatric fractures. *Pediatr Emerg Care*. 2010;26:594–603 quiz 4-6.
24. Al-Ansari K, Howard A, Seeto B, Yoo S, Zaki S, Boutis K. Minimally angulated pediatric wrist fractures: is immobilization without manipulation enough? *CJEM*. 2007;9:9–15.
25. Alffram PA, Bauer GC. Epidemiology of fractures of the forearm. A biomechanical investigation of bone strength. *J Bone Joint Surg Am*. 1962;44-A:105–114.
26. Krabbe S, Christiansen C, Rodbro P, Transbol I. Effect of puberty on rates of bone growth and mineralisation: with observations in male delayed puberty. *Arch Dis Child*. 1979;54:950–953.
27. Rizzoli R, Bonjour JP, Ferrari SL. Osteoporosis, genetics and hormones. *J Mol Endocrinol*. 2001;26:79–94.
28. Henry YM, Fatayerji D, Eastell R. Attainment of peak bone mass at the lumbar spine, femoral neck and radius in men and women: relative contributions of bone size and volumetric bone mineral density. *Osteoporos Int*. 2004;15:263–273.
29. Faulkner RA, Davison KS, Bailey DA, Mirwald RL, Baxter-Jones AD. Size-corrected BMD decreases during peak linear growth: implications for fracture incidence during adolescence. *J Bone Miner Res*. 2006;21:1864–1870.
30. Price CT, Scott DS, Kurzner ME, Flynn JC. Malunited forearm fractures in children. *J Pediatr Orthop*. 1990;10:705–712.
31. Fuller DJ, McCullough CJ. Malunited fractures of the forearm in children. *J Bone Joint Surg (Br)*. 1982;64:364–367.

32. Arunachalam VS, Griffiths JC. Fracture recurrence in children. *Injury.* 1975;7:37–40.
33. Vince KG, Miller JE. Cross-union complicating fracture of the forearm. Part I: adults. *J Bone Joint Surg Am.* 1987;69:640–653.
34. Court-Brown CM, Caesar B. Epidemiology of adult fractures: a review. *Injury.* 2006;37:691–697.
35. Griffin MR, Ray WA, Fought RL, Melton 3rd LJ. Black-white differences in fracture rates. *Am J Epidemiol.* 1992;136:1378–1385.
36. Baron JA, Barrett J, Malenka D, et al. Racial differences in fracture risk. *Epidemiology.* 1994;5:42–47.
37. Flinkkila T, Sirnio K, Hippi M, et al. Epidemiology and seasonal variation of distal radius fractures in Oulu, Finland. *Osteoporos Int.* 2011;22:2307–2312.
38. Sigurdardottir K, Halldorsson S, Robertsson J. Epidemiology and treatment of distal radius fractures in Reykjavik, Iceland, in 2004. Comparison with an Icelandic study from 1985. *Acta Orthop.* 2011;82:494–498.
39. Imai N, Endo N, Shobugawa Y, et al. Incidence of four major types of osteoporotic fragility fractures among elderly individuals in Sado, Japan, in 2015. *J Bone Miner Metab.* 2019;37:484–490.
40. Xu W, Ni C, Yu R, Gu G, Wang Z, Zheng G. Risk factors for distal radius fracture in postmenopausal women. *Orthopade.* 2017;46:447–450.
41. Kanterewicz E, Yanez A, Perez-Pons A, Codony I, Del Rio L, Diez-Perez A. Association between Colles' fracture and low bone mass: age-based differences in postmenopausal women. *Osteoporos Int.* 2002;13:824–828.
42. Lofman O, Hallberg I, Berglund K, et al. Women with low-energy fracture should be investigated for osteoporosis. *Acta Orthop.* 2007;78:813–821.
43. Oyen J, Rohde GE, Hochberg M, Johnsen V, Haugeberg G. Low-energy distal radius fractures in middle-aged and elderly women-seasonal variations, prevalence of osteoporosis, and associates with fractures. *Osteoporos Int.* 2010;21:1247–1255.
44. Oyen J, Brudvik C, Gjesdal CG, Tell GS, Lie SA, Hove LM. Osteoporosis as a risk factor for distal radial fractures: a case-control study. *J Bone Joint Surg Am.* 2011;93:348–356.
45. Cuddihy MT, Gabriel SE, Crowson CS, O'Fallon WM, Melton 3rd LJ. Forearm fractures as predictors of subsequent osteoporotic fractures. *Osteoporos Int.* 1999;9:469–475.
46. Saarelainen J, Hassi S, Honkanen R, et al. Bone loss and wrist fractures after withdrawal of hormone therapy: the 15-year follow-up of the OSTPRE cohort. *Maturitas.* 2016;85:49–55.
47. Marchewka J, Glodzik J, Marchewka W, Golec E. Higher mortality in men compared with women following distal radius fracture in population aged 50 years or above: are common distal radius fracture classifications useful in predicting mortality? *Biomed Res Int.* 2019;2019:5359204.
48. Chung KC, Shauver MJ, Yin H, Kim HM, Baser O, Birkmeyer JD. Variations in the use of internal fixation for distal radial fracture in the United States medicare population. *J Bone Joint Surg Am.* 2011;93:2154–2162.
49. Wu JC, Strickland CD, Chambers JS. Wrist fractures and osteoporosis. *Orthop Clin North Am.* 2019;50:211–221.
50. Mauck BM, Swigler CW. Evidence-based review of distal radius fractures. *Orthop Clin North Am.* 2018;49:211–222.
51. Lutz K, Yeoh KM, MacDermid JC, Symonette C, Grewal R. Complications associated with operative versus nonsurgical treatment of distal radius fractures in patients aged 65 years and older. *J Hand Surg [Am].* 2014;39:1280–1286.
52. Sander AL, Leiblein M, Sommer K, Marzi I, Schneidmuller D, Frank J. Epidemiology and treatment of distal radius fractures: current concept based on fracture severity and not on age. *Eur J Trauma Emerg Surg.* 2020;46:585–590.
53. Huetteman HE, Zhong L, Chung KC. Cost of surgical treatment for distal radius fractures and the implications of episode-based bundled payments. *J Hand Surg [Am].* 2018;43:720–730.

CHAPTER 3

Surgical Anatomy of the Distal Radius

FRANÇOIS LOISEL • LAURENT OBERT
Orthopaedics, Traumatology, Plastic and Reconstructive Surgery Unit, Hand Surgery Unit,
University Hospital J. Minjoz, Besançon, France

KEY POINTS

- The precise knowledge of the evolution of the anatomy of the radius is essential to understand the main points of the treatment decision and the surgical principles.
- General anatomy of the distal radius subdivides it in a diaphysis, metaphysis, and epiphysis. Each surface of different shape is covered by a different structure, mostly tendoninous. The angulations of the ulnar and the radial columns are different. The watershed line is the most distal limit that a standard osteosynthesis plate must not exceed.
- The "radiographic check list" of the distal radius include:
  - radial inclination (frontal plain)
  - volar tilt
  - teardrop angle
  - AP distance
  - articular depth
  - dorsal rim line
  - coronal shift

IMPORTANCE OF THE PROBLEM

A distal radius fracture (DRF) is a very frequent pathology, involving 15% of women after age of 50 years, in relation with decrease of bone mineral density (85% low BMD, 51% osteoporosis).[1] Development and innovation of not only the anatomy's comprehension, but also of the implants and approaches have considerably improved the function of these patients.

CURRENT OPINION

Advanced knowledge of basic anatomy and individual variations are deemed mandatory for the anatomic reduction of distal radius fractures (mainly in case of comminution) as well as to obtain fracture fixation while "staying out of trouble," hence avoiding iatro-genic tendinous/ligamentous injuries when anatomic principles are violated.

Finding the Evidence

- Cochrane search: Distal Radius Fracture
- Pubmed (Medline): distal radius fracture*[tiab] AND anatom*[tiab]
- Bibliography of eligible articles
- Articles that were not in the English or French language were excluded.

Quality of the Evidence

For purposes of this chapter, the authors assembled the full bibliography of articles published by our unit since 2004 on the current subject. Furthermore, we included the most recent metaanalyses, reviews, and international expert

---

Distal Radius Fractures. https://doi.org/10.1016/B978-0-323-75764-5.00019-6

21

Panel 1: Case Scenario: A "Simple" Distal Radius Fracture

A 63-year-old woman fell on her left upper limb 10 days ago and was immobilized in a sugar tong splint (Fig. 1). What radio-anatomic aspects of the radius are important to improve in this patient?

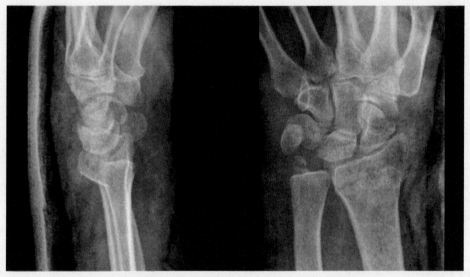

FIG. 1 Radiographs showing a mildly displaced distal radius fracture.

recommendations (AAOS), as well as the main hand surgery reference book (i.e., Green Surgery, 7th edition).

Findings

***Distal radius anatomy: general aspects[2]** (Fig. 2)*
The distal portion of the radius is quadrilateral in cross-section, including the metaphyseal and epiphyseal regions.

Anatomic features of distal radius include four surfaces (anterior, lateral, posterior, and medial), the styloid process and the dorsal tubercle.

The three concave articular surfaces are the scaphoid fossa, the lunate fossa, and the sigmoid notch.

The anterior surface is concaved, palmary directed and covered by the pronator quadratus (Fig. 2A). The surface is rough for the attachment of the palmar

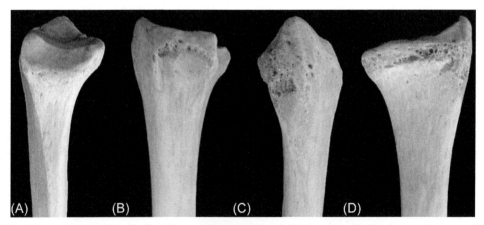

(A)   (B)   (C)   (D)

FIG. 2 From left to right A, B, C, D the osseous anatomy of distal radius with the four surfaces (medial, posterior, lateral, and anterior), the styloid process and the dorsal tubercle.

radiocarpal ligaments extending radially form the radial styloid ulnarly to the TFCC. The lateral surface extends along the lateral margin to form the styloid process (Fig. 2B). The styloid process is conical and projects 10–12 mm distal to the articular surface for the proximal scaphoid and lunate. The radial styloid area may have a flat groove for the tendon of the first dorsal compartment (abductor pollicis longus and extensor pollicis brevis tendons).

The dorsal surface of the distal radius is irregular, convex, and acts as a fulcrum for extensor tendon function (Fig. 2C).

The prominent dorsal tubercle (Lister's tubercle) lies from 5 to 10 mm from the distal joint surface. On the medial aspect of the dorsal tubercle is a smooth groove for passage of the extensor pollicis longus tendon. Ulnar to the dorsal tubercle, are grooves for passage of the extensor indicis which passes deeper than the extensor digitorum communis. The posterior interosseous nerve courses along the dorsal margin and adjacent to the cortex.

The medial surface of the distal radius consists of the ulnar notch and the articular surface for the ulnar head (Fig. 2D). The distal radius rotates about the ulnar head via the sigmoid notch which is concave, with a well-defined dorsal, palmar, and distal margin but variation in the depth of the articulation with the ulnar head.

The height of the ulna in respect to the radius varies with pronation and supination. There are various degrees of positive or negative ulna variance which affect the amount of force transmitted to the distal radius and to the triangular fibrocartilage complex (TFCC). Between the distal radioulnar joint and the radiocarpal joint there is a ridge, located in the ulnar notch, which provides the radial attachment for the triangular fibrocartilage. In various degrees of radio-ulnar deviation there is greater or lesser contact with the TFCC.

FRESH LOOK AT ANATOMY OF THE DISTAL RADIUS

Few studies of the anatomy of radial epiphysis have been published in the past 15 years. However, with the availability of new implants (intra- or extramedullary) and the recent rash of avoidable iatrogenic injuries, there is an increased need for a more detailed description of the metaphysis-epiphysis region in the distal radius. Studies on this topic are scarce and its clinical applications may be difficult to interpret.

The review by Herzberg et al. performed in 1998 on regional and bony anatomy is one of those examples.[3] They found the anterior cortex to be thicker than the

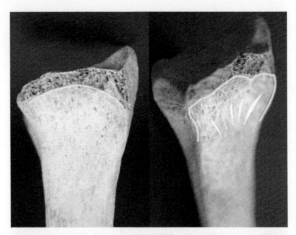

FIG. 3 Two oblique views of the distal radius showing the more proximal pronator quadratus line *(solid line)* and the watershed line *(dashed line)*.

posterior cortex and the tendons and nerves to run along the dorsal side.

In 2005, Nelson characterized the most distal edge of the epiphysis and described the watershed and pronator quadratus lines (Fig. 3).[4]

The pronator quadratus line marks the highest part of the epiphysis and helps the surgeon visualize the patient-specific radius curvature. If an implant goes beyond this line when viewed on lateral radiographs, there is a potential for impingement with the thumb and finger flexor tendons. The watershed line marks the most distal edge of the epiphysis; sometimes it is as high as the pronator quadratus line, sometimes it is higher. A small 3–5 mm thick strip of bone separates these two lines. **If you go past the watershed line, you will be in the joint!**

Imatani et al. studied the volar aspect of the distal radius macroscopically and histologically in 20 distal forearms of 10 cadavers. The watershed line might not be a distinct line, corresponding to the distal margin of the pronator fossa in the lateral half of the volar radius and to a hypothetical line between the distal and proximal lines in the medial half.[5]

Windish et al. defined the protuberance as the radial part of the radial epiphysis. The geometry of this protuberance varies greatly.[6] Two recent studies from the same team provide an even better description of the distal radius. Pichler et al. found large variability in the measurements about the Lister tubercle and the extensor pollicis longus groove (cadaver study with 30 forearms) and also found a difference between the radial and ulnar slopes (cadaver study with 100 radiuses).[7, 8]

Buzzell et al. evaluated eight distal radius volar plates and found that the area between the plate and distal radius is very thin and varies by 3%–6%.[9] Gasse et al. have shown in their anatomic study that the ulnar column had an average angle of 155.3 degrees and the intermediate column 144.9 degrees.[10]

Based on this data, it seems logical to imagine using a plate of varying curvature for optimal fit on the wrist. However, because the radial epiphysis actually has two slopes (due to its two columns), it is more difficult to develop anatomical plates.

Plates that are currently available on the market have a slope of approximately 155 degrees. However, their slope is constant and does not change over the width of the radius. Four generations of plates are now available on the market.[11] The last generation with polyaxial screw and special design of the plate in order to apply it on the ulnar column which is further forward than the radial column (Fig. 4).

If we look at the more ulnar side, the sigmoid notch was more extensively studied, and was shown to be important for the stability of the distal radioulnar joint. Tollat et al. described in 1996[12] four types of sigmoid notch, classified as A, B, C or D (Fig. 5).

More recently, it was shown that the flatter and less angulated the sigmoid notch is, the greater the risk of TFCC injury as it would make the ulnar head less contained hence more prone to anteroposterior dislocation.[13]

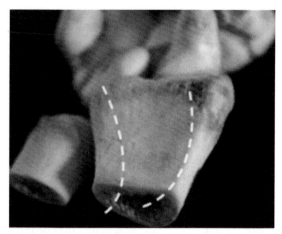

FIG. 4 The area of application of a plate is more ulnar than radial. Plate design should be based on this principle and should not be too radial because the ulnar column is further forward than the radial column.

LIGAMENT ANATOMY

The progress of knowledge in the field of extrinsic ligament anatomy of the wrist has implications in the understanding of the different models of articular fractures of the distal radius,[14] and also in highlighting the importance of these ligaments in the stability of the first carpal row.[15, 16] Although this anatomy is subject to variation, it has been extensively described previously.[17–21]

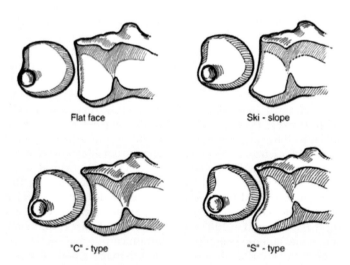

Flat face   Ski - slope

"C" - type   "S" - type

FIG. 5 Classification of four different shapes of the sigmoid notch by Tolat et al.

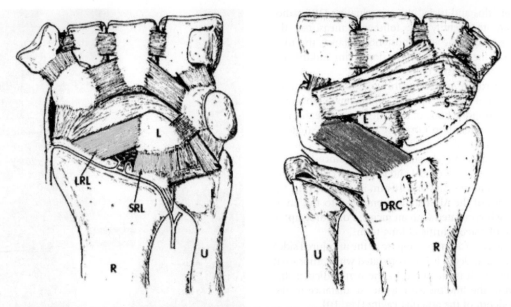

FIG. 6 Main extrinsic ligaments of the wrist: on the left, LRL *(blue)*, SRL *(green)*, on the right (dorsal side), DRC *(red)*. (Images modified from Berger RA. Arthroscopic anatomy of the wrist and distal radioulnar joint. *Hand Clin* 1999;15:393–413.)

On the dorsal part of the radius, the dorsal radio-carpal (DRC) ligament spans the ulnar aspect of the dorsal rim from the ulnar margin of the dorsal tubercle (Lister's tubercule) to the sigmoid notch.

On the volar side, the radioscaphocapitate (RSC) ligament origin spans from the radial styloid to the volar rim at the level of the scaphoid fossa.

The long radiolunate ligament (LRL) ligament originates from the volar rim of the scaphoid fossa.

The short radiolunate ligament (SRL) ligament originates from the volar rim of the lunate fossa (Fig. 6).

RADIOGRAPHIC PATHOANATOMY

The distal articular surface of the radius has a radial inclination averaging 22 degrees and tilts palmary an average of 11 degrees (Fig. 7). The sigmoid notch angles distally and medially an average of 22 degrees.

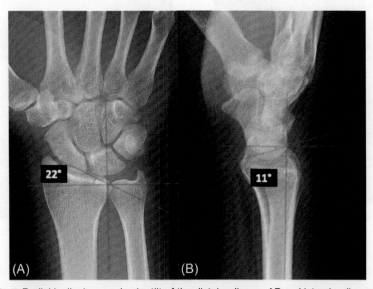

FIG. 7 Radial inclinaison and volar tilt of the distal radius on AP and lateral radiographs.

Other "tips and tricks" when evaluating DRF radiograph are to identify the following measures: the "teardrop" angle, the anteroposterior distance, the articular depth, the projection of the dorsal rim and the coronal shift of the distal radius.[22]

The "teardrop" represents the volar projection of the lunate facet of the distal radius. A line drawn tangential to the subchondral bone of the articular surface through the tip of the teardrop normally subtends an angle of 70 degrees (Fig. 8).

The average anteroposterior (AP) distance between the distal apex of the dorsal and volar rims of the lunate facet is 20 mm in males and 18 mm in females (Fig. 9). An increase of the AP distance compared to the uninjured side is correlated with an increase of radiographic evidence of osteoarthritis at long term.

The increase (>2 mm compare to the uninjured side) of the articular depth is also correlated with radiocarpal osteoarthritis: it is measured by the perpendicular distance from the line measuring the AP distance to the greatest depth of the articular cavity (Fig. 10).

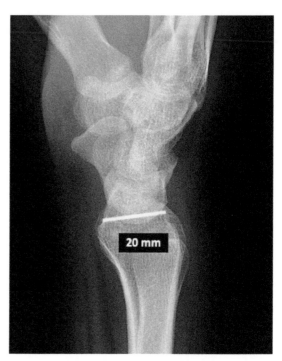

FIG. 9 Anteroposterior distance.

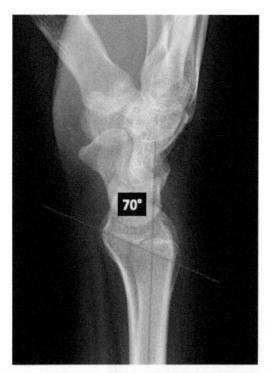

FIG. 8 Angle between the "teardrop" and the axis of the radius.

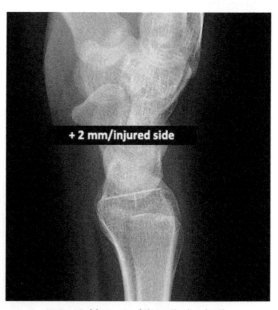

FIG. 10 Measure of the articular depth.

On normal anteroposterior view, the normal dorsal rim of the radius projects 3–5 mm beyond the dense subchondral bone of the volar rim. Displaced fractures may perturb this relationship as well as breaks in the dense subchondral bone (step-offs, gaps) (Fig. 11).

The radial translation or coronal shift has been shown to cause radioulnar instability through its slackening effect on the distal oblique bundle of the interosseous membrane. The measurement is performed by extending a line along the ulnar diaphysis of the radius

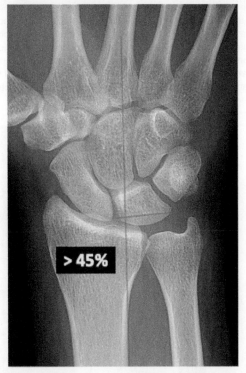

FIG. 12 A line along the ulnar diaphysis of the radius distally cross the transverse line drawn across the lunate at its widest point: more than average 45% of the lunate is ulnar to the intersection point.

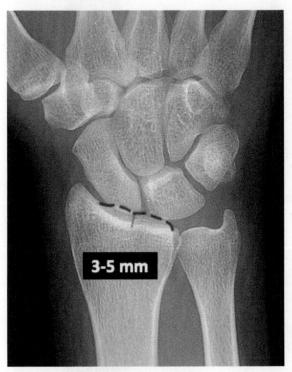

FIG. 11 Dorsal rim line.

distally across the carpus (Fig. 12). A transverse line is drawn across the lunate at its widest point. The percentage of the lunate radial to the intersection point of the line averages 45% (if less than half of the lunate projects ulnar to this intersection point, this indicates a coronal shift risk).

Panel 2: Case Scenario

In the light of the parameters studied, the following are those that have been improved, in this case by an anterior plate osteosynthesis. At the beginning there were no alterations concerning the anterioposterior measurement, nor the articular depth (extra articular fracture) or radial translation of the fracture. However, the following pathoanatomic parameters were:

–   decrease of the radial inclination
–   increased dorsal tilt
–   increased tear drop angle

Although these last parameters have not returned to a physiological norm, they have been improved by open reduction and internal fixation (Figs. 13 and 14).

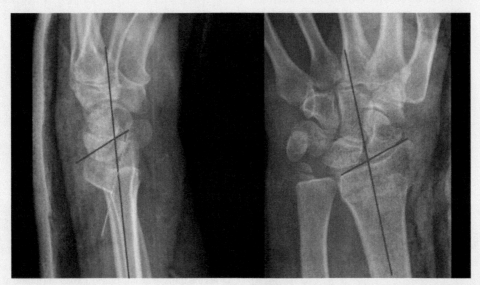

FIG. 13 Increase of the teardrop angle *(green)* on the left. Pathological radial inclination *(in red)* on the right, and dorsal tilt *(in red)* on the left.

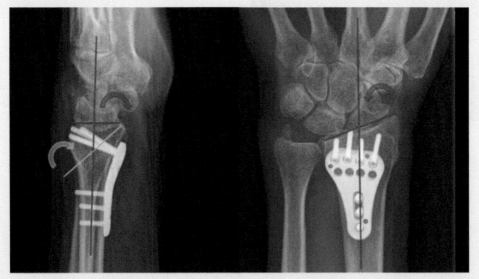

FIG. 14 After ORIF, improvement of the radial inclination, achievement of a neutral tilt and improvement of the tear drop angle.

CONCLUSION

The precise anatomy of the distal radius has now been well established and recent work has improved our ability to specify the fracture parameters that need to be corrected. The knowledge and verification of an anatomical checklist on radiographs may help guide us toward the best selection of complementary exams and choice of treatment.

REFERENCES

1. Gehrmann SV, Windolf J, Kaufmann RA. Distal radius fracture management in elderly patients: a literature review. *J Hand Surg [Am]*. 2008; 33(3):421–429.
2. Obert L, Uhring J, Rey PB, et al. Anatomy and biomechanics of distal radius fractures: a literature review. *Chir Main*. 2012; 31(6):287–297.
3. Herzberg G, Garret J, Ehrard L. Anatomie du radius distal. In: ESF, ed. *Cahiers d'enseignement de la SOFCOT*. Expansion Scientifique Francaise; 1998:1–13. vol. 67.
4. Nelson D. Anatomy Notes and Their Clinical Significance for the Volar Approach By David L. Nelson, MD. [cité 28 mai 2014]. Disponible sur:(). http://www.davidlnelson.md/articles/Radius_Anatomy_Annotated.htm.
5. Imatani J, Akita K, Yamaguchi K, Shimizu H, Kondou H, Ozaki T. An anatomical study of the watershed line on the volar, distal aspect of the radius: implications for plate placement and avoidance of tendon ruptures. *J Hand Surg [Am]*. 2012; 37(8):1550–1554.
6. Windisch G, Clement H, Tanzer K, et al. Promontory of radius: a new anatomical description on the distal radius. *Surg Radiol Anat*. 2007; 29(8):629–633.
7. Pichler W, Windisch G, Schaffler G, Rienmüller R, Grechenig W. Computer tomography aided 3D analysis of the distal dorsal radius surface and the effects on volar plate osteosynthesis. *J Hand Surg Eur Vol*. oct 2009; 34 (5):598–602.
8. Pichler W, Clement H, Hausleitner L, Tanzer K, Tesch NP, Grechenig W. Various circular arc radii of the distal volar radius and the implications on volar plate osteosynthesis. *Orthopedics*. 2008; 31(12).
9. Buzzell JE, Weikert DR, Watson JT, Lee DH. Precontoured fixed-angle volar distal radius plates: a comparison of anatomic fit. *J Hand Surg [Am]*. 2008; 33(7):1144–1152.
10. Gasse N, Lepage D, Pem R, et al. Anatomical and radiological study applied to distal radius surgery. *Surg Radiol Anat*. 2011; 33(6):485–490.
11. Obert L, Rey P-B, Uhring J, et al. Fixation of distal radius fractures in adults: a review. *Orthop Traumatol Surg Res*. 2013; 99(2):216–234.
12. Tolat AR, Stanley JK, Trail IA. A cadaveric study of the anatomy and stability of the distal radioulnar joint in the coronal and transverse planes. *J Hand Surg (Br)*. 1996; 21(5):587–594.
13. Jung H-S, Park MJ, Won Y-S, Lee GY, Kim S, Lee JS. The correlation between shape of the sigmoid notch of the distal radius and the risk of triangular fibrocartilage complex foveal tear. *Bone Joint J*. 2020; 102-B(6):749–754.
14. Zumstein MA, Hasan AP, McGuire DT, Eng K, Bain GI. Distal radius attachments of the radiocarpal ligaments: an anatomical study. *J Wrist Surg*. 2013; 2(4):346–350.
15. Pérez AJ, Jethanandani RG, Vutescu ES, Meyers KN, Lee SK, Wolfe SW. Role of ligament stabilizers of the proximal carpal row in preventing dorsal intercalated segment instability: a cadaveric study. *J Bone Joint Surg Am*. 2019; 101(15):1388–1396.
16. Elsaidi GA, Ruch DS, Kuzma GR, Smith BP. Dorsal wrist ligament insertions stabilize the scapholunate interval: cadaver study. *Clin Orthop Relat Res*. 2004; 425:152–157.
17. Berger RA. The ligaments of the wrist. A current overview of anatomy with considerations of their potential functions. *Hand Clin*. 1997; 13(1):63–82.
18. Berger RA. The anatomy of the ligaments of the wrist and distal radioulnar joints. *Clin Orthop Relat Res*. 2001; 383:32–40.
19. Nagao S, Patterson RM, Buford WL, Andersen CR, Shah MA, Viegas SF. Three-dimensional description of ligamentous attachments around the lunate. *J Hand Surg [Am]*. 2005; 30(4):685–692.
20. Viegas SF, Yamaguchi S, Boyd NL, Patterson RM. The dorsal ligaments of the wrist: anatomy, mechanical properties, and function. *J Hand Surg [Am]*. 1999; 24(3):456–468.
21. Mizuseki T, Ikuta Y. The dorsal carpal ligaments: their anatomy and function. *J Hand Surg (Br)*. 1989; 14 (1):91–98.
22. Garcia-Elias M, Lluch AL. Wrist instabilities, misalignments, and dislocations. In: Wolfe SW, Hotchkiss RN, Pederson WC, Kozin SH, Cohen MS, eds. *Green's Operative Hand Surgery*. 7th ed. Philadelphia, PA: Elsevier; 2017.

CHAPTER 4

Biomechanics of Distal Radius Fractures

FRANÇOIS LOISEL • LAURENT OBERT
Orthopaedics, Traumatology, Plastic and Reconstructive Surgery Unit, Hand Surgery Unit, University Hospital J. Minjoz, Besançon, France

---

KEY POINTS

- The ideal classification meets three objectives: to describe the lesion, to guide treatment choice, and to predict the functional outcome.
  - An example of such is the Patient Accident Fracture (PAF) classification as it allows an exhaustive analysis that also puts into perspective patient and mechanism of injury characteristics.
- An altered anatomy of the distal radius leads to biomechanical disorders such as altered load transfer, decreased joint amplitudes, carpal instability, stiffness, or instability of the distal radioulnar joint.
  - An important example of this is the fragmented discontinuity of the volar intermediate column—also referred to as the critical corner—with high risk of biomechanical construct failure when inadequately fixated.
- The most recent biomechanical works on anterior plate osteosynthesis can be summarized by variable angulation plates with 3 to 4 unicortical epiphyseal locking screws in a single row, with 2 or 3 bicortical diaphyseal screws.

IMPORTANCE OF THE PROBLEM

Based on the knowledge of the anatomical "key points" of the distal radius, it is possible to classify the fracture in order to guide the treatment and explain the subsequent functional prognosis to the patient. It is also essential to know the biomechanical factors applied to distal radius fractures (DRF), which influence the decision of the type of treatment envisaged.

Panel 1: Case Scenario 1

A 72-year-old woman who fell directly on her left arm sustained an open DRF with an anterior displacement. How can this DRF best be classified? And based on biomechanical principles of DRFs, which type and configuration of osteosynthesis would be most adequate for this osteopenic fracture? (Fig. 1)

Continued

Distal Radius Fractures. https://doi.org/10.1016/B978-0-323-75764-5.00039-1

Panel 1: Case Scenario 1—cont'd

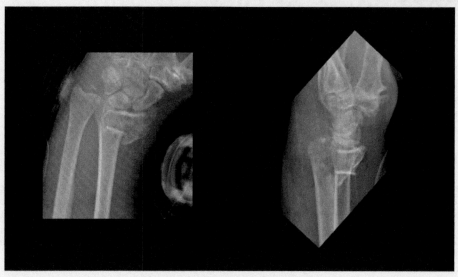

FIG. 1 Open comminuted articular DRF.

Panel 1: Case Scenario 2

A 51 year-old women was brought the emergency department with multiple fractures after sustaining a motor cycle accident. Her radiographs and reconstructed CT body scan of the left wrist show a displaced volar rim fragment of the distal radius (Fig. 2). From a biomechanical point of view, what type of plate fixation would be most adequate for this type of fracture: a standard distal radius plate or a volar rim plate?

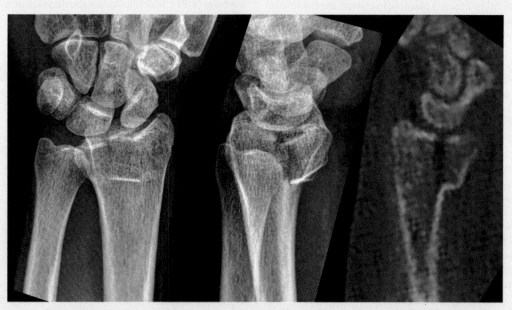

FIG. 2 Radiographs showing a displaced volar rim fragment of the distal radius. (Courtesy of Benjamin Degeorge.)

CURRENT OPINION

Advanced knowledge of distal radius biomechanics is mandatory to choose the adequate treatment strategy, whether operative or conservative. Multiple risk factors of fracture instability and fixation construct failure have been identified and should be considered during decision-making.

Finding the Evidence

- Cochrane search: Distal Radius Fracture biomechanics
- Pubmed (Medline): distal radius fracture*[tiab] AND biomechanic*[tiab]
- Bibliography of eligible articles
- Articles that were not in the English or French language were excluded.

Findings

Biomechanical studies of distal radius fractures are numerous. It is important to take into consideration that some in vitro studies are limited by the use of synthetic bone,[1] or postulate boundary conditions that are different from one team to another, raising the question of the validity of comparing them with each other (strong heterogeneity bias).[2, 3] Finally, some biomechanically validated hypotheses still lack validation or clinical relevance. The emergence of new tools such as finite element models should not make us forget that these numerical models must be validated in vitro before valid conclusions can be drawn.[4]

CLASSIFICATION: WHY AND WHICH ONE?

Energy and Fracture[5]

There is no "typical DRF" but an injury spectrum, a consequence of hyperextension. Pechlaner[6] reported the results of a cadaveric study in which 63 forearms were used in machine hyperextension. Depending on the position of the first row during the impact, the pressures applied on the articular surface of the radius will generate fractures rather dorsal, central, or palmar. In each of the three localizations, there is an increasing injury severity with pure metaphyseal fractures, followed by epiphyseal metaphysis (articular resection) and finally with dislocation. The most common form was the articular and metaphyseal form with dorsal displacement.[6] In two-thirds of cases there were associated injuries at the level of the triangular complex (with or without avulsion of the ulnar styloid) or interosseous ligaments. This work legitimizes Laulan's work and the MEU classification[7] (Fig. 3). Some particular lesions have been identified and are often described as specific entities:

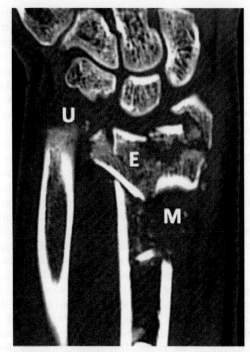

FIG. 3 MEU classification of Laulan. Each fracture is composed of the three associated injury components: **M**etaphyseal involvement, **E**piphyseal joint involvement, (distal radio-)**U**lnar joint involvement.

the fracture with a Die Punch fragment (postero-medial fragment) described by Scheck in 1962, and the radial styloid fracture (Chauffeur's fracture).[8]

The "Best" Classification

The large number of classifications published over time did not allow one of them to become a relevant management tool. Classifications are closely linked to an era and a type of treatment. The ideal classification must meet three objectives: **to describe the injury**, to **guide decision-making**, and to reliably **predict the functional outcome**.[9]

Unfortunately, none of the classifications fulfill the three conditions defined above. Most only take into account the fractures of the radius, and on the radius only few parameters differ from one classification to another.

In addition, intra- and interobserver reliability are often poor and objectify the limits of these classifications where the observer has cannot readily "box" the fracture. Using both AP and lateral views, the AO classification was moderately reproducible in an interobserver and weakly in an intraobserver reliability analysis.[10] Only type A (extraarticular), B (intraarticular partial) and C (intraarticular) of AO was reproducible.[11] Using a scanner to complete the analysis, the AO classification lost any interobserver reproducibility.[12] Similarly, the Frykman, Melone, and Mayo Clinic classifications were unreliable, both intra- and interobserver.[10, 13, 14] Moreover, several studies have shown the lack of prognostic interest of these classifications, proving that the criteria studied are not the right ones to describe the fracture. After 5 years, the AO and Frykman classifications did not predict the clinical course of 652 patients.[12] Older's classification, tested on 633 patients, was also insufficient in terms of prognosis.[14] Lenoble's study also found no prognostic value in Casting, Frykman, Gartland, Older, Lindström, and Jenkins' classifications.[15] The so-called universal classification proposed by Cooney[16] tries to propose a therapeutic strategy but its recently tested validity remains debatable.[17] Thus, the classifications studied are neither reproducible nor prognostic. Their usefulness is hence questionable. And more than a classification, a system of description of the injuries must prevail to compare the fractures.[7] That of Laulan is validated and allows to "tidy up" in all cases the fracture of the radius. This classification describes the fracture with sufficient intra- and interobserver reproducibility to become a useful tool for treatment and functional prognosis. It consists in the description of three parameters allowing to know if the fracture is "serious" or not, each parameter having been validated as related to the prognosis. Metaphysis (comminution), epiphysis (articular fracture) and ulna involvement are different in each fracture, but each fracture case is a combination of these three parameters (Figs. 3 and 4).[7]

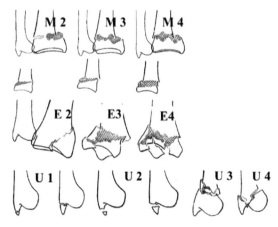

FIG. 4 MEU classification of Laulan.

Analysis of the **metaphyseal** component (presence of comminution and/or corticospongious impaction at the metaphysis level):
- M 0: absent metaphyseal line, and.
- M 1: simple metaphyseal line, without comminution.
- M 2: metaphyseal trait displaced with localized comminution. Comminution is less than hemicircumference (postero-external scale).
- M 3: metaphyseal line with comminution of at least one hemicircumference (all the posterior cortical with respect for the opposite hemicircumference (antero-medial console allowing a reduction).
- M 4: metaphyseal line with circumferential comminution. The instability after reduction is multidirectional.

The parameter "prime" is assigned to the parameter M if the metaphyseal line ends definitively in the distal radioulnar joint.

Analysis of the **epiphyseal** component of the fracture (presence of articular features with or without displacement).
- E 0: absent joint line and.
- E 1: articular line (s), not displaced.
- E 2: articular fragment (s) displaced by shearing. There is no subchondral embedding component. The displacement concerns only a part of the articular surface with one or two epiphyseal fragments (radial styloid fracture, volar rim fracture, etc.)
- E 3: articular fragment (s) displaced by localized compression. There is subchondral depression localized to a part of the articular surface which can involve up to three fragments.
- E 4: articular fragments displaced by extended compression. Subchondral depression involves almost the entire articular surface with a bursting appearance. The small size of the fragments prevents their reduction and/or fixation.

Analysis of the **ulnar** line, according to its location and its displacement:
- U 0: absence of ulnar fracture.
- U 1: nondisplaced fracture of the ulnar styloid (distal or proximal).
- U 2: displaced fracture of the ulnar styloid (distal or proximal).
- U 3: metaphysio-diaphyseal ulnar fracture (+/– styloid).
- U 4: metaphysio-epiphyseal ulnar fracture (+/– styloid).

Fracture Analysis by the PAF System (Patient, Accident, Fracture)

The "analysis method" presented for the first time at the French Orthopaedic Society (SOFCOT) by Herzberg and Dumontier,[9] then modified and improved by Herzberg,[18, 19] is a simple way of understanding the DRF in order to identify and therefore to treat all injuries without forgetting them (Fig. 5). This is a list of essential elements whose anatomy is to be restored because it is related to the functional prognosis. There are four specific parameters of the distal radius (radial inclination, volar tilt, articular impaction, and the shortening of the radius by metaphyseal compression) as well as intracarpal and distal radioulnar (RUD) joint injury. The three parameters of the MEU classification finally become part of it (Fig. 4). This "checklist" is filled out using a standard emergency radiographic assessment consisting of anteroposterior (AP), lateral and oblique

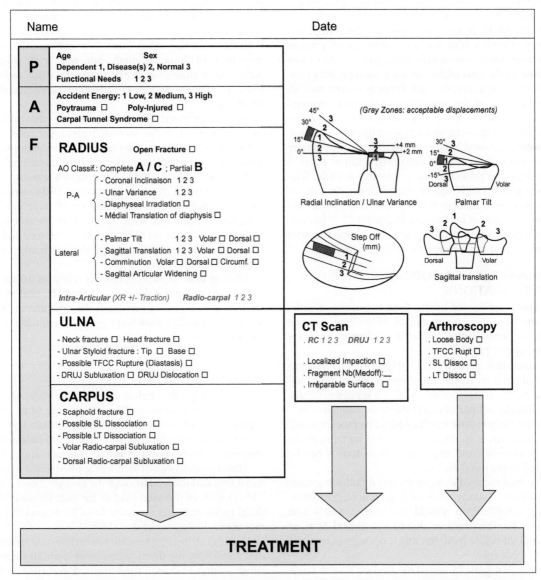

FIG. 5 Herzberg's proposed analysis system that stratifies patients and provides the best treatment option for different fracture parameters and estimated patient needs.

views. These allow to analyze the presence and importance of a posteromedial fragment. In the event of a high-energy fracture, a CT scan will analyze all articular injuries at the radiocarpal level and at the radioulnar level. Intraoperatively, under anesthesia radiographs under traction allow a better analysis (especially comminution) and often relativize large displacement. In two thirds of cases they provided information to the operator that make him modify his strategy.[9] In this analysis, arthroscopy is an additional tool to complete the assessment, in a contemporary way to fixation. Ligament and osteocartilaginous injuries will be perfectly visualized.[20] With regard to ligamentous injuries, their high frequency contrasts with the small number of patients who secondarily require ligament repair.[6, 21] As Laulan showed, at the level of the interosseous ligaments (scapholunate), ligamentous injury is not synonymous with incompetence of the structure and therefore synonymous with repair.[22] In a 1-year radiographic prospective study, 43% of dissociative intracarpal ligamentous injuries were diagnosed but these ligamentous injuries were not found to influence the functional result at 1 year.[22] With regard to osteochondral injuries, in articular fractures in patients with high functional demands, arthroscopy remains a modern tool for the visualization and optimal fixation of inaccessible fragments.[20, 23] But seeing and better understanding intraarticular injuries does not mean that they always can or should be fixed.

GENERAL BIOMECHANICAL CONSIDERATIONS

The loads experienced by the distal radius vary greatly. Wrist motion during activities of daily living generate loads of nearly 100 N, while finger flexion produces an average of 250 N.[24]

Putnam et al. showed that a 10 N grip force translates to an axial force of 26.3 N in the metaphysis of the distal radius. For each 10 N applied, 26–52 N is applied to the distal radius, depending on hand position and radius length.[25]

When the grip force reaches 450 N (average for men), a 2410 N load is applied on the radial metaphysis. In certain positions and grips, more than 3000 N can be applied to the distal radius.[26]

The load required to break the distal radius is greater than 2500 N.[27] Many advocate grip tightening exercises during rehabilitation should not exceed 169 N and range-of-motion exercises should not exceed 50% of the implant failure load. But this is not easy to extrapolate to a patient.

Loads that cause failure of the fixation system range from 55 to 825 N and are directly related to the type of hardware used and its inherent features.[26]

Regarding the cortical thickness, several papers have been published. Mueller et al. analyzed age and gender differences in architectural measures of bone quality and their correlation to bone mechanical competence in the human radius of an elderly population. In this study women had considerably thinner trabeculae in subchondral regions. Cortical thickness was relatively low for both genders at the distal region: 0.38 mm (0.41 mm in men, 0.36 mm in women).[28]

It is important to notice and to inform the patient about the higher risk of controlateral DRF. Indeed, as reported by de Jong in 2017, in 15 postmenopausal women a stable fracture at the distal radius is associated with accelerated cortical bone loss and concomitant reduction of bone strength but not with microarchitectural changes at the contra-lateral distal radius, even in the presence of adequate antiresorptive treatment.[29]

In another point of view, a team has shown in a cadaver study that the increased ulnar variance and decreased cortical bone mineral density correlates with decreased load to failure under axial compression.[30]

Daniels et al. in 2019, have shown among 251 patient that type C (complete articular) DRFs were significantly older and more frequently of male gender compared to patients with a type A (extra-articular) DRF, but there was no difference in body mass index, bone mineral density, smoking, alcohol intake, and 25(OH) vitamin D levels.[31]

Dhillon et al. reported a cadaver study on 10 specimens to compare the thickness of the volar and distal cortices at 0, 5 and 10 mm from the articular surface: at each level volar cortex was significantly thicker than the dorsal cortex.[32]

LOAD DISTRIBUTION

Physiologically, the radius withstands 80% of the mechanical stress compared to 20% for the ulna: 60% for the scaphoid surface and 20% for the lunate surface.

During an articular fracture of the distal radius this distribution and the contact surface may be disturbed.[33]

After a predetermined load was applied to the wrist it was found that the load through the ulna increased from 21% to 67% of the total load as the angulation of the distal radial fragment increased from 10 degrees of palmar tilt to 45 degrees of dorsal tilt.[34]

Pogue et al. in 1990 have shown on five cadaver arms that angulating the distal radius more than 20 degrees either palmar or dorsal, there was a dorsal shift in the scaphoid and lunate high pressure areas, and the loads were more concentrated, but there was no change in the load distribution between the scaphoid and lunate. Decreasing the radial inclination shifted the load distribution so that there was more load in the lunate fossa and less load in the scaphoid fossa.[35]

FRACTURE SPECIFIC BIOMECHANICAL CONSIDERATIONS: THE CRITICAL CORNER

The lunate facet is a central element with the dual role of transmitting force and allowing he wrist's pivotal motion. Thus, the restoration of stability and anatomical reduction of the intermediate column plays a major role in the final result. Lunate facet fractures displaced by more than 5 mm are a risk factor for failure with traditional anterior plates. The inability to reduce and properly fix the volar lunar facet fragment, commonly referred to as the "critical corner", is well described by Harness et al.[36] and others. Some authors also propose a fragment specific hook plate solution.[37] Loss of reduction of this key fragment may result in a radiocarpal dislocation despite otherwise successful reduction.

SPECIAL CASE OF ANTERIOR PLATES FOR DRF

There are many therapeutic solutions for the management of distal radius fractures. Today, even if the latest generation anterior plates seem to be the most suitable solution for the treatment of the most frequent fractures,[38] it is essential to adapt the therapeutic solution to the type of fracture, its displacement and the patient. The biomechanical elements concerning anterior plates are as follows.

The first question is related to the screw types. There is controversy over the use of "pegs" compared to traditional screws. While pegs theoretically have the advantage of reducing the risk of intraarticular penetration and having more resistance during bending stress, this is not highlighted in the different works: locked screws are preferable with regard to torsion and compression resistance.[1] In any case, there is no superiority in using locked screws in proximal holes, even in osteoporotic subjects.[39]

The second question is about the screw length. Baumach et al. in 2015, on a cadaveric study on 11 paired arms, have shown that 75% distal locking screw length provides similar primary stability to 100% unicortical locking screw length.[40] This study, for the first time, provided the biomechanical basis to choose distal screws significantly shorter then measured.

Consistently, Wall et al. in 2012, in 30 osteoporotic radius model have shown that locked unicortical distal screws of at least 75% length produce construct stiffness

similar to bicortical fixation.[41] In both studies, no torsional forces were applied to the models.

For the question related to the number of screws, most of the studies compared the use of 7 locked screws compared to 4: although there was a trend toward greater rigidity for the greater number of screws, the differences were not significant. Note that in these studies, more failures were seen as the plate deformed before the screws cut out.[1] In the diaphysis, a minimum of two screws seems to be sufficient in a nonosteoporotic context.[42]

For the placement of the distal screws, it is proven that the subchondral plate-screw-bone constructs present significantly greater rigidity, indicating higher resistance to postoperative loads and displacement forces.[43] The placement of distal screws in the two distal rows is also controversial. While some studies show increased stability for the first solution, this is not always significant or clinically relevant.[1] Some authors have even shown that two distal screw rows do not add to construct rigidity and resistance against loss of reduction.[44]

And finally, concerning the plate's type: it seems that the variable angle plate is more advantageous than the fixed angle plate, whether it is ideally positioned or not (offset of 3 mm). Studies comparing the latest generation plates show equivalent results between them, biomechanically and clinically,[1] with locked screw plates being better at maintaining the anatomical parameters than unlocked plates.[45]

CONSEQUENCES OF FRACTURE DISPLACEMENT

Chung et al. recently showed in a randomized prospective study that precise restoration of wrist anatomy is not associated with better patient outcomes in a group of 2190 patients over 60 years with a DRF at 12 months following treatment. However, for younger patients, or for educational purposes, it is important to recall the main theoretical biomechanical consequences of poor anatomical parameter reduction.

An anteriorly displaced extraarticular fracture (greater than 10 degrees) results in RUD joint stiffness if the TFCC is intact.[46]

In the same way, it is important to correct distal radius volar angulation deformatity to less than 20 degrees to maintain normal forearm rotation amplitude and to less than 10 degrees to maintain normal DRUJ kinematics when the TFCC is ruptured.[47]

A dorsally angulated extraarticular fracture caused the radiocarpal joint to have an increased contribution to wrist motion in both flexion and extension. With progressive dorsal angulated displacement, the midcarpal motion range of motion (ROM) decreased and contributed less to wrist ROM. This demonstrate changes to radiocarpal biomechanics, load transfer mechanisms, and a potential increase in strain among the radiocarpal articulation.[48]

In other study, in both dorsal and palmar translations in all forearm positions at 10 and 20 degrees of dorsal tilt, distal radioulnar joint stiffness decreased significantly. The authors recommend that dorsal angulation of the distal radius should be corrected to less than 10 degrees of dorsal tilt to prevent DRUJ instability, when there is no radioulnar ligament (RUL) rupture.[49]

In addition, radial inclination deformities of the distal radius should be corrected within 10 degrees when the RUL is intact, to reduce the risk of symptomatic DRUJ instability.[50]

Panel 2: Case Scenario 1 Continued

The authors prefer to classify this fracture as a M3 E3 C2, according to Laulan's classification.

Open lavage, reduction and volar plate osteosynthesis with a second radial plate with locking screws was performed: intraoperative observations highlighted important anterior and posterior comminution, with a styloid in four main fragments. It should be noted that the material chosen does not solve the problem of the posterior metaphysio-epiphyseal comminution: the plates were able to obtain a neutral tilt, a slightly underreduced radioulnar variance and a reduced radial inclination in the frontal plane, without translation.

At 2 months after the surgery, the patient presented 35 degrees of flexion, 50 degrees of extension, fully restored pronosupination, and minimal pain (Fig. 6).

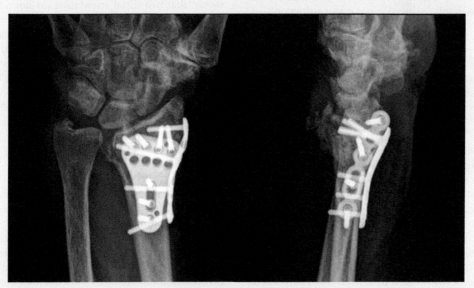

FIG. 6 Dual anterior and radial plating of the DRF.

Panel 2: Case Scenario 2 Continued

In this case the fracture was stabilized with a standard volar plate (Fig. 7A). However, in case of a fracture involving the "volar critical corner" such as the present one (Fig. 1), the important biomechanical forces of the lunate and proximal carpal row can destabilize a volar rim fragment and cause secondary fracture malreduction/displacement when it is not secured by fragment-specific fixation (Fig. 7B)

Upon radiographic follow-up showing loss of reduction, the patient was successfully revised to a volar rim plate (Fig. 7C).

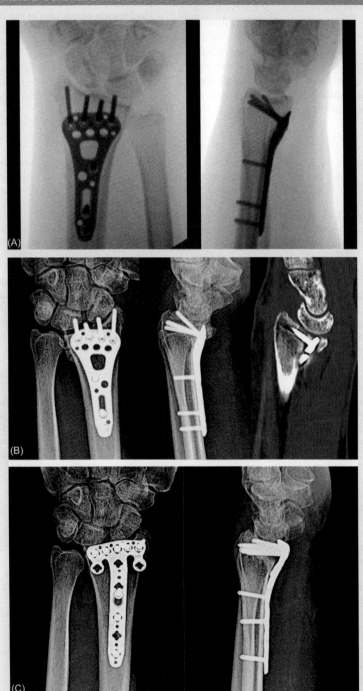

FIG. 7 (A) Intraoperative fluoroscopy of a standard volar plate fixation. (B) Secondary loss of fixation of the critical corner fragment, where one can notice the carpal malalignment. (C) Revision to a volar rim plate. (Courtesy of Benjamin Degeorge.)

CONCLUSION

Solid knowledge of the biomechanical disorders caused by an altered anatomy in the context of a DRF is fundamental: classifying the patient and his fracture, analyzing the key anatomical parameters to be corrected, selecting the best therapeutic strategy (surgical or not) and finally, depending on the short-term clinical and radiographic obtained results, being able to predict at best the patient's future outcome.

REFERENCES

1. Ramavath A, Howard N, Lipscombe S. Biomechanical considerations for strategies to improve outcomes following volar plating of distal radius fractures. *J Orthop.* 2019;16(5):445–450.
2. Edwards WB, Troy KL. Simulating distal radius fracture strength using biomechanical tests: a Modeling study examining the influence of boundary conditions. *J Biomech Eng.* 2011;133(11):114501.
3. Synek A, Chevalier Y, Schröder C, Pahr DH, Baumbach SF. Biomechanical testing of distal radius fracture treatments: boundary conditions significantly affect the outcome of in vitro experiments. *J Appl Biomech.* 2016;32(2):210–214.
4. Burkhart TA, Quenneville CE, Dunning CE, Andrews DM. Development and validation of a distal radius finite element model to simulate impact loading indicative of a forward fall. *Proc Inst Mech Eng H.* 2014;228(3):258–271.
5. Obert L, Lepage D, Saadnia R, Mille F, Rey P-B, Loisel F. Distal radius fractures: which classification is the right one? *Hand Surg Rehabil.* 2016;35S:S24–S27.
6. Pechlaner S, Kathrein A, Gabl M, et al. Distal radius fractures and concomitant lesions. Experimental studies concerning the pathomechanism. *Handchir Mikrochir Plast Chir.* 2002;34(3):150–157.
7. Laulan J, Bismuth J-P, Clément P, Garaud P. An analytical classification of fractures of the distal radius: the "M.E.U." classification. *Chir Main.* 2007;26(6):293–299.
8. Garcia-Elias M, Lluch AL. Wrist instabilities, misalignments, and dislocations. In: Wolfe SW, Hotchkiss RN, Pederson WC, Kozin SH, Cohen MS, eds. *Green's Operative Hand Surgery.* 7th ed. Philadelphia, PA: Elsevier; 2017.
9. Herzberg G, Dumontier C. Les fractures fraiches du radius distal chezl'adulte. *Rev Chir Orthop Reparatrice Appar Mot.* 2001;IS 136–IS 141.
10. Illarramendi A, González Della Valle A, Segal E, De Carli P, Maignon G, Gallucci G. Evaluation of simplified Frykman and AO classifications of fractures of the distal radius. Assessment of interobserver and intraobserver agreement. *Int Orthop.* 1998;22(2):111–115.
11. Kreder HJ, Hanel DP, McKee M, Jupiter J, McGillivary G, Swiontkowski MF. Consistency of AO fracture classification for the distal radius. *J Bone Joint Surg (Br).* 1996;78(5):726–731.
12. Flikkilä T, Nikkola-Sihto A, Kaarela O, Pääkkö E, Raatikainen T. Poor interobserver reliability of AO classification of fractures of the distal radius. Additional computed tomography is of minor value. *J Bone Joint Surg (Br).* 1998;80(4):670–672.
13. Andersen DJ, Blair WF, Steyers CM, Adams BD, el-Khouri GY, Brandser EA. Classification of distal radius fractures: an analysis of interobserver reliability and intraobserver reproducibility. *J Hand Surg [Am].* 1996;21(4):574–582.
14. Dóczi J, Fröhlich P. Classification of distal radius fractures and its diagnostic value. *Unfallchirurg.* 1996;99(5):323–326.
15. Lenoble E, Dumontier C, Goutallier D, Apoil A. Fractures of the distal radius with dorsal displacement: a comparative study of the predictive value of 6 classifications. *Rev Chir Orthop Reparatrice Appar Mot.* 1996;82(5):396–402.
16. Cooney WP. Fractures of the distal radius. A modern treatment-based classification. *Orthop Clin North Am.* 1993;24(2):211–216.
17. Jin W-J, Jiang L-S, Shen L, et al. The interobserver and intraobserver reliability of the cooney classification of distal radius fractures between experienced orthopaedic surgeons. *J Hand Surg Eur Vol.* 2007;32(5):509–511.
18. Herzberg G, Izem Y, Al Saati M, Plotard F. "PAF" analysis of acute distal radius fractures in adults. Preliminary results. *Chir Main.* 2010;29(4):231–235.
19. Burnier M, Herzberg G, Izem Y. Patient-accident-fracture (PAF) classification of distal radius fractures. *Hand Surg Rehabil.* 2016;35S:S34–S38.
20. Cognet J-M, Martinache X, Mathoulin C. Arthroscopic management of intra-articular fractures of the distal radius. *Chir Main.* 2008;27(4):171–179.
21. Fontès D. Arthroscopic management of recent or chronic lesions of triangular fibrocartilage complex of the wrist. *Chir Main.* 2006;25(Suppl. 1):S178–S186.
22. Laulan J, Bismuth JP. Intracarpal ligamentous lesions associated with fractures of the distal radius: outcome at one year. A prospective study of 95 cases. *Acta Orthop Belg.* 1999;65(3):418–423.
23. Barbary S, Pozetto M, Segret J, Delétang F, Dederichs A, Dap F. Fracture du radius distal. In: Fontaine C, Liverneaux P, Masmejean E, eds. *Cours Européen de Pathologie Chirurgicale du Membre Supérieur.* Montpellier: Sauramps Médical; 2010:435–453.
24. Osada D, Viegas SF, Shah MA, Morris RP, Patterson RM. Comparison of different distal radius dorsal and volar fracture fixation plates: a biomechanical study. *J Hand Surg [Am].* 2003;28(1):94–104.
25. Putnam MD, Meyer NJ, Nelson EW, Gesensway D, Lewis JL. Distal radial metaphyseal forces in an extrinsic grip model: implications for postfracture rehabilitation. *J Hand Surg [Am].* 2000;25(3):469–475.
26. Mathiowetz V, Kashman N, Volland G, Weber K, Dowe M, Rogers S. Grip and pinch strength: normative data for adults. *Arch Phys Med Rehabil.* 1985;66(2):69–74.

27. Augat P, Iida H, Jiang Y, Diao E, Genant HK. Distal radius fractures: mechanisms of injury and strength prediction by bone mineral assessment. *J Orthop Res.* 1998;16(5): 629–635.

28. Mueller TL, van Lenthe GH, Stauber M, Gratzke C, Eckstein F, Müller R. Regional, age and gender differences in architectural measures of bone quality and their correlation to bone mechanical competence in the human radius of an elderly population. *Bone.* 2009;45 (5):882–891.

29. de Jong JJA, Arts JJC, Willems PC, et al. Contra-lateral bone loss at the distal radius in postmenopausal women after a distal radius fracture: a two-year follow-up HRpQCT study. *Bone.* 2017;101:245–251.

30. Casagrande DJ, Morris RP, Carayannopoulos NL, Buford WL. Relationship between ulnar variance, cortical bone density, and load to failure in the distal radius at the typical site of fracture initiation. *J Hand Surg [Am].* 2016;41(12):e461–e468.

31. Daniels AM, Theelen LMA, Wyers CE, et al. Bone microarchitecture and distal radius fracture pattern complexity. *J Orthop Res.* 2019;37(8):1690–1697.

32. Dhillon SS, Kumar AJS, Sadaiyyappan V, Bassi RS, Shanahan D, Deshmukh SC. Anatomical study comparing the thickness of the volar and dorsal cortex of cadaveric adult distal radii using digital photography. *Arch Orthop Trauma Surg.* 2007;127(10):975–977.

33. Baratz ME, Des Jardins JD, Anderson DD, Imbriglia JE. Displaced intra-articular fractures of the distal radius: the effect of fracture displacement on contract stresses in a cadaver model. *J Hand Surg [Am].* 1996;21(2):183–188.

34. Short WH, Palmer AK, Werner FW, Murphy DJ. A biomechanical study of distal radial fractures. *J Hand Surg [Am].* 1987;12(4):529–534.

35. Pogue DJ, Viegas SF, Patterson RM, et al. Effects of distal radius fracture malunion on wrist joint mechanics. *J Hand Surg [Am].* 1990;15(5):721–727.

36. Harness NG. Fixation options for the volar lunate facet fracture: thinking outside the box. *J Wrist Surg.* 2016;5 (1):9–16.

37. O'Shaughnessy MA, Shin AY, Kakar S. Volar marginal rim fracture fixation with volar fragment-specific hook plate fixation. *J Hand Surg [Am].* 2015;40(8):1563–1570.

38. Chaudhry H, Kleinlugtenbelt YV, Mundi R, Ristevski B, Goslings JC, Bhandari M. Are volar locking plates superior to percutaneous K-wires for distal radius fractures? A meta-analysis. *Clin Orthop Relat Res.* 2015;473(9):3017–3027.

39. Bockmann B, Budak C, Figiel J, et al. Is there a benefit of proximal locking screws in osteoporotic distal radius fractures?—a biomechanical study. *Injury.* 2016;47(8): 1631–1635.

40. Baumbach SF, Synek A, Traxler H, Mutschler W, Pahr D, Chevalier Y. The influence of distal screw length on the primary stability of volar plate osteosynthesis—a biomechanical study. *J Orthop Surg Res.* 2015;10(1):139.

41. Wall LB, Brodt MD, Silva MJ, Boyer MI, Calfee RP. The effects of screw length on stability of simulated osteoporotic distal radius fractures fixed with volar locking plates. *J Hand Surg [Am].* 2012;37(3):446–453.

42. Jung H-S, Jung HS, Baek S-H, Lee JS. How many screws are needed for reliable stability of extra-articular nonosteoporotic distal radius fractures fixed with volar locking plates? *Clin Orthop Surg.* 2020;12(1):22.

43. Drobetz H, Bryant AL, Pokorny T, Spitaler R, Leixnering M, Jupiter JB. Volar fixed-angle plating of distal radius extension fractures: influence of plate position on secondary loss of reduction—a biomechanic study in a cadaveric model. *J Hand Surg [Am].* 2006;31(4):615–622.

44. Drobetz H, Weninger P, Grant C, et al. More is not necessarily better. A biomechanical study on distal screw numbers in volar locking distal radius plates. *Injury.* 2013;44(4):535–539.

45. Kumar S, Chopra RK, Sehrawat S, Lakra A. Comparison of treatment of unstable intra articular fractures of distal radius with locking plate versus non-locking plate fixation. *J Clin Orthop Trauma.* 2014;5(2):74–78.

46. Bessho Y, Nakamura T, Nagura T, Nishiwaki M, Sato K, Toyama Y. Effect of volar angulation of extra-articular distal radius fractures on distal radioulnar joint stability: a biomechanical study. *J Hand Surg Eur Vol.* 2015;40(8): 775–782.

47. Nishiwaki M, Welsh MF, Gammon B, Ferreira LM, Johnson JA, King GJW. Effect of volarly angulated distal radius fractures on forearm rotation and distal radioulnar joint kinematics. *J Hand Surg [Am].* 2015;40 (11):2236–2242.

48. Padmore CE, Stoesser H, Nishiwaki M, et al. The effect of dorsally angulated distal radius deformities on carpal kinematics: an in vitro biomechanical study. *J Hand Surg [Am].* 2018;43(11):1036.e1–1036.e8.

49. Saito T, Nakamura T, Nagura T, Nishiwaki M, Sato K, Toyama Y. The effects of dorsally angulated distal radius fractures on distal radioulnar joint stability: a biomechanical study. *J Hand Surg Eur Vol.* 2013;38(7): 739–745.

50. Bessho Y, Nakamura T, Nishiwaki M, et al. Effect of decrease in radial inclination of distal radius fractures on distal radioulnar joint stability: a biomechanical study. *J Hand Surg Eur Vol.* 2018;43(9):967–973.

CHAPTER 5

Radiographic Parameters of Distal Radius Fractures

ROBERT J. MEDOFF[a] • STEVEN M. KOEHLER[b]

[a]John A Burns School of Medicine, University of Hawaii, Kailua, HI, United States, [b]Department of Orthopaedic Surgery, SUNY Downstate Medical Center, Brooklyn, NY, United States

KEY POINTS

1. Radiographs are essential for evaluation and treatment of distal radius fractures.

2. Complete radiographic assessment requires proper technique and all projections necessary to fully evaluate the injury.

3. Interpretation of distal radius fracture radiographs requires more than simple identification of radial inclination, volar tilt, and radial length; routine assessment of several other essential landmarks and parameters is needed to avoid missed pathology and unrecognized malreduction.

4. Radiographs of distal radius fractures provides important information that helps identify the injury mechanism, type, and direction of principle instability, and pattern and components of peri-articular fragmentation.

Panel 1: Case Scenario

A 60 year-old, right-handed female seamstress/artist fell on her outstretched left arm. She was treated in a splint and now complains that anytime she loads her wrist in dorsiflexion she experiences intense pain. Radiographs show dorsal angulation of the distal fragment and her examination shows moderate deformity with limited forearm rotation (Fig. 1). Other than the dorsal angulation of the distal fragment, what other significant abnormalities require correction in order to alleviate her symptoms?

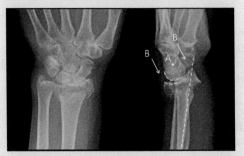

FIG. 1 Radiographs show dorsal angulation of the distal fragment with clear dorsal translation of the center of the head of the capitate (A).

IMPORTANCE OF THE PROBLEM

Of all the joints in the human body, there are none as complex as the wrist. The wrist coordinates synchronous movement of 10 independent bones, allowing rotational motion along all three cardinal axes as well as providing gliding motion in the coronal and sagittal plane. Fractures of the distal radius are the most common fractures of the wrist and represent 17% of all fractures.[1, 2] Although adjunctive modalities such as CT and MRI are certainly helpful in providing detailed information about the morphology of distal radius fractures at a single point in time, there is no question that plain radiographic studies remain the workhorse for the evaluation of wrist injuries, especially at the initial presentation, during operative treatment, and with the routine assessments that are necessary for follow-up care.

Panel 2: Teardrop Angle

The teardrop is best visualized on the 10 degrees lateral radiograph, but can also be identified on the standard lateral radiograph. It represents the outline of the cortical and subchondral bone surfaces of the volar rim of the lunate facet, and is important in maintenance of the sagittal position of the carpus.

Continued

Distal Radius Fractures. https://doi.org/10.1016/B978-0-323-75764-5.00010-X

The teardrop angle (defined as the angle between the central axis of the radial shaft and the central axis of the teardrop) in normal wrist is 70±10 degrees.

Axial instability patterns of the volar rim can be recognized by depression of the teardrop angle below 45 degrees along with pathologic dorsal subluxation of the central rotational axis of the base of the capitate. Stable reduction includes correction of the dorsiflexed position along with restoration of carpal alignment to a line extended from the volar shaft of the radius.

Volar instability patterns of the volar rim typically present with a normal teardrop angle, but show palmar displacement and shortening of the volar rim. Stable reduction of this pattern of instability should include restoration of length to the volar rim as well as palmar support of the volar fragment.

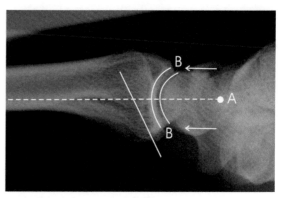

FIG. 3 On a lateral radiograph, one can appreciate the normal teardrop angle and the centralized head of the capitate (A) aligned with the inner volar cortex.

Interpretation of standard radiographs requires more than simple assessment of radial inclination, volar tilt, and radial length. For instance, the teardrop angle of the volar rim of the lunate facet, loss of congruency of the radii of curvature of adjacent articulating surfaces, identification of the position and displacement of the carpal facet horizon, assessment of the lateral carpal alignment, AP distance, pathologic widening of the distal radioulnar joint (DRUJ), coronal fragment shift, and carpal malalignment are examples of some of the other landmarks and parameters used to identify pathologic conditions that otherwise can be overlooked (Figs. 2 and 3).[3]

The importance of these additional landmarks and parameters has only been recognized relatively recently.

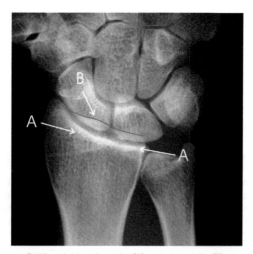

FIG. 2 Distinguishing the volar (A) and dorsal rim (B) on anteroposterior radiographs.

Because of this, large numbers of studies in the literature omit recognition of these important radiographic features and should be interpreted with caution as conclusions may be based on incomplete information.

Fernandez and Jupiter characterized distal radius fractures according to the mechanism of injury: (1) bending, (2) shear, (3) axial load, (4) carpal avulsions, and (5) high energy.[4] The character and personality of injuries in each of these groups varies considerably, and it is probably not reasonable to lump these different fracture mechanisms together when evaluating clinical results related to a specific parameter or treatment. Moreover, the expectations and demands in a low demand patient population are considerably different from those in a very active patient population. For this reason, additional caution should be exercised when reaching conclusion from clinical evaluations that are based on clinical data based on a nonuniform population.

MAIN QUESTION

What is the significance of the features of radiographic assessment in the management of distal radius fractures?

CURRENT OPINION

There is an overwhelming consensus of opinion that radiographs are necessary as part of the evaluation and management of distal radius fractures, and the AO classification is the established standard in the literature for identifying the various types of injury. Despite this, there are differences of opinion on our ability to consistently recognize radiographic pathology and the relative significance of specific abnormalities to clinical outcomes.

FINDING THE EVIDENCE

- Cochrane search: distal radius lateral carpal alignment; distal radius teardrop; distal radius radiographs; distal radius DTV.
- Pubmed (Medline): ("distal radius") AND ("radiograph") AND ("teardrop" OR "alignment" OR "parameters").
- Articles not in English were excluded from review.
    Level I:
        Randomized controlled trials: 4
    Level II:
        Randomized controlled trials with methodological limitations: 5
    Level IV:
        Case series: 14
    Lever V:
        Expert opinion: 1

FINDINGS

Three level-one studies examined radiographic criteria in cadaveric specimens and volunteers. One study evaluated the ability of an anatomic tilt view to assess screw penetration in the radiocarpal and distal radioulnar joints in 24 cadavers; this view showed high levels of specificity (0.93) and sensitivity (0.98) of articular screw penetration (Fig. 4).[5] Another study reviewed anthropomorphic variability between left and right specimens

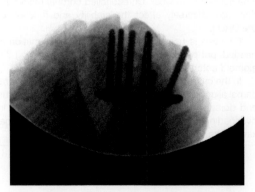

FIG. 4 The dorsal tangential view.

with 3D CT scans; no significant difference in radial height, radial inclination, or volar tilt was noted.[6] Another study evaluated the effect of rotational position of the forearm specifically on the dorsal tangential view (DTV) for determining alignment of the distal radioulnar joint.[7] Four transhumeral specimens were used and observers correctly identified abnormalities of DRUJ position as reduced, volarly malreduced, or dorsally malreduced on 94% of the DTV images (97%, 95%, and 92% in the neutral, supinated, and pronated forearm positions, respectively) with high intraobserver and interobserver reliability.

A fourth level-one study reported the sensitivity and specificity of dorsal tangential view and carpal shoot-through fluoroscopic views in cadavers. They assessed the ability of the radiographic views to capture dorsal cortex penetration and then 64 orthopedic surgeons view randomized fluoroscopic images to assess for penetration. Sensitivity for the DTV and carpal shoot-through views were 76% and 89%, respectively. Specificities were 85% and 84%, respectively.[8]

Five level-two studies were included in the evaluation. In one, 22 consecutive patients undergoing open reduction for distal radius fractures were prospectively studied with a dorsal tangential view intraoperatively and correlated with postoperative CT scan; observers were blinded in measuring the screw tip to cortical distance with the two methods.[9] Eleven screws were changed on the basis of this assessment, with good inter- and intraobserver correlation with CT scan. Another study compared evaluation with traction views to CT scan; poor interobserver reliability was noted but intraobserver variability was not found to be significant.[10] In another study, 163 patients were prospectively studied with univariate analysis to determine whether radiographic abnormalities were predictive of distal radioulnar instability; they determined that only coronal or sagittal malposition was associated with pathologic instability of the DRUJ.[11] Two additional studies examined the reliability and reproducibility of radiographic measurements of distal radius fractures.[12, 13] Both studies found that inter- and intraobserver reliability was high for radial height, inclination and volar tilt and poor for articular step-off.

Fourteen level-four studies were included. In early literature, Altissimi et al. and McQueen and Caspers demonstrated in retrospective cohorts that significant radiological abnormalities are associated with poor functional outcomes.[14, 15]

In another study, reliability of radiographic assessment between 25 general orthopedic surgeons and residents showed a poor correlation with a musculoskeletal trained radiologist.[16] Another study showed a poor prognosis associated with an adaptive carpal instability pattern and loss of radial inclination but not volar tilt.[17] However, contrary to this finding, Perugia et al. Reported a retrospective evaluation of 51 intraarticular distal radius fractures finding that ulnar variance and volar tilt correlate with good functional outcomes and are the most important radiographic parameters to be restored.[18] This supported Rubinovich and Rennie's early study that found patient's had poor function and grip strength when normal volar tilt was not restored.[19]

The study by Dias et al. in a prospective cohort of 252 distal radius fractures provides insight into the relation of dorsal tilt in aggravation of lateral carpal alignment. With reduction of the capitate with the volar axis of the radius, carpal malalignment was corrected.[20]

A review of 36 patient in another study showed that pathologic changes in the teardrop angle showed a high association with anterior lunate facet displacement, and that residual postoperative abnormalities of the AP distance were associated with residual incongruity of the articular surface.[21] Other studies confirm the significance of an unreduced teardrop angle and residual coronal malreduction. In one, evaluation of the teardrop angle in 24 injured and 24 uninjured wrists showed a high intra and inter observer reliability and association with step-off and articular incongruity on CT scan.[22]

In another study, 29 patients that underwent open reduction and arthroscopy were studied retrospectively to determine whether any radiographic parameters were associated with the finding of a foveal-based TFCC tea and DRUJ instability; univariate analysis revealed that increased radial translation, decreased radial inclination, increased radial shortening, and an ulnar styloid fragment radially displace by more than 4 mm were significant predictors of radioulnar ligament avulsion at the fovea.[23]

An additional study defines the full range of landmarks and parameters used for assessing radiographs of the distal radius.[3] Other articles are included for reference.[24–32]

RECOMMENDATIONS

In patients with an intraarticular displaced distal radius fracture, evidence suggests:

Recommendations	Overall Quality
• The inclusion of supplemental views such as the 10 degrees lateral view and dorsal tangential view (skyline, horizon, or carpal shoot-through) view can provide useful and significant information to supplement radiographic assessment of distal radius fractures.	⊕⊕⊕⊕ High
• Routine evaluation for abnormalities of the teardrop angle, coronal position, and lateral carpal alignment (sagittal position) has clinical significance and should always be included as part of the assessment of distal radius fractures in both clinical and research settings.	⊕⊕⊕○ Moderate
• The AO classification system forms the basis of a majority of studies but has low intra- and interobserver reliability.	⊕⊕⊕○ Moderate

---

Panel 3: Author's Preferred Technique

The standard radiographic evaluation for fractures of the distal radius includes a standard PA, lateral and 10 degrees lateral radiograph; the 10 degrees radiograph is tilted to orient the beam parallel to the inclination of the ulnar two-thirds of the joint. If necessary, additional oblique views may be warranted. The lateral X-ray is performed with the forearm in neutral rotation with the pisiform superimposed over the distal pole of the scaphoid.

For intraarticular fractures, particular attention is focused on the teardrop angle, lateral carpal alignment, uniformity and width of both the radiocarpal and distal radioulnar joint intervals. Incomplete correction of the lateral carpal alignment and or teardrop angle suggests residual dorsal instability and can compromise the normal kinematics of the wrist. Unreconciled coronal malreduction may adversely affect the stability and function of the DRUJ.

CT scan is used whenever additional information is needed, but particularly with fragmentation involving the sigmoid notch and articular comminution.

In the case provided, the marked dorsal shift of lateral carpal alignment coupled with the shortening of the radius and dorsal angulation of the distal fragment resulted in overloading of the dorsal rim and abnormal carpal kinematics.

CONCLUSION

Because radiographic interpretation of distal radius fractures has such profound impact on the approach to treatment, accurate assessment of radiographs is essential for appropriate management. Subtle abnormalities of a variety of radiographic landmarks and parameters can provide critical information in the recognition of the pattern and extent of injury. Inclusion of the 10 degrees lateral projection and assessment of parameters such as the teardrop angle, AP distance, lateral carpal alignment and others should be a routine part of the evaluation and treatment of these injuries and will help us better define the behavior and outcomes of these injuries in the future.

Panel 4: Pearls and Pitfalls

PEARLS

- Axial instability of the volar rim is identified by depression of the teardrop angle (less than 45 degrees) and dorsal sagittal shift of the lateral carpal alignment; correction of a dorsiflexed volar rim and reduction of the abnormal dorsal shift of the capitate is necessary for reduction.

- Volar instability of the volar rim is identified by shortening and volar translation of the lunate facet and volar subluxation of the carpus; it is corrected by restoration of length and palmar buttress of the volar rim fragment and realignment of the carpus.

- A nonuniform joint interval on the 10 degrees lateral view may suggest incomplete reduction of the articular surface.

PITFALL

- Widening of the DRUJ joint interval and/or offset on the radial cortex of the fracture site can indicate unrecognized coronal malreduction; this can adversely affect the function and stability of the DRUJ and should be corrected.

Editor's Tips & Tricks: Carpal Shoot Through
Geert Alexander Buijze

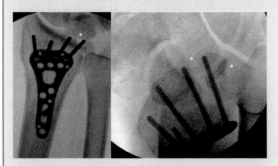

Fig. 1. As the authors of this chapter explained, use of the dorsal tangential view or—in reversed—the carpal shoot through view can also help to identify incongruency of the dorsal radial rim and the sigmoid notch (asterisks), for instance when a dorsoradial fragment remains unreduced. © Dr Buijze 2020.

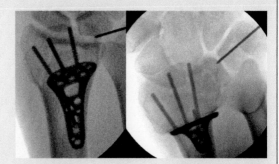

Fig. 2. Removing the most ulnar screw and reducing the dorsoradial fragment percutaneously with a K-wire improves the previously existent step-off and gap of the dorsal radial rim and the sigmoid notch. © Dr Buijze 2020.

Continued

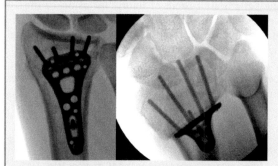

Fig. 3. The carpal shoot through view best appreciates the restored congruency of the dorsal radial rim and the sigmoid notch after reinserting a 2 mm shorter screw while maintaining reduction. © Dr Buijze 2020.

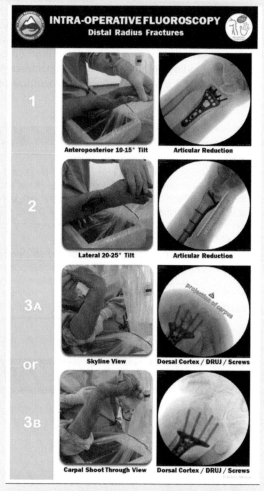

Fig. 4. I recommend to always record the following three standard intraoperative views for each case: (1) an anteroposterior view with 10–15 degrees tilt to better appreciate articular reduction, (2) a lateral view with 20–25 degrees tilt to assess plate positioning (ideally beneath the watershed line) and best appreciate articular reduction, and (3A) the skyline view or (3B) the carpal shoot-through view to assess reduction of the dorsal cortex and DRUJ as well as, importantly, screw length. A practical open-source smartphone-sized pdf guide can be downloaded at education.pbma.fr © Dr. Buijze 2020.

REFERENCES

1. Singer BR, McLauchlan GJ, Robinson CM, Christie J. Epidemiology of fractures in 15000 adults: the influence of age and gender. *J Bone Joint Surg (Br)*. 1998;80B: 243–248.
2. Kopvulov P, Johnell O, Redlund-Johnell L, Bengner U. Fractures of the distal end of the radius in young adults: a 30-year follow-up. *J Hand Surg (Br)*. 1993;18B: 45–49.
3. Medoff RJ. Essential radiographic evaluation for distal radius fractures. *Hand Clin*. 2005;21(3):279–288.
4. Jupiter JB, Fernandez DL. Comparative classification for fractures of the distal end of the radius. *J Hand Surg [Am]*. 1997;22(4):563–571.
5. Boyer M, Korcek KJ, Gelberman R, Gilula L, Ditsios K, Evanoff B. Anatomic tilt x-rays of the distal radius: an ex vivo analysis of surgical fixation. *J Hand Surg [Am]*. 2004;29(1):116–122.
6. Gray R, Thorn M, Riddle M, Sug N, Burkhart T, Lalone E. Image-based comparison between the bilateral symmetry of the distal radii through established measures. *J Hand Surg [Am]*. 2019;44(11):966–972.
7. El Naga AN, Jordan M, Netscher D, Adams BD, Mitchell S. Reliability of the dorsal tangential view in assessment of distal radioulnar joint reduction in the neutral, pronated, and supinated positions in a cadaver model. *J Hand Surg [Am]*. 2019. https://doi.org/10.1016/j.jhsa.2019.08.004. pii: S0363-5023(18)31196-1.
8. Stoops TK, Santoni BG, Clark NM, Bauer AA, Shoji C, Schwartz-Fernandes F. Sensitivity and specificity of skyline and carpal shoot-through fluoroscopic views of volar plate fixation of the distal radius: a cadaveric investigation of dorsal cortex screw penetration. *Hand*. 2017;12(6):551–556.
9. Brunner A, Siebert C, Stieger C, Kastius A, Link B-C, Babst R. The dorsal tangential x-ray view to determine dorsal screw penetration during volar plating of distal radius fractures. *J Hand Surg [Am]*. 2015;40(1):27–33.
10. Avery 3rd DM, Matullo KS. Distal radial traction radiographs: interobserver and intraobserver reliability compared with computed tomography. *J Bone Joint Surg Am*. 2014;96(7):582–588.
11. Fujitani R, Omokawa S, Akahane M, Iida A, Ono H, Tanaka Y. Predictors of distal radioulnar joint instability in distal radius fractures. *J Hand Surg [Am]*. 2011;36(12):1919–1925.
12. Watson NJ, Asadollahi S, Parrish F, Ridgway J, Tran P, Keating J. Reliability of radiographic measurements for acute distal radius fractures. *BMC Med Imaging*. 2016; 16:44.
13. Stirling E, Jeffery J, Johnson N, Dias J. Are radiographic measurements of the displacement of a distal radius fracture reliable and reproducible? *Bone Joint J*. 2016;98-B:1069–1073.
14. McQueen M, Caspers J. Colles fracture: does the anatomical result affect the final function? *J Bone Joint Surg (Br)*. 1988;70(4):649–651.
15. Altissimi M, Antenucci R, Fiacca C, Mancini GB. Long-term results of conservative treatment of fractures of the distal radius. *Clin Orthop Relat Res*. 1986;206:202–210.
16. O'Malley MP, Rodner C, Ritting A, Cote MP, Leger R, Stock H. Radiographic interpretation of distal radius fractures; visual estimations versus digital measuring techniques. *Hand*. 2014;9:488–493.
17. Batra S, Gupta A. The effect of fracture-related factors on the functional outcome at 1 year in distal radius fractures. *Injury*. 2002;33:499–502.
18. Perugia D, Guzzini M, Civitenga C, et al. Is it really necessary to restore radial anatomic parameters after distal radius fracture? *Injury*. 2014;45S:S21–S26.
19. Rubinovich RM, Rennie WR. Colles' fracture: end results in relation to radiologic parameters. *Can J Surg*. 1983;26: 361–363.
20. Dias R, Johnson NA, Dias JJ. Prospective investigation of the relationship between dorsal tilt, carpal malalignment, and capitate shift in distal radius fractures. *Bone Joint J*. 2020;102-B1:137–143.
21. Teunis T, Meijer S, Jupiter JB, Rikli D. The correlation between the teardrop angle and anterior lunate facet displacement in plating distal radial fractures. *J Hand Surg Eur Vol*. 2019;44(5):462–467.
22. Fujitani R, Omokawa S, Iida A, Santo S, Tanaka Y. Reliability and clinical importance of teardrop angle measurement in intra-articular distal radius fracture. *J Hand Surg [Am]*. 2012;37(3):454–459.
23. Nakamura T, Iwamoto T, Matsumura N, Sato K, Toyama Y. Radiographic and arthroscopic assessment of DRUJ instability due to foveal avulsion of the radioulnar ligament in distal radius fractures. *J Wrist Surg*. 2014;3(1):12–17.
24. Andersen DJ, Blair WF, Steyers CMJ, Adams BD, El-Khouri GY, Brandser EA. Classification of distal radius fractures: an analysis of interobserver reliability and intraobserver reproducibility. *J Hand Surg [Am]*. 1996;21(4):574–582.
25. Arealis G, Galanopoulos I, Nikolaou VS, Lacon A, Ashwood N, Kitsis C. Does the CT improve inter- and intra-observer agreement for the AO, Fernandez and universal classification systems for distal radius fractures? *Injury*. 2014;45(10):1579–1584.
26. Broadbent M, Stevenson I, Maceachern C, Johnstone A. Investigation of radiolunate relations in normal and fractured wrists. *Hand Surg*. 2009;14(2–3):105–112.
27. Jordan M, El Naga AN, Mitchell S, Adams BD, Netscher D. Assessment of distal radioulnar joint reduction with the dorsal tangential view in the neutral, pronated, and supinated positions. *J Hand Surg [Am]*. 2018;43(9):S29–S30.
28. Kuhnel SP, Bigham AT, McMurtry RY, Faber KJ, King GJW, Grewal R. The capitate-to-axis-of-radius distance (CARD): a new radiographic measurement for wrist and carpal alignment in the sagittal plane. *J Hand Surg [Am]*. 2019;44(9):797.e1–797.e8.
29. Pennock AT, Phillips CS, Matzon JL, Daley E. The effects of forearm rotation on three wrist measurements; radial inclination, radial height and palmar tilt. *Hand Surg*. 2004;10(1):17–22.

30. Ranjeet N, Estrella EP. Distal radius fractures: does a radiologically acceptable reduction really change the result? *J Clin Diagn Res.* 2012;6(8):1388–1392.

31. Ross M, Di Mascio L, Peters S, Cockfield A, Taylor F, Couzens G. Defining residual radial translation of distal radius fractures: a potential cause of distal radioulnar joint instability. *J Wrist Surg.* 2014;3(1):22–29.

32. Slutsky DJ. Predicting the outcome of distal radius fractures. *Hand Clin.* 2005;21(3):289–294.

CHAPTER 6

Advanced Imaging in Distal Radius Fractures

WILLIAM F. PIENTKA, II[a] • MICHAEL J. SANDOW[b] • SARA F. HAYNES[a]
[a]John Peter Smith Hospital, Department of Orthopaedic Surgery, Fort Worth, TX, United States,
[b]Wakefield Orthopaedic Clinic, Adelaide, SA, Australia

KEY POINTS

- CT scan can allow for improved identification of intraarticular fracture fragments in distal radius fractures.
- Use of CT scan for preoperative planning can allow for improved guidance of fracture fragment fixation intraoperatively.
- Utilization of CT in association with 3D printing can allow for improvement in the surgical treatment of distal radius malunions.
- Currently available 3D CT reconstruction technology has significant limitations as it is only a 2D projection of the 3D data set. True 3D modeling allows for virtual preoperative planning and can provide invaluable information to the surgeon.

Panel 1: Case Scenario

A 48 year-old, right-handed female visited the emergency department with a right wrist deformity after a fall on the out-stretched hand. Radiographs shows an intraarticular distal radius fracture with 25 degrees of dorsal angulation and dorsal metaphyseal as well as intraarticular comminution (Fig. 1A–C). What is the most effective approach to preoperative planning for this fracture?

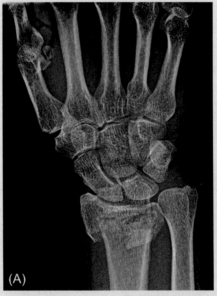

(A)

FIG. 1 Injury PA (A), oblique (B), and lateral (C) radiograph of a 48-year-old female with an intraarticular distal radius fracture.

Continued

Panel 1: Case Scenario—cont'd

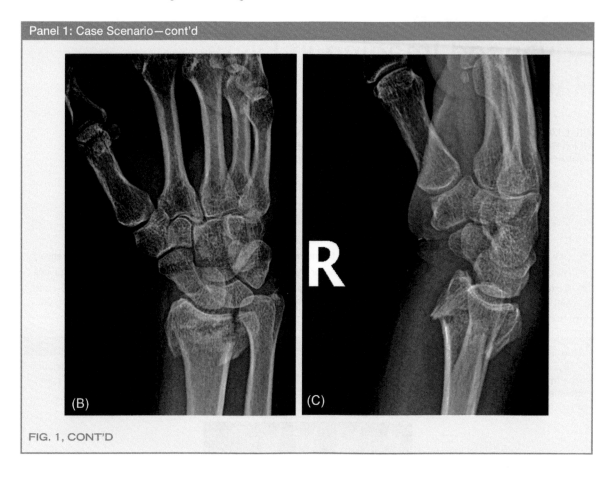

FIG. 1, CONT'D

IMPORTANCE OF THE PROBLEM

Distal radius fractures are a common injury, and diagnosis of fracture patterns and stability are critical factors in the management of these fractures. Identification of fracture patterns in intraarticular fractures can affect the determination of optimal fixation technique. Preoperative computed tomography (CT) can aid in the identification of intraarticular fracture patterns and guide treatment. CT can also be a beneficial adjunct in the treatment of distal radius malunion correction, especially when combined with 3D modalities.

Confusion over the functionality of the various forms of 3D imaging has created challenges in expanding the use of such technology, with cost, time, and access convenience being potential issues. Sandow[1] has detailed some of the technical aspects of both volume rendering (which is the predominant 3D modality in medical CT) and surface rendering (which is the predominant 3D modality use outside of the field of medicine).

3D printing technology is an advanced preoperative planning tool that can be utilized to decrease operative time, blood loss, and fluoroscopy use (Fig. 2). However, improved surgeon access to computer based digital 3D simulation may improve the contribution and utility of such advanced imaging techniques to improve preoperative planning, implant selection, and optimal technique in malunion correction.

MAIN QUESTION

What is the utility of advanced imaging techniques in the diagnosis, preoperative planning, and treatment of distal radius fractures?

CURRENT OPINION

Displaced intraarticular distal radius fractures are often treated surgically. Current opinion is variable with regard to preoperative imaging and the utility of advanced imaging (CT scan, 3D reconstruction, etc.) in surgical decision making.

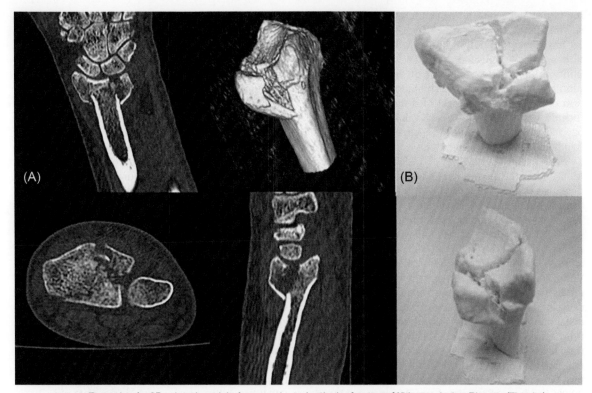

FIG. 2 Example of a 3D printed model of a comminuted articular fracture. (With permission Bizzotto/Elsevier)

FINDING THE EVIDENCE

- Cochrane search: Distal Radius Fracture CT Scan; Distal Radius Fracture MRI; Distal Radius Fracture 3D CT Scan.
- Pubmed (Medline): ("distal radius fracture") AND ("CT Scan" OR "MRI" OR "3D").
- Articles not in English were excluded from review.

QUALITY OF THE EVIDENCE

Levels of Evidence—Sackett

Level	Description	Included Studies
1	Randomized controlled Trial	1
2B	Cohort study or randomized controlled trial with methodological limitations	1
3B	Case-controlled study	21
4	Case series	27
5	Expert opinion	5

FINDINGS

One level-1 and one level-2 studies were identified and met inclusion criteria for review, the first describing the

utilization of a 3D printed wrist model based on CT images for preoperative planning in distal radius malunion correction,[2] and the second with the finding that traction radiographs are a suitable alternative to CT in determining a treatment strategy in acute distal radius fractures.[3] Buijze et al. identified a potential for improved accuracy and consistency of malunion correction with computer assisted surgical planning and patient-specific osteotomy guides.[2]

Twenty level-3 studies and 25 level-4 studies met inclusion criteria, covering a range of topics related to the identification and treatment of both acute distal radius fractures, as well as malunion correction.

Eight level-3 studies[4–11] including 429 distal radius fractures and 13 level 4 studies[12–24] including 516 fractures, describe the advantage of CT in the diagnosis and treatment of acute distal radius fractures when compared to plain radiographs alone. Each of these studies describe the benefit of preoperative CT in patients with a distal radius fracture, allowing for improved identification of intraarticular fracture propagation into both the radiocarpal and distal radioulnar joint. Multiple studies[7–9, 11, 13, 14, 17–19] identify the addition of CT as clearly superior to radiographs alone in the identification of intraarticular fracture propagation, especially into the sigmoid notch. Intraoperative CT has been reported useful in the identification of intraarticular screw penetration as well as articular step-offs.[12, 16] CT also has utility in preoperative planning of distal radius malunion correction.[15] Identified limitations of the utilization of CT in the assessment of distal radius fractures include cost[19, 25] and limited valuable information beyond the identification of intraarticular fracture fragments.[23]

Four level-3 studies[11, 26–28] and four level 4 studies[29–32] describe the utility of advanced imaging in the diagnosis of concurrent injuries with distal radius fractures. Freedman et al.[26] identified a 45% occurrence of TFCC pathology with an acute distal radius fracture, identified on MRI of 60 patients with an acute distal radius fracture, with higher prevalence in Frykman VI and VII fractures compared to other grade injuries. Von Schnieder-Egestorf et al.[27] reviewed 603 distal radius fracture CT scans, and identified injury to the extensor tendon sheath in 71% of patients with an acute distal radius fracture, most commonly of the second or third extensor compartment. This was identified as fat-fluid levels or fatty effusions with the extensor compartments as seen on CT. In a review of 313 distal radius fracture CT scans, retrospectively, Heo et al.[28] identified a 20.9% incidence of associated carpal fracture not identified on plain radiographs, thus identifying an additional benefit of CT scan in the assessment of complex distal radius fractures. Further reports suggest MRI allows for assessment of the TFCC and scapholunate complex,[29–31] and can assist in the diagnosis of subtle concurrent osseous lesions,[29, 32] but does not improve functional outcome and appears to be of limited utility.[30]

Seven studies (four level 3,[33–36] four level 4[37–40]), including 295 wrists, report the utility of 3D printing technology in the surgical treatment of distal radius fractures. 3D digital planning or 3D printing allows for advanced preoperative planning including implant selection[33, 37, 39] and screw lengths.[34] 3D printing technology in preoperative planning reduces intraoperative fluoroscopy, blood loss, and operative time but did not lead to an improvement in final wrist function compared to fractures that did not undergo 3D fracture printing for surgical planning.[35, 36] At present, a distal radius fracture model takes approximately 4 hours to print and has a cost of $10.[37] Furthermore, 3D printed models were used in the preoperative planning of distal radius malunion correction in 24 patients[38, 39] and intraoperatively in 20 patients.[2]

Six additional level-3 studies were identified which did not match any of the above subcategorizations. There are conflicting reports on the utility of arthroscopy in the treatment of distal radius fractures. Christiaens et al.[41] found arthroscopy as a useful adjunct in improving intraarticular distal radius fracture reduction, but did not identify a benefit of arthroscopy in extraarticular distal radius fracture treatment. Saab et al.[42] identified no functional benefit to intraarticular reduction with the addition of arthroscopy in the surgical treatment of a distal radius fracture. Sivrikaya et al.[43] describes the use of ultrasonography in the emergency department as a diagnostic tool, with 100% specificity in identifying a distal radius fracture in a cohort of 93 patients. On CT imaging after distal radius fractures, Kim et al.[44] did not find a correlation between DRUJ alignment on CT and DRUJ stability on physical exam. Other identified studies include the utility of MRI in improving the measurement of distal radius fracture displacement on lateral radiographs[45] and the observation that the rate of CT utilization in the assessment and treatment of distal radius fractures did not increase over a 5-year period.[46]

Furthermore, eight additional studies were identified with level-4 evidence outside of the above topics. Chatzikonstaninou et al.[47] and Arealia et al.[48] were unable to identify an improvement in the reproducibility of fracture classification by the addition of a CT scan to radiographs. In 46 patients after a distal radius fracture, Van Leerdam et al.[49] found CT unreliable in diagnosing DRUJ instability. Murase et al.[50] found 3D virtual simulation beneficial in the preoperative planning of growth arrest correction after a distal radius fracture. In a case series of three distal radius fractures, Atesok et al.[51] found intraoperative CT adds 7.5 min to case length but did not identify the need for any reduction or screw revision. Das Graças Nascimento et al.[52] found that CT did not influence the treatment proposed by experienced hand surgeons but was beneficial for less experienced surgeons in fracture pattern determination. Wijffels et al.[53] noted fair interobserver reliability in identifying a coronal fracture line in the lunate facet with both radiographs and 2-dimensional CT.

Five level-5 studies were identified and included for completeness of Ref. 54–58.

RECOMMENDATION

In patients with an intraarticular displaced distal radius fracture, evidence suggests:

Recommendations	Overall Quality
• The addition of CT to radiographs aids in the identification of fracture pattern and in the determination of optimal fixation strategy	⊕⊕⊕○ MODERATE

- 3D modeling for preoperative planning of distal radius fracture fixation and malunion correction may decrease fluoroscopy usage, blood loss, and operative time ⊕○○○ VERY LOW
- MRI can aid in the diagnosis of concurrent osseous and soft tissue injuries but is of limited utility in the treatment of acute distal radius fractures ⊕⊕○○ LOW

CONCLUSION

The use of advanced imaging, including CT scan, 3D modeling, and MRI in the treatment of distal radius fractures is of variable utility based on the current available literature. CT scan allows for improved identification of intraarticular fracture fragments, as well as DRUJ incongruity, but does not appear to improve surgical outcomes. Advanced imaging does increase the identification of concomitant injuries in distal radius fractures, but the utility of MRI in the assessment of distal radius fractures is limited. Access to a computer-based interactive 3D imaging environment may avoid some of the difficulties experience with 3D printing but is not currently routinely available. Such surgeon access may be the next expansion in advance imaging that will facilitate the assessment, therapeutic planning, and management of distal radial fractures.

Panel 2: Author's Preferred Technique

In the case of a highly comminuted intraarticular distal radius fracture, such as in the patient in Panel 1, the authors prefer to obtain a preoperative CT scan (Fig. 3A–C) with 3D image reconstruction (Fig. 4A–C) for preoperative planning to more accurately identify fracture fragments and guide fracture fixation decisions. CT is not routinely utilized for extraarticular distal radius fractures or fractures that do not have significant intraarticular comminution due to the reliability of plain radiographs in these fracture patterns as well as the cost of advanced imaging. Traction radiographs are also utilized in cases where CT is not obtained or available to assist in fracture fragment identification and determination of treatment strategy.

Standard CT, and even 3D CT reconstructions, are actually two-dimensional projections of a three-dimensional data set. When available, a fully interactive 3D virtual reconstruction allows for virtual preoperative planning, including reduction techniques and 3D templating of fixation strategies.

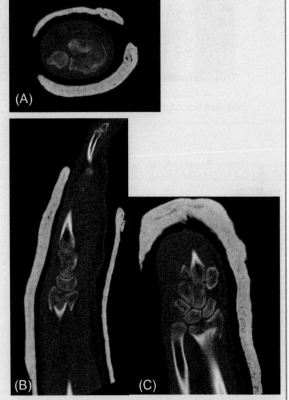

FIG. 3 Axial (A), sagittal (B), and coronal (C) CT images of the same 48-year-old female showing a comminuted intraarticular distal radius fracture.

Continued

Panel 2: Author's Preferred Technique—cont'd

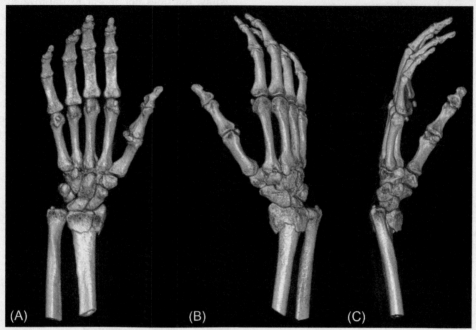

FIG. 4 (A–C) 3D CT reconstructions of the same 48-year-old female showing a displaced intraarticular distal radius fracture.

Panel 3: Pearls and Pitfalls

PEARLS:

- In the case of significant intraarticular comminution, CT +/ − 3D modeling improves fracture fragment identification.
- CT allows for improved visualization of sigmoid notch involvement of distal radius fractures when compared to radiographs.
- CT and 3D modeling can provide beneficial information in preoperative planning for the treatment of distal radius malunions.
- The use of advanced imaging (CT, MRI, 3D modeling) can improve the diagnosis of concomitant injuries, including adjacent carpal fractures, DRUJ instability, and ligamentous injuries.

- Traction radiographs can be an adequate substitute for CT in comminuted intraarticular fractures, and can be done more economically and with lower radiation exposure.

PITFALLS:

- The use of advanced imaging in the treatment of distal radius fractures has variable impact on clinical outcomes in surgically treated fractures.
- Using currently available systems, there is a significant increase in cost of treatment of distal radius fractures when advanced imaging is utilized, without a clearly documented advantage.

CONFLICT OF INTEREST

Associate Professor Sandow has been involved in the development of interactive 3D imaging (www.truelifeanatomy.com.au and www.rubamas.com) and has a potential conflict of interest in the subject of the paper.

REFERENCES

1. Sandow M. The why, what, how and where of 3D imaging. *J Hand Surg Eur Vol.* 2014;39(4):343–345.
2. Buijze GA, Leong NL, Stockmans F, et al. Three-dimensional compared with two-dimensional preoperative planning of corrective osteotomy for extra-articular distal radial

malunion: a multicenter randomized controlled trial. *J Bone Joint Surg Am.* 2018;100(14):1191–1202.

3. Avery DM, Matullo KS. Distal radial traction radiographs: interobserver and intraobserver reliability compared with computed tomography. *J Bone Joint Surg Am.* 2014;96(7): 582–588.

4. Cole RJ, Bindra RR, Evanoff BA, Gilula LA, Yamaguchi K, Gelberman RH. Radiographic evaluation of osseous displacement following intra-articular fractures of the distal radius: reliability of plain radiography versus computed tomography. *J Hand Surg [Am].* 1997;22(5): 792–800.

5. Kleinlugtenbelt YV, Hoekstra M, Ham SJ, et al. Spectrum bias, a common unrecognised issue in orthopaedic agreement studies: do CT scans really influence the agreement on treatment plans in fractures of the distal radius? *Bone Joint Res.* 2015;4(12):190–194.

6. Hunt JJ, Lumsdaine W, Attia J, Balogh ZJ. AO type-C distal radius fractures: the influence of computed tomography on surgeon's decision-making. *ANZ J Surg.* 2013;83(9): 676–678.

7. Nakanishi Y, Omokawa S, Shimizu T, Nakano K, Kira T, Tanaka Y. Intra-articular distal radius fractures involving the distal radioulnar joint (DRUJ): three dimensional computed tomography-based classification. *J Orthop Sci.* 2013;18(5):788–792.

8. Rozental TD, Bozentka DJ, Katz MA, Steinberg DR, Beredjiklian PK. Evaluation of the sigmoid notch with computed tomography following intra-articular distal radius fracture. *J Hand Surg [Am].* 2001;26(2):244–251.

9. Dahlen HC, Franck WM, Sabauri G, Amlang M, Zwipp H. Incorrect classification of extra-articular distal radius fractures by conventional X-rays. Comparison between biplanar radiologic diagnostics and CT assessment of fracture morphology. *Unfallchirurg.* 2004;107(6):491–498.

10. Wijffels M, Stomp W, Krijnen P, Reijnierse M, Schipper I. Computed tomography for the detection of distal radioulnar joint instability: normal variation and reliability of four CT scoring systems in 46 patients. *Skelet Radiol.* 2016;45(11):1487–1493.

11. Arora S, Grover SB, Batra S, Sharma VK. Comparative evaluation of postreduction intra-articular distal radial fractures by radiographs and multidetector computed tomography. *J Bone Joint Surg Am.* 2010;92(15):2523–2532.

12. Jakubietz MG, Mages L, Zahn RK, Kenn W, Jakubietz RG, Meffert RH. The role of CT scan in postoperative evaluation of distal radius fractures: retrospective analysis in regard to complications and revision rates. *J Orthop Sci.* 2017;22(3):434–437.

13. Kleinlugtenbelt YV, Madden K, Groen SR, et al. Can experienced surgeons predict the additional value of a CT scan in patients with displaced intra-articular distal radius fractures. *Strategies Trauma Limb Reconstr.* 2017;12 (2):91–97.

14. Zhang X, Zhang Y, Fan J, Yuan F, Tang Q, Xian CJ. Analyses of fracture line distribution in intra-articular distal radius fractures. *Radiol Med.* 2019;124(7):613–619.

15. Rieger M, Gabl M, Gruber H, Jaschke WR, Mallouhi A. CT virtual reality in the preoperative workup of malunited distal radius fractures: preliminary results. *Eur Radiol.* 2005;15(4):792–797.

16. Mehling I, Rittstieg P, Mehling AP, Küchle R, Müller LP, Rommens PM. Intraoperative C-arm CT imaging in angular stable plate osteosynthesis of distal radius fractures. *J Hand Surg.* 2013;38(7):751–757.

17. Heo YM, Roh JY, Kim SB, et al. Evaluation of the sigmoid notch involvement in the intra-articular distal radius fractures: the efficacy of computed tomography compared with plain X-ray. *Clin Orthop Surg.* 2012;4(1):83–90.

18. Souer JS, Wiggers J, Ring D. Quantitative 3-dimensional computed tomography measurement of volar shearing fractures of the distal radius. *J Hand Surg [Am].* 2011;36 (4):599–603.

19. Pruitt DL, Gilula LA, Manske PR, Vannier MW. Computed tomography scanning with image reconstruction in evaluation of distal radius fractures. *J Hand Surg [Am].* 1994;19(5):720–727.

20. Katz MA, Beredjiklian PK, Bozentka DJ, Steinberg DR. Computed tomography scanning of intra-articular distal radius fractures: does it influence treatment? *J Hand Surg [Am].* 2001;26(3):415–421.

21. Neubauer J, Benndorf M, Reidelbach C, et al. Comparison of diagnostic accuracy of radiation dose-equivalent radiography, multidetector computed tomography and cone beam computed tomography for fractures of adult cadaveric wrists. *PLoS ONE.* 2016;11(10), e0164859.

22. Johnston GH, Friedman L, Kriegler JC. Computerized tomographic evaluation of acute distal radial fractures. *J Hand Surg [Am].* 1992;17(4):738–744.

23. Flikkilä T, Nikkola-Sihto A, Kaarela O, Pääkkö E, Raatikainen T. Poor interobserver reliability of AO classification of fractures of the distal radius. Additional computed tomography is of minor value. *J Bone Joint Surg (Br).* 1998;80(4):670–672.

24. Harness NG, Ring D, Zurakowski D, Harris GJ, Jupiter JB. The influence of three-dimensional computed tomography reconstructions on the characterization and treatment of distal radial fractures. *J Bone Joint Surg Am.* 2006;88(6):1315–1323.

25. Bombaci H, Polat A, Deniz G, Akinci O. The value of plain X-rays in predicting TFCC injury after distal radial fractures. *J Hand Surg Eur Vol.* 2008;33(3):322–326.

26. Freedman DM, Dowdle J, Glickel SZ, Singson R, Okezie T. Tomography versus computed tomography for assessing step off in intraarticular distal radial fractures. *Clin Orthop Relat Res.* 1999;361:199–204.

27. Von Schneider-Egestorf A, Meyer B, Wacker F, Rosenthal H, Von Falck C. Systematic evaluation of concomitant extensor tendon sheath injury in patients with distal intra-articular radial fractures in MDCT using the floating fat sign. *Eur Radiol.* 2017;27(10):4345–4350.

28. Heo YM, Kim SB, Yi JW, et al. Evaluation of associated carpal bone fractures in distal radial fractures. *Clin Orthop Surg.* 2013;5(2):98–104.

29. Spence LD, Savenor A, Nwachuku I, Tilsley J, Eustace S. MRI of fractures of the distal radius: comparison with conventional radiographs. *Skelet Radiol.* 1998;27(5): 244–249.

30. Deniz G, Kose O, Yanik S, Colakoglu T, Tugay A. Effect of untreated triangular fibrocartilage complex (TFCC) tears on the clinical outcome of conservatively treated distal radius fractures. *Eur J Orthop Surg Traumatol.* 2014;24(7): 1155–1159.

31. Yan B, Xu Z, Chen Y, Yin W. Prevalence of triangular fibrocartilage complex injuries in patients with distal radius fractures: a 3.0T magnetic resonance imaging study. *J Int Med Res.* 2019;47(8):3648–3655.

32. Pierre-Jerome C, Moncayo V, Albastaki U, Terk MR. Multiple occult wrist bone injuries and joint effusions: prevalence and distribution on MRI. *Emerg Radiol.* 2010;17(3):179–184.

33. Yoshii Y, Kusakabe T, Akita K, Tung WL, Ishii T. Reproducibility of three dimensional digital preoperative planning for the osteosynthesis of distal radius fractures. *J Orthop Res.* 2017;35(12):2646–2651.

34. Totoki Y, Yoshii Y, Kusakabe T, Akita K, Ishii T. Screw length optimization of a volar locking plate using three dimensional preoperative planning in distal radius fractures. *J Hand Surg Asian Pac Vol.* 2018;23(4):520–527.

35. Chen C, Cai L, Zhang C, Wang J, Guo X, Zhou Y. Treatment of die-punch fractures with 3D printing technology. *J Investig Surg.* 2017;31(5):385–392.

36. Chen C, Cai L, Zheng W, Wang J, Guo X, Chen H. The efficacy of using 3D printing models in the treatment of fractures: a randomised clinical trial. *BMC Musculoskelet Disord.* 2019;20(1):65.

37. Bizzotto N, Tami I, Santucci A, et al. 3D Printed replica of articular fractures for surgical planning and patient consent: a two years multi-centric experience. *3D Print Med.* 2015;2(1):2.

38. Shintani K, Kazuki K, Yoneda M, et al. Computer-assisted three-dimensional corrective osteotomy for malunited fractures of the distal radius using prefabricated bone graft substitute. *J Hand Surg Asian Pac Vol.* 2018;23(4): 479–486.

39. Gehweiler D, Teunis T, Varjas V, et al. Computerized anatomy of the distal radius and its relevance to volar plating, research, and teaching. *Clin Anat.* 2019;32(3):361–368.

40. Byrne AM, Impelmans B, Bertrand V, Van haver A, Verstreken F. Corrective osteotomy for malunited diaphyseal forearm fractures using preoperative 3-dimensional planning and patient-specific surgical guides and implants. *J Hand Surg [Am].* 2017;42(10): 836.e1–836.e12.

41. Christiaens N, Nedellec G, Guerre E, et al. Contribution of arthroscopy to the treatment of intraarticular fracture of the distal radius: retrospective study of 40 cases. *Hand Surg Rehabil.* 2017;36(4):268–274.

42. Saab M, Wunenburger P-E, Guerre E, et al. Does arthroscopic assistance improve reduction in distal

articular radius fracture? A retrospective comparative study using a blind CT assessment. *Eur J Orthop Surg Traumatol.* 2018;29(2):405–411.

43. Sivrikaya S, Aksay E, Bayram B, Oray NC, Karakasli A, Altintas E. Emergency physicians performed point-of-care-ultrasonography for detecting distal forearm fracture. *Turk J Emerg Med.* 2016;16(3):98–101.

44. Kim JP, Park MJ. Assessment of distal radioulnar joint instability after distal radius fracture: comparison of computed tomography and clinical examination results. *J Hand Surg [Am].* 2008;33(9):1486–1492.

45. Welling RD, Jacobson JA, Jamadar DA, Chong S, Caoili EM, Jebson PJ. MDCT and radiography of wrist fractures: radiographic sensitivity and fracture patterns. *AJR Am J Roentgenol.* 2008;190(1):10–16.

46. Lumsdaine W, Enninghorst N, Hardy BM, Balogh ZJ. Patterns of CT use and surgical intervention in upper limb periarticular fractures at a level-1 trauma Centre. *Injury.* 2013;44(4):471–474.

47. Chatzikonstantinou M, Theodoraki K, Arealis G, et al. Evaluation of the reliability of three classification systems for the distal radius fractures along with CT imaging. *Int J Surg.* 2014;12.

48. Arealis G, Galanopoulos I, Nikolaou VS, Lacon A, Ashwood N, Kitsis C. Does the CT improve inter- and intra-observer agreement for the AO, Fernandez and Universal classification systems for distal radius fractures? *Injury.* 2014;45(10):1579–1584.

49. Van Leerdam RH, Wijffels MME, Reijnierse M, Stomp W, Krijnen P, Schipper IB. The value of computed tomography in detecting distal radioulnar joint instability after a distal radius fracture. *J Hand Surg Eur Vol.* 2017;42(5):501–506.

50. Murase T, Oka K, Moritomo H, Goto A, Sugamoto K, Yoshikawa H. Correction of severe wrist deformity following physeal arrest of the distal radius with the aid of a three-dimensional computer simulation. *Arch Orthop Trauma Surg.* 2009;129(11):1465–1471.

51. Atesok K, Finkelstein J, Khoury A, et al. The use of intraoperative three-dimensional imaging (ISO-C-3D) in fixation of intraarticular fractures. *Injury.* 2007;38(10): 1163–1169.

52. Das Graças Nascimento V, Da costa AC, Falcochio DF, Lanzarin LD, Checchia SL, Chakkour I. Computed tomography's influence on the classifications and treatment of the distal radius fractures. *Hand (N Y).* 2015;10(4):663–669.

53. Wijffels MM, Guitton TG, Ring D. Inter-observer variation in the diagnosis of coronal articular fracture lines in the lunate facet of the distal radius. *Hand (N Y).* 2012;7(3): 271–275.

54. Brink PR, Rikli DA. Four-corner concept: CT-based assessment of fracture patterns in distal radius. *J Wrist Surg.* 2016;5(2):147–151.

55. Kataoka T, Oka K, Murase T. Rotational corrective osteotomy for Malunited distal diaphyseal radius

fractures in children and adolescents. *J Hand Surg [Am]*. 2018;43(3):286.e1–286.e8.

56. Kovler I, Joskowicz L, Weil YA, et al. Haptic computer-assisted patient-specific preoperative planning for orthopedic fractures surgery. *Int J Comput Assist Radiol Surg*. 2015;10(10):1535–1546.

57. Metz VM, Gilula LA. Imaging techniques for distal radius fractures and related injuries. *Orthop Clin North Am*. 1993;24(2):217–228.

58. Catalano LW, Barron OA, Glickel SZ. Assessment of articular displacement of distal radius fractures. *Clin Orthop Relat Res*. 2004;423:79–84.

CHAPTER 7

Closed Reduction and Immobilization of Displaced Distal Radius Fractures

HYOUNG-SEOK JUNG • JAE-SUNG LEE
Department of Orthopedic Surgery, Hospital of Chung-Ang University of Medicine, Seoul, Republic of Korea

KEY POINTS

- Despite the popularity of surgical treatment, most displaced distal radius fractures (DRFs) are initially managed with closed reduction and immobilization.
- Radiological outcomes were not significantly different between mechanical reduction using finger-trap traction and manual reduction.
- Compared to procedural sedation, local anesthesia (hematoma block) is a safe and effective alternative anesthesia for reduction of DRFs, which provides excellent pain relief in adult and pediatric patients.
- Immobilization using a sugar-tong or above-the-elbow splint is equivalent to a short-arm splint for maintaining the reduction and quality of molding has more influence on maintaining reduction than the length of the cast.
- The evidence of the benefit of routinely repeating reduction or routine preoperative reduction in DRFs is insufficient
- Repeated reduction should be reserved for experienced teams in selected patients, such as those with minimal comminution, those who fail to get appropriate reduction due to inadequate anesthesia or those who have relative contraindications to surgery.

Panel 1: Case Scenario

A 46-year-postmenopausal woman visited the emergency department with a swollen and deformed right wrist after falling on an outstretched hand. Radiographs showed a displaced distal radius fracture with a 40 degrees dorsal angulation and metaphyseal comminution (Fig. 1). How is her fracture most effectively reduced and maintained?

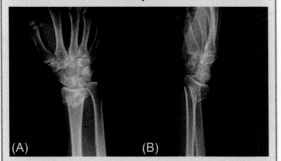

FIG. 1 Radiographs showing an extraarticular displaced distal radius fracture: (A) anteroposterior view. (B) Lateral view.

IMPORTANCE OF THE PROBLEM

Distal radius fractures (DRFs) are a common orthopedic condition among adults and high incidence is reported worldwide.[1-3] Multiple treatment options are available for patients with DRFs, including cast immobilization, percutaneous pinning, external fixation, and open reduction with internal fixation (ORIF) using a plate. The optimal choice depends on several factors such as patient age, fracture pattern, displacement, fracture instability, and surgeon preference. Over the recent decades, surgical approaches such as ORIF have been increasingly used.[2, 4, 5] Despite the popularity of ORIF, most displaced DRFs are initially managed with closed reduction and subsequent orthosis. Closed reduction of DRFs is commonly performed in the emergency department to obtain acceptable fracture alignment and maintain stability. In some cases, two or more reduction attempts are performed to achieve these goals.[6]

Distal Radius Fractures. https://doi.org/10.1016/B978-0-323-75764-5.00025-1

MAIN QUESTION

What is the most effective technique for closed reduction and immobilization in the treatment of DRFs?

CURRENT OPINION

The initial management of DRFs typically consists of closed reduction and immobilization in the emergency department. The quality of reduction can influence definitive management; thus, some authors have suggested that significant efforts should be made to obtain anatomical reduction when possible. Therefore, a combination of closed reduction and cast immobilization remains a preferred treatment option in most cases. However, the optimal method for closed reduction remains to be determined.

Closed reduction of a fracture is considered acceptable when the following radiologic conditions are obtained: radial inclination ≥15 degrees, loss of radial height ≤ 5 mm, dorsal angulation ≤15 degrees and palmar angulation ≤20 degrees.[7] The classic method of closed reduction for DRFs requires two people pulling in opposite directions to produce and maintain longitudinal traction. This is termed *manual reduction*. The mechanical methods of reduction usually include the use of "finger traps." In finger-trap traction, the injured arm is suspended using finger traps attached to two or more fingers, and a counterweight is suspended over the upper arm.[8] Although manual manipulation is widely used, several studies have recommended finger-trap traction as a more gentle method of reduction.[9, 10] Finger-trap traction can be applied without the need for an assistant, and it allows for easier application of the plaster cast. However, during molding of the plaster, the traction tends to pull the wrist straight, making ulnar deviation, and flexion difficult to achieve.

To reduce the pain during reduction, regional anesthesia (hematoma block) or procedural sedation is commonly performed.[7, 11, 12] After closed reduction, a sugar-tong splint or above-elbow cast is commonly used to prevent pronation and supination, although a short-arm cast is deemed to be equivalent.[8, 12, 13] It has been suggested that the quality of molding has more influence on maintaining reduction than the length of the cast.

FINDING THE EVIDENCE

A literature search was conducted in PubMed, Embase, and the Cochrane Library. The following search terms were used: (*colles, fracture* OR *colles fracture* OR *colles fractures* OR *colles* OR *distal radius fracture* OR *distal radius fractures* OR *distal radial fracture* OR *distal radial fractures*) AND (*traction jig* OR *finger stretch* OR *finger stretch traction* OR *finger trap* OR *finger trap traction* OR *manual reposition* OR *manual repositioning* OR *reposition* OR *repositioning* OR *manual reduction* OR *reduction* OR *closed reduction* OR *closed manual reduction*). A manual search for additional eligible studies that were not found during the abovementioned search was performed using the reference lists of the included studies and relevant review articles.

- Bibliographies of the eligible articles
- Articles that were not in the English, French, or German were excluded.
- The search of the abovementioned databases was performed by a trained Cochrane librarian.

QUALITY OF THE EVIDENCE

Level I

Systematic Reviews/Metaanalyses: 2
Randomized trials: 8

Level II

Randomized trials with methodological limitations: 1

Level III

Retrospective comparative studies: 6

FINDINGS

Finger-Trap Versus Manual Reduction

Kongsholm et al.[10] performed a prospective randomized study to compare finger-trap and manual reductions for DRFs. They reported that finger-trap reduction was significantly less painful than manual reduction, even without anesthesia. However, the radiological outcomes of both reduction techniques were similar, and both techniques resulted in acceptable reduction in terms of volar angle and radial length.

Holkenborg et al.[9] also performed a randomized study and reported that the mean visual analog scale (VAS) score, satisfaction level, and radiological outcomes after reduction did not differ between the finger-trap and manual reduction groups. Although finger-trap traction seemed more technically challenging, they reported a significantly better Quick Disabilities of the Arm, Shoulder, and Hand (DASH) score, and reduced incidence of carpal tunnel syndrome and complex regional pain syndrome in the finger-trap reduction group.

Earnshaw et al.[14] conducted a prospective randomized study to compare the results of conventional manipulation with those of finger-trap traction for closed reduction of DRFs on the basis of radiographic outcome. Two hundred and 23 patients with 225 displaced DRFs were randomized to treatment groups of closed reduction with either finger-trap traction (112 patients) or manual manipulation (111 patients). Dorsal angulation, radial shortening, and radial angulation were reported to have no differences between the two groups either at initial presentation or after reduction. No significant difference in VAS scores between the two groups were found. When the dorsal tilt less than 10 degrees and radial shortening less than 5 mm are considered as acceptable, both techniques resulted in 87% of satisfactory reductions. However, the percentages of fracture that showed an acceptable alignment were only 57% and 50% at 1 week and only 27% and 32% at 5 weeks in the finger-trap traction and manual manipulation groups, respectively. The failure rates did not differ significantly between the two groups.

A recent systematic review and metaanalysis reported that closed reduction using finger-trap traction seems better than manual manipulation in restoring radial length, whereas a manual reduction technique seems better in restoring dorsal tilt (Figs. 2 and 3).[13] However, finger-trap reduction seemed to provide less pain and fewer complications.

IMAGE-ASSISTED REDUCTION

Dailey et al.[15] conducted a prospective randomized controlled study on the effectiveness of mini C-Arm fluoroscopy for closed reduction of DRFs. Standard reductions were performed in 34, and fluoroscopically aided reductions in 29 patients. No significant differences in postreduction radial height, radial inclination, ulnar variance, and volar tilt were observed. The overall reduction attempts and subjective difficulty of fracture reduction increased when fluoroscopy was performed. The rate of initial operative management did not differ between the groups.

Kazum et al.[16] also compared the radiological outcomes of adult closed DRF reductions with and without fluoroscopy. In this retrospective study, 90 and 84 patients underwent reduction with and without fluoroscopy, respectively. According to the accepted radiographic guidelines, nonsurgical treatment was indicated for 62% of the patients in the reduction without fluoroscopy group and for 56% of the patients in the fluoroscopy-assisted reduction group ($P = .44$). In addition, no significant difference in any postreduction radiographic parameters or alignment of unstable fractures was observed between the groups.

Kodama et al.[17] compared ultrasonography-assisted closed reduction between a retrospective cohort of blind and fluoroscopy-assisted reduction and a blind

Study or Subgroup	Finger–trap Mean	SD	Total	Manual Mean	SD	Total	Weight	Std. Mean Difference IV, Fixed, 95% CI
Earnshaw 2002	−2.5	1.95	112	−3.6	2.15	111	45.8%	0.53 [0.27, 0.80]
Holkenborg 2013	5.3	9.3	66	2.7	9.6	78	30.2%	0.27 [−0.06, 0.60]
Kongsholm 1987	−0.2	4.3	62	−1.9	3.8	54	24.0%	0.41 [0.05, 0.78]
Total (95% CI)			**240**			**243**	**100.0%**	**0.43 [0.25, 0.61]**

Heterogeneity. Chi² = 1.45, df = 2 (P = 0.48); I² = 0%
Test for overall effect: Z = 4.62 (P < 0.00001)

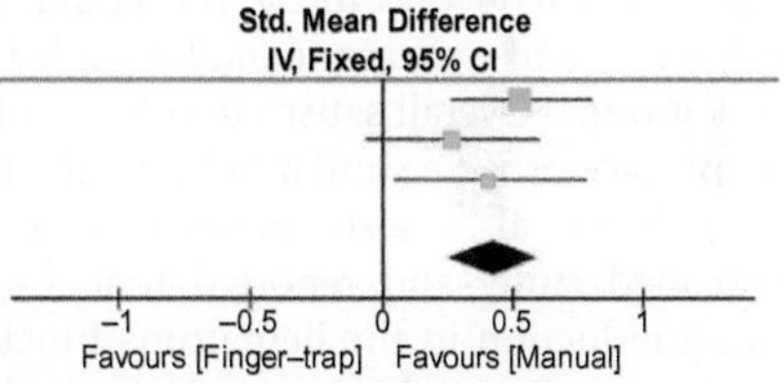

FIG. 2 Radiological outcomes (dorsal tilt) of finger-trap and manual reductions of distal radius fractures. (From Sosborg-Wurtz H, Corap Gellert S, Ladeby Erichsen J, Viberg B. Closed reduction of distal radius fractures: a systematic review and meta-analysis. *EFORT Open Rev* 2018;3:114–120; with permission.)

Study or Subgroup	Finger–trap Mean	SD	Total	Manual Mean	SD	Total	Weight	Std. Mean Difference IV, Fixed, 95% CI
Earnshaw 2002	1.86	1	112	1.98	1	112	46.6%	−0.12 [−0.38, 0.14]
Holkenborg 2013	0.19	2.8	66	0.8	2.9	78	29.6%	−0.21 [−0.54, 0.12]
Kongsholm 1987	1.3	2.5	62	2	2.4	54	23.8%	−0.28 [−0.65, 0.08]
Total (95% CI)			**240**			**244**	**100.0%**	**−0.19 [−0.37, −0.01]**

Heterogeneity. Chi² = 0.54, df = 2 (P = 0.76); I² = 0%
Test for overall effect: Z = 2.04 (P = 0.04)

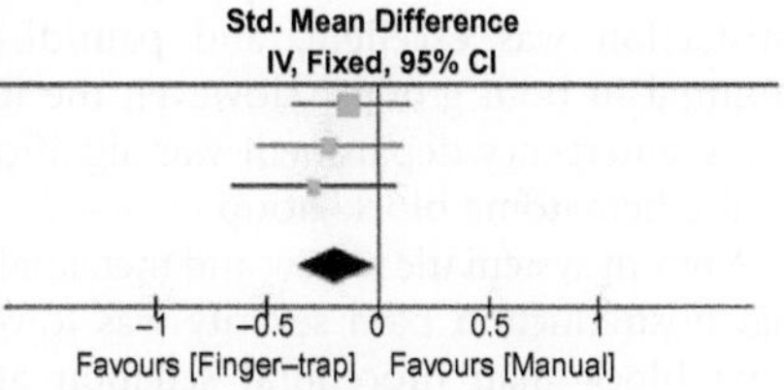

FIG. 3 Radiologic outcomes (radial shortening) of finger-trap versus manual reduction of distal radius fractures. (From Sosborg-Wurtz H, Corap Gellert S, Ladeby Erichsen J, Viberg B. Closed reduction of distal radius fractures: a systematic review and meta-analysis. *EFORT Open Rev* 2018;3:114–120; with permission.)

reduction control group. The ultrasonography-guided group consisted of 43 patients, and the control group consisted of 57 patients, including 35 who underwent fluoroscopic reduction and 22 who underwent reduction unaided by imaging. They found no significant displacement differences between the radiographic and ultrasonographic measurements. Ultrasonography-guided reduction took longer than the other two methods. The criteria for successful reduction were defined as radial shortening of less than 1 mm and the volar tilt of 0 degree or greater in postreduction radiographs. The success rates were similar between the ultrasonography and fluoroscopy groups (95% and 94%, respectively). However, fluoroscopy-assisted reduction had a higher success rate than blinded closed reduction (94% vs 68%), but both reduction methods provided similar radiographic results. They suggest that both ultrasonographic and fluoroscopic assistance can aid in the reduction of DRFs.

COMPARISON BETWEEN HEMATOMA BLOCK AND PROCEDURAL SEDATION

Fathi et al.[18] compared the efficacy and safety of ultrasonography-guided hematoma block with those of procedural sedation and analgesia in patients with acute DRF reduction pain control. This randomized clinical trial demonstrated that pain scores did not differ significantly before and during reduction, and at 5 and 15 min after reduction in the procedural sedation and analgesia, and ultrasonography-guided hematoma block groups. Overall satisfaction levels of the patients and physicians were similar between the two groups.

Singh et al.[19] also performed a randomized controlled study and reported that the pain scores during reduction in the hematoma block group were significantly lower than those in the sedation group.

Bear et al.[20] conducted a prospective study for DRF reduction in children. They reported no significant difference in pre- and postreduction angulations between the hematoma block and sedation groups, and reductions maintained satisfactory alignment. The overall satisfaction was excellent, and pain/discomfort was minimal in both groups. However, the length of stay in the emergency department was significantly shorter for the hematoma block group.

A recent systematic review and metaanalysis reported that postreduction pain severity was lower for hematoma block than procedural sedation and analgesia (95% confidence interval [CI], 1.170–0.029; $P=.039$), although there was no difference in pain severity during reduction between these two groups (95% CI,

1.101–1.812; $P=.632$).[21] Most of the reported side effects include nausea, vomiting, and respiratory distress in adult patients treated with procedural sedation and analgesia. The incidence rates of the reported side effects did not significantly differ between the groups of pediatric patients.

IMMOBILIZATION AFTER REDUCTION

The sugar-tong splint is a long-arm plaster construct that prevents pronation and supination while allowing some flexion and extension at the elbow. It is commonly used in the acute setting of DRFs; however, the sugar-tong splint is a heavy and cumbersome splint that typically requires patients to use an arm sling. Bong et al.[22] performed a prospective randomized study to compare the sugar-tong splint with the short-arm splint in terms of patient satisfaction and the ability to maintain reduction of DRFs. They found that 16 out of 38(%) fractures immobilized with the short-arm splint, and 17 out of 47(%) fractures immobilized with a sugar-tong splint were displaced, indicating no significant difference. When the splint constructs were evaluated based on fracture stability, no significant differences were found between the splints in terms of the ability to maintain fracture reduction in both stable and unstable displaced fractures. The patients in the short-arm splint group had significantly better DASH scores than those in the sugar-tong group at 1 week.

Park et al.[23] also conducted a prospective randomized multicenter study to compare short- and long-arm plaster casts for the treatment of stable distal radius fractures in patients aged older than 55 years. There were no significant differences in radiological parameters between the groups, except for volar tilt. Volar tilt is superior for the patients in the long arm cast group at each follow-up. However, the mean score for disability caused by plaster cast immobilization and the incidence rate of shoulder pain were significantly higher in the patients who had a long plaster cast.

Chess et al. demonstrated a cast index to determine the quality of the molding of the cast to the normal contours of the child's forearm. The index was determined by dividing the sagittal width of the cast by the coronal width of the cast at the fracture site and was shown to be 0.7 for a cast used on the distal part of a normal forearm of a child. They reported that 10% of the fractures in their series had reduction loss which were related to poor cast-molding as demonstrated by the cast index. These results suggest that short arm casts, if applied with appropriate molding, can be effective in the treatment of fractures of the distal third of the forearm in children.[24]

Webb et al. performed prospective randomized study to compare short and long arm casts for displaced fractures in the distal third of the forearm in children and demonstrated there were no significant differences between the two groups with regard to the change in displacement, angulation, or deviation during the treatment. However, fractures that lost reduction in the cast had significantly higher cast indices, indicating poor cast molding. Thus, either a long or a short arm cast can be used, but proper molding of either is mandatory.[25]

REPEATED REDUCTION

Repeated attempts of closed reduction of DRFs are occasionally performed in the emergency department or outpatient clinical setting to optimize fracture alignment and avoid surgery. However, additional manipulation of the fracture may increase dorsal comminution and lead to loss of reduction in the cast. Schermann et al.[6] found that repeated reduction attempts worsen dorsal comminution, however, they improve immediate fracture alignment. Only 5.2% of patients who underwent two reduction attempts had acceptable final alignment without requiring any surgery. Another study investigated whether re-manipulation of DRFs 1–2 weeks after the initial closed reduction was beneficial, at the time of the first follow-up.[26] They found that repeated reduction attempts improved dorsal angulation in only 32% of the patients, all of whom were aged less than 60 years. This suggests that re-manipulation and optimal molded casting is best reserved for experienced teams in selected patients, such as those with minimal comminution, those who fail to get appropriate reduction due to inadequate anesthesia or those who have relative contraindications to surgery. In experienced hands, satisfactory rates of maintained reduction can be achieved in order to avoid surgery.

PREOPERATIVE REDUCTION

When the decision is made to operate, based on the initial fracture radiographs, controversy exists whether the fracture should be reduced before surgery. Reduction can relieve soft tissue tension, reduced pressure on the median nerve and might reduce discomfort. However, the hypothetical risks of soft tissue problems, median neuropathy related to deformity, and increased pain remain controversial as routinely manipulating the reduction provides discomfort to the patient and takes considerable time and resources

for medical personnel without evident benefit. ANY EVIDENCE ON CASES WITH SIGNS OF ACUTE CARPAL TUNNEL SYNDROME? ASSUME THEY SHOULD BE REDUCED ASAP? (Although it is generally agreed that closed reduction should be performed in patient who had skin tenting or acute carpal tunnel syndrome due to distal radius fractures, no clear consensus exists about the appropriate indication for closed reduction.)

Based on the study by Fan et al.[27] who retrospectively evaluated 128 patients with unstable DRFs, there were no significant differences between the patients who did and did not undergo closed reduction in terms of surgery time, complication rate, and functional outcomes. Teunis et al.[28] performed a retrospective cohort study to assess unreduced fractures before surgery in the cases without any wound, skin tenting, or neuropathy. They reported no significant differences in rates of adverse events or number of subsequent surgeries within the first year after surgery between the reduced and unreduced fractures before surgery. Jung et al.[29] also performed retrospective comparative study between the acceptable reduction and nonacceptable reduction group. They reported that there were no significant differences in the preoperative pain VAS score, mean length of stay, operation time, and postoperative complications between the groups. In addition, radiologic parameters and the DASH score at a 1-year follow-up were also not significantly different between the groups.

RECOMMENDATION

In patients with an intraarticular displaced distal radius fracture, evidence suggests:

Recommendation	Overall Quality
• Radiological outcomes do not significantly differ between finger-trap and manual reductions	⊕⊕⊕⊕ HIGH
• Finger-trap reduction may be associated with less pain and fewer complications	⊕⊕⊕◯ MODERATE
• Radiological outcomes do not differ significantly between the fluoroscopy-assisted and conventional reduction methods	⊕⊕⊕◯ MODERATE
• Ultrasonographic and fluoroscopic assistance can aid the reduction of DRFs	⊕⊕◯◯ LOW
• Hematoma block may be a safe and effective alternative to procedural sedation and analgesia with low complication rates	⊕⊕⊕⊕ HIGH

- A short-arm cast appears to be less functionally limiting but equally effective at maintaining reduction when compared with a standard sugar-tong or above-elbow splint   ⊕⊕⊕◯ MODERATE
- SOME RECOMMENDATION ABOUT OPTIMAL MOLDING BASED ON YOUR FINDINGS
- Either a long or a short arm cast can be used, but proper molding of either based on cast index is mandatory   ⊕⊕⊕◯ MODERATE
- Repeated reduction is reserved for selected patients such as those with minimal comminution and those who failed to achieve adequate reduction due to inadequate anesthesia   ⊕◯◯◯ VERY LOW
- Routine preoperative reduction does not have any benefit on surgical outcomes in cases without wound, skin tenting, or neuropathy   ⊕⊕◯◯ LOW

CONCLUSION

No universally agreed consensus has been reached on the optimal technique and anesthetic approach for closed reduction of DRFs as various methods seem equally effective. In addition, the reduction technique does not appear to influence radiological outcomes. Patient characteristics and preferences, fracture type, local expertise, and resources influence treatment choices. Thus, there is sufficient argument to support that surgeons should continue to use the technique that they have been trained on and perform best in their institution with local facilities. Evidence regarding the benefit of routine repeated or preoperative reduction in patients with DRFs is insufficient. A future prospective randomized study is necessary to investigate the need for repeated or preoperative reduction in terms of radiological or surgical outcomes and patient comfort.

Panel 2: Author's Preferred Technique

In this case scenario, primary manual reduction without C-arm guidance was performed to relieve soft tissue tension and reduce discomfort. To reduce pain during reduction, a hematoma block with 10 mL of 1% lidocaine without epinephrine was performed before reduction. Traction was applied along the axis of the limb to disimpact the fracture, and counter-traction was applied to the elbow by an assistant. Next, the wrist was deviated ulnarly and flexed to approximately 15 degrees. After manual reduction, sugar-tong plaster immobilization was applied using the three-point fixation technique and radiographs were repeated (Fig. 4). Subsequently, the patient was rescheduled to visit the outpatient clinic within a week. After checking the radiographs on the second visit, the decision to proceed with surgery for DRFs was made. The decision to proceed with surgery was determined together by the patient and the surgeon based of the factors related to expected instability, such as old age, female sex, ulnar variance, and dorsal comminution, even if the patients maintain a satisfactory reduction at second visit.[30, 31]

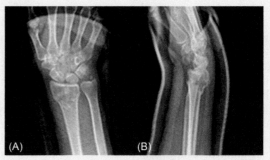

FIG. 4 Radiological appearance after closed reduction and application of a sugar-tong splint for a displaced distal radius fracture: (A) anteroposterior and (B) lateral views. Note the slight volar bending of the cast according to the three-point fixation principles and the position of ulnar deviation with care taken not to immobilize the metacarpophalangeal joint.

Panel 3: Pearls and Pitfalls

PEARLS:

- When the patient and surgeon decide upon surgical treatment, primary reduction can be performed as gently as possible to relieve soft tissue tension and reduce swelling and patient discomfort. Although acceptable radiological parameters are generally not achieved, preoperative repeated reduction is not recommended.

- The decision for repeated reduction to achieve acceptable radiological parameters should be made carefully. Repeated reduction was performed by experienced hand surgeons in the outpatient clinic only for patients with high wrist function demands who prefer conservative treatment.

PITFALLS:

- Reduction with brute force should be avoided, especially in patients with thin skin or severe osteoporosis.

- Positions of extreme flexion and ulnar deviation should be avoided because of the risk of carpal tunnel syndrome (Fig. 5).

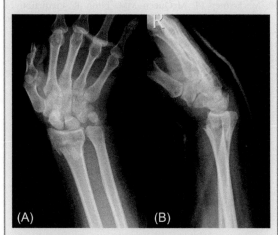

(A)   (B)

FIG. 5 Radiographs of extreme ulnar deviation and flexion of the wrist after closed reduction of an unstable distal radius fracture: (A) anteroposterior and (B) lateral views. This should be avoided because of the risk of carpal tunnel syndrome.

REFERENCES

1. Jo YH, Lee BG, Kim HS, et al. Incidence and seasonal variation of distal radius fractures in Korea: a population-based study. *J Korean Med Sci*. 2018;33(7):e48.
2. Jo YH, Lee BG, Kim JH, et al. National surgical trends for distal radius fractures in Korea. *J Korean Med Sci*. 2017;32 (7):1181–1186.
3. Diamantopoulos AP, Rohde G, Johnsrud I, Skoie IM, Hochberg M, Haugeberg G. The epidemiology of low- and high-energy distal radius fracture in middle-aged and elderly men and women in Southern Norway. *PLoS ONE*. 2012;7(8):e43367.
4. Chaudhry H, Kleinlugtenbelt YV, Mundi R, Ristevski B, Goslings JC, Bhandari M. Are volar locking plates superior to percutaneous K-wires for distal radius fractures? A meta-analysis. *Clin Orthop Relat Res*. 2015;473(9):3017–3027.
5. Kandemir U, Matityahu A, Desai R, Puttlitz C. Does a volar locking plate provide equivalent stability as a dorsal nonlocking plate in a dorsally comminuted distal radius fracture?: a biomechanical study. *J Orthop Trauma*. 2008;22(9):605–610.
6. Schermann H, Kadar A, Dolkart O, Atlan F, Rosenblatt Y, Pritsch T. Repeated closed reduction attempts of distal radius fractures in the emergency department. *Arch Orthop Trauma Surg*. 2018;138(4):591–596.
7. Mulders MAM, Walenkamp MMJ, van Dieren S, Goslings JC, Schep NWL, Collaborators VT. Volar plate fixation versus plaster immobilization in acceptably reduced extra-articular distal radial fractures: a multicenter randomized controlled trial. *J Bone Joint Surg Am*. 2019;101(9):787–796.
8. Handoll HH, Madhok R. Closed reduction methods for treating distal radial fractures in adults. *Cochrane Database Syst Rev*. 2003;(1):Cd003763.
9. Holkenborg J, Napel SJT, Kolkman K. Closed reduction of distal radius fractures: is finger trap traction superior to manual traction? *Ann Emerg Med*. 2013;62(4).
10. Kongsholm J, Olerud C. Reduction of Colles' fractures without anaesthesia using a new dynamic bone alignment system. *Injury*. 1987;18(2):133–136.
11. Myderrizi N, Mema B. The hematoma block an effective alternative for fracture reduction in distal radius fractures. *Med Arh*. 2011;65(4):239–242.
12. Tabrizi A, Mirza Tolouei F, Hassani E, Taleb H, Elmi A. Hematoma block versus general anesthesia in distal radius fractures in patients over 60 years in trauma emergency. *Anesth Pain Med*. 2017;7(1):e40619.
13. Sosborg-Wurtz H, Corap Gellert S, Ladeby Erichsen J, Viberg B. Closed reduction of distal radius fractures: a systematic review and meta-analysis. *EFORT Open Rev*. 2018;3(4):114–120.
14. Earnshaw SA, Aladin A, Surendran S, Moran CG. Closed reduction of colles fractures: comparison of manual manipulation and finger-trap traction: a prospective, randomized study. *J Bone Joint Surg Am*. 2002;84(3):354–358.
15. Dailey SK, Miller AR, Kakazu R, Wyrick JD, Stern PJ. The effectiveness of mini-C-arm fluoroscopy for the closed reduction of distal radius fractures in adults: a randomized controlled trial. *J Hand Surg [Am]*. 2018;43 (10):927–931.
16. Kazum E, Kadar A, Sharfman ZT, et al. Adult closed distal radius fracture reduction: does fluoroscopy improve alignment and reduce indications for surgery? *Hand (N Y)*. 2017;12(6):557–560.

17. Kodama N, Takemura Y, Ueba H, Imai S, Matsusue Y. Ultrasound-assisted closed reduction of distal radius fractures. *J Hand Surg [Am].* 2014;39(7):1287–1294.

18. Fathi M, Moezzi M, Abbasi S, Farsi D, Zare MA, Hafezimoghadam P. Ultrasound-guided hematoma block in distal radial fracture reduction: a randomised clinical trial. *Emerg Med J.* 2015;32(6):474–477.

19. Singh GK, Manglik RK, Lakhtakia PK, Singh A. Analgesia for the reduction of Colles fracture. A comparison of hematoma block and intravenous sedation. *Online J Curr Clin Trials.* 1992; Doc No 23:[3614 words; 3643 paragraphs].

20. Bear DM, Friel NA, Lupo CL, Pitetti R, Ward WT. Hematoma block versus sedation for the reduction of distal radius fractures in children. *J Hand Surg [Am].* 2015;40(1):57–61.

21. Tseng PT, Leu TH, Chen YW, Chen YP. Hematoma block or procedural sedation and analgesia, which is the most effective method of anesthesia in reduction of displaced distal radius fracture? *J Orthop Surg Res.* 2018;13(1):62.

22. Bong MR, Egol KA, Leibman M, Koval KJ. A comparison of immediate postreduction splinting constructs for controlling initial displacement of fractures of the distal radius: a prospective randomized study of long-arm versus short-arm splinting. *J Hand Surg [Am].* 2006;31 (5):766–770.

23. Park MJ, Kim JP, Lee HI, Lim TK, Jung HS, Lee JS. Is a short arm cast appropriate for stable distal radius fractures in patients older than 55 years? A randomized prospective

24. Chess DG, Hyndman JC, Leahey JL, Brown DC, Sinclair AM. Short arm plaster cast for distal pediatric forearm fractures. *J Pediatr Orthop.* 1994;14(2):211–213.

25. Webb GR, Galpin RD, Armstrong DG. Comparison of short and long arm plaster casts for displaced fractures in the distal third of the forearm in children. *J Bone Joint Surg Am.* 2006;88(1):9–17.

26. McQueen MM, MacLaren A, Chalmers J. The value of remanipulating Colles' fractures. *J Bone Joint Surg.* 1986;68(2):232–233.

27. Fan J, Yuan F, Li S-Z, Tang Q, Xian CJ. Is the preoperative closed reduction irreplaceable for distal radius fracture surgical treatment?—a retrospective clinical study. *Int J Clin Exp Med.* 2017;10(1):1309–1314.

28. Teunis T, Mulder F, Nota SP, Milne LW, Dyer GS, Ring D. No difference in adverse events between surgically treated reduced and unreduced distal radius fractures. *J Orthop Trauma.* 2015;29(11):521–525.

29. Jung HS, Chun KJ, Kim JY, Lee JS. Necessity of acceptable radiologic alignment by preoperative closed reduction for unstable distal radius fractures treated with volar locking plates. *Eur J Trauma Emerg Surg.* 2020; Online ahead of print.

30. Mackenney PJ, McQueen MM, Elton R. Prediction of instability in distal radial fractures. *J Bone Joint Surg Am.* 2006;88(9):1944–1951.

31. Walenkamp MM, Aydin S, Mulders MA, Goslings JC, Schep NW. Predictors of unstable distal radius fractures: a systematic review and meta-analysis. *J Hand Surg Eur Vol.* 2016;41(5):501–515.

multicentre study. *J Hand Surg Eur Vol.* 2017;42 (5):487–492.

CHAPTER 8

Surgical Versus Conservative Interventions for Displaced Distal Radius Fractures

NATSUMI SAKA[a] • YUKICHI ZENKE[b]
[a]Department of Orthopaedics, Teikyo University School of Medicine, Tokyo, Japan, [b]Department of Orthopaedics, University of Occupational and Environmental Health School of Medicine, Fukuoka, Japan

---

KEY POINTS

- Treatment is based on radiographical fracture pattern, bone quality, and functional demand.
- Evidence suggests that functional recovery may be faster in volar locking plating compared to conservative treatment, whereas there is not enough study of external fixation and percutaneous pinning compared to conservative treatment regarding patient-reported outcome.
- Evidence suggests that regarding the complication rate, which needed secondary surgery, there is no statistical difference in percutaneous pinning and volar plating compared to conservative treatment. The risk of having secondary surgery may be lower in external fixation compared to conservative treatment.
- When performing the surgical treatment, care should be taken to prevent nerve and tendon injury.

Panel 1: Case Scenario

A 48-year-old, right-handed female who works in the agricultural industry visited the orthopedics clinic with a swollen and deformed right wrist after a fall on the outstretched hand while riding a bicycle. Radiographs showed an extraarticular distal radius fracture with 25 degrees of dorsal tilt (Fig. 1). What is the most effective approach for the treatment of her fracture?

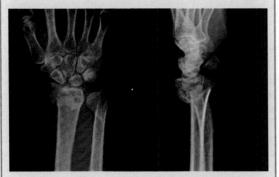

FIG. 1 A 48-year-old female case. The radiographs show distal radius fracture at the time of injury.

IMPORTANCE OF THE PROBLEM

Distal radius fracture (DRF) is one of the most common types of fracture, and the pediatric and geriatric population have a higher risk of sustaining this injury.[1] Most of the fractures can be treated by closed reduction and casting. However, conservative treatment can be associated with redisplacement and subsequent malunion of the distal radius, which may lead to the pain and disability. Besides, especially among the elderly population, there is a growing need for faster recovery of limb function.

As surgical treatment of distal radius fractures, percutaneous pinning by K-wires, external fixation, or internal fixation by a volar locking plate (VLP) are widely performed. Conservative treatment is more cost-effective, and there is no risk of complication associated with surgery but can be complicated by malunion or wrist contracture. On the other hand, patients can start the range of motion exercises earlier with a stable surgical fixation, especially with VLP. However, it can be complicated with other adverse events such as tendonitis and tendon ruptures.

Distal Radius Fractures. https://doi.org/10.1016/B978-0-323-75764-5.00016-0

The objective of this chapter is to clarify the current evidence comparing surgical treatment and conservative treatment of distal radius fractures.

MAIN QUESTION

What is the relative effect of conservative treatment versus surgical treatment on functional outcome and complication rates in the management DRFs?

P: patient with distal radius fracture.

I: surgical treatment (percutaneous pinning, volar locking plating, external fixation).

C: conservative treatment (reduction and fixation by cast).

O: patient-reported outcome and complications.

CURRENT OPINION

Surgical indication differs based on the patient's age, demand, and type of fracture. Generally, surgical treatment is recommended if there is the following one or more parameters on radiographs after reduction.[2]

(1) More than 10 degrees of dorsal angulation on the lateral view
(2) Ulnar variance (UV) of more than 2 mm
(3) Articular step-off or gap of more than 2 mm
(4) Incongruity of the distal radioulnar joint
(5) Dorsal loss of substance and comminution of the fracture

FINDING THE EVIDENCE

- Cochrane search: "Distal radius fracture," "Distal radial fracture"
- Pubmed (Medline):
  (((((((("radius fractures"[MeSH Terms] OR "forearm injuries"[MeSH Terms] OR "wrist injuries" [MeSH Terms]))) OR ((distal radius fracture*[tiab]) OR distal radial fracture* [tiab])))) OR ("Broken wrist*"[tiab] OR "Colles fracture*" [tiab])) AND (((conservative treatment[tiab] OR nonoperative treatment [tiab]) OR nonoperative treatment[tiab] OR splint[tiab] OR cast[tiab] OR casting[tiab] OR closed treatment[tiab] OR closed management [tiab] OR "closed reduction"[tiab])))
- Articles that were not in English were excluded.
- For the pooled analysis of the functional outcome, data from studies that reported the mean and standard deviation of the validated patient-reported outcomes such as Disability of the Arm, Shoulder, and Hand questionnaire (DASH), Patient-Rated Wrist

Evaluation (PRWE), Short Form Health Survey-36 (SF-36). If these outcomes were not reported, a result of other functional outcomes that report the functional grade such as Gartland and Werley system were extracted.

- For the article which reported only median and interquartile, mean, and standard deviation were estimated using the method by developed by Wan.[3]
- For percutaneous pinning and external fixation, the complication was defined as the redisplacement of fracture which required the surgery.
- For volar plating, the complication was defined as the condition which requires the surgery, such as carpal tunnel release for carpal tunnel syndrome, tendon rupture, tendonitis which requires plate removal, refixation of the fracture due to redisplacement or malposition of the plate, osteotomy due to malunion, infection requiring lavage, and debridement.
- Data abstraction for the metaanalysis was based on the published studies.
- Due to the nature of the intervention, all studies lacked blinding of the study population and health care providers, as such an overall risk of bias was high.
- Metaanalysis was conducted using StataCorp 2019 (*Stata Statistical Software: Release 16*. College Station, TX: StataCorp LLC).

PERCUTANEOUS PINNING VS CONSERVATIVE TREATMENT

Quality of the Evidence

Level I:
1A: Metaanalyisis: 1[4]
1B: Randomized controlled trials: 3[5–7]
Level II:
2B: Randomized controlled trials with methodological limitations: 3[8–10]

Findings

There is no study that reported DASH or PRWE regarding pinning versus conservative treatment. Only one study reported the SF-36.[5] This study reported a mean physical score of SF-36 at 4 months as 42.2 (SD 9.7) for pinning and 38.2 (SD 11.2) for conservative treatment. For the mental health component score at 4 months, the mean score was 51 (SD 13.2) for pinning and 50.4 (SD 8.6) for conservative treatment. The difference was not statistically significant.[5] Several studies reported the functional grading, the risk ratio of developing fair or poor grading was 0.45 in favor of percutaneous pinning (95% CI: 0.21–0.97, $I^2 = 13.9\%$)

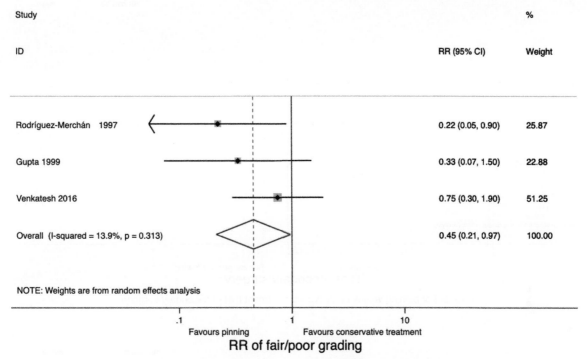

FIG. 2 For pinning versus conservative treatment (RR of fair/poor grading).

(Fig. 2).[7,8,10] For the complication rate, there was no difference in the rate of redisplacement requiring surgical treatment (RR 0.09, 95% CI: 0.01–1.03, $I^2 = 25.5\%$) (Fig. 3).[5,8]

EXTERNAL FIXATION VS CONSERVATIVE TREATMENT

Quality of the Evidence

Level I:

1A: Metaanalysis: 1[11]

1B: Randomized controlled trials: 1[12]

Level II:

2B: Randomized controlled trials with methodological limitations: 12[13–24]

Findings

Most studies were randomized controlled trials comparing conservative treatment and external fixation but did not mention the randomization protocol, hence were categorized as level 2B. In addition, none of the studies included DASH or PRWE as an outcome. Moroni et al. reported that the mean SF-36 score was 66.2 (SD 13.1) for conservative treatment and 67.1 (SD 13.1) for external fixation, and the result was not statistically significant.[22] The risk ratio of developing fair or poor

grading was not statistically significant (RR 0.73, 95% CI: 0.45–1.18, $I^2 = 60.1\%$) (Fig. 4).[13–21,23,24] For the complication rate, the risk ratio of redisplacement, which needed surgical treatment was 0.24 (95% CI: 0.08–0.68, $I^2 = 37.6\%$) in favor of external fixation (Fig. 5)[12–14,16,17,21] (Figs. 6 and 7).

VOLAR LOCKING PLATING VS CONSERVATIVE TREATMENT

Quality of the Evidence

Level I:

1A: Systematic Reviews/Metaanalyses: 1[25]

1B: Randomized controlled trials: 6[26–31]

Level II:

2B: Randomized controlled trials with methodological limitations: 2[20,32]

Findings

Most of the studies which compared volar plating and conservative treatment included only elderly patients, except for two studies.[29,32] In addition, there is heterogeneity in the inclusion criteria of the fracture type. Studies by Arora et al., Mulders et al., and Saving et al. excluded patients with an intraarticular fracture, whereas an inclusion criteria of the studies from Bartl et al., and Marinez-Mendez et al.

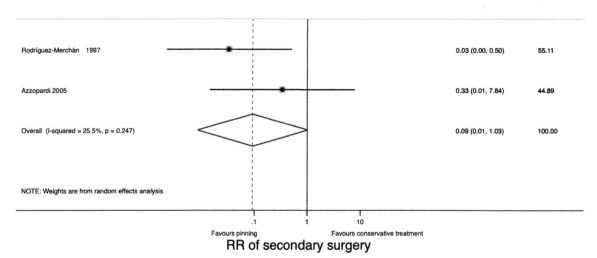

FIG. 3 For pinning versus conservative treatment (RR of secondary surgery).

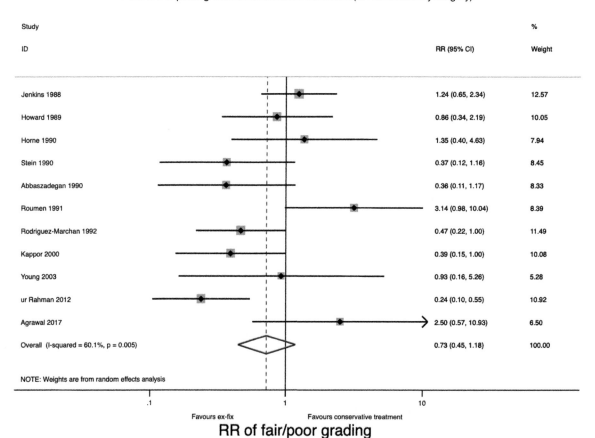

FIG. 4 For ex-fix versus conservative treatment (RR of fair/poor grading).

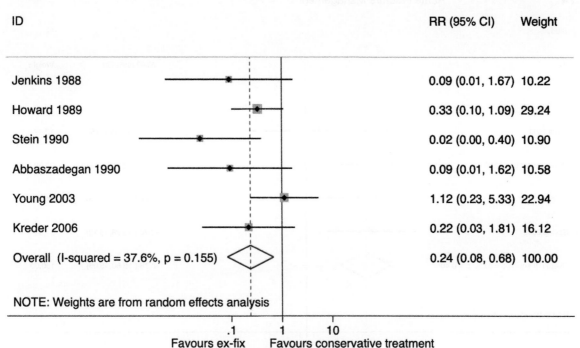

Study ID		RR (95% CI)	% Weight
Jenkins 1988		0.09 (0.01, 1.67)	10.22
Howard 1989		0.33 (0.10, 1.09)	29.24
Stein 1990		0.02 (0.00, 0.40)	10.90
Abbaszadegan 1990		0.09 (0.01, 1.62)	10.58
Young 2003		1.12 (0.23, 5.33)	22.94
Kreder 2006		0.22 (0.03, 1.81)	16.12
Overall (I-squared = 37.6%, p = 0.155)		0.24 (0.08, 0.68)	100.00

NOTE: Weights are from random effects analysis

.1   1   10

Favours ex-fix   Favours conservative treatment

RR of secondary surgery

FIG. 5 For ex-fix versus conservative treatment (RR of secondary surgery).

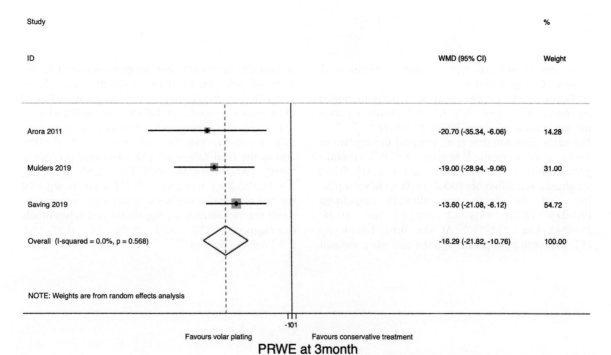

Study ID		WMD (95% CI)	% Weight
Arora 2011		-20.70 (-35.34, -6.06)	14.28
Mulders 2019		-19.00 (-28.94, -9.06)	31.00
Saving 2019		-13.60 (-21.08, -6.12)	54.72
Overall (I-squared = 0.0%, p = 0.568)		-16.29 (-21.82, -10.76)	100.00

NOTE: Weights are from random effects analysis

-10   1

Favours volar plating   Favours conservative treatment

PRWE at 3month

FIG. 6 For volar plating versus conservative treatment (PRWE at 3 months).

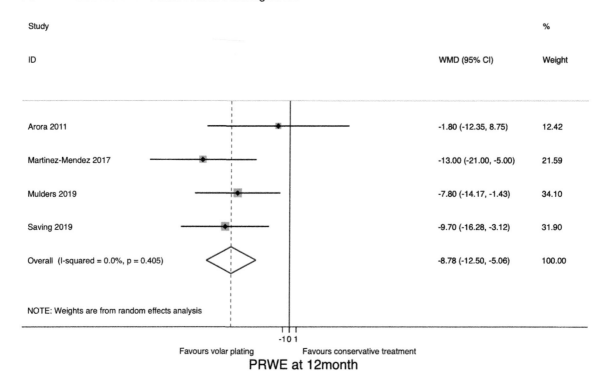

FIG. 7 For volar plating versus conservative treatment (PRWE at 12 months).

were patients with AO type C fractures. Sirniö et al. excluded C3 type fractures.

Regarding the pooled analysis of patient-reported outcome, five out of eight selected studies reported the mean score of either PRWE or DASH.[26–28, 30, 32] The study from Mulders et al. reported the median of the functional outcome.[29] In terms of PRWE, 3 months postoperatively, the analysis revealed a significant weighted mean difference (WMD) in favor of volar plating, and the result was clinically significant (WMD = −16.29, 95% CI: −21.82 to −10.76, $I^2 = 0\%$) (Fig. 2).[26,29,30] At the final follow up (12–24 month postoperatively), the difference was still

statistically significant, but smaller compared to the result of 3 months (WMD = −8.78, 95% CI: −12.50 to −5.06, $I^2 = 0\%$) (Fig. 3).[26, 28–30] The analysis showed the statistically significant difference of the DASH score in favor of volar plating both at 3 month postoperatively (WMD = −6.81, 95% CI: −10.18 to −3.45, $I^2 = 0\%$) and at the final follow up (12–24 month, postoperatively) (WMD = −6.26, 95% CI: −8.97 to −3.55, $I^2 = 31.2\%$) (Figs. 8 and 9).[26–30, 32] Six studies reported the rate of overall complications requiring surgery. The result was not statistically significant and substantially heterogeneous (RR 0.74, 95% CI: 0.27–2.02, $I^2 = 76.9\%$) (Fig. 10).[26–31]

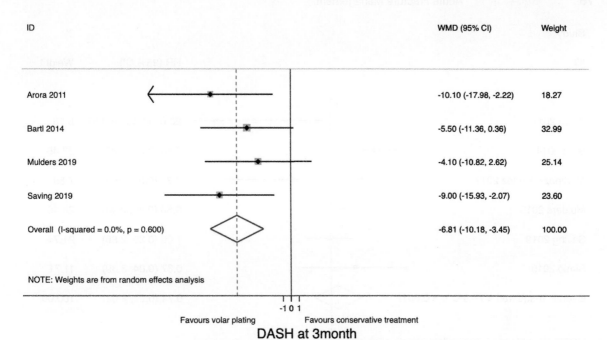

FIG. 8 For volar plating versus conservative treatment (DASH at 3 months).

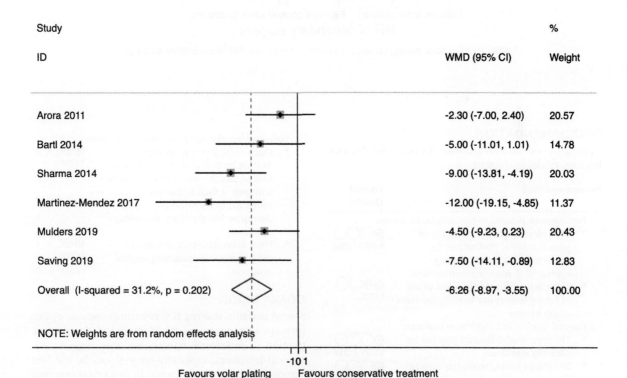

FIG. 9 For volar plating versus conservative treatment (DASH at 12 months).

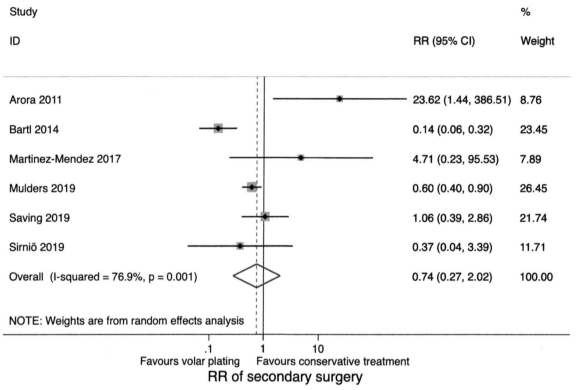

FIG. 10 For volar plating versus conservative treatment (RR of secondary surgery).

RECOMMENDATION

In patients with an intraarticular displaced distal radius fracture, evidence suggests:

Recommendation	Overall Quality
– Percutaneous pinning vs conservative treatment	
• The risk ratio of developing fair or poor functional grading may be lower in percutaneous pinning compared to conservative treatment	⊕○○○ VERY LOW
• There is no difference in terms of risk of having surgery due to redisplacement of the fracture	⊕⊕○○ LOW
– External fixation vs conservative treatment	
• The functional difference may not be clinically significant	⊕○○○ VERY LOW
• The risk of having secondary surgery due to redisplacement may be lower in external fixation compared to conservative treatment	⊕○○○ VERY LOW
– Volar locking plating vs conservative treatment	
• Open reduction and internal fixation by VLP may provide better functional outcome both in the early term and at final follow-up compared to conservative treatment, but the effect diminishes over time	⊕⊕○○ LOW
• There is no difference in terms of complication rate requiring surgical treatment	⊕⊕○○ LOW

CONCLUSION

Shared decision making is a key component in opting for surgical management. If patients prefer an earlier restoration of functional activity, evidence suggests that surgical treatment, especially by VLP can be the best choice. However, the difference in functional outcome favoring surgical over conservative treatment diminishes over time.

Panel 2: Author's Preferred Technique

In case of a highly unstable extraarticular distal radius fracture such as in this relatively young patient with an injury on the dominant side, we prefer primary open reduction and internal fixation by VLP, since functional recovery is faster and patients can return to work sooner. The surgical technique of VLP for the distal radius extraarticular fracture is relatively simple. However, there have been reports of complications such as flexor and extensor tendon ruptures.[33, 34]

We have standardized this surgical procedure for VLP similar to procedures as arthroplasty for knee osteoarthritis. In order to reduce complications and stabilize postoperative clinical results, the procedure is standardized as "step by step" so that a predictable result can be obtained regardless of who operates.[35]

Step1: Approach; We perform the surgery using the modified Henry approach, then the pronator quadratus (PQ) muscle attached to the distal end of the radius is detached to expose the intermediate fibrous zone (IMF). Next, the IMF is sharply cut at the center of the wrist using a sharp scalpel to expose the volar cortex (Fig. 11A).

Step2: Reduction and temporary fixation; we first correct the overall alignment by percutaneous pinning using the intrafocal pinning method.[36]

Step3: Plate and screw fixation; Even after alignment of the fracture is corrected by intrafocal pinning, the correction of volar tilt is often insufficient. In this case, we use the so-called condylar stabilizing method (Fig. 11B) in which the screw is fixed on the distal side of the plate first, with the proximal side of the plate floating above the volar cortex.[37] Care should be taken to flex the wrist when screwing the distal end of the plate and using compression forceps so that the plate can obtain close contact with the volar cortex.

Step4: Coverage of the plate; Once dissected, the IMF is repaired at the distal end of the plate, and the detached PQ muscle is sutured. It may not be possible to suture all of the PQ, depending on the muscle's quality and integrity.

Repairing PQ may prevent (long term) flexor tendon injury at the distal end of the plate.

The optimal timing of surgery remains unclear, but we generally perform surgery on the day of visit unless there is a particular reason not to. Our colleagues Yamashita et al. compared patients with an extraarticular distal radius fracture who underwent VLP fixation as early surgery (0 or 1 day after injury) and delayed surgery (1 week or more after injury).[38] According to this study, the patients in the early surgery group had better short-term outcomes (such as grip strength and Q-DASH score until 12 weeks).

We sometimes perform percutaneous pinning for fixation, especially for middle-aged patients with an injury on the nondominant side. At first, we perform a bone mineral density (BMD) test to evaluate bone quality. Our colleagues Oshige et al. reported that in patients with an UV of more than 5 mm or bone mineral density (BMD) with less than 70% of the young adult mean (YAM) at first examination, UV increased again at final follow-up by pinning, while UV was maintained by volar plating, independent of the degree of baseline UV and BMD.[39] In other words, these results indicate that in cases where the UV is 5 mm or less, and the YAM is 70% or larger at the time of injury, shortening can be avoided even with percutaneous pinning. Fig. 12A shows the radiographical finding at the time of injury, and Fig. 12B shows the finding just after operation. We apply conservative treatment for the patients with minor displacement at the time of injury when the volar cortex of the fracture site is clearly reduced after manual reduction, especially for the nondominant hand. In the previous study, we divided the type of reduction into three groups; intramedullary, anatomical, and extramedullary (Fig. 13A–C) in patients with dorsally displaced distal radius fracture who underwent cast immobilization.[40] We found that the correction loss of UV at final follow up was significantly larger in the intramedullary group, suggesting that converting to surgical treatment may be beneficial for patients with intramedullary fractures.

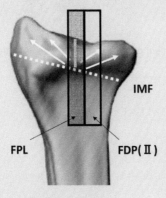

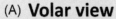

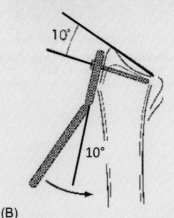

(A) **Volar view**   (B)

FIG. 11 (A) The view of distal radius volar side. (B) How to perform the condylar stabilizing technique.

Continued

Panel 2: Author's Preferred Technique—cont'd

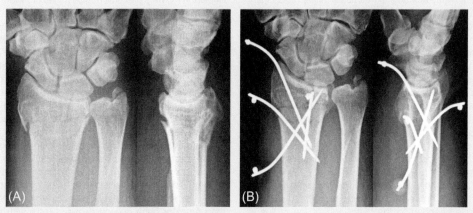

FIG. 12 (A) The radiographs show distal radius fracture at the time of injury. (B) The radiographs show the finding just after operation using pinning technique.

Intramedullary Anatomical Extramedullary

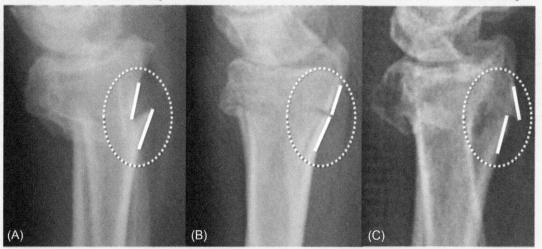

FIG. 13 Our classification about volar cortex displacement of distal radius fracture. (A) Intramedullary type, (B) anatomical type, (C) extramedullary type.

Panel 3: Pearls and Pitfalls

PEARLS:

- In the case of comminution and poor bone stock, the fracture could be highly unstable. After closed reduction using ligamentotaxis principles, one or multiple temporary 1.8mm K-wires can be placed through the radial styloid to stabilize the fracture while applying the plate. We believe/assume that K-wire insertion from the distal dorsal side of the radius may be a risk of postoperative pain and extensor tendon injury. Therefore, we insert K-wires from the proximal radial/volar side to the distal ulnar/dorsal side.

- It is essential to fix the distal end of the locking plate in close contact with the volar cortex. Therefore, we secure the plate using a dedicated compression device; reduction forceps to ensure the procedure (Fig. 14A). This procedure prevents the distal end of the plate from being lifted (Fig. 14B), reducing the risk of postoperative flexor tendon rupture.

- After plate and screw fixation, we assess the fluoroscopic skyline or dorsal tangential view to evaluate adequate screw length (Fig. 15A and B).[41, 42] However, in cases where the wrist has initial stiffness and depending on the angle between the wrist and elbow joints, over projection of the line of the dorsal cortex and the line of the carpal bones may be difficult to comprehend. Even in the group confirmed by the skyline view, 11.8% of cases had a protrusion of 1mm, and 12/40 cases (30%) had tendon sheath inflammation.[43]

- For conservative treatment, we recommend dorsiflexion casts. This method, as described by Gupta et al., is reported to be better in maintaining the repositioning point and cause less impairment in activities of daily living.[44, 45] In addition, it has been reported that volar translation is improved/enhanced as a mechanism of stabilization of a fractured part by dorsiflexion cast fixation.[46] An important point in the casting is to substantially trim the thenar muscle portion so that the thumb can be mobilized fully (Fig. 16A and B).

PITFALLS:

- When using radial sided provisional K-wires, be sure to protect the sensory branch of the radial nerve. Nerve injury in this area can be uncomfortable for the patient. A small incision is made on the skin with a sharp blade before inserting the K-wire, and the soft tissue should be sufficiently peeled off using mosquito forceps till the bone is exposed.

- When using a temporary external fixator, be careful not to fix it for more than 2 weeks or using excessive traction, since there is a risk of CRPS and joint contracture. At our department, the number of external fixation is limited because of these risks and inconvenience of its management. We only perform primary external fixation for open fractures.

- In the case of internal fixation using VLP, attention should be paid whether the patient can perform flexion and extension of the thumb without pain during postoperative follow-up observation. By these check-ups, we can examine the irritation on the flexor pollicis longus tendon. Pain is an important finding and don't overlook crepitations, noise, and discomfort as well. In these cases, it is prudent to examine the tendon using ultrasonography.

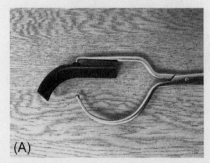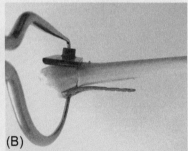

(A)   (B)

FIG. 14 (A) The reduction forceps. (B) How to use the reduction forceps for distal radius fracture model.

Continued

Panel 3: Pearls and Pitfalls—cont'd

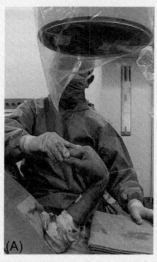
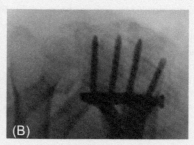

FIG. 15 (A) The position of the wrist for the skyline view using fluoroscopy. (B) The radiograph of skyline view after the volar plate fixation.

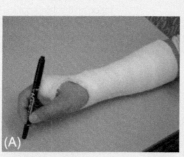
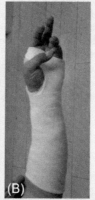

FIG. 16 (A) After the casting for distal radius fracture. (B)The thenar muscle portion was trimed so that the thumb can be mobilized fully.

Editor's Tips & Tricks: Simple Fracture but Difficult Reduction
Geert Alexander Buijze

Even simple fractures can at times be recalcitrant to reduce, such as the present example with persistent radial translation despite brachioradialis release and external maneuvers. © Dr Buijze 2020.

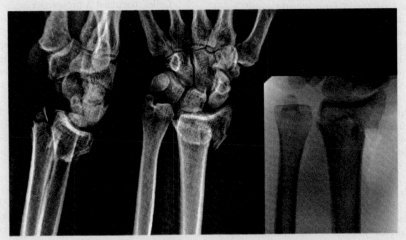

Several options exist including Orbay's maneuver (see Chapter 13) and maneuvers including intrafocal Kapandji pinning using K-wires sizes of 1.5–2.0 mm. © Dr Buijze 2020.

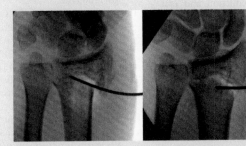

The intrafocal pin is bent and held together with thumb in the nondominant hand while stabilizing the fragment with a second temporary K-wire before screwing on the plate. © Dr Buijze 2020.

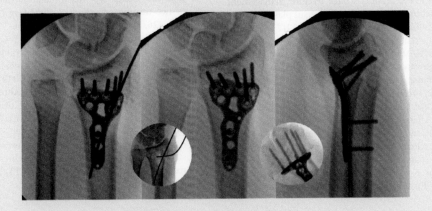

REFERENCES

1. Court-Brown CM, Caesar B. Epidemiology of adult fractures: a review. *Injury.* 2006;37(8):691–697. https://doi.org/10.1016/j.injury.2006.04.130.
2. Danish Health Authority. *National Clinical Guideline on the Treatment of Distal Radial Fractures*; 2016.
3. Wan X, Wang W, Liu J, Tong T. Estimating the sample mean and standard deviation from the sample size, median, range and/or interquartile range. *BMC Med Res Methodol.* 2014;14:135. https://doi.org/10.1186/1471-2288-14-135.
4. Karantana A, Handoll HH, Sabouni A. Percutaneous pinning for treating distal radial fractures in adults. *Cochrane Database Syst Rev.* 2020;2(2). https://doi.org/10.1002/14651858.CD006080.pub3, CD006080.
5. Azzopardi T, Ehrendorfer S, Coulton T, Abela M. Unstable extra-articular fractures of the distal radius. *J Bone Joint Surg.* 2005;87(6):837–840. https://doi.org/10.1302/0301-620X.87B6.15608.
6. Wong TC, Chiu Y, Tsang WL, Leung WY, Yam SK, Yeung SH. Casting versus percutaneous pinning for extra-articular fractures of the distal radius in an elderly Chinese population: a prospective randomised controlled trial. *J Hand Surg Eur Vol.* 2010;35(3):202–208. https://rsm.idm.oclc.org/login?url=https://www.rsm.ac.uk?url=http://dialog.proquest.com/professional/docview/736112151?accountid=138535.
7. Venkatesh RB, Maranna GK, Narayanappa RKB. A comparative study between closed reduction and cast application versus percutaneous K-wire fixation for extra-articular fracture distal end of radius. *J Clin Diagn Res.* 2016;10(2):RC05–RC9. https://doi.org/10.7860/JCDR/2016/18266.7220.
8. Rodríguez-Merchán EC. Plaster cast versus percutaneous pin fixation for comminuted fractures of the distal radius in patients between 46 and 65 years of age. *J Orthop Trauma.* 1997;11(3):212–217. https://doi.org/10.1097/00005131-199704000-00013.
9. Stoffelen DV, Broos PL. Closed reduction versus Kapandji-pinning for extra-articular distal radial fractures. *J Hand Surg (Br).* 1999;24(1):89–91. https://doi.org/10.1016/s0266-7681(99)90045-1.
10. Gupta R, Raheja A, Modi U. Colles' fracture: management by percutaneous crossed-pin fixation versus plaster of Paris cast immobilization. *Orthopedics.* 1999;22(7):680–682. https://pubmed.ncbi.nlm.nih.gov/10418864.
11. Handoll HHG, Madhok R, Huntley JS. External fixation versus conservative treatment for distal radial fractures in adults. *Cochrane Database Syst Rev.* 2006;4. https://doi.org/10.1002/14651858.CD006194.
12. Kreder HJ, Agel J, McKee MD, Schemitsch EH, Stephen D, Hanel DP. A randomized, controlled trial of distal radius fractures with metaphyseal displacement but without joint incongruity: closed reduction and casting versus closed reduction, spanning external fixation, and optional percutaneous K-wires. *J Orthop Trauma.* 2006;20(2):115–121. https://doi.org/10.1097/01.bot.0000199121.84100.fb.
13. Jenkins NH, Jones DG, Mintowt-Czyz WJ. External fixation and recovery of function following fractures of the distal radius in young adults. *Injury.* 1988;19(4):235–238. https://doi.org/10.1016/0020-1383(88)90033-2.
14. Howard PW, Stewart HD, Hind RE, Burke FD. External fixation or plaster for severely displaced comminuted Colles' fractures? A prospective study of anatomical and functional results. *J Bone Joint Surg (Br).* 1989;71(1):68–73. https://pubmed.ncbi.nlm.nih.gov/2915010.
15. Horne JG, Devane P, Purdie G. A prospective randomized trial of external fixation and plaster cast immobilization in the treatment of distal radial fractures. *J Orthop Trauma.* 1990;4(1):30–34. https://doi.org/10.1097/00005131-199003000-00005.
16. Stein H, Volpin G, Horesh Z, Hoerer D. Cast or external fixation for fracture of the distal radius. A prospective study of 126 cases. *Acta Orthop Scand.* 1990;61(5):453–456. https://www.ncbi.nlm.nih.gov/pubmed/2239172.
17. Abbaszadegan H, Jonsson U. External fixation or plaster cast for severely displaced Colles' fractures? Prospective 1-year study of 46 patients. *Acta Orthop Scand.* 1990;61(6):528–530. https://doi.org/10.3109/17453679008993575.
18. Roumen RM, Hesp WL, Bruggink ED. Unstable Colles' fractures in elderly patients. A randomised trial of external fixation for redisplacement. *J Bone Joint Surg (Br).* 1991;73(2):307–311. https://pubmed.ncbi.nlm.nih.gov/2005162.
19. Merchan EC, Breton AF, Galindo E, Peinado JF, Beltran J. Plaster cast versus Clyburn external fixation for fractures of the distal radius in patients under 45 years of age. *Orthop Rev.* 1992;21(10):1203–1209. https://www.ncbi.nlm.nih.gov/pubmed/1437248.
20. Kapoor H, Agarwal A, Dhaon BK. Displaced intra-articular fractures of distal radius: a comparative evaluation of results following closed reduction, external fixation and open reduction with internal fixation. *Injury.* 2000;31(2):75–79. https://rsm.idm.oclc.org/login?url=https://www.rsm.ac.uk?url=http://dialog.proquest.com/professional/docview/690573075?accountid=138535.
21. Young CF, Nanu AM, Checketts RG. Seven-year outcome following Colles' type distal radial fracture. A comparison of two treatment methods. *J Hand Surg (Br).* 2003;28(5):422–426. https://doi.org/10.1016/s0266-7681(02)00394-7.
22. Moroni A, Vannini F, Faldini C, Pegreffi F, Giannini S. Cast vs external fixation: a comparative study in elderly osteoporotic distal radial fracture patients. *Scand J Surg.* 2004;93(1):64–67. https://doi.org/10.1177/145749690409300114.
23. ur Rahman O, Khan MQ, Rasheed H, Ahmad S. Treatment of unstable intraarticular fracture of distal radius: POP casting with external fixation. *J Pak Med Assoc.* 2012;62(4):358–362.
24. Agrawal V, Rohit K. Distal radius fractures—a comparative study between conservative management and external fixation. *J Evol Med Dent Sci.* 2017;6(14):2–7. https://doi.org/10.14260/Jemds/2017/237.

25. Yu GS, Lin YB, Le LS, Zhan MF, Jiang XX. Internal fixation vs conservative treatment for displaced distal radius fractures: a meta-analysis of randomized controlled trials. *Ulus Travma Acil Cerrahi Derg.* 2016;22(3):233–241. https://doi.org/10.5505/tjtes.2015.05995.

26. Arora R, Lutz M, Deml C, Krappinger D, Haug L, Gabl M. A prospective randomized trial comparing nonoperative treatment with volar locking plate fixation for displaced and unstable distal radial fractures in patients sixty-five years of age and older. *J Bone Joint Surg Am.* 2011;93 (23):2146–2153. https://doi.org/10.2106/JBJS.J.01597.

27. Bartl C, Stengel D, Bruckner T, Gebhard F, ORCHID Study Group. The treatment of displaced intra-articular distal radius fractures in elderly patients. *Dtsch Arztebl Int.* 2014;111(46):779–787. https://doi.org/10.3238/arztebl. 2014.0779.

28. Martinez-Mendez D, Lizaur-Utrilla A, De-Juan-Herrero J. Intra-articular distal radius fractures in elderly patients: a randomized prospective study of casting versus volar plating. *J Hand Surg Eur Vol.* 2018;43(2):142–147. https://doi.org/10.1177/1753193417727139.

29. Mulders MAM, Walenkamp MMJ, van Dieren S, Goslings JC, Schep NWL, Collaborators VT. Volar plate fixation versus plaster immobilization in acceptably reduced extra-articular distal radial fractures: a multicenter randomized controlled trial. *J Bone Joint Surg Am.* 2019;101(9):787–796. https://doi.org/10.2106/JBJS.18.00693.

30. Saving J, Severin Wahlgren S, Olsson K, et al. Nonoperative treatment compared with volar locking plate fixation for dorsally displaced distal radial fractures in the elderly: a randomized controlled trial. *J Bone Joint Surg (Am Vol).* 2019;101(11):961–969. https://doi.org/10.2106/JBJS.18. 00768.

31. Sirnio K, Leppilahti J, Ohtonen P, Flinkkila T. Early palmar plate fixation of distal radius fractures may benefit patients aged 50 years or older: a randomized trial comparing 2 different treatment protocols. *Acta Orthop.* 2019. https://doi.org/10.1080/17453674.2018.1561614.

32. Sharma H, Khare GN, Singh S, Ramaswamy AG, Kumaraswamy V, Singh AK. Outcomes and complications of fractures of distal radius (AO type B and C): volar plating versus nonoperative treatment. *J Orthop Sci.* 2014. https://doi.org/10.1007/s00776-014-0560-0.

33. Stepan JG, Marshall DC, Wessel LE, et al. The effect of plate design on the flexor pollicis longus tendon after volar locked plating of distal radial fractures. *J Bone Joint Surg Am.* 2019;101(17):1586–1592. https://doi.org/10.2106/ JBJS.18.01087.

34. Zenke Y, Oshige T, Menuki K, et al. Analysis of tendon injuries accompanying distal radius fractures using volar locking plates. *J UOEH.* 2014;36(4):257–264. https://doi.org/10.7888/juoeh.36.257.

35. Imatani J, Kondo H, Moritani S, et al. "Standard" volar locking plate fixation for distal radius fractures. *J Jpn Hand Surg.* 2014;30(4):487–491 [in Japanese].

36. Kapandji A. Intra-focal pinning of fractures of the distal end of the radius 10 years later. *Ann Chir Main.* 1987;6(1):57–63. https://doi.org/10.1016/s0753-9053 (87)80011-x.

37. Kiyoshige Y. Condylar stabilizing technique with AO/ASIF distal radius plate for Colles' fracture associated with osteoporosis. *Tech Hand Up Extrem Surg.* 2002;6 (4):205–208. https://doi.org/10.1097/00130911-20021 2000-00009.

38. Yamashita K, Zenke Y, Sakai A, Oshige T, Moritani S, Maehara T. Comparison of functional outcome between early and delayed internal fixation using volar locking plate for distal radius fractures. *J UOEH.* 2015;37 (2):111–119. https://doi.org/10.7888/juoeh.37.111.

39. Oshige T, Sakai A, Zenke Y, Moritani S, Nakamura T. A comparative study of clinical and radiological outcomes of dorsally angulated, unstable distal radius fractures in elderly patients: intrafocal pinning versus volar locking plating. *J Hand Surg [Am].* 2007;32(9):1385–1392. https://doi.org/10.1016/j.jhsa.2007.07.005.

40. Zenke Y, Furukawa K, Furukawa H, et al. Radiographic measurements as a predictor of correction loss in conservative treatment of Colles' fracture. *J UOEH.* 2019;41 (2):139–144. https://doi.org/10.7888/juoeh.41.139.

41. Riddick AP, Hickey B, White SP. Accuracy of the skyline view for detecting dorsal cortical penetration during volar distal radius fixation. *J Hand Surg Eur Vol.* 2012;37(5):407–411. https://doi.org/10.1177/1753193411426809.

42. Ozer K, Wolf JM, Watkins B, Hak DJ. Comparison of 4 fluoroscopic views for dorsal cortex screw penetration after volar plating of the distal radius. *J Hand Surg [Am].* 2012;37(5):963–967. https://doi.org/10.1016/j.jhsa.2012. 02.026.

43. Herisson O, Delaroche C, Maillot-Roy S, Sautet A, Doursounian L, Cambon-Binder A. Comparison of lateral and skyline fluoroscopic views for detection of prominent screws in distal radius fractures plating: results of an ultrasonographic study. *Arch Orthop Trauma Surg.* 2017;137(10):1357–1362. https://doi.org/10.1007/ s00402-017-2759-y.

44. Gupta A. The treatment of Colles' fracture. Immobilisation with the wrist dorsiflexed. *J Bone Joint Surg (Br).* 1991;73 (2):312–315.

45. Takahata S. Fracture of the distal end of the forearm. *Clin Calcium.* 2003;13(10):1311–1316 [in Japanese].

46. Taylor KF, Gendelberg D, Lustik MB, Drake ML. Restoring volar tilt in AO type C2 fractures of the distal radius with unilateral external fixation. *J Hand Surg [Am].* 2017;42 (7):511–516. https://doi.org/10.1016/j.jhsa.2017.03.020.

CHAPTER 9

Predictors of Instability and Secondary Displacement After Conservatively Managed Distal Radius Fractures

Katrina R. Bell[a,b] • Timothy O. White[a] • Samuel G. Molyneux[a] • Andrew D. Duckworth[a,b]

[a]Edinburgh Orthopaedics, Royal Infirmary of Edinburgh, Edinburgh, United Kingdom, [b]University of Edinburgh, Edinburgh, United Kingdom

KEY POINTS

- Up to two-thirds of distal radius fractures re-displace after initial reduction or from a minimally displaced position at presentation.
- Increasing age and the presence of comminution, particularly dorsal, are the most commonly significant predictors of secondary displacement.
- Other factors proposed to increase displacement risk are female gender, as well as dorsal tilt >5 degrees, ulnar variance >0 mm, loss of radial inclination, and increasing radial shortening on initial trauma radiographs, as well as the absence of volar cortical continuity (the "volar hook") on postreduction radiographs.

Panel 1: Case Scenarios

A 65-year-old woman falls on an outstretched hand whilst gardening, sustaining a right distal radius fracture. She is right hand-dominant and works as a shop assistant. Fig. 1A and B demonstrate her presentation radiographs. Fig. 2A and B are her satisfactory postreduction radiographs following manipulation under regional anesthesia.

1. Which aspects of this case are concerning regarding the risk of secondary displacement?

2. How would this influence decision-making in terms of when to follow her up in clinic?

The same patient is seen in the out-patient department 8 days postreduction. Fig. 3A and B show her repeat radiographs.

3. What are the available management options for this patient and how would a definitive decision be made?

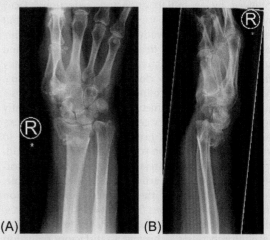

(A) (B)

FIG. 1 Radiographs showing a severely displaced distal radius fracture.

Continued

Distal Radius Fractures. https://doi.org/10.1016/B978-0-323-75764-5.00022-6

Panel 1: Case Scenarios—cont'd

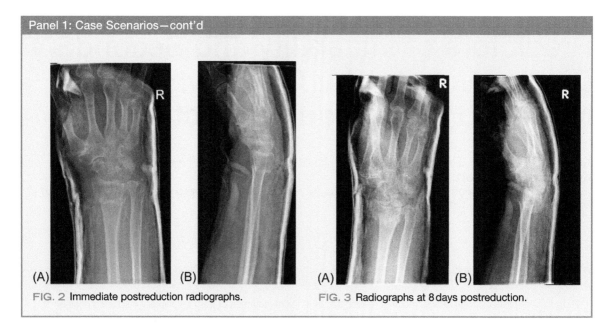

FIG. 2 Immediate postreduction radiographs.

FIG. 3 Radiographs at 8 days postreduction.

IMPORTANCE OF THE PROBLEM

This chapter examines factors that result in an unstable fracture that subsequently displaces. The literature suggests that anything from 10% to 62% of distal radius fractures (DRFs) become displaced, either after being initially minimally displaced or after early displacement followed by an initial satisfactory reduction.[1] Exact management strategies vary between institutions, but in many centers conservative management with casting forms the mainstay of treatment for undisplaced and minimally displaced fractures. Fractures that are initially displaced can undergo closed reduction and casting. Patients require clinic follow-up to monitor for subsequent fracture displacement, and this most frequently occurs within the first 2 weeks of injury.[2] If loss of position does occur, there needs to be a decision as to whether the new position is felt to be acceptable, considering important patient-related factors including comorbidities and preinjury activity levels. If unacceptable, treatment options can then include re-manipulation and casting, percutaneous fixation with Kirschner wires, plate fixation or external fixation. As the time from initial injury increases, achieving a satisfactory reduction can be more technically challenging and time consuming, especially with closed techniques and poorer bone quality. The ability to predict subsequent fracture

displacement would avoid this and allow patients to begin rehabilitation as soon as is possible.

MAIN QUESTION

Which injury characteristics predict fracture instability and secondary displacement in a distal radius fracture that is being managed conservatively?

CURRENT OPINION

Historically, Lafontaine's criteria of dorsal tilt (referred to as angulation in the original paper) of more than 20 degrees, dorsal comminution, intraarticular radiocarpal fracture, associated ulnar fracture and age of over 60 years have been the most widely accepted predictors of secondary displacement.[3] It is acknowledged that displacement results in inferior outcomes in young active patients, although some studies have demonstrated that this may not be the case in older lower demand patients.[4–6] There is evidence to suggest that radiological parameters correlate poorly with functional and patient-reported outcomes.[7] As with any orthopedic procedure, the risks of the proposed intervention must be considered against the perceived benefits. Decision making as to whether operative or nonoperative management is selected in the presence of a displaced fracture is highly dependent on patient factors, such as functional demand and medical comorbidities.

FINDING THE EVIDENCE

A literature search was carried out using the terms "distal" and "radius fractures" plus "instability" and subsequently plus "unstable" and "displacement." Titles and abstracts were reviewed, and articles not written in English or carried out in those under the age of 16 were excluded. Databases searched included the Cochrane Database of Systematic Reviews, Cochrane Central Register of Controlled Trials, MEDLINE, and EMBASE. Bibliographies of suitable articles were also examined.

QUALITY OF EVIDENCE

Level I:
Prospective cohort studies: 5[1, 8–11]
Level II:
Systematic Reviews/Metaanalyses: 1[12]
Level III:
Systematic Reviews/Metaanalyses: 1[13]
Retrospective comparative studies: 5[3, 14–17]

FINDINGS

Level-I Evidence

Zenke et al. prospectively studied 60 patients with a dorsally displaced distal radius fracture.[8] Fractures were reduced with local anesthetic hematoma block before immobilization in a sugar-tong (above-elbow) splint. Seventy-eight percent were female and the mean age was 72 years (range 55–96). By AO/OTA classification, patients with A2, A3, C1, C2, and C3 were included, with more than half of patients falling into the A3 category. The authors classified fractures into three types based on the volar cortex on the lateral postreduction radiograph. Fractures were classed as "intramedullary" when the volar cortex of the distal fragment was translated and impacted dorsally to the proximal part (in the medulla), "anatomical" when the proximal and distal parts of the volar cortex met, and "extramedullary" when the volar cortex of the distal fragment was translated and impacted volarly to the proximal fragment. They evaluated subsequent displacement based on volar tilt, radial inclination, and ulnar variation. There was a loss of volar tilt and radial inclination correction in all three groups, but no significant differences between

them. However, although there was a loss of ulnar variance correction in all three groups, this was significantly greater in the intramedullary group ($P = .012$). The authors suggest that, based on this, conservative management should be avoided in patients in the intramedullary group. However, given the small sample size, this classification can only be used as one factor to aid in the prediction of secondary displacement.

Jung et al. prospectively studied 132 displaced distal radius fractures after closed reduction and stabilization with a sugar-tong splint followed by a below-elbow cast.[9] Seventy-eight percent were female and the mean age was 58 years (range 21–89). By AO/OTA classification, 90 were type A, 33 type B, and 9 type C. Secondary displacement was divided into early (occurring before the first follow-up visit at 1 week) and late (occurring after 1 week). Early displacement was significantly associated with the presence of initial displacement ($P < .001$). Initial acceptable alignment was defined as dorsal tilt <10 degrees, volar tilt 15 ± 10 degrees, radial inclination ≥17 degrees and translation <2.0 mm. It is not clear from the study if the volar tilt includes, or is in addition to, the normal anatomical volar tilt. Late secondary displacement was only significantly associated with age ($P = .005$).

Wadsten et al. conducted a prospective multicenter study involving 398 fractures.[10] The mean age was 56 years (range 15–74) and 78% were female. Minimally displaced fractures were casted in a dorso-radial slab and displaced fractures were reduced under hematoma block or intravenous regional anesthesia and similarly casted. The Buttazzoni classification (Table 1), which primarily focuses on comminution, formed the basis of the analysis.[18] There was a significant difference in frequency of displacement between each type as the classification ascended ($P < .001$), except for B2 versus B3 ($P = .92$), with B1 least likely to displace and B4 most likely. A similar relationship was observed in relation to late displacement at 10–14 days postinjury. Many studies focus on dorsal or generalized comminution, whereas *Wadsten* and colleagues specified this as being dorsal or volar. The Buttazzoni classification does seem to be useful in risk stratification of secondary displacement, but in several of their analyses the B2 and B3 results did not concur with the overall trend of increased displacement risk as the classification progressed.

Tahrininian et al. conducted a prospective cohort study including 157 patients.[11] The mean age was 51 years (20–86) and 68% were female. Displaced fractures were treated with 5 kg of finger-trap traction and then manual

TABLE 1
The Buttazzoni Classification.[18, 19]

Buttazzoni 1 (B1)	Extraarticular DRF with no cortical (metaphyseal) comminution
Buttazzoni 2 (B2)	Extraarticular DRF with comminution of the dorsal cortex
Buttazzoni 3 (B3)	Intraarticular (radio-carpal joint) DRF with or without metaphyseal comminution
Buttazzoni 4 (B4)	DRF with comminution of the volar cortex regardless of other coexisting fracture lines
Buttazzoni 0 (B0)	DRF that cannot be classified according to the above types such as intraarticular fractures without metaphyseal comminution (partially articular fractures), e.g., Barton or Chauffeur fractures; carpal fracture-dislocation

(Reproduced with permission from SAGE Publications.)

closed reduction under intravenous sedation followed by below-elbow casting. Fracture type was not classified. Patients were divided into two groups based on whether they maintained or lost the primary acceptable reduction. These groups were subsequently compared. Gender ($P = .13$), presence of dorsal comminution ($P = .08$) and the presence of ulna fracture ($P = .21$) were not significantly associated with secondary displacement. The presence of an intraarticular fracture was significantly more likely in the group that maintained reduction ($P = .01$), which contrasts with the general findings and consensus in the literature. Loss of radial height ($P < .001$), loss of radial inclination ($P < .001$) and age ($P < .001$) were the most important factors in predicting secondary displacement after an initially satisfactory closed reduction. A receiver operating characteristic (ROC) curve was used to try and predict secondary

displacement. A 6.5 mm loss of radial height (sensitivity 68.5% and specificity 81.5%) and 6.5 degrees loss of radial inclination (sensitivity 80.4% and specificity 67.7%) were felt to be the most appropriate cut-off values for likelihood of displacement. The contralateral uninjured wrist was evaluated radiographically to assess radial shortening and inclination.

Mackenney et al. prospectively recorded data on 4000 distal radius fractures.[1] Seventy-nine percent of patients were female and the mean age was 64 (range 14–100). They divided instability into:
1. Early: displacement (or re-displacement following reduction) within 2 weeks of injury
2. Late: displacement at the time of union (6 weeks) but not before

Minimally displaced fractures were described as having dorsal tilt of ≤10 degrees and ulnar variance of <3 mm.

Displaced fractures had dorsal tilt of >10 degrees and/or ulnar variance of >3 mm. Carpal malalignment was defined as failure of the long axes of the radius and the capitate to intersect within the carpus (Fig. 4). Metaphyseal comminution was judged qualitatively from the radiographs. Ten percent of minimally displaced fractures at presentation demonstrated early instability and this was significantly associated with age ($P<.001$), comminution, dorsal tilt >5 degrees ($P<.01$) and ulnar variance >0 mm ($P<.01$). A total of 22% of minimally displaced fractures demonstrated late instability with patient age ($P<.001$), the presence of comminution ($P<.01$), the dorsal angle ($P<.001$) and ulnar variance ($P<.001$) being significant. Forty-three percent of fractures that were displaced at presentation went on to further early displacement. Age ($P<.001$), ulnar variance at presentation ($P<.001$) and comminution ($P<.01$) were significantly associated. Overall, 47% of displaced fractures at presentation subsequently re-displaced, either early or late, with age ($P<.001$), 1-week dorsal tilt ($P<.001$) and ulnar variance ($P<.001$) being significant. The

authors also produced a formula to predict instability and carpal malalignment. This is referred to as "the McQueen equation" in subsequent literature.[21] *Mackenney et al.* do provide further information to aid the prediction of secondary displacement, although in terms of age, they simply describe that the risk of displacement increases with age and do not further explain this. However, quantification of instability is suggested, e.g., early instability is $10 \times$ more common in those over 80 years old than in those under 30 years of age.

Level-II Evidence

Walenkamp et al. published a systematic review in 2015 and a systematic review with metaanalysis in 2016.[12, 13] Their systematic review with metaanalysis from 2016 included 27 studies.[12] Dorsal comminution, female gender, and an age greater than 60–65 years were found to be significant predictors of secondary displacement. AO/OTA type 3 fractures (A3, B3, C3) were significantly associated with displacement. Contrary to Lafontaine's findings, an ulnar fracture or an intraarticular fracture were not significantly associated with secondary displacement. Additionally, dorsal tilt was not felt to be associated with secondary displacement, with both >15 degrees or >20 degrees from neutral assessed for significance. Again, a lack of standardization of definitions was one of the limitations of this review.

Level-III Evidence

Walenkamp et al.'s 2015 systematic review included 479 studies, although only 149 studies stated that patients with unstable distal radius fractures were recruited.[13] Only 54% of these 149 studies went on to define what they meant by an unstable fracture, and these definitions were heterogenous. The most common description was secondary displacement after an initial anatomical closed reduction. Lafontaine's definition of an unstable fracture was second most common. This is the presence of three or more of the following parameters present on initial trauma radiographs: dorsal tilt ("angulation") >20 degrees, dorsal comminution, intraarticular fracture, associated ulnar fracture, as well as age over 60 years.[3] Third and fourth most common were a volarly displaced fracture, followed by an irreducible fracture. The AO/OTA classification was the mostly commonly used classification system. *Walenkamp et al.* concluded that there needed to be more consensus on the definition of unstable fracture to allow standardization of future research.

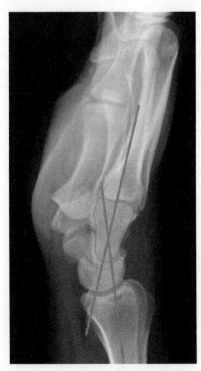

FIG. 4 Lateral radiograph demonstrating the assessment of carpal alignment.[20] (Reproduced with permission from Elsevier.)

Lafontaine et al. studied 112 consecutive distal radius fractures aiming to identify risk factors for secondary displacement despite adequate initial anatomical reduction.[3] The mean age was 54 years (range 13–93) and 77% were female. Patients were managed with fracture reduction under local anesthesia and immobilization in a below-elbow cast. Fractures were classified using the Frykmann classification. The presence of three or more of the following factors were felt to prompt closer radiological follow-up to detect and act upon displacement: dorsal tilt >20 degrees, dorsal comminution, intraarticular fracture, associated ulnar fracture, and age over 60 years. Each risk factor significantly increased the probability of secondary displacement ($P < .05$). It is not fully described how the presence of three or more "gravity," or instability, factors was decided upon. However, they do reference the Stewart score, which is graded from 0 to 12 according to the severity of displacement; with scores of less than three equating to a "good" anatomical reduction. They state that the mean Stewart score of fractures with two instability factors was less than three, and those with three factors was more than three.[22] This is illustrated in Fig. 5.

Makhni et al. retrospectively analyzed 124 conservatively managed distal radius fractures, looking specifically at dorsal metaphyseal comminution.[14] Seventy-four percent were female and the mean age was 56 years (range 19–93). Fractures were managed by casting alone or by reduction using hematoma block with local anesthesia or procedural sedation, followed by casting. The type of casting was not specified. Sixty-two percent of fractures had dorsal comminution; these were significantly more likely to displace than those without comminution (75% vs 45%, $P < .001$). Patients were classified into young (<44), middle aged (45–64) and elderly (≥65). Dorsal comminution tended to be more frequent with increasing age ($P = .05$). There was no significant difference related to gender in terms of displacement in patients with dorsal comminution ($P = .20$).

Lamartina et al. prospectively studied 168 distal radius fractures to validate the McQueen equation (*MacKenney et al.*) and Lafontaine's criteria to predict secondary displacement.[1, 3, 15] They also predicted that restoring the volar cortex, which they describe as the presence of the "volar hook" on postreduction radiographs, would be protective in terms of preventing displacement. This is defined as a "collinear alignment of the cortical edges of the fracture at the volar surface." There are some similarities to the classification later used by *Zenke* et al in 2019.[8] The mean age was 52 years (range 18–96) and 69% of patients were females. Fractures were reduced with weighted traction and closed reduction before below-elbow circumferential casting using three-point molding. The AO/OTA classification was used and only A1, A3, C1, or C2 fractures were included. The McQueen equation and the number of Lafontaine's criteria were significant in the prediction of ulnar variance, radial height, and radial inclination at

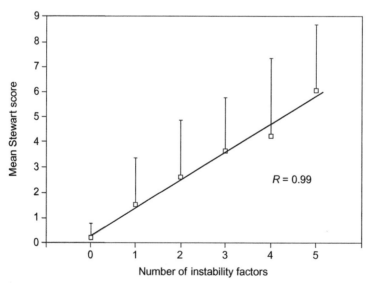

FIG. 5 Conservatively treated distal radius fractures divided into groups according to the number of instability factors present then plotted according to their mean Stewart score.[3] (Reproduced with permission from Elsevier.)

union ($P < .01$) for all parameters but did not predict dorsal tilt. This was, however, predicted by absence of volar hook ($P = .05$) and dorsal comminution ($P = .05$). Both the absence of a volar hook ($P < .01$) and increasing age ($P = .03$) predicted carpal malalignment.

Nesbitt et al. retrospectively reviewed 50 fractures that met three or more of Lafontaine's criteria.[3, 16] Eighty-six percent of patients were female, and the mean age was 60 years (range 16–87). Fractures were reduced using a hematoma block followed by 10 pounds of finger-trap traction and closed reduction held in a well-molded sugar-tong splint. A total of 54% of fractures went on to a secondary displacement. The only significant factor predicting secondary displacement was age ($P = .012$). Risk of displacement increased with increasing age, with a 76-year old having a 50% risk of displacement at 1 week after reduction ($P = .041$). Dorsal tilt greater than 20 degrees, dorsal comminution, intraarticular fracture or an associated ulna fracture were not found to be statistically associated with secondary displacement.

Leone et al. retrospectively analyzed 71 extraarticular distal radius fractures.[17] Displaced fractures underwent closed reduction under local anesthesia before being placed in a below-elbow plaster cast. The mean age was 64.9 years and 87% of patients were female. Again, instability was divided into early (1 week) and late (6 weeks). In terms of early displacement, radial shortening, and dorsal tilt on initial radiographs were significantly predictive of secondary displacement ($P < .01$). This was not quantified. Dorsal comminution was more common in fractures that subsequently displaced, although this did not reach significance ($P = .06$). Radial shortening, radial inclination and age were all significant in predicting late displacement ($P < .05$). However, as with a number of these studies, there were no cut-off values to predict likely displacement.

RECOMMENDATIONS

In patients with an intraarticular displaced distal radius fracture, evidence suggests:

Recommendations	Overall Quality
• Increasing age (especially above age 60 years) and dorsal comminution are the most common predictors of secondary displacement	⊕⊕⊕⊕ HIGH
• Other factors proposed to increase displacement risk include female gender, dorsal tilt >5 degrees, ulnar variance >0 mm, loss of radial inclination, and increasing radial shortening on initial trauma radiographs, as well as the absence of volar cortical continuity (the "volar hook") and an "intramedullary" fracture configuration on postreduction radiographs	⊕⊕⊕◯ MODERATE
• Two of Lafontaine's criteria (intraarticular radiocarpal fracture and ulnar fracture) are not widely supported by other literature as increasing displacement risk	⊕⊕⊕◯ MODERATE
• There is no established and validated scoring system or tool to aid in the prediction of instability, but as the number of risk factors increase, so should the surgeon's index of suspicion	⊕⊕⊕◯ MODERATE

CONCLUSION

There is no clear consensus on the predictors of instability with regards to secondary displacement for fractures of the distal radius. Increasing age, especially above 60 years of age, and the presence of dorsal comminution are the most widely reported and recognized predictors. However, patients who have had a degree of displacement at any point still require radiological follow-up, particularly in the first 2 weeks postinjury, to detect subsequent displacement in patients who are suitable for operative intervention. Further research, particularly into classification or clinical prediction models, could allow the reliable identification of those at risk of secondary displacement and would simplify risk stratification. This could also potentially allow for early intervention in appropriate patients, as well as avoiding unnecessary clinical reviews in patients where the fracture is unlikely to displace.

Panel 2: Authors' Preferred Treatment

Risk of secondary displacement is best considered in terms of patient factors and injury factors. Based on these determining factors, we have adopted a decision-making algorithm (Fig. 6). We have also published an open-source predictor formula based on the above—describe "McQueen equation"[21] to estimate the risk of displacement (https://www.trauma.co.uk/wristcalc).The patient presented in Case Scenario 1 is both female and elderly, increasing the risk of displacement. Following our predictor formula, her chances of redisplacement are 72%. In terms of the fracture characteristics on initial trauma radiographs, there is evidence of dorsal comminution, dorsal tilt >5 degrees, ulnar variance >0mm and radial shortening. Moreover, postreduction radiographs show an intramedullary translation of the volar

cortex. Given the presence of several factors increasing the risk of secondary displacement, this patient would routinely be followed up at both 1- and 2-weeks post-injury with repeated radiographs. This allows timely intervention should the position deteriorate.

At follow-up, the past medical history and functional demands of the patient are now key in determining the definitive management. In this case, there is the option of continued conservative management, but the fracture will go on to a malunion, which may have functional consequences for the patient. The patient was a keen tennis-player and gardener and decided to proceed with operative intervention in the form of volar plate fixation.

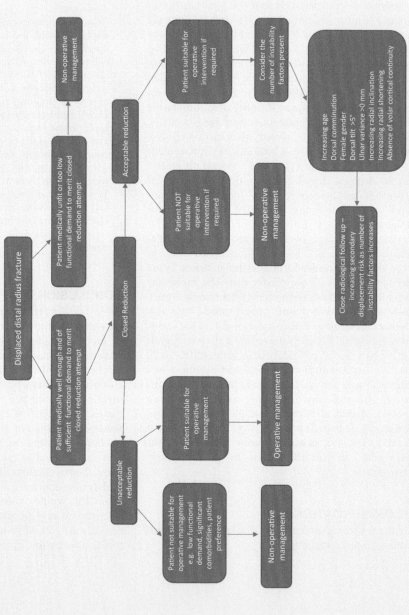

FIG. 6 Suggested algorithm for the management of a displaced distal radius fracture.

REFERENCES

1. Mackenney PJ, McQueen MM, Elton R. Prediction of instability in distal radial fractures. *J Bone Joint Surg.* 2006; 88(9):1944–1951.

2. Solgaard S. Early displacement of distal radius fracture. *Acta Orthop.* 1986; 57(3):229–231.

3. Lafontaine M, Hardy D, Delince P. Stability assessment of distal radius fractures. *Injury.* 1989; 20(4):208–210.

4. McQueen M, Caspers J. Colles fracture: does the anatomical result affect the final function? *J Bone Joint Surg.* 1988; 70(4):649–651.

5. Saving J, Severin Wahlgren S, Olsson K, et al. Nonoperative treatment compared with volar locking plate fixation for dorsally displaced distal radial fractures in the elderly. *J Bone Joint Surg.* 2019; 101(11):961–969. Available from: (2019). http://insights.ovid.com/crossref?an=00004623-201906050-00002.

6. Blakeney WG. Stabilization and treatment of Colles' fractures in elderly patients. *Clin Interv Aging.* 2010; 5:337–344.

7. Plant CE, Parsons NR, Costa ML. Do radiological and functional outcomes correlate for fractures of the distal radius? *Bone Joint J.* 2017; 99B(3):376–382.

8. Zenke Y, Furukawa K, Furukawa H, et al. Radiographic measurements as a predictor of correction loss in conservative treatment of Colles' fracture. *J UOEH.* 2019; 41(2):139–144.

9. Jung H-W, Hong H, Jung HJ, et al. Redisplacement of distal radius fracture after initial closed reduction: analysis of prognostic factors. *Clin Orthop Surg.* 2015; 7(3):377. Available from: (2015). https://synapse.koreamed.org/DOIx.php?id=10.4055/cios.2015.7.3.377.

10. Wadsten MÅ, Sayed-Noor AS, Englund E, Buttazzoni GG, Sjödén GO. Cortical comminution in distal radial fractures can predict the radiological outcome: a cohort multicentre study. *Bone Joint J.* 2014; 96-B(7):978–983. Available from: (2014). http://online.boneandjoint.org.uk/doi/10.1302/0301-620X.96B7.32728.

11. Tahririan MA, Javdan M, Nouraei MH, Dehghani M. Evaluation of instability factors in distal radius fractures. *J Res Med Sci.* 2013; 18(10):892–896.

12. Walenkamp MMJ, Aydin S, Mulders MAM, Goslings JC, Schep NWL. Predictors of unstable distal radius fractures: a systematic review and meta-analysis. *J Hand Surg Eur Vol.* 2016; 41(5):501–515.

13. Walenkamp M, Vos L, Strackee S, Goslings J, Schep N. The unstable distal radius fracture—how do we define it? A systematic review. *J Wrist Surg.* 2015; 04(04):307–316.

14. Makhni EC, Taghinia A, Ewald T, Zurakowski D, Day CS. Comminution of the dorsal metaphysis and its effects on the radiographic outcomes of distal radius fractures. *J Hand Surg Eur Vol.* 2010; 35(8):652–658.

15. Lamartina J, Jawa A, Stucken C, Merlin G, Tornetta P. Predicting alignment after closed reduction and casting of distal radius fractures. *J Hand Surg [Am].* 2015; 40 (5):934–939. https://doi.org/10.1016/j.jhsa.2015.01.023.

16. Nesbitt KS, Failla JM, Les C. Assessment of instability factors in adult distal radius fractures. *J Hand Surg [Am].* 2004; 29(6):1128–1138.

17. Leone J, Bhandari M, Adili A, McKenzie S, Moro JK, Dunlop RB. Predictors of early and late instability following conservative treatment of extra-articular distal radius fractures. *Arch Orthop Trauma Surg.* 2004; 124 (1):38–41.

18. Wadsten MÅ, Sayed-Noor AS, Sjödén GO, Svensson O, Buttazzoni GG. The Buttazzoni classification of distal radial fractures in adults: Interobserver and intraobserver reliability. *Hand.* 2009; 4(3):283–288.

19. Wadsten M, Sjödén GO, Buttazzoni GG, Buttazzoni C, Englund E, Sayed-Noor AS. The influence of late displacement in distal radius fractures on function, grip strength, range of motion and quality of life. *J Hand Surg Eur Vol.* 2018; 43(2):131–136.

20. White TO, Mackenzie SP, Gray AJ. *McRae's Orthopaedic Trauma and Emergency Fracture Management.* 3rd ed. Edinburgh: Elsevier; 2016232.

21. No authors listed. Wristcalc. [cited 12 May 2020]. Available from:(2020). https://www.trauma.co.uk/wristcalc; 2020.

22. Stewart HD, Innes AR, Burke FD. Factors affecting the outcome of Colles' fracture: an anatomical and functional study. *Injury.* 1985; 16(5):289–295.

Minimally Invasive Plate Osteosynthesis of Distal Radius Fractures

PAUL VERNET • STÉPHANIE GOUZOU • SYBILLE FACCA •
PHILIPPE LIVERNEAUX
Department of Hand Surgery, SOS Hand, University Hospital of Strasbourg, FMTS, University of
Strasbourg, Strasbourg, France

KEY POINTS

- The minimally invasive approach of the flexor carpi radialis can be used for volar plate fixation of distal radius fractures.
- The upsides of this technique are the preservation of the ligamentotaxis to facilitate the reduction of the fracture and the small size of the incision to improve the cosmetic results of the procedure.
- The incision can always be extended in case of difficulties of reduction.

Panel 1: Case Scenario

A 49-year-old, left-handed female director of a cosmetic enterprise sustained a dorsally displaced extraarticular distal radius fracture when walking her dog. Radiographs show 25 degrees of dorsal angulation and dorsal metaphyseal comminution. In your office she immediately states that she refuses surgery as she does not accept any large scar on her wrist. You esteem that casting nor K-wire fixation will yield sufficient stability in her mild osteoporotic bone and comminutive fracture, for which you recommend plate fixation. What are the advantages and drawbacks for minimal invasive plate fixation?

IMPORTANCE OF THE PROBLEM

Since the year 2000, the fixation of distal radius fractures by volar locking plate has become the gold standard.[1, 2] Three surgical approaches have been described: conventional, extended,[3] and minimally invasive.[4]

The conventional approach of the flexor carpi radialis (FCR) (Fig. 1A) has been developed to treat volar tilt fractures.[5] It corresponds to the distal part of the Henry Approach[6] and is less aggressive for the extensor tendons than dorsal approaches.[7] It also enables the fixation of dorsal tilt fractures where the reduction is facilitated by ligamentotaxis.[8]

The extended approach of the FCR (Fig. 1B) is used for dorsal tilt fractures. The incision is 8–10 cm long.[3] The distal edge of the pronator quadratus (PQ) forms a transverse line on the surface of the radius called the watershed line beyond which the plate should not be positioned to avoid conflicts with the flexor tendons. The PQ is elevated to expose the fracture site without risk of necrosis for some authors,[3] and with a risk of necrosis for others.[9] MIPO enables the mobilization of the proximal end of the radius in pronation through the fracture site giving a large exposure.[8] Ligamentotaxis is limited with this technique.

Minimally invasive plate osteosynthesis (MIPO) techniques were developed for hip,[10] knee,[11, 12] ankle,[13] shoulder,[14, 15] and elbow surgeries.[16] They aim at preserving bone vascularization,[17] improve bone healing,[18] reduce the rate of infections, ease the reduction of the fracture using ligamentotaxis,[19] and meet the cosmetic expectations of the patients.[10]

For the wrist, the concept is raised in 2000.[20] It has been reported to improve bone healing[21] because of the preservation of the periosteum and PQ at the

---

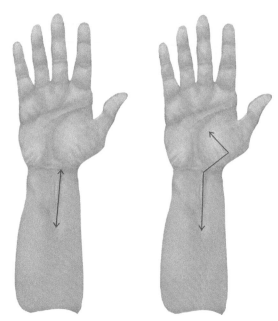

FIG. 1 Flexor carpi radialis (FCR) approaches.
(A) Conventional FCR approach. (B) Extended FCR approach.

fracture site unlike in the traditional approach.[6, 22] The cosmetic benefit is notable.[23]

MAIN QUESTION

What is the additional value of a Minimal Invasive Approach for plate fixation of simple distal radius fractures?

CURRENT OPINION

Minimal invasive plate fixation is a cosmetically attractive treatment option with the potential drawback of adding intraoperative difficulty due to lesser visualization of the fracture. Being considered in developmental phase, its superiority remains to be proven.

FINDING THE EVIDENCE

- Cochrane search: Distal Radius Fracture
- Pubmed (Medline): ("Radius Fractures" [Mesh] OR distal radius fracture*[tiab]) AND (minim* invasive plate OR MIPO)
- Bibliography of eligible articles
- Articles that were not in the English, French or German language were excluded.

QUALITY OF THE EVIDENCE

Level II:
Systematic Reviews/Metaanalyses: 1
Randomized trials with methodological limitations: 1
Level III:
Retrospective comparative studies: 3
Level IV:
Case series: 12

FINDINGS

Minimally invasive techniques are growing stronger in all surgical specialties. They are not only justified for cosmetic reasons, but also for technical and physiological reasons.

From a technical point of view, it has been proven that an approach of a limited size preserved ligament and muscle insertions of the distal radius and carpus thus facilitating the reduction of the fracture and contributing to its stability thanks to ligamentotaxis.[20, 24, 25] The concept is opposed to the concept of the extended approach of the FCR that requires to almost "strip" the distal radius.[3] From a physiological point of view, a limited approach should, theoretically, limit bone ischemia, source of necrosis of small articular fragment or nonunion, sometimes observed in extensive approaches with extensive deperiosting in patients with comorbidities.[26] Finally, a limited approach preserves the hematoma of the fracture site leading to faster bone healing.[27]

Lee et al. recently performed a systematic review and metaanalysis of four studies comparing conventional distal radius plating to MIPO.[28] They included one randomized controlled trial with methodological limitations and three retrospective comparative series. All studies reported patient-reported outcome scores (PROMs) at the final follow-up of 139 patients in the conventional group and 149 patients in the MIPO group. There were no significant differences in PROMS, grip strength or range of motion between the conventional and MIPO groups. However, there was a significant higher patient satisfaction in the MIPO group compared to the conventional plating group at final follow-up reported in three studies (123 patients in the conventional group and 134 patients in the MIPO group) (standard mean difference −0.54; 95% confidence interval −0.79 to −0.29). It should be acknowledged that this difference being inferior to 1 out of 10 points is likely nonclinically relevant.

With almost 500 cases published to date (Table 1), indications of MIPO techniques in distal radius fractures are growing. Some consider they can only be used for simple extraarticular fractures.[29] While others extend

TABLE 1
Overview of Studies on Volar Locking Plate Fixation of the Distal Radius Using a Minimally Invasive Technique (MIPO).

| Authors | Date | Incision | | | Arthroscopy (Y/N) | Respect PQ (Y/N) | Patients | Result | | |
		Number (N)	Size (mm)	Orientation (T/L)			Number (N)	Clinical	Complications	Radiological
Geissler et Fernandes	2000	2	?	L (Pl) L (Dl)	N	N	?	?	?	?
Imatani et al.	2005	2	50 (20+30)	L (Ds) L (Pr)	N	Y	5	F59° E55° P85° S82° Grip 88%	N	Volar tilt 13° Radial inclination 24° Ulnar variance 0.6 mm
Yoshikawa et al.	2008	2	40 (25+15)	T (Ds) L (Pr)	N	Y	13	Cooney score 92.7 F+E = 122° P+S = 157° Grip 86%	N	Volar tilt 8.6° Radial inclination 22.5° Ulnar variance 0.4 mm
Sen et al.	2008	2	50 (20+30)	L (Ds) L (Pr)	N	Y	?	?	?	?
Zenke et al.	2011	2	40 (30+10)	T (Ds) L (Pr)	N	Y	30	F86° E67° P89° S89° Grip 94%	Intraarticular screw (1)	Volar tilt 9.4° Radial inclination 24° Ulnar variance 1.1 mm
Abe et al.	2013	1	30 (25–30)	L	Y	Y	153	Score Mayo 89.5% DASH 4.1 F60° E63° P83° S86° Grip 88%	Secondary displacement (3) EPL rupture (2) CPRS type I (1)	Volar tilt 5.6° Radial inclination 26.1° Ulnar variance 0.1 mm

Continued

TABLE 1
Overview of Studies on Volar Locking Plate Fixation of the Distal Radius Using a Minimally Invasive Technique (MIPO).—cont'd

Authors	Date	Number (N)	Size (mm)	Incision Orientation (T/L)	Arthroscopy (Y/N)	Respect PQ (Y/N)	Patients Number (N)	Result Clinical	Result Complications	Result Radiological
Zemirline et al.	2014	1	15	L	Y	Y	20	Pain 1.9/10 DASH 24.6 F71° E72° P86° S86° Grip 67%	CPRS type I (3)	Volar tilt 8.8° Radial inclination 20.7° Ulnar variance −1 mm
Rey et al.	2014	1	26	L	N	Y	31	DASH 10 Grip 80%	Secondary displacement (1)	Volar tilt 4.8° Ulnar variance 0.3 mm
Lebailly et al.	2014	1	15	L	Y	Y	144	DASH 25 F86° E86° P96° S91° Grip 67%	CPRS type I (9) Secondary displacement (2) tenosynovitis (9) Intraarticular screw (2) Distal screw displacement (1)	Volar tilt 8.3 Radial inclination 22° Ulnar variance 0.4 mm
Wei et al.	2014	2	40 (20+20)	T (Ds) L (Pr)	N	Y	22	?	Anesthesia of thenar eminence (1) Delayed healing (1) Pain of ulnar aspect of wrist (2) Limited function (2)	?
Chmielnicki et Prokop	2015	2	30 (25+5)	T (Ds) L (Pr)	N	Y	11	F45° E45° P85° S85° Grip 96%	?	?

Chen et al.	2015	2	30 (20+10)	T (Ds) L (Pr)	N	Y	21	N	Mayo wrist score 95.0	Volar tilt 9.86° Radial inclination 22.43° Ulnar variance 0.29 mm
Naito et al.	2016	1	10	L	N	Y	18	CPRS type I (1)	F67° F67° P88° S88° DASH 0.7 Mayo wrist score 93.3	Complete union
Wei et al.	2016	2	40 (20+20)	T (Ds) L (Pr)	N	N	9	Delayed healing (1)	DASH 5.8 F76° E77° P79° S81° Grip 89%	Volar tilt 10.7° Radial inclination 18.2° Ulnar variance 2.3 mm
Zhang X et al.	2017	1	18	L	N	Y	182	?	F75° E65° P80° S85° Grip 94% DASH 3.5 Mayo wrist Score 81%	Volar tilt 12° Radial inclination 22° Ulnar variance 1 mm

PQ, pronator quadratus; Pl, palmaire; DI, dorsal; Ds, distal; Pr, proximal; F, flexion; E, extension; S, supination; P, pronation; T, transverse; L, longitudinal; Grip strength is expressed in percentage compared to the contralateral healthy side; Y, yes; N, no; EPL, extensor pollicis longus; FPL, flexor pollicis longus; CRPS, complex regional pain syndrome. "?" means that the difference is significative.

their indications to articular fractures[21] and diaphysio-metaphyseal fractures.[30] Others recommend arthroscopy for articular fractures with fragments that are not spontaneously reduced when the plate is put in place.[31] A double approach, proximal and distal, is recommended for fractures with a diaphyseal extension.[32]

Several authors consider that beside acute complications (skin opening, signs of nerve or vascular compression and severe displacement) distal radius fractures do not need to be operated in emergency surgery but can be attended to a few days after the injury.[21, 33] The procedure can be performed as outpatient surgery in most cases. Some authors use a MIPO technique for osteotomies of distal radius malunions.[34, 35] A MIPO technique has been developed with two incisions using bicolumnar locking plates.[36]

Noncomparative studies report comparable clinical and radiological results to conventional techniques (Table 1).

For extraarticular fractures, some authors have compared the results of two types of minimally invasive approaches: longitudinal vs transverse. The longitudinal approach gives similar functional results to the transverse approach but leads to smaller incisions.[37]

Among the 477 published cases, 42 complications are reported (8.8%) (Table 1). This rate of complications is equivalent to the rates published for other techniques. No complication is specific of the MIPO technique. Pain is the most frequent complication with 14 cases of type I complex regional pain syndromes and 2 cases of unexplained painful syndromes of the ulnar aspect of the wrist. Tendon lesions come in second place with 9 cases of flexor tendon tenosynovitis and 2 cases of tendon ruptures of the flexor pollicis longus. Some authors insist on the importance of ensuring peroperatively that the flexor tendons are not trapped under the plate.[21, 33] Flexor tendons should be checked for signs of entrapment at the beginning and at the end of the procedure and be identified on vessel loops if necessary. An article reports the case of a flexor pollicis longus tendon trapped under the plate.[38] Osteoarticular complications have been reported: 3 cases of intraarticular screws, 2 cases of joint stiffness, 1 case of displacement of one distal screw and 6 cases of secondary displacements. It is essential to make regular

fluoroscopic controls after each step of a MIPO technique, especially to make sure of the absence of intraarticular screws and in particular in the distal radio-ulnar joint, using for example a fluoroscopic skyline view.[39] There were 2 cases of delayed healing reported in the flexion crease of the wrist probably due to maceration.[30] A case of anesthesia of the thenar eminence was reported, probably due to a lesion of the cutaneous branch of the median nerve, which can be avoided by drawing the incision on the lateral aspect of the FCR tendon.[40]

All minimally invasive techniques are learned following a learning curve.[41] The minimally invasive FCR approach is not an exception to this rule and prior training on anatomical parts is recommended to avoid tendon and/or articular complications. It is wise to start using this technique for simple extraarticular fractures, starting with a 50 mm FCR approach and then diminishing the size of the incision every five fractures, all the way down to 15 mm and even 10 mm.[42] It is important to remember that it is always possible to convert to a longer incision in case of a difficult reduction, which is not possible with an extended FCR approach.

RECOMMENDATION

In patients with an intraarticular displaced distal radius fracture, evidence suggests:

Recommendation	Overall Quality
• MIPO techniques are equally effective for patients with distal radius fractures.	⊕⊕◯◯ LOW
• MIPO technique may result in a slightly higher patient satisfaction and better cosmesis	⊕⊕◯◯ LOW

CONCLUSION

In conclusion, volar plate fixation of distal radius fractures using a minimally invasive FCR approach seems reliable, reproducible, with few complications. Preservation of ligamentotaxis facilitates fracture reduction and the small size of the incision improves the cosmetic results of the procedure. It is always possible to convert the incision to a more extensive approach in case of a difficult reduction.

Panel 2: Author's Preferred Technique

The author's series to date included 710 patients, aged 58 years in average (min 18; max 95), among which 512 women. Two groups were defined, group I (AO type A and B fractures) and group II (AO type C fractures). All patients were operated under locoregional anesthesia, using a pneumatic tourniquet as an outpatient procedure. The procedure was performed in emergency only in cases of complications (open fracture, signs of acute compression of the median nerve). A 15-mm line was drawn on the lateral aspect of the tendon of the FCR, about 20 mm proximal to the tip of the radial styloid process (Fig. 2A). After incision of the skin, the subcutaneous tissues were dissected 50 mm proximal to the incision and 20 mm distally. The superficial (Fig. 2B) and deep aspect of the sheath of the FCR (Fig. 2C) were opened likewise. All muscle, nerve and vascular structures were reclined on the ulnar aspect of the wrist at the exception of the radial artery that was reclined on the radial aspect. A transverse incision of the distal edge of the PQ was performed and the PQ was then elevated preserving its radial and ulnar attachments (Fig. 2D). A volar locking plate was prepared by attaching four aiming guides or a specific jig to its distal end. The plate was then introduced under the PQ by its proximal end (Fig. 2E). The distal end of the plate was introduced by its radial aspect and then its ulnar aspect, making sure of the absence of interpositions of noble structures between the plate and the radius. The plate was positioned just proximal to the watershed line and secured temporarily to the radial epiphysis using two 1.8 mm K-wires, one through the most ulnar aiming guide and then through the most radial. A fluoroscopy ensured the good positioning of the plate (Fig. 2F). This step was repeated until optimal positioning was reached. The two central distal epiphyseal screws are put in place. The two temporary K-wires are removed and replaced by screws (Fig. 2G). The proximal part of the plate was exposed by maximum flexion of the wrist to take advantage of skin elasticity, and the two proximal screws were put in place (Fig. 2H). The skin was closed by a running subcuticular suture of absorbable 3/0 suture thread, pulling on its extremities to reduce the size of the incision. No postoperative immobilization was used, and the patients were encouraged to use their upper limb, without strength, as soon as the effects of the anesthesia have worn off.[43]

In the case of more complex fractures of the distal radius, some tips and tricks could help resolve difficult situations. When the classic technique of reduction of the epiphysiometaphyseal fragment had failed, it could be obtained by using the "tyre changer" effect of a periosteal elevator inserted on the volar aspect of the fracture site, or by using a "leverage" effect by inserting a percutaneous K-wire on the dorsal or radial aspect of the fracture site, like it is done in the technique of intrafocal pinning of dorsal tilt fractures.[44] When the reduction of osteochondral fragments had failed after the distal screws were put in place, it could be obtained either by putting pressure on the fragments with an intra focal K-wire, or by traction on the fragments using an arthroscopic hook probe. When it came to metaphysiodiaphyseal extraarticular or articular fractures, a second minimally invasive incision at the level of the proximal screws could be useful.[32] When the reduction was unstable, a direct temporary pinning was useful to stabilize the fragments while the plate was put in place.

Hardware removal could be performed, if needed, using a similar minimally invasive approach.[45]

The size of the incision was 17 mm in average (range, 10–40 mm) (Fig. 3). The time of tourniquet was 41 min in average (11–120 min).

At the last follow-up, the average pain was 1.13 (0–8). The quick-D.A.S.H. was 13.3 in average (0–86). The P.R.W.E. was 11.5 on average (0–91). The grip strength was at 80% in average (18%–360%). The flexion of the wrist was at 87% on average (0%–133%). The extension of the wrist was at 89% on average (25%–133%). The ulnar deviation was at 92% on average (25%–150%). The radial deviation was at 96% on average (0%–167%). The pronation was at 96% on average (40%–133%). The supination was at 93% on average (13%–130%).

We noted 16 cases of secondary displacements among which 3 cases required a surgical revision, 1 case of sepsis at 6 months postoperative (in a context of general sepsis), 10 cases of type I complex regional pain syndrome and 14 cases of paresthesia in the median nerve territory of which 4 cases had a carpal tunnel release. The hardware was removed in 46% of cases using the same incision. There were no case of tendon rupture.

There was no significant difference in terms of quick-DASH or PRWE between group I and group II.

Continued

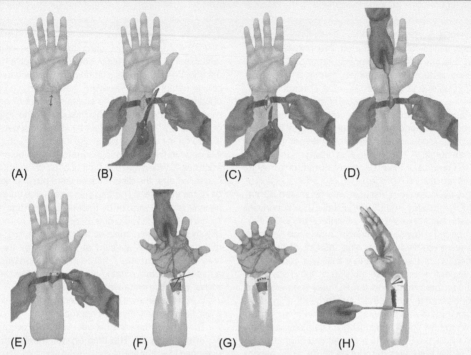

FIG. 2 Minimally invasive volar plate fixation of distal radius fractures. (A) Drawing of the incision on the lateral aspect of the FCR. (B) Longitudinal incision of the sheath of the FCR on its lateral aspect. (C) The FCR is reclined on the ulnar aspect of the wrist. Longitudinal incision of the deep aspect of the sheath of the FCR. (D) A transverse incision is performed on the distal edge of the PQ. The PQ is then elevated while preserving its radial and ulnar attachments. (E) The plate is placed under the PQ by its proximal end. (F) The plate is positioned just proximal to the watershed line and secured temporarily by two K-wires. (G) Two central epiphyseal screws are put in place. The two K-wires are removed and replaced by screws. (H) The proximal end of the plate is exposed in maximal flexion of the wrist using the elasticity of the skin and the two proximal screws put in place.

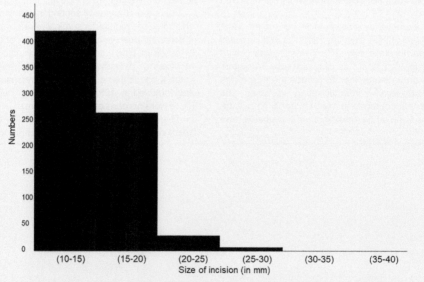

FIG. 3 Size of the incision in 710 cases of minimally invasive volar plate fixation.

Panel 3: Pearls and Pitfalls

PEARLS:

- MIPO may better preserve ligamentotaxis to facilitate the reduction.
- A standard but smaller sized FCR approach can be used and easily extended if necessary. Hence cosmetics may be improved.

PITFALLS:

- There is a risk of tendon interposition under the plate. The operator should always assess the absence of tendon entrapment after positioning the plate and at the end of the surgery.
- The correct position of the plate is difficult to assess though the incision. Fluoroscopy should be used until the plate is positioned correctly on AP and lateral views.

ACKNOWLEDGMENT

Pr François Severac, Marie Mielcarek, Public Health Department and Statistics, Strasbourg University Hospitals, France.

CONFLICTS OF INTEREST

Philippe Liverneaux has conflicts of interest with Argomedical, Newclip Technics. None of the other authors have conflicts of interest.

REFERENCES

1. Orbay JL. The treatment of unstable distal radius fractures with volar fixation. *Hand Surg.* 2000;5:103–112.
2. Orbay JL, Fernandez DL. Volar fixation for dorsally displaced fractures of the distal radius: a preliminary report. *J Hand Surg [Am].* 2002;27:205–215.
3. Wijffels MM, Orbay JL, Indriago I, Ring D. The extended FCR approach for partially healed malaligned fractures of the distal radius. *Injury.* 2012;43:1204–1208.
4. Liverneaux P, Ichihara S, Facca S, Hidalgo Diaz JJ. Outcomes of minimally invasive plate osteosynthesis (MIPO) with volar locking plates in distal radius fractures: a review. *Hand Surg Rehabil.* 2016;35S:S80–S85.
5. Smith RS, Crick JC, Alonso J, Horowitz M. Open reduction and internal fixation of volar lip fractures of the distal radius. *J Orthop Trauma.* 1988;2:181–187.
6. Henry AK. Complete exposure of the radius. In: *Exposures of Long Bones and Other Surgical Methods.* Bristol: John Wright & Sons Ltd; 1927:9–12.
7. Mares O, Coulomb R, Lazerges C, Bosch C, Kouyoumdjian P. Surgical exposures for distal radius fractures. *Hand Surg Rehabil.* 2016;35S:S39–S43.
8. Orbay JL, Infante A, Khouri RK, Fernandez DL. The extended FCR approach: a new perspective for the distal radius fracture. *Tech Hand Up Extrem Surg.* 2001;5:204–211.
9. Placzek JD, Sobol GV, Arnoczky SP, Quinn M, Magnell T. The effect of an extended FCR approach on blood flow to the distal radius: a cadaveric study. *Orthopedics.* 2005;28:1364–1367.
10. Krettek C, Schandelmaier P, Miclau T, Tscherne H. Minimally invasive percutaneous plate osteosynthesis (MIPPO) using the DCS in proximal and distal femoral fractures. *Injury.* 1997;28:20–30.
11. Kim JJ, Oh HK, Bae JY, Kim JW. Radiological assessment of the safe zone for medial minimally invasive plate osteosynthesis in the distal femur with computed tomography angiography. *Injury.* 2014;45:1964–1969.
12. Bhat R, Wani MM, Rashid S, Akhter N. Minimally invasive percutaneous plate osteosynthesis for closed distal tibial fractures: a consecutive study based on 25 patients. *Eur J Orthop Surg Traumatol.* 2015;25:563–568.
13. Pires RE, Mauffrey C, de Andrade MA, et al. Minimally invasive percutaneous plate osteosynthesis for ankle fractures: a prospective observational cohort study. *Eur J Orthop Surg Traumatol.* 2014;24:1297–1303.
14. Gao YB, Tong SL, Yu JH, Lu WJ. Case control study on open reduction internal fixation (ORIF) and minimally invasive percutaneous plate osteosynthesis (MIPPO) for the treatment of proximal humerus fractures in aged. *Zhongguo Gu Shang.* 2015;28:335–339.
15. Zhang Y, Xu J, Zhang C, Sun Y. Minimally invasive plate osteosynthesis for midshaft clavicular fractures using superior anatomic plating. *J Shoulder Elb Surg.* 2016;25:7–12.
16. Zogbi DR, Terrivel AM, Mouraria GG, Mongon ML, Kikuta FK, Filho AZ. Fracture of distal humerus: MIPO technique with visualization of the radial nerve. *Acta Ortop Bras.* 2014;22:300–303.
17. Helfet DL, Shonnard PY, Levine D, Borrelli Jr. J. Minimally invasive plate osteosynthesis of distal fractures of the tibia. *Injury.* 1997;28:42–48.
18. Wagner M. General principles for the clinical use of the LCP. *Injury.* 2003;34:31–42.
19. Agee JM. Distal radius fractures. Multiplanar ligamentotaxis. *Hand Clin.* 1993;9:577–585.
20. Geissler WB, Fernandes D. Percutaneous and limited open reduction of intra-articular distal radial fractures. *Hand Surg.* 2000;5:85–92.
21. Zenke Y, Sakai A, Oshige T, et al. Clinical results of volar locking plate for distal radius fractures: conventional versus minimally invasive plate osteosynthesis. *J Orthop Trauma.* 2011;25:425–431.
22. Heim U, Pfeiffer KM. *Internal Fixation of Small Fractures.* 3rd ed. Berlin: Springer Verlag; 1987.
23. Yoshikawa Y, Saito T, Matsui H. A new cosmetic approach for volar fixed-angle plate fixation to treat distal radius fractures. *J Jpn Soc Surg Hand.* 2008;24:889–893.

24. Bindra RR. Biomechanics and biology of external fixation of distal radius fractures. *Hand Clin.* 2005;21:363–373.

25. Kapandji A. Biomechanics of the carpus and the wrist. *Ann Chir Main.* 1987;6:147–169.

26. Segalman KA, Clark GL. Un-united fractures of the distal radius: a report of 12 cases. *J Hand Surg [Am].* 1998; 23:914–919.

27. Kolar P, Schmidt-Bleek K, Schell H, et al. The early fracture hematoma and its potential role in fracture healing. *Tissue Eng Part B Rev.* 2010;16:427–434.

28. Lee DY, Park YJ, Park JS. A meta-analysis of studies of volar locking plate fixation of distal radius fractures: conventional versus minimally invasive plate osteosynthesis. *Clin Orthop Surg.* 2019;11:208–219.

29. Imatani J, Noda T, Morito Y, Sato T, Hashizume H, Inoue H. Minimally invasive plate osteosynthesis for comminuted fractures of the metaphysis of the radius. *J Hand Surg (Br).* 2005;30:220–225.

30. Wei XM, Sun ZZ, Rui YJ, Song XJ, Jiang WM. Minimally invasive percutaneous plate osteosynthesis for distal radius fractures with long-segment metadiaphyseal comminution. *Orthop Traumatol Surg Res.* 2016; 102:333–338.

31. Zemirline A, Taleb C, Facca S, Liverneaux P. Minimally invasive surgery of distal radius fractures: a series of 20 cases using a 15mm anterior approach and arthroscopy. *Chir Main.* 2014;33:263–271.

32. Pire E, Hidalgo Diaz JJ, Salazar Botero S, Facca S, Liverneaux PA. Long volar plating for metadiaphyseal fractures of distal radius: study comparing minimally invasive plate osteosynthesis versus conventional approach. *J Wrist Surg.* 2017;6:227–234.

33. Zemirline A, Naito K, Lebailly F, Facca S, Liverneaux P. Distal radius fixation through a mini-invasive approach of 15 mm. Part 1: feasibility study. *Eur J Orthop Surg Traumatol.* 2014;24:1031–1037.

34. Taleb C, Zemirline A, Lebailly F, et al. Minimally invasive osteotomy for distal radius malunion: a preliminary series of 9 cases. *Orthop Traumatol Surg Res.* 2015; 101:861–865.

35. Viegas SF. A minimally invasive distal radial osteotomy for treatment of distal radius fracture malunion. *Tech Hand Up Extrem Surg.* 1997;1:70–76.

36. Chen AC, Chou YC, Cheng CY. Distal radius fractures: minimally invasive plate osteosynthesis with dorsal bicolumnar locking plates fixation. *Indian J Orthop.* 2017; 51:93–98.

37. Galmiche C, Rodríguez GG, Xavier F, Igeta Y, Hidalgo Diaz JJ, Liverneaux P. Minimally invasive plate osteosynthesis for extra-articular distal radius fracture in postmenopausal women: longitudinal versus transverse incision. *J Wrist Surg.* 2019;8:18–23.

38. Chiu YC, Kao FC, Tu YK. Flexor pollicis longus tendon entrapment after performing minimally invasive plate osteosynthesis of a distal radius fracture: a case report. *Hand Surg.* 2013;18:403–406.

39. Vaiss L, Ichihara S, Hendriks S, Taleb C, Liverneaux P, Facca S. The utility of the fluoroscopic skyline view during volar locking plate fixation of distal radius fractures. *J Wrist Surg.* 2014;3:245–249.

40. Wei XM, Sun ZZ, Rui YJ, Song XJ. Minimally invasive plate osteosynthesis for distal radius fractures. *Indian J Orthop.* 2014;48:20–24.

41. Thornhill TS. The mini-incision hip: proceed with caution. *Orthopedics.* 2004;27:193–194.

42. Naito K, Zemirline A, Sugiyama Y, Obata H, Liverneaux P, Kaneko K. Possibility of fixation of a distal radius fracture with a volar locking plate through a 10 mm approach. *Tech Hand Up Extrem Surg.* 2016;20:71–76.

43. Duprat A, Hidalgo Diaz JJ, Vernet P, et al. Volar locking plate fixation of distal radius fractures: splint versus immediate mobilization. *J Wrist Surg.* 2018;7:237–242.

44. Kapandji A. Internal fixation by double intrafocal plate. Functional treatment of non-articular fractures of the lower end of the radius. *Ann Chir.* 1976;30:903–908.

45. Medda PL, Matheron AS, Hidalgo Diaz JJ, et al. Minimally invasive hardware removal after minimally invasive distal radius plate osteosynthesis (MIPO): feasibility study in a 388-case series. *Orthop Traumatol Surg Res.* 2017; 103:85–87.

CHAPTER 11

Volar, Dorsal, and/or Radial Plating

K.R. ESPOSITO • S.C. SHOAP • C.E. FREIBOTT • R.J. STRAUCH
Columbia University, Department of Orthopedic Surgery, New York, NY, United States

KEY POINTS

- Volar plating is the workhorse of internal fixation for unstable distal radius fractures (DRFs)
- Dorsal plate technology has improved, decreasing associated hardware-related complications
- Combination plating is a viable option for highly unstable fracture patterns
- Fixation strategy should ultimately be chosen based on fracture pattern and stability

Panel 1: Case Scenario

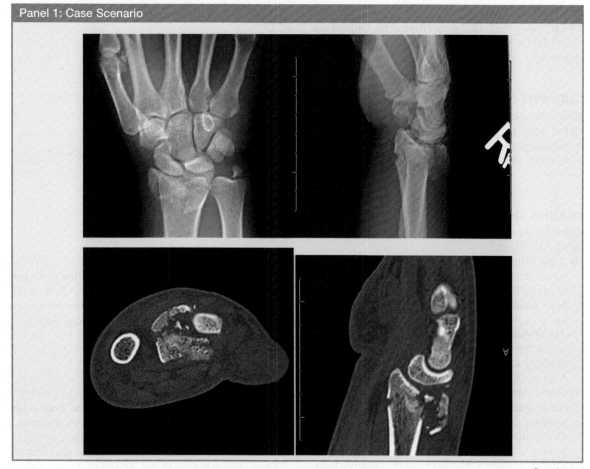

Continued

Distal Radius Fractures. https://doi.org/10.1016/B978-0-323-75764-5.00027-5

A 27-year-old right hand dominant male fell on his outstretched hand and sustained a highly comminuted intraarticular DRF. The fracture had dorsal, palmar, and radial comminution, with pieces of the articular surface impacted.

He agreed to have surgical treatment. Which plating method is the most effective for this fracture: volar, dorsal, radial plating, or a combination plating configuration?

IMPORTANCE OF THE PROBLEM

DRFs are a common clinical problem with many treatment options available. Unstable and displaced or angulated DRFs are commonly treated with plate osteosynthesis. When considering options for fixation of DRFs, the optimal strategy will maximize function while minimizing complications. This chapter will explore the evidence for different types of plate fixation along with associated tradeoffs and complications.

MAIN QUESTION

Which plating method is most effective for ORIF of displaced DRFs: volar, dorsal, radial, or a combination approach?

CURRENT OPINION

Most unstable or displaced DRFs are treated with a locked volar plate. However, it is important that the treating surgeon be able to recognize situations in which a different fixation strategy is necessary to achieve stability.

FINDING THE EVIDENCE

Below is a list of Pubmed search algorithms used to construct this chapter:

For Volar Plating: ("Radius Fractures" [Mesh] OR distal radius fracture*[tiab]) AND ("classification" [Subheading] OR displace* OR dislocat*) AND ((volar AND plating) OR "volar locking" OR "volar plating")- (199 results)

For Dorsal Plating: ("Radius Fractures" [Mesh] OR distal radius fracture*[tiab]) AND ("classification" [Subheading] OR displace* OR dislocat*) AND (dorsal AND plating)- (83 results)

For Radial Plating: ("Radius Fractures" [Mesh] OR distal radius fracture*[tiab]) AND ("classification" [Subheading] OR displace* OR dislocat*) AND ((radial AND plating) OR "radial plating" OR "radial column plating" OR "radial styloid")- (128 results)

For Combined Plating: ("Radius Fractures" [Mesh] OR distal radius fracture*[tiab]) AND ("classification" [Subheading] OR displace* OR dislocat*) AND

((combination AND plating) OR dual OR "fragment specific" OR "ulnar column")- (32 results)

Pubmed Clinical Queries: systematic[sb] AND (Distal radius plating) (6 results), systematic[sb] AND (Distal radius classification) (10 results), systematic[sb] AND (displaced distal radius) (19 results)

Cochrane Database of Systematic Reviews: Displaced distal radius (19 results), distal radius plating (12 results), distal radius classification (26 results)

QUALITY OF THE EVIDENCE

Level I:
Randomized Controlled Trial: 1
Level II:
Prospective Cohort Studies: 5
Systematic Review of Cohort Studies: 1
Randomized Trial with methodological limitations: 1
Outcomes Research: 1
Level III:
Retrospective Cohort Studies: 14
Systematic Review of Case-Controlled Studies: 1
Level IV:
Case Series: 1
Level V:
Expert Opinion: 1

FINDINGS

Volar Plating

Volar plating has risen to prominence as the preferred choice among most surgeons for internal fixation of DRFs. The technique has been applied to a wide variety of fracture patterns and patient populations with successful radiographic and functional outcomes and a low complication rate.[1-4]

Fracture Pattern and Displacement

Volar plating can be used successfully to treat a variety of fracture types and patterns of displacement. Both volar and dorsal displacement are amenable to volar plating, as are extraarticular, partial articular, and intraarticular patterns. Erhart et al. studied whether the direction of fracture displacement, dorsal or volar, affected radiographic and clinical outcomes following volar plating.[3] They evaluated 50 patients who underwent volar plating, half of whom had dorsally displaced (Colles) and half with volarly displaced (Smith) fractures. At a mean follow-up of 5 years postoperatively, they found no significant clinical difference between the groups. All patients had progression of arthrosis thought to be secondary to the injury itself. The dorsally displaced group had a trend toward restriction of flexion if the final position had residual dorsal tilt, although this did not affect function.[3]

Braziulis et al. found that all fracture types (AO Types A, B, and C) had improved function and radiographic parameters at 6-months of follow-up following volar plating.[2] Patients with complete articular fractures had worse DASH scores and radiographic parameters than the other two groups, but all were improved from their preoperative status.[2]

Function and Radiographic Parameters

Volar plating is an excellent choice with respect to patient function postoperatively, and the available evidence supports that volar plating successfully maintains reduction through standard follow-up intervals. Lattmann et al. prospectively followed 245 patients through 1-year follow-up following volar locking plate treatment of an unstable distal radius fracture.[5] Range of motion and function all improved throughout the 1-year follow-up period with excellent maintenance of reduction.[5] The authors noted an overall complication rate of 15%, with 4% of the cohort requiring a second operation, which is consistent with other studies.[6]

Jose et al. looked at radiographic and functional outcomes of 53 patients with unstable DRFs treated with locked volar plating at 1 year.[4] Of the 53 patients included, 46 had excellent or good radiographic parameters and 37 patients had excellent or good functional outcomes. One case developed a superficial infection that resolved with oral antibiotics. The authors concluded that volar plating is an effective treatment for unstable distal radius fractures in that it allows early motion and return to function while preventing loss of reduction.[4]

Lee et al. prospectively studied 89 patients with dorsally displaced DRFs that were treated with locked volar plates. They assessed functional outcomes at 1 year, including wrist motion, grip strength, and DASH score. Among surgeon-modifiable factors, only positive ulnar variance was associated with lower DASH scores at 1 year.[7]

Patient Demographics

Volar plating has been shown to be a viable treatment option for a wide variety of patients with respect to age, gender, and comorbidities. Martinez-Mendez et al. prospectively studied 66 patients with a mean age of 68 (range 60–81) to ascertain radiographic parameters over time in the setting of complex intraarticular fractures.[1] They examined the association of fracture type, age, and gender with hand function at 6-month follow-up following distal radius volar plating. The authors retrospectively examined the records of 120 patients, with 28 extraarticular fractures, 70 partial articular fractures, and 22 complete articular fractures. They found no demographic differences between the groups, and found that patients with complete articular fractures had worse function (lower DASH scores and worse radiographic parameters) at 6-month follow-up than the other two groups. In this study, fracture type was associated with function after distal radius plating at 6 months while age and gender were not.[2]

Lee et al. found that patient age was the only significant factor affecting grip strength and range of motion, and diabetes was significantly associated with lower DASH scores.[7]

Complications

Despite the widespread familiarity with volar plating and its wide variety of successful applications, surgeons must be cognizant that this treatment modality is not without complications. Alter et al. performed a systematic review of complications of volar plating of DRFs which included 55 studies comprising 3911 patients.[6] They found an overall 15% complication rate, with 5% qualifying as major complications requiring reoperation.[6] The most common complications encountered were nerve dysfunction (including carpal tunnel syndrome and complex regional pain syndrome) in 5.7% of patients. Tendon injury occurred in 3.5% of patients in this study, and of these, extensor tendon issues such as rupture (0.6%) and synovitis (1%) were more common than flexor tendon complications. Hardware-related issues were found in 1.6%, the most common of which was malunion at 0.6%. Hardware prominence, intraarticular screws, and screw loosening were rare.[6]

Although rare, flexor tendon injury, in particular FPL rupture, is a dreaded complication of volar plating. Asadollahi et al. performed a systematic review examining the demographics, clinical characteristics, treatment, and outcome of flexor tendon injuries following volar plating of DRFs.[8] In a total of 47 cases reported in the literature, the FPL was the most commonly ruptured tendon (57% of cases), followed by the FDP to the index finger (15%). The median interval to rupture after surgery was 9 months, and mean age of the affected patients was 61. Most patients had prodromal symptoms of crepitus, pain with finger motion, clicking or a rubbing sensation prior to rupture.[8] The authors recommend careful plate positioning proximal to the watershed line and early removal of the plate in cases with suboptimal positioning or symptomatic warning signs.

It is important to note that although the prevention of flexor tendon injuries deserves significant attention, surgeons must remain cognizant that extensor tendon problems were actually found to be more common overall than flexor tendon problems. These are likely related to dorsal hardware prominence (long screws).[6]

Dorsal Plating

Dorsal plating has historically been associated with higher complication rates, primarily related to prominent hardware. More recently, advances in plate design have been associated with better postoperative outcomes. Low-profile plates, which are thinner than the original dorsal plates, were developed to address the extensor tendon complications often seen with dorsal plating. With the advent of these low-profile plate designs, there is increasing evidence supporting dorsal plating for the treatment of dorsally comminuted DRFs.

Plate Selection

Low-profile plating systems have largely alleviated the problems with extensor tendon irritation that historically plagued dorsal plating of DRFs. Rozental et al. assessed a cohort of 28 patients with a comminuted, dorsally displaced DRF treated operatively with dorsal plating.[9] Nineteen patients had a Synthes Pi plate, whereas nine received a low-profile plate. In this cohort, all 28 fractures were satisfactorily reduced. All patients achieved good or excellent functional outcome at final follow-up, regardless of fixation type.

Simic et al. retrospectively reviewed 60 consecutive unstable distal radius fractures that were treated with a low-profile dorsal plating system.[10] 50 (85%) patients (51 fractures) returned for outcome assessment after at least 1 year. The authors reported successful fixation of all fractures, with excellent postoperative radiographic parameters, range of motion, and grip strength. There were no instances of extensor tendon irritation or rupture, and the patients reported minimal dorsal implant tenderness. The mean DASH score in this patient cohort was 11.9. Using the Gartland and Werley scoring system (GWS), 31 (62%) patients had an excellent rating and 19 (38%) patients had a good rating.

Kamath et al. retrospectively reviewed 30 patients who were treated with low profile, stainless steel plates for dorsally angulated DRFs.[11] The authors reported that

there were no instances of malunion, plate breakage, infection, compressed neuropathy, soft-tissue complications, or extensor tendon ruptures. The authors reported satisfactory radiographic reduction when comparing preoperative to postoperative radiographs for all but one patient. The mean DASH score in this cohort was 15. When using the GWS, 16 (53%) patients had an excellent outcome, 12 (40%) had a good outcome, and 2 (4%) had a fair outcome.

In the largest cohort included in this chapter, Matzon et al. retrospectively reviewed 110 patients that were treated with dorsal plating for a DRF.[12] All patients received a low-profile titanium plate. At final follow-up (mean 2.25 years), satisfactory reduction was obtained and there were no reported instances of nonunion, hardware failure, or compression neuropathy. The mean flexion extension arc was 138 degrees, with 85 degrees of pronation and 85 degrees of supination. The average DASH at final follow-up in this cohort was 6.3. Using the GWS, 82 (75%) patients had an excellent outcome, 22 (20%) had a good outcome, 5 (4%) had a fair outcome, and 1 (1%) had a poor outcome.

Chen et al. retrospectively reviewed 24 patients with unilateral DRF who were treated with bicolumnar plate fixation via a minimally invasive dorsal approach.[13] At 1 year postoperatively, all patients achieved radiographic union with all anatomical parameters effectively restored. On average, range of motion of the injured side was restored to 85% of extension, 75% of flexion, 93% pronation, and 85% supination of the contralateral side. Patients regained 83% of their grip strength.

Fracture Pattern

In general, patients treated with dorsal plating in the studies outlined in this chapter had dorsally comminuted fractures, which ostensibly dictated the plating strategy. Hamada et al. further subdivided the fracture patterns in their cohort. They retrospectively assessed 24 patients who received low-profile dorsal plates for dorsally displaced, unstable DRFs.[14] Of the 24 included patients, 9 had type 1 fractures and 15 had type 2 fractures. Type 1 was defined as having a volar fracture line distal to the watershed line in the dorsally displaced fragment, and type 2 consisted of a displaced dorsal die-punch fragment along with a minimally displaced styloid shear fracture or transverse volar fracture line. At 6 months postoperatively, both types had similar range of motion and mean grip strength was within 82.5% of the uninjured hand. There were no instances of tendon rupture, neurovascular complication, or prolonged tenderness or discomfort. Mean time to union was 2.7 months, with no nonunions.

Complications and Limitations

While the studies included in this chapter reported mostly positive results when using low-profile plating for dorsally comminuted DRFs, some complications were encountered.

Rozental et al. compared a cohort of patients with a Synthes Pi plate to those treated with a low-profile plate.[9] Nine patients underwent reoperation secondary to postoperative complications, all of whom had a Synthes pi plate placed in their index procedure. Seven of these patients had isolated extensor tenosynovitis, while two had extensor tendon rupture. Plate type was significantly in favor of patients treated with the low-profile plate who had no postoperative complications ($P < .025$).

The cohort in the study published by Simic et al. received low-profile dorsal plates.[10] There were no instances of extensor tendon irritation or rupture. However, hardware removal was performed for one patient who was experiencing dorsal wrist pain at 1 year postoperatively. Intraoperative examination in this case did not reveal evidence of tendon irritation or tenderness over the plate. Plate removal did not relieve the patient's symptoms.

Similarly, the Kamath et al. cohort was treated with low-profile plates exclusively.[11] One patient had loss of anatomic reduction, but reported fair functional outcome at 25 months. Three patients underwent a second operation (10%), one for superficial scarring on the extensor retinaculum, and two for the removal of a single metaphyseal screw as a result of loosening. No patients required plate removal and there were no extensor tendon ruptures.

The cohort in the study by Matzon et al. received low-profile titanium plates.[12] While satisfactory alignment was achieved in all cases, nine patients (8%) had hardware removed. Intraoperative evidence of extensor tenosynovitis was found in six patients (5%). These six complications comprised the fair ($n=5$) and poor ($n=1$) GWS.

Hamada et al. reported only one serious complication, one patient who experienced a collapse of the dorsal ulnar fragment because of a lack of distal locking screws in the buttress plate.[14] As a result, the patient underwent implant removal and an ulnar shortening osteotomy 1 year after the index procedure. Clinical outcomes improved in this patient 3 months after revision

surgery, and ultimately, the patient had a positive outcome. They also reported three cases of mild discomfort of the dorsum of the wrist, however all resolved within 6 months postoperatively. Two patients (8%) lost reduction of their fracture within 1 month.

Chen et al. reported a 13% complication rate (3 of 24 patients).[15] One complication was screw loosening in an elderly, osteoporotic patient. By 6 months, the patient went on to osseous union with pain-free range of motion. Two patients with soft tissue complications reported extensor tendon irritation, with only one requesting removal of all implants. There were no cases of wound infection or extensor tendon ruptures.

Radial Column Plating

Radial column plates typically serve as an adjunct to volar or dorsal locking plates in severely comminuted DRFs, or in fracture patterns that displace large fragments of the radial styloid. They can also be used in isolation, although much less frequently than either volar or dorsal plating alone. A number of retrospective reviews examining both objective and subjective outcome scores, as well as radiographic evaluation of reduction and union, have stated that dual radial styloid and volar plating achieved acceptable clinical and radiographic outcomes.[16–19]

Function and Radiographic Parameters

The evidence available for radial column plating as an adjunct to volar plating shows favorable results with regard to patient function and maintenance of reduction. Helmerhorst et al. conducted a retrospective review on 14 patients treated with locked volar plate fixation and an additional radial column plate with an average follow-up of 30 months.[16] They found that 13 of the patients achieved union within 7 weeks after surgery, and all 14 had either good or excellent functional outcome scores.[16] This is also reflected in the findings of Tang et al., who conducted a case series on eight patients treated with dual plating, with an average follow-up of 35 weeks.[17] All patients went on to union and had an average DASH of 19.9.[17] Similarly, a retrospective chart review of 10 patients treated using a similar plating technique by Jacobi et al. with an average follow-up of 4 months found that all patients achieved anatomic reduction and bony union. 90% of these patients had outcome scores rated as either excellent or good.[18] Garner et al. conducted a retrospective review of 36 patients treated with radial column and volar locking plates with an average follow-up of 15.6 months.[19] These patients had an average DASH of 20.7, and all had acceptable radial height, radial inclination, and volar tilt at final follow-up.[19]

The evidence supporting radial column plating alone is limited, as clinical scenarios in which a radial column plate alone is sufficient for fixation are rare. A randomized controlled trial by Wei et al. looked at 46 patients with unstable DRFs who were treated with a locked volar plate, external fixation, or a locked radial column plate. Outcome measures, including DASH, grip strength, range of motion and pinch strength, were collected at 3 months, 6 months, and 1 year. They found that within the first 3 months, the use a locked volar plate resulted in better outcome measures than external fixation and radial column plates. However, at 6 months and 1 year, all three fixation methods were found to have satisfactory outcome measures.[20]

Biomechanical Evidence

Biomechanical studies of radial column plating have also demonstrated favorable results. Grindel et al. compared the stability and construct strength of volar plating alone to a combination of volar and radial styloid plating in eight matched pairs of cadaveric arms.[21] Load-to-failure testing revealed that dual plating resulted in a 50% increase in construct rigidity and a 76% increase in failure strength compared to volar plating alone.[21] In a similar comparison, Blythe et al. found a significantly higher construct rigidity in a cadaveric fracture model fixed with a combination of volar and styloid plating when compared to one fixed with volar plating alone.[22]

Complications

Radial column plating does have some associated complications unique to the position of the hardware. If the radial plate is too prominent, it predictably will irritate tendons in the first dorsal compartment, creating a De Quervain-like clinical picture.[17] Among the 10 patients evaluated by Jacobi et al., 5 of them had De Quervain symptoms, and benefitted from the plate being removed.[18] Galle et al. retrospectively analyzed functional outcomes of 63 patients who underwent radial column plating.[23] Of the 17 patients that had their hardware removed, 8 were because of De Quervain's symptoms. Although this did not reach statistical significance, it was the leading cause of hardware removal in this study, followed by hardware removal for activity-related pain.

Radial column plating has a higher hardware removal rate than other types of plating. Although they reported no complications or wound infections in their cohort, Garner et al. performed hardware removal in 13 of their 36 patients within the average follow-up time of 15.6 months.[19] In the Galle et al. cohort, 17 patients had their plates removed and 44 retained their hardware, but ultimately there were no clinically or statistically significant differences between the two groups in DASH, VAS, and grip strength.[23] Although reoperation is burdensome, these findings suggest that hardware removal has no long-term adverse effect on outcome. Patients undergoing radial column plating should be counseled about potential hardware-related symptoms and a roughly 25% chance of needing hardware removal.[23]

Combined Plating

For the majority of surgeons performing open reduction and internal fixation for unstable DRFs, volar plating is the workhorse technique.[24, 25] However, in some injuries with complex fracture patterns, a volar plate alone may not provide adequate stability. Surgeons must be able to recognize when volar plating alone is not sufficient and the construct may require multiple plates to achieve satisfactory fixation. The most common combinations of plates for severely comminuted, intraarticular DRFs include radial column/volar plating and dorsal/volar plating.[11, 17–19, 23, 24, 26, 27] The instances in which these strategies are employed are highly dependent on both the fracture pattern and surgeon discretion.

The evidence for dorsal/volar combination plating is described in this section. For radial column/volar combination plating, please refer to the Radial Column Plating section of this chapter.

Dorsal/Volar Combination Plating

A number of studies examining combination plating have determined that this technique achieves satisfactory outcomes, and have advocated for its use in the setting of complex fractures of the distal radius. A case series by Ring et al. examined 25 patients that received combined dorsal/volar plate fixation with an average follow-up of 26 months.[27] They found an average grip of 78% compared to the contralateral side, a GWS of good or excellent in 98% of patients, and satisfactory union achieved in all patients. In addition, average extension was 54 degrees, flexion was 51 degrees, pronation was 79 degrees, and supination was 74 degrees. They concluded that this fixation technique can achieve a stable, mobile wrist in patients with very complex fractures.[27]

Day et al. retrospectively analyzed the data of 10 patients that had received dorsal/volar combination plating with an average follow-up time of 17 months.[28] Their cohort had an average grip of 72% compared to the contralateral side, a GWS of good or excellent in 70% of patients, DASH of 16, and satisfactory union in all, without any tendon ruptures. Extension was 46 degrees, flexion was 46 degrees, pronation was 80 degrees, and supination was 71 degrees. This study concluded that this "sandwich" plating technique is an effective method of regaining near-anatomic reconstruction of intraarticular, volarly, and dorsally comminuted DRFs.[11]

A retrospective review by Farhan et al. examined 24 patients receiving combined dorsal/volar locked plating with an average follow-up of 17 months.[26] They reported an average grip strength of 69% compared to the contralateral side, satisfactory union in all patients, extension of 52 degrees, flexion of 49 degrees, pronation of 77 degrees, and supination of 86 degrees. This study concluded that combined dorsal/volar plating enables early mobilization and good outcomes for certain complex comminuted DRFs.[26] A retrospective cohort study by Sagerfors et al. reviewed 102 consecutive patients receiving combined dorsal/volar plating with an average

follow-up of 27 months.[25] Compared to the contralateral side, they found grip strength to be 80%, extension 74%, flexion 70%, pronation 94%, and supination 90%. Average DASH was 19.4, and VAS scores were 0 at rest and 3 with activity. They concluded that a good outcome can be expected after combined dorsal/volar plating.[25] This data can be found in Table 1.

Complications

Complication rates for combined dorsal/volar plating are relatively low. The most frequently reported complications are tendon problems (irritation and ruptures) and hardware removal. Ring et al. reported plate removal in 21/25 (84%) of patients and tendon ruptures in two patients.[27] The authors explained the high rate of hardware removal as related to the complexity of the injuries.[27] However, two studies that reported using more low-profile plates had lower rates of tendon injury and hardware removal. Compared to the traditional plates used by Ring et al. (2–3.5 mm in thickness),[27] Day et al. used anatomically designed stainless steel plates ranging from 1.2 to 1.5 mm in thickness.[28] In their cohort of 10 patients, they reported no tendon ruptures and no hardware removals.[11] Farhan et al., who used 2.4 mm locked compression plates in their study, reported a similar complication rate.[26] They removed hardware in 4/24 of their patients, and had no tendon

TABLE 1
Table Comparing Data Across Five Different Studies That Examined Outcomes of Patients Receiving Dorsal and Volar Combined Plating.

	DASH	Good or Excellent Gartland and Werley Scores	Good or Excellent Green and O'Brien Scores	Grip Strength (Compared to Contralateral Side)	Extension	Flexion	Pronation	Supination	Hardware Removals
Ring et al.	X	98%	40%	78%	54	51	79	74	84%
Day et al.	16	70%	X	72%	46	46	80	71	0%
Farhan et al.	X	X	X	69%	52	49	77	86	17%
Medlock et al.	30	39%	55%	71%	42	36	78	81	X
Sagerfars et al.	19.4	X	X	80%	X	X	X	X	19%

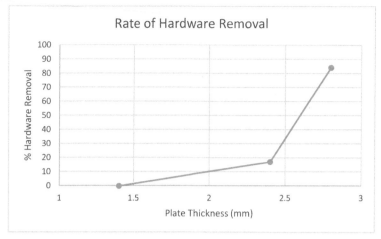

FIG. 1 The rate of hardware removal relative to the thickness of the plates used across the following three studies respectively: Day et al., Farhan et al., and Ring et al.

ruptures.[26] When comparing these three studies, there seems to be a correlation between the plate thickness and the rate of hardware removal (see Fig. 1). Other complications mentioned throughout these studies did not achieve statistical significance.

RECOMMENDATIONS

In patients receiving plating for DRFs, evidence suggests:

Recommendation	Overall Quality
• Volar plating is a workhorse treatment option for a wide variety of DRF patterns across many patient populations, although approximately 5% of patients require reoperation. Surgeons must optimize plating technique to minimize complication risk and be vigilant in monitoring for warning signs in the postoperative period.	⊕⊕⊕⊕ HIGH
• Dorsal plating is a viable option for fracture patterns with significant dorsal comminution or die-punch patterns. As hardware technology has improved, particularly with the advent of thinner plates, complications involving extensor tendons have become less common.	⊕⊕⊕◯ MODERATE

• Radial column plating can be used as a reliable tool to achieve union and favorable clinical outcomes for more complicated fractures when combined with additional plating. There is a high rate of hardware removal, although this does not seem to adversely affect long-term outcomes.   LOW

CONCLUSIONS

Volar plating is an appropriate choice for the treatment of many unstable DRFs. It can be employed across a diverse range of patients and fracture patterns with predictably good outcomes in radiographic parameters and function. Wrist surgeons are generally comfortable with the surgical approach and fixation techniques of volar plating, and are able to reliably employ the technique in a majority of cases.

However, it is paramount that the treating surgeon is able to recognize situations in which a volar plate is inadequate for fixation of an unstable distal radius fracture. In some situations, combining a volar plate with an additional radial column or dorsal plate may be necessary to provide adequate stability to the construct. In other scenarios, the fracture may require a dorsal or radial column plate alone and a volar plate may add no benefit.

Panel 2: Author's Preferred Technique

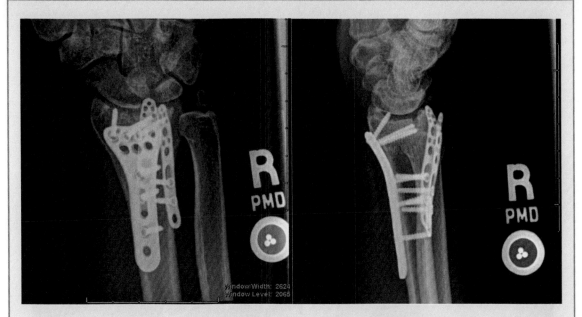

In the case of this severely comminuted DRF, the author's preference was to perform ORIF utilizing a combination plating technique. This included a volar plate and two dorsal low-profile plates, as well as cancellous allograft chips. Radiographs above obtained at 1 year post-op demonstrated consolidation and stable fixation. The following data were collected at this time: VAS both at rest and activity: 0, flexion: 20 degrees, extension: 35 degrees, supination: 90 degrees, pronation: 90 degrees. In all plating configurations, we do not remove hardware as a matter of routine. We do remove hardware if there are symptoms of tendon irritation.

Panel 3: Pearls and Pitfalls[29]

PEARLS

- The senior author typically uses a volar plate for most DRFs in which the volar cortex of the radius has fractured. The dorsally directed screws are depth gauged off the dorsal cortex so as not to be prominent and are rarely longer than 18 mm.

- In the event of significant radial comminution not able to be captured by the plate, K-wires are placed through the fragments and into stable radius bone to maintain position, as opposed to a radial plate.

- Dorsal plates are used in stand-alone fashion for dorsal Barton's fractures, or in combination with a volar plate in the case of dorsal and volar comminution which cannot be stabilized by the volar plate alone.

PITFALLS

- In the case of extreme comminution, volar and dorsal plates can be used to realign the joint surface and neutralized with an external fixator for 6 weeks, or a dorsal spanning plate for 3 months.

- Care should be taken to avoid screws impinging on the extensor tendons from a volar plate, and the volar plate should be adequately covered with soft tissue to lessen the chance of soft tissue irritation. The senior author's preferred method of soft tissue coverage is a distally based segment of the brachioradialis tendon, rotated to cover the distal aspect of the hardware.

In a high-energy polytrauma case like this, goals are anatomical articular reduction with buttressing of the volar critical corner (*) and the highly comminuted dorsal rim (**). © Dr. Buijze 2020.

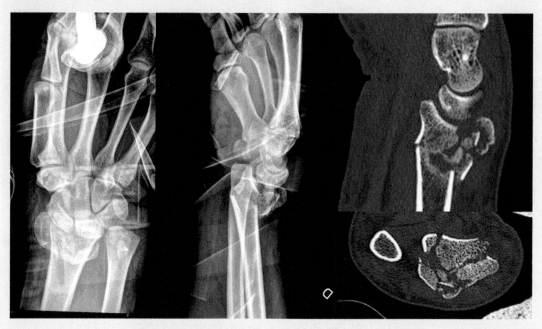

In case of difficulty in maintaining the volar "Die punch" impaction reduced with K-wires and/or an elevator, a drill hole can be made in the desired screw direction through a volar rim plate. © Dr. Buijze 2020.

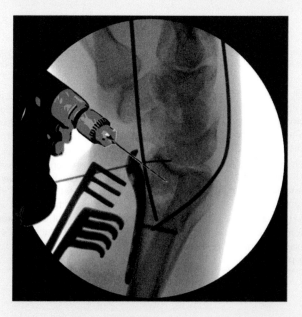

A short locking screw is then used to lift the fragment and lock it in the variable angle plate without purchasing the dorsal fragments. © Dr. Buijze 2020.

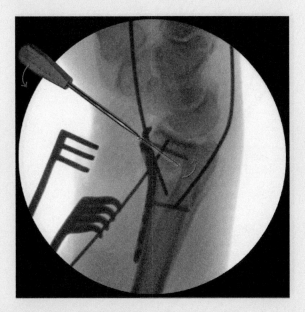

Arthroscopic assistance can help to achieve adequate artic-ular reduction of the radiodorsal fragments using a probe and K-wires. © Dr. Buijze 2020.

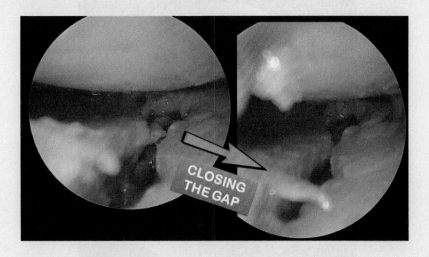

CLOSING THE GAP

Continued

Editor's Tips & Tricks: Double Plating—cont'd

Multiple dorsal and radial K-wires may be necessary in case of high degree of comminution. Kapandji-type intrafocal pinning is a helpful technique to buttress small fragments. © Dr. Buijze 2020.

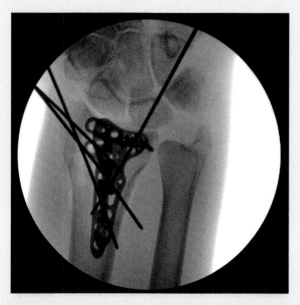

A low-profile plate is applied to buttress the dorsal rim of the radius as the volar screws don't offer sufficient grip. The short critical corner screw of the volar plate can now be replaced by a longer one. © Dr. Buijze 2020.

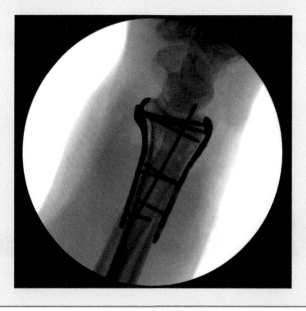

Additional radial column (triple) plating is in the editor's opinion seldom necessary. Leaving one or two additional K-wires instead for 6 weeks (and/or screws) through the radial styloid can be sufficient to complete a stable osteosynthesis.

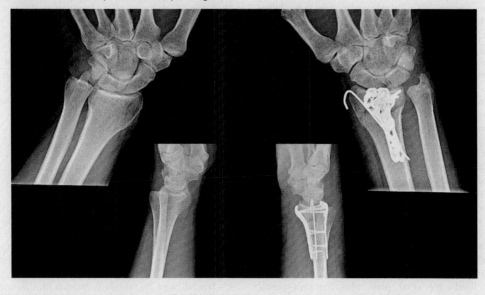

REFERENCES

1. Martinez-Mendez D, Lizaur-Utrilla A, de Juan-Herrero J. Prospective study of comminuted articular distal radius fractures stabilized by volar plating in the elderly. *Int Orthop.* 2018;42:2243–2248.
2. Braziulis K, Rimdeika R, Kregzdyte R, Tarasevicius S. Associations between the fracture type and functional outcomes after distal radial fractures treated with a volar locking plate. *Medicina (Kaunas).* 2013;49:399–402.
3. Erhart S, Toth S, Kaiser P, Kastenberger T, Deml C, Arora R. Comparison of volarly and dorsally displaced distal radius fracture treated by volar locking plate fixation. *Arch Orthop Trauma Surg.* 2018;138:879–885.
4. Jose A, Suranigi SM, Deniese PN, Babu AT, Rengasamy K, Najimudeen S. Unstable distal radius fractures treated by volar locking anatomical plates. *J Clin Diagn Res.* 2017;11, Rc04-rc8.
5. Lattmann T, Meier C, Dietrich M, Forberger J, Platz A. Results of volar locking plate osteosynthesis for distal radial fractures. *J Trauma.* 2011;70:1510–1518.
6. Alter TH, Sandrowski K, Gallant G, Kwok M, Ilyas AM. Complications of volar plating of distal radius fractures: a systematic review. *J Wrist Surg.* 2019;8:255–262.
7. Lee S-J, Park JW, Kang BJ, Lee JI. Clinical and radiologic factors affecting functional outcomes after volar locking plate fixation of dorsal angulated distal radius fractures. *J Orthop Sci.* 2016;21:619–624.
8. Asadollahi S, Keith PP. Flexor tendon injuries following plate fixation of distal radius fractures: a systematic review of the literature. *J Orthop Traumatol.* 2013;14:227–234.
9. Rozental TD, Beredjiklian PK, Bozentka DJ. Functional outcome and complications following two types of dorsal plating for unstable fractures of the distal part of the radius. *J Bone Joint Surg Am.* 2003;85:1956–1960.
10. Simic PM, Robison J, Gardner MJ, Gelberman RH, Weiland AJ, Boyer MI. Treatment of distal radius fractures with a low-profile dorsal plating system: an outcomes assessment. *J Hand Surg [Am].* 2006;31:382–386.
11. Day CS, Kamath AF, Makhni E, Jean-Gilles J, Zurakowski D. "Sandwich" plating for intra-articular distal radius fractures with volar and dorsal metaphyseal comminution. *Hand (N Y).* 2008;3:47–54.
12. Matzon JL, Kenniston J, Beredjiklian PK. Hardware-related complications after dorsal plating for displaced distal radius fractures. *Orthopedics.* 2014;37:e978–e982.
13. Chen AC, Chou YC, Cheng CY. Distal radius fractures: minimally invasive plate osteosynthesis with dorsal bicolumnar locking plates fixation. *Indian J Orthop.* 2017;51:93–98.
14. Hamada Y, Gotani H, Hibino N, et al. Surgical strategy and techniques for low-profile dorsal plating in treating dorsally displaced unstable distal radius fractures. *J Wrist Surg.* 2017;6:163–169.

15. Chen CH, Zhou RK, Zhen HQ, Huang L, Jiao YJ. Efficacy of volar and dorsal plate fixation for unstable dorsal distal radius fractures. *Int J Clin Exp Med.* 2015;8:4375–4380.

16. Helmerhorst GT, Kloen P. Orthogonal plating of intra-articular distal radius fractures with an associated radial column fracture via a single volar approach. *Injury.* 2012;43:1307–1312.

17. Tang P, Ding A, Uzumcugil A. Radial column and volar plating (RCVP) for distal radius fractures with a radial styloid component or severe comminution. *Tech Hand Up Extrem Surg.* 2010;14:143–149.

18. Jacobi M, Wahl P, Kohut G. Repositioning and stabilization of the radial styloid process in comminuted fractures of the distal radius using a single approach: the radio-volar double plating technique. *J Orthop Surg Res.* 2010;5:55.

19. Garner MR, Schottel PC, Thacher RR, Warner SJ, Lorich DG. Dual radial styloid and volar plating for unstable fractures of the distal radius. *Am J Orthop (Belle Mead NJ).* 2018;47.

20. Wei DH, Raizman NM, Bottino CJ, Jobin CM, Strauch RJ, Rosenwasser MP. Unstable distal radial fractures treated with external fixation, a radial column plate, or a volar plate. A prospective randomized trial. *J Bone Joint Surg Am.* 2009;91:1568–1577.

21. Grindel SI, Wang M, Gerlach M, McGrady LM, Brown S. Biomechanical comparison of fixed-angle volar plate versus fixed-angle volar plate plus fragment-specific fixation in a cadaveric distal radius fracture model. *J Hand Surg [Am].* 2007;32:194–199.

22. Blythe M, Stoffel K, Jarrett P, Kuster M. Volar versus dorsal locking plates with and without radial styloid locking plates for the fixation of dorsally comminuted distal radius fractures: a biomechanical study in cadavers. *J Hand Surg [Am].* 2006;31:1587–1593.

23. Galle SE, Harness NG, Hacquebord JH, Burchette RJ, Peterson B. Complications of radial column plating of the distal radius. *Hand (N Y).* 2018. https://doi.org/10.1177/1558944718760861.

24. Medlock G, Smith M, Johnstone AJ. Combined volar and dorsal approach for fixation of comminuted intra-articular distal radial fractures. *J Wrist Surg.* 2018;7:219–226.

25. Sagerfors M, Bjorling P, Niklasson J, Pettersson K. Combined volar T-plate and dorsal pi-plate for distal radius fractures: a consecutive series of 80 AO type C2 and C3 cases. *J Wrist Surg.* 2019;8:180–185.

26. Farhan MF, Wong JH, Sreedharan S, Yong FC, Teoh LC. Combined volar and dorsal plating for complex comminuted distal radial fractures. *J Orthop Surg (Hong Kong).* 2015;23:19–23.

27. Ring D, Prommersberger K, Jupiter JB. Combined dorsal and volar plate fixation of complex fractures of the distal part of the radius. *J Bone Joint Surg Am.* 2004;86:1646–1652.

28. Day CS, Franko OI. Low-profile dorsal plating for dorsally angulated distal radius fractures. *Tech Hand Up Extrem Surg.* 2007;11:142–148.

29. Jew NB, Karl JW, Trupia E, Strauch RJ, Calandruccio JH. Brachioradialis tendon coverage in volar distal radius plating. *Tech Hand Up Extrem Surg.* 2016;20:151–154.

CHAPTER 12

Comminuted Articular Distal Radius Fractures

JASON A. STRELZOW

University of Chicago, Department of Orthopaedic Surgery and Rehabilitation Medicine, University of Chicago Medicine, Chicago, IL, United States

KEY POINTS

- A number of treatment strategies exist for successful management of complex intraarticular distal radius fractures including: immobilization, external fixation, open reduction, and volar or fragment-specific plating as well as dorsal bridging plating. No well-controlled, methodologically strong studies have compared all treatment modalities and thus there is a paucity of evidence to support the use of one treatment modality over another.

- Careful diagnosis, an appropriate understanding of the fracture pattern and the patient physiological requirements will facilitate the selection of a personalized and optimal treatment strategy for each patient.

- Computer tomography facilitates an understanding and appreciation for the fracture pattern and involvement of the articular fracture.

- Final functional outcomes may be similar between treatment options. Radiographic outcomes appear to be improved with more invasive techniques such as open reduction and internal fixation.

- Overall, there is a high rate of posttraumatic arthrosis regardless of treatment modality; however, persistent articular mal-reduction may increase the rate of radiographic degenerative changes present.

Panel 1: Case Scenario

A 33-year-old male, right hand dominant, falls off his motorbike at high speed while performing a bike stunt maneuver. Evaluation in the Emergency Department demonstrates a visibly deformed, swollen neurovascularly intact wrist and hand. He has associated long bone, chest and head injuries that require surgical management. Radiographic imaging demonstrates a highly comminuted intraarticular distal radius fracture. The patient is eager for a full return to normal function in his wrist and to avoid development of wrist arthritis. A friend of his was placed in an external fixator for a similar injury and the patient would like to know if he will need something similar. He also wants to know what the ideal type of treatment. Would an alternative treatment strategy be more effective?

IMPORTANCE OF THE PROBLEM

Comminuted, intraarticular distal radial fractures present a substantial management challenge.[1, 2] Typically, the result of higher energy injuries they can also occur during fractures in osteopenic bone. Although frequently the focus of our efforts is directed at the bony injury, the surgeon must consider associated bon and soft-tissue injuries and their impact on the patients overall clinical picture.[3, 4] While all injuries have the potential for ongoing disability and functional impairment, overall fracture severity of the distal radius has been shown to be correlated with inferior health-related quality of life and radiographic outcomes.[5, 6] During the assessment of these injuries, radiography remains the mainstay of initial management. Radiographic examination alone,

Distal Radius Fractures. https://doi.org/10.1016/B978-0-323-75764-5.00021-4

however, may inaccurately predict the amount and location of intraarticular pathology and thus additional cross-sectional imaging modalities may provide valuable information to guide management.[7–10] Computer tomographic (CT) evaluation improves assessment of the articular involvement and provides a more reliable, reproducible assessment of the fracture pattern[7, 11, 12] (Fig. 1).

Once diagnosed treatment goals are to restore the wrist to as near anatomic as possible. Ultimately radiographic parameters for reconstruction focus on[13]:

- Radial tilt between 20 degrees volar and 15 degrees dorsal
- Restoration of radial inclination >15 degrees
- Minimized radial shortening <5 mm
- Minimized radiocarpal articular step-off or gap <2 mm
- Minimized sigmoid notch articular congruency <2 mm

In the setting of complex articular fracture pattern, a number of approaches and techniques have been described.[4, 14] Regardless of treatment modality, surgical goals remain the restoration of alignment, length, and re-establishing articular congruency. Additionally, the congruity and stability of the articular component of the lunate facet fragment and sigmoid notch generate a stable central column for reconstruction.[15–17] The lunate facet serves as the central component for force transmission and fulcrum of motion for the wrist.[4, 18, 19] In this role, the re-establishment of stability and alignment of the intermediate column plays a critical role in eventual outcome.[16, 17] Despite a variety of available surgical techniques to aid in the management of these complex intraarticular distal radius fractures, strong evidence to support the superiority of any one technique remains limited, however. Each technique brings with it specific advantages and complications. Despite a lack of scientific consensus, volar plating has become the mainstay of conventional treatment for distal radius fractures. However, highly comminuted articular fractures may present specific challenges for this technique.[2, 6, 20] This is particularly the case when complex articular comminution, and shear patterns are present where higher rates of complications and poorer radiographic outcomes have been reports.[6]

Interestingly, despite evidence to support improved radiological restoration of articular congruency using many of these techniques, inferior functional outcomes regardless of reduction are common in these complex injuries. This finding likely represents the inherent chondral injury present despite radiographic osseous reduction. Further complicating the issue is the lack of clear a relationship between radiographic outcome and functional/clinical outcomes, particularly in the elderly.

MAIN QUESTION

How are comminuted articular DRF most effectively treated?

CURRENT OPINION

Comminuted intraarticular fractures can be successfully managed with a number of techniques each with specific advantages and disadvantages. While no single technique has documented superiority, an understanding of the merits of each technique allows the surgeon to select the most appropriate strategy for a particular fracture pattern and patient.

FINDING THE EVIDENCE

- Cochrane Database search: Comminuted intraarticular Distal Radius fracture
- PUBMED: ("Complex intra-articular distal radius" [Mesh] OR "Distal radius articular fracture")
- Bibliography of eligible articles
- Foreign language articles not written in English were excluded from review
- Nonscientific review manuscripts were excluded

QUALITY OF THE EVIDENCE

Level I:
Metaanalysis/Systematic Reviews: 3
Level II:
Randomized trials with methodological limitations: 6
Level III:
Retrospective/Cohort studies: 66
Level IV:
Consecutive case series/Bio-mechanical studies: 35

FINDINGS

Multiple treatment options are reported in the literature including nonoperative cast immobilization, K-wire fixation, external fixation, internal bridging fixation, conventional volar plating, and fragment-specific techniques. The overall management of distal radius fractures has continued to evolve.[21] Predicting which technique is superior for each injury pattern requires an understanding of the reported risks and benefits of each technique as well as the individual patient

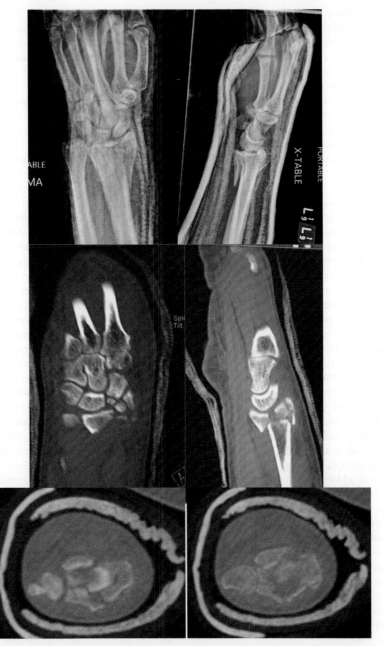

FIG. 1 Isolated intraarticular distal radius fracture with appreciable comminution of the articular surface better appreciated with cross-sectional imaging (CT scan). No associated injuries.

characteristics and comorbidities. Despite an exhaustive list of publications on distal radius fractures, high-level well-constructed randomized controlled trials and metaanalyses are lacking. Additionally, the majority of the published literature does not substratify distal radius fractures by severity or pattern making larger conclusions regarding the impact of intraarticular fracture patterns difficult. As a result, Cochrane and other metaanalyses evaluating operative and nonoperative strategies for complex intraarticular distal radius fractures have failed to detect differences in functional outcomes between treatment modalities.[22] Intraarticular distal radius fractures are associated with a high rate of post-traumatic arthrosis (65% at 7 years), however the clinical importance of this radiographic finding is unclear.[23] Any residual articular step-off, regardless of fixation technique, leads to early radiographic posttraumatic arthritis.[24] Given the lack of consensus within the literature, it is paramount that the surgeon considers patient, fracture, and technical factors in the determination of an overall treatment plan for an individual patient.

Cast Immobilization

Only two large randomized trials have formally evaluated cast immobilization for the treatment of intraarticular distal radius fractures.[25, 26] One additional randomized trial compared plate fixation with cast immobilization in all variations of distal radius fractures. They included a significant proportion (70%) of patients with intraarticular fracture patterns and reported modest early advantages in patient reported outcomes which were not maintained beyond 3 months.[27] Complications however were significantly higher in the operative group. A number of retrospective reviews have also addressed the same question with similar results suggesting cast immobilization for intraarticular distal radius fractures may produce similar clinical outcomes when compared to surgical fixation technique.[28-30] Importantly, many of these studies have focused on the elderly population (over 60 years old) and no evidence currently evaluates the use of this technique in younger age groups, although an ongoing randomized trial hopes to address this in the near future.[31] Predictive models for re-displacement and the effect of articular reduction on functional outcome following distal radius fractures appear to have limited reliability which further cloud the picture for an evidence-based treatment algorithm.[32, 33] However, the current evidence does suggest that in the older, low-demand patient population deformity appears to be well tolerated often despite articular involvement.[34-37] Final healed position frequently mimics that of their initial displacement. Malunion is therefore an expected outcome.[27, 38]

External Fixation

External fixation once a commonly employed tool in the management for distal radius fractures has largely fallen out of contemporary use except in specific circumstances.[39] Despite this, the clinical and radiographic outcomes have been well described and objectively reported as similar to other techniques.[40-42] Although a reliable and simple tool for the management of complex wrist injuries, the complication rate (24%-62%) has been well described and contributes to the limited widespread adoption.[43-49] Despite these concerns and recent trends toward alternative fixation methods, a number of randomized control trials have demonstrated no difference in outcomes when external fixation was compared to volar locked plating, and fragment-specific fixation when used in the management of complex articular fractures of the distal radius.[2, 45, 50-52] In comparison to nonoperative management small cohort and retrospective series have demonstrated improved radiographic and clinical outcomes with the use of external fixation.[53, 54] In complex comminuted articular fractures bridging external fixators are traditionally used over nonbridging techniques. For nonarticular fractures nonbridging external fixation have been shown in two well performed studies to have improved function and radiographic outcomes. In articular fractures, bridging fixation through distraction and ligamentotaxis obtain the alignment and allow for the reduction to be maintained.[55] When compared to volar plate fixation there is conflicting evidence regarding the differences in clinical and radiograph outcomes between these modalities.[2, 41, 42, 50, 53, 56-61] Overall measurable clinical outcomes appear similar, however, there may be an improved range of motion when plate fixation is utilized. A secondary advantage of external fixation is the use of additional augmentation of fixation which can be employed to achieve and maintain reduction such as K-wires, direct reduction, and supplemental plate fixation (Fig. 2). Overall, it appears that external fixation continues to remain a suitable option for the treatment of complex intraarticular distal radius management. Despite this a number of complications are well documented that merit careful attention. Care must be used to prevent overdistraction which can lead to complex regional pain syndrome (CRPS) and pin-site irritation or infection requires frequent pin-checks.[46, 62] If percutaneous K-wires are utilized, they should be promptly removed at 6-8 weeks to prevent the development of pin-track infection.[16]

Dorsal Bridge Plating/Dorsal Distraction Plate

Originally described as a technique to provide the soft tissue benefits of external fixation and internal fixation in the poly-trauma patient.[39, 63-66] This technique provides immediate stability while minimizing soft tissue disruption and avoiding the complications associated with external fixation, such as pin-site infection and stiffness.[63, 67] The dorsal plate can be applied percutaneously and generates a buttress type effect for complex

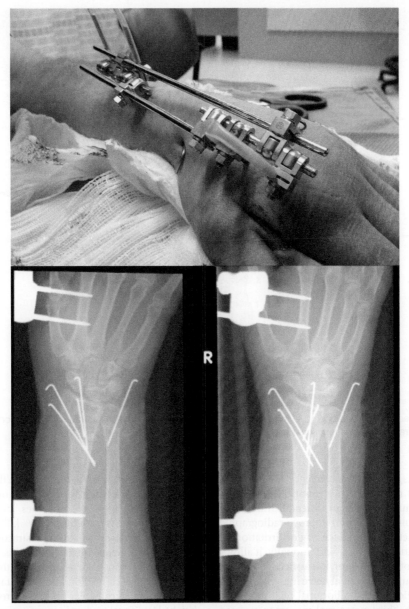

FIG. 2 Example of an external fixator with percutaneous adjuvant fixation with K-wires of a complex intraarticular distal radius fracture.

comminution of the dorsal cortex (Fig. 3). This technique has demonstrated similar clinical outcomes to those of other fixation methods.[1, 64, 68, 69] As a tool it is particularly useful in fractures with severe articular comminution when traditional plate fixation may be deemed inadequate. In this technique the plate is placed within the second or the fourth extensor compartment

floor and traction is applied. Distraction provides ligamentotaxis and helps restore the anatomic relationships of the distal radius through indirect reduction. Distal fixation can then be placed on the second or third metacarpal with the plate fixed proximally after distraction. Traditionally, the location of distal fixation was surgeon's choice. More recently a number of studies have

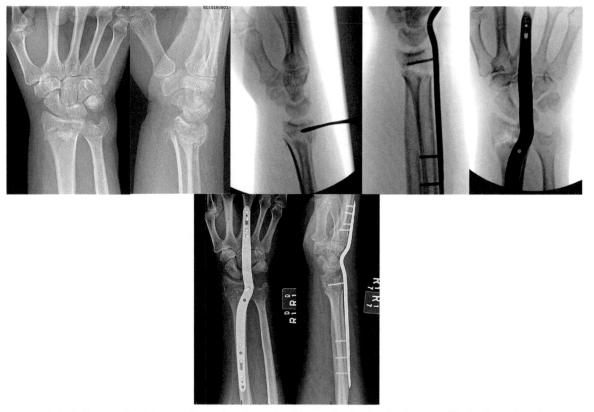

FIG. 3 Preoperative, intraoperative and postoperative images of a distal radius fracture with significant dorsal cortical intraarticular comminution managed with dorsal bridge plating.

suggested advantages and disadvantages for both the second and third metacarpal.[70–72] Fixation to the second metacarpal may facilitate grip strength if the wrist is positioned in ulnar deviation, improve radiographic alignment parameters, and reduce tendon irritation in the fourth compartment.[67, 73, 74] Additionally, it allows for a straight line of pull however, it is associated with an increased risk of superficial radial nerve injury and a less anatomic restoration of the radiocarpal relationship.[75] Plate fixation to the third metacarpal appears to increase the stiffness of the construct however, there is a greater risk of tendon entrapment.[70] Overall stability of the bridging locked plate appears more stable than traditional external fixation biomechanically.[73] Wolf et al. also demonstrated adequate stability of the construct requires only three locking screws proximally and three distally in a biomechanical model. Additional construct rigidity may be obtained with screw fixation into the lunate facet.[76] Typically, the bridging plate is removed at approximately 12 weeks when consolidation is demonstrated.[66] Overall, outcomes in the setting of distraction bridge plating for complex intraarticular fracture patterns suggests outcomes can be good to excellent in most patients [>80%].[64, 68, 69, 77, 78] A recent metaanalysis of dorsal distraction plating suggests most patients treated with this technique gain nearly 80% of contralateral grip strength with functional return of range of motion and radiographic restoration of alignment (mean volar tilt [3.6 degrees], mean radial height [10.5 mm] and radial inclination [19.4 mm]).[79] While most complications associated with dorsal bridge plating are minor, extensor lag and finger stiffness are well documented and specific complications from the technique.[66, 69, 77] Rates of infections [~1.6%] appears to be significantly lower than that seems in external fixation or volar plating techniques.[79, 80] Although this evidence suggests dorsal bridge plating may be a useful tool, the evidence remains limited to predominantly small case series and retrospective reviews. Further high-level comparative studies are needed.

Arthroscopic Techniques

Wrist arthroscopy techniques may help provide additional evaluation of intraarticular fractures and minimize soft tissue trauma.[81-84] Only one study has compared reduction using arthroscopic evaluation with conventional fluoroscopy.[83] Burnier et al. in this small consecutive series found a statistically significant improvement in reduction when arthroscopy was employed intraoperative. Our understanding and appreciation of intraarticular reduction and fracture morphology is poor when compared to advanced imaging modalities (computer tomography) and arthroscopy may prove to be a useful intraoperative adjunct to evaluate reduction.[7] Various arthroscopic techniques are described to improve articular reduction beyond that which can be obtained with fluoroscopy however robust studies have yet to confirm any clinical or long-term benefits to these techniques.

Volar Locking Plate Fixation

Volar locking plate fixation is currently the mainstay of surgical management for distal radius fractures and good results have been reported in the setting of complex intraarticular distal radius fracture[85-88] (Fig. 4). Locking technology allows for the generation of a stable fixed angled construct. With more complex fracture patterns however, the standard volar approach and fixation technique may need to be augmented with additional extensile exposures and techniques.[89] In the context of comminuted articular fractures, a small number of randomized and numerous retrospective studies have evaluated volar plating for comminuted intraarticular fractures.[27, 90] When compared to conservative management with cast immobilization volar locked plating offers improved articular congruity, and reduced rates of mal-union radiographically.[26, 35, 36] Chaudhry et al. demonstrated the superiority of volar locking plate techniques statistically but not in a clinically relevant capacity in a recent metaanalysis on the topic.[80] Marcheix et al. documented excellent wrist motion and good radiographic results in a randomized controlled trial of comminuted articular fractures managed with volar plating.[91] In their study there was less loss of reduction and improved clinical motion in those treated with volar locking plates compared to K-wire fixation, which has also been demonstrated by others.[15, 92] This finding was similarly demonstrated by Lutz et al. who demonstrated a reduction in postoperative arthritic changes (Grade I and II) in those patients with improved articular reduction as a result of volar plating.[33] This finding has also been demonstrated by a number of other authors.[93, 94] Despite promising radiographic improvements, the

evidence for any potentially improved clinical outcomes is mixed as radiographic arthrosis does not appear to correlate with functional outcomes.[27, 90] Challenges with locked volar plating are well documented. In more heavily comminuted intraarticular fractures difficulties in obtaining a reduction or maintaining a reduction can occur with a single plate.[6, 95-97] Finally, volar plate fixation of the distal radius appears to be associated with a documented higher complication rate compared to nonoperative and other modalities.[89, 90]

Fragment-Specific Fixation

More recently fragment-specific fixation has been employed to address the issues identified with other more traditional techniques particularly in the face of more complex fracture patterns. Beck et al. identified the presence of extremely distal (<15 mm remaining distal bone stock) or significantly depressed (>5 mm) lunate facet fractures as a risk factor for failure with conventional volar locked plating.[98] The presence of and failure to adequately capture the volar lunate facet fragment, commonly referred to as the "critical corner" is well described by Harness et al. and others.[99-102] Loss of reduction of this key fragment may lead to radiocarpal dislocation despite otherwise successful reduction. With fragment-specific techniques plates may be placed in multiple planes and locations on the distal radius and frequently orthogonal plating is used to increase rigidity of the fixation[14, 103-105] (Fig. 5). However, biomechanical data suggests this presumed increased rigidity may only be theoretical.[106] Fragment-specific fixation specifically applied focus on the reduction of the intermediate column, sigmoid notch and volar lunate facet allowing for the restoration of carpal alignment and congruity through limited open techniques.[107] Alternatively, dorsal buttress plating has a number of potential benefits in the management of complex articular distal radius fractures.[108, 109] The dorsal approach to the distal radius can facilitate intraarticular visualization and reduction of fragments while a dorsal based plate provides a stabilizing force against dorsal collapse and shear.[108] Ring, Benson, and others have evaluated outcomes using combined fragment-specific fixation for complex distal radius fractures and documented successful clinically and radiological outcomes.[21, 78, 110, 111] Volar rim plating techniques have gained increased interest for dealing with complex fracture patterns, particularly those involving the volar lunate facet of the distal radius.[102] Volar rim plating provides more distal fixed angle support to both capture and hold the reduced critical corner (volar lunate facet) rim fractures. Additionally, these lower profile plates may reduce the complications associated with

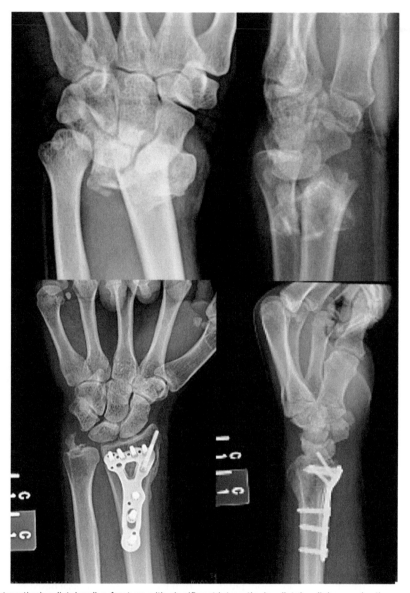

FIG. 4 Intraarticular distal radius fracture with significant intraarticular distal radial comminution successfully managed with volar plate fixation.

fixation distal to the watershed line.[104, 112] Although strong evidence is lacking to determine if this technique offers clinically important outcome differences small case and cohort series offer strong support for the techniques potential.[102, 104, 112–115] Unfortunately, the rate of metalwork irritation can be high and despite combining surgical approaches and the use of multiple plates, congruent and satisfactory articular reduction may not be achieved in a significant proportion (upwards of 30%) of patients.[21, 109] Although no specific fracture patterns have evidence-based indications to endorse the use of fragment-specific plates this technique continues to be a well-described method for the management of complex articular radial fractures.

Complications

The treatment of distal radius fractures using either non-operative strategies or surgical techniques is associated

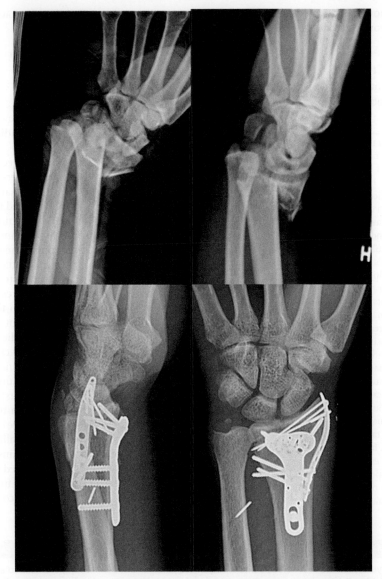

FIG. 5 Fragment-Specific Fixation of a complex intraarticular distal radius fracture. (A) Preoperative images demonstrate gross instability and articulate comminution. (B) Postoperative imaging demonstrates a concentric reduction with restoration of the articular congruency with early radio-lunate joint narrowing suggestive of arthrosis.

with a number of complications. In the setting of complex intraarticular distal radius fractures the complications are no less frequent.[16, 66, 116] Metalwork prominence, failure or patient preference may necessitate removal. Additional consideration should be given to CRPS which appears to be linked to excessive distraction through external fixation, bridge plating or conventional plating strategies.[16, 66] Pin tract infections,

posttraumatic arthritic change, intraarticular placement of fixation and loss of reduction are all possible complications. Although a common mild symptom pronounced stiffness, a common concern after articular fracture fixation, does not appear to be affected by more prolonged periods of wrist immobilization typically required in higher-energy injuries.[117] Despite these issues, functional improvements overall are typically for most patients; however, they appear more reliable and quicker in the younger patient population.[118]

RECOMMENDATIONS

In patients with an intraarticular displaced distal radius fracture, evidence suggests:

Recommendations	Overall Quality
• External fixation for the management of intraarticular distal radius fracture remains a successful option in the management of the intraarticular distal radius fracture, particularly in the setting of soft tissue trauma or when alternative techniques are not available	⊕⊕⊕◯ MODERATE
• Closed reduction and cast immobilization results in functionally equivalent outcomes to other treatment modalities despite higher rates of malunion and poor radiographic outcomes in patients over the age of 60	⊕⊕⊕◯ MODERATE
• Residual articular mal-reduction is associated with increased rates of radiographic arthrosis	⊕⊕⊕⊕ HIGH
• Failure to reduce and adequately stabilize a volar lunate fragment may result in loss of fixation and volar subluxation of the carpus	⊕⊕◯◯ LOW
• Malunion and residual radiographic deformity after management of intraarticular distal radius fractures does not appear to affect functional outcome	⊕⊕⊕◯ MODERATE
• There is conflicting evidence to demonstrate the superiority of one treatment modality over another in the management of intraarticular distal radius fractures	⊕⊕◯◯ LOW

• Open reduction and internal fixation of complex intraarticular fractures is associated with a higher rate of complications than other treatment techniques ⊕⊕⊕◯ MODERATE

CONCLUSION

Multiple treatment options are available for the management of intraarticular distal radius fractures, all of which have potential advantages and disadvantages. Individual factors including surgeon familiarity, and an understanding of the fracture personality and patient factors may help in the determination of a preferred technique. For heavily comminuted intraarticular distal radius fractures, internal distraction bridge plating appears to offer satisfactory outcomes with a low rate of complications compared to more conventional treatment techniques. Despite substantial literature evaluating techniques and management strategies for complex intraarticular distal radius fractures, strong evidence-based guidelines are lacking. From the available literature, well selected patients without complications can achieve good functional and radiographic outcomes through the use of multiple techniques including bridging external fixation, volar and fragment-specific plating, and distraction bridge plating. It behooves the surgeon to ensure a carefully understanding of the benefits and potential pitfalls of each technique allowing them to customize care to maximize outcome. Although extensive low and moderate quality literature exists for specific techniques there remains a paucity of reliable, methodologically standardized studies to evaluate the available techniques and thus further investigation is warranted before definitive conclusions can be formed.

Panel 2: Author's Preferred Technique

In the case of our 33-year-old male with a closed extensively comminuted intraarticular distal radius fracture there are a number of possible treatment modalities available for management of this injury.

Cross-section imaging with fine-cut CT scan is recommended to further delineate fracture morphology and intraarticular involvement. Once this confirms and defines the displaced articular fracture pattern an informed discussion can be undertaken with the patient. Given his injury pattern he has a high rate of posttraumatic arthritis regardless of management strategy.[21, 24]

Current evidence would suggest that in the presence of a high energy, grossly displaced intraarticular fracture with distal extension of the fracture pattern locked volar plating is at higher risk of failure.[119] Additionally, given his multiple injuries a device allowing for immediate weightbearing, with comparable clinical outcomes would be preferred. Thus, a spanning bridging distraction dorsal plate would be suggested. An informed discussion regarding the advantages and disadvantages would be performed reviewing the many viable alternative options including cast immobilization, external fixation, volar plating, and fragment-specific plate techniques. He underwent bridging internal plate fixation, was immediately made weightbearing as tolerated through his arm. The plate was removed at 10 weeks and a manipulation was performed at the time of the removal of metalwork. ROM at 12 weeks was Flexion 65 degrees, extension 60 degrees, Ulnar deviation 20 degrees, Radial deviation 20 degrees. Motion was pain free (Fig. 6).

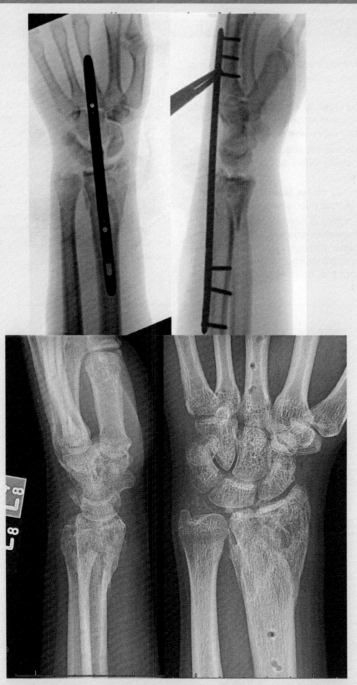

FIG. 6 Intraoperative and postmetalwork removal radiographs after Bridging fixation of a heavily comminuted intraarticular distal radius fracture in a poly-traumatized patient. The patient was immediately weightbearing postoperatively after fixation. The metalwork was removed at 10 weeks and therapy started immediately. Radiographically there is restoration of the alignment with residual posttraumatic changes at the radio-carpal joint that are asymptomatic for the patient at 1-year post injury.

Panel 3: Pearl's and Pitfalls

PEARLS

- Intraarticular distal radius fractures are complex injuries without well defined, evidence-based algorithms to guide practice.
- A patient and surgeon-specific approach to each case is warranted until additional evidence demonstrates the superiority of one technique over another.
- Cross-sectional imaging provides an opportunity to understand and reliability detect fracture fragments at the articular surface.
- Radiographic outcomes do not predict functional outcomes particularly in older populations (>60 years).
- Articular reduction quality is associated with onset of posttraumatic radiographic arthrosis. Thus, younger patients may be better managed with more invasive techniques, such as open reduction and internal fixation in an effort to prevent this, however, additional data is required in this field.

PITFALLS

- Careful decision making to maximize outcome and minimize complications is critical particularly in the older population as radiographic outcome does not appear to predict functional outcome. Increasingly invasive techniques do appear to improve radiographic outcomes but have yet to demonstrate clinical benefit and there is an increased rate of complications with these techniques.
- Conventional volar plating may not adequately stabilize a volar lunate fragment and may result in loss of fixation and volar subluxation of the carpus.
- In the setting of bridging or closed reduction and internal fixation techniques distraction at the wrist and fracture site should be avoided during treatment to minimize the risk of CRPS.

Editor's Tips and Tricks: Fragment Specific Fixation for Articular DRF
Robert J. Medoff, Geert Alexander Buijze

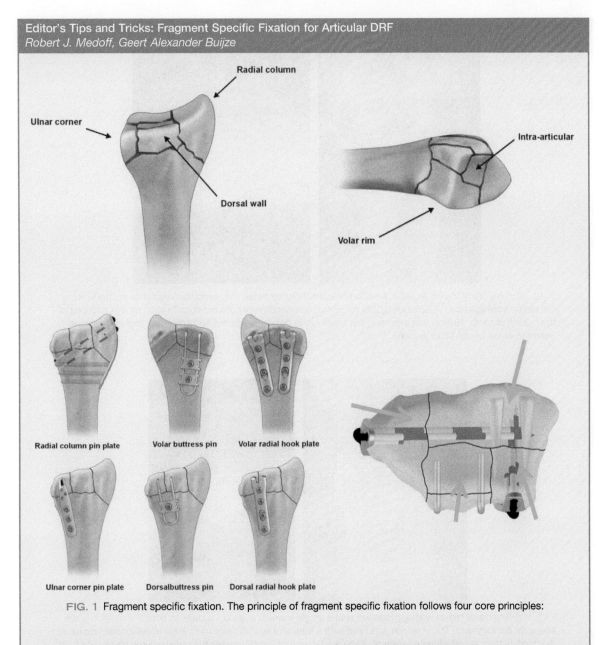

FIG. 1 Fragment specific fixation. The principle of fragment specific fixation follows four core principles:

1. Identify the primary fracture components
2. Obtain independent fixation using implants specific to each fracture component
3. Utilize semielastic fixation mechanisms, avoiding dependence on thread purchase in peri-articular fragments.
4. Create a load sharing construct.

    Treatment is individualized to the specific combination of fracture components present in a particular injury. The goal of this approach is to achieve a reconstruction that is load sharing.

Continued

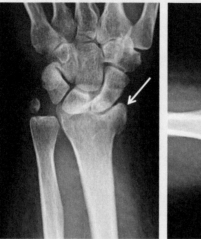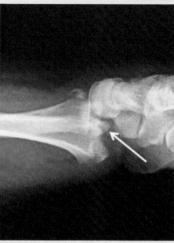

FIG. 2A This injury shows a carpal avulsion characterized by small, peri-articular fragments avulsed by the radiocarpal ligament. Restoring stability requires a combination of both osseous fixation as well as repair of the volar ligaments. Note in this example, the small radial column fragment and small, but highly displaced volar rim of the lunate facet (arrows).

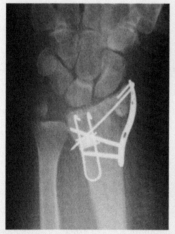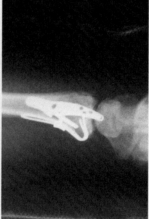

FIG. 2B The distal radius was approached with a single incision allowing access to both the radial column and volar rim fragment. The volar rim was fixed with a fragment specific wire form in combination with repair of the origin of the long radiolunate ligament. Bone graft was applied underneath the radial column fragment which was fixed with a fragment specific radial column plate to close and compressed the fracture across the coronal plane.

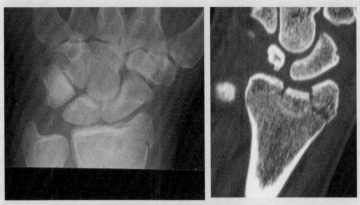

FIG. 3A This example is of a 22-year-old flight instructor who sustained an intraarticular dorsal shear fracture which included a depressed, central free articular fragment, a dorsal wall fragment, and a radial column fragment.

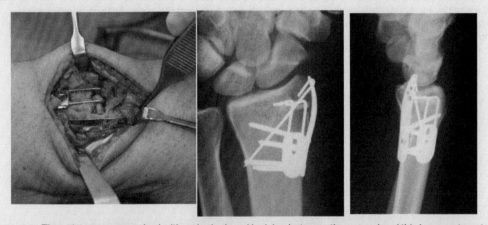

FIG. 3B The wrist was approached with a single dorsal incision between the second and third compartments, allowing simultaneous exposure of the dorsal wall and radial column. An arthrotomy was used to visualize congruous restoration of the joint surface, and the fracture was secured using bone graft behind the articular fragment and fragment specific implants as shown. Fixation was strong enough to allow immediate motion after surgery.

Continued

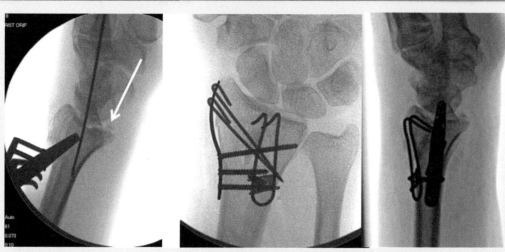

FIG. 4 This injury demonstrates a more extensive dorsal shear fracture involving the radial column, doral wall, and included a free intraarticular fragment. Note the intact articular portion of the volar rim but the presence of a small avulsed bone fleck off the volar rim indicating disruption of the origin of the volar radiocarpal ligaments (arrow). An impactor placed through the metaphyseal defect dorally was used to reduce the free intraarticular piece to the proximal carpal row (left); the fracture was then secured with bone graft to the metaphyseal defect, a dorsal wire form, and a fragment specific radial column plate.

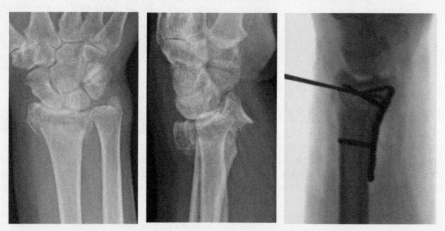

FIG. 5A This intraarticular fracture shows a radial column, ulnar corner, dorsal wall, and volar rim fragment. Note the extreme dorsiflexion of the volar rim (depressed teardrop angle) associated with sagittal shift of lateral carpal alignment. In these types of highly unstable, multiarticular patterns, the volar rim of the lunate facet is usually addressed first and helps reduce and support the unstable carpus. In this case, a volar hook plate was used to correct dorsiflexion of the teardrop and secure the volar rim; next, a dorsal approach was added to stabilize the ulnar corner and dorsal wall.

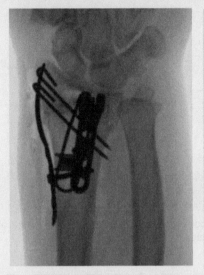
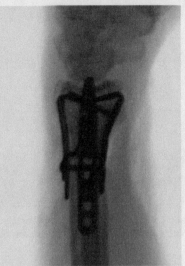

FIG. 5B Fixation was completed with bone graft to the metaphyseal defect and application of a radial column fragment specific plate.

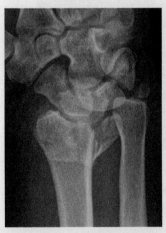
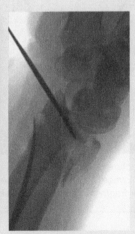
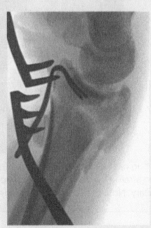

FIG. 6A Another example of a highly comminuted intraarticular fracture of the distal radius. The approach starts with a volar exposure and using K-wires to reduce the dorsiflexed volar rim, allowing reduction and fixation of this fragment and helps correct the sagittal shift of the lateral carpal alignment.

Continued

Editor's Tips and Tricks: Fragment Specific Fixation for Articular DRF—cont'd

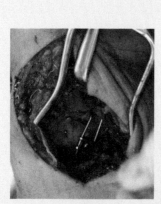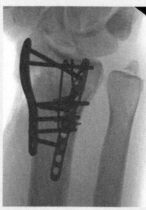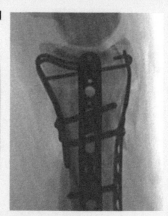

FIG. 6B Fixation of the volar rim is completed and a dorsal approach is added to secure the dorsal portion of the sigmoid notch and dorsal wall. A radial column plate is added to complete the fixation.

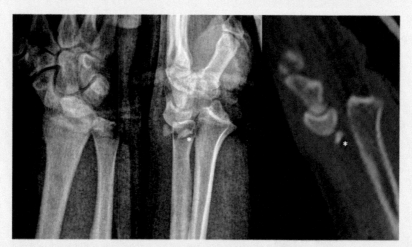

FIG. 7 In case of (open) radiocarpal fracture dislocations, one can opt for a one-stage or two-stage fixation strategy, with debridement and lavage, carpal tunnel release and temporary external fixation as necessary. Note the small critical corner fragment (*) including the short radiolunate ligament.

Editor's Tips and Tricks: Fragment Specific Fixation for Articular DRF—cont'd

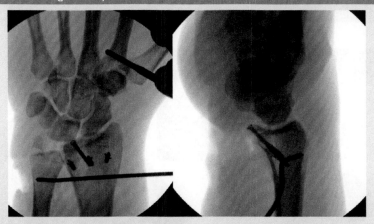

FIG. 8 Definitive fixation requires anatomic reduction and fixation of the critical corner fragment to provide stable carpal alignment (buttressing the lunate), and suturing of the (volar) radiocarpal ligaments with several anchors.

Editors' Tips and Tricks: Innovative Suture Technique to Fix a Dorsal Rim Fragment Through a Volar Plate in Comminuted Articular DRFs

Márcio Aurélio Aita

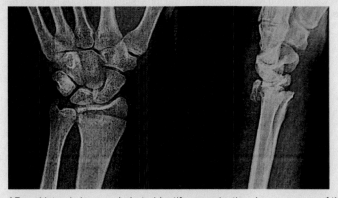

FIG. 1 Use of the AP and lateral view can help to identify comminution, incongruency of the palmar/dorsal radial rim, for instance, when a dorsoradial fragment remains unreduced.

Continued

Editors' Tips and Tricks: Innovative Suture Technique to Fix a Dorsal Rim Fragment Through a Volar Plate in Comminuted Articular DRFs—cont'd

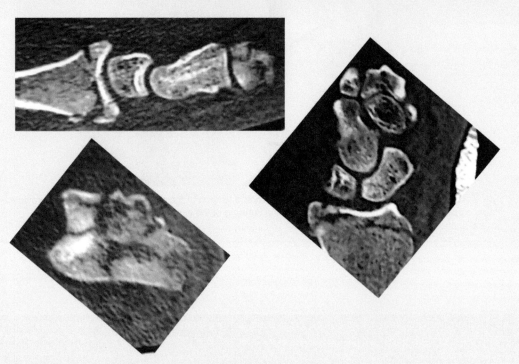

FIG. 2 Use of CT scanning with reconstructions in the three standard planes can also help to identify comminution, incongruency of the palmar/dorsal radial rim.

Editors' Tips and Tricks: Innovative Suture Technique to Fix a Dorsal Rim Fragment Through a Volar Plate in Comminuted Articular DRFs—cont'd

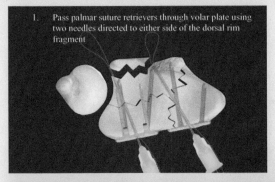

1. Pass palmar suture retrievers through volar plate using two needles directed to either side of the dorsal rim fragment

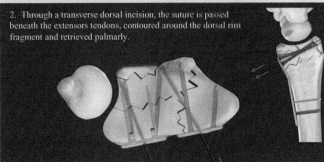

2. Through a transverse dorsal incision, the suture is passed beneath the extensors tendons, contoured around the dorsal rim fragment and retrieved palmarly.

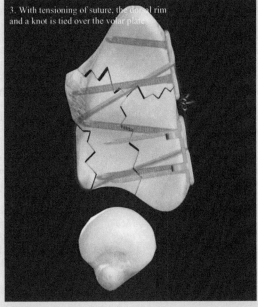

3. With tensioning of suture, the dorsal rim and a knot is tied over the volar plate.

FIG. 3 Three steps to reduce and fix a dorsal rim fragment with a suture through a volar plate (see Video 1 from https://www.elsevier.com/books-and-journals/book-companion/9780323757645).

Continued

Editors' Tips and Tricks: Innovative Suture Technique to Fix a Dorsal Rim Fragment Through a Volar Plate in Comminuted Articular DRFs—cont'd

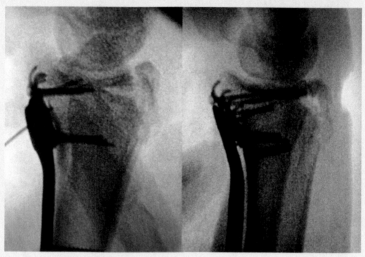

FIG. 4 The lateral view appreciates the restored congruency of the dorsal rim before and after transradial suture reduction and knot tying.

REFERENCES

1. Grewal R, MacDermid JC, King GJW, Faber KJ. Open reduction internal fixation versus percutaneous pinning with external fixation of distal radius fractures: a prospective, randomized clinical trial. *J Hand Surg [Am].* 2011;36(12):1899–1906. https://doi.org/10.1016/j.jhsa.2011.09.015.

2. Roh YH, Lee BK, Baek JR, Noh JH, Gong HS, Baek GH. A randomized comparison of volar plate and external fixation for intra-articular distal radius fractures. *J Hand Surg [Am].* 2014;40(1):34–41. https://doi.org/10.1016/j.jhsa.2014.09.025.

3. Fowler TP, Fitzpatrick E. Simultaneous fractures of the ipsilateral scaphoid and distal radius. *J Wrist Surg.* 2018;7 (4):303–311. https://doi.org/10.1055/s-0038-1641719.

4. Kennedy SA, Hanel DP. Complex distal radius fractures. *Orthop Clin North Am.* 2013;44(1):81–92. https://doi.org/10.1016/j.ocl.2012.08.008.

5. Tsitsilonis S, Machó D, Manegold S, Krapohl BD, Wichlas F. Fracture severity of distal radius fractures treated with locking plating correlates with limitations in ulnar abduction and inferior health-related quality of life. *J Wrist Surg.* 2016;5. https://doi.org/10.3205/iprs000099, Doc20.

6. Yoon JO, You SL, Kim JK. Intra-articular comminution worsens outcomes of distal radial fractures treated by open reduction and palmar locking plate fixation. *J Hand Surg Eur Vol.* 2016;42(3):260–265. https://doi.org/10.1177/1753193416682943.

7. Cole RJ, Bindra RR, Evanoff BA, Gilula LA, Yamaguchi K, Gelberman RH. Radiographic evaluation of osseous displacement following intra-articular fractures of the distal radius: reliability of plain radiography versus computed tomography. *J Hand Surg [Am].* 1997;22(5):792–800. https://doi.org/10.1016/s0363-5023(97)80071-8.

8. das Nascimento VG, da Costa AC, Falcochio DF, Lanzarin LD, Checchia SL, Chakkour I. Computed tomography's influence on the classifications and treatment of the distal radius fractures. *Hand N Y.* 2015;10(4):663–669. https://doi.org/10.1007/s11552-015-9773-8.

9. Nakamura R, Horii E, Tanaka Y, Imaeda T, Hayakawa N. Three-dimensional CT imaging for wrist disorders. *J Hand Surg (Br).* 1989;14(1):53–58. https://doi.org/10.1016/0266-7681(89)90016-8.

10. Catalano LW, Barron OA, Glickel SZ. Assessment of articular displacement of distal radius fractures. *Clin Orthop Relat Res.* 2004;423:79–84. https://doi.org/10.1097/01.blo.0000132884.51311.28.

11. Pruitt DL, Gilula LA, Manske PR, Vannier MW. Computed tomography scanning with image reconstruction in evaluation of distal radius fractures. *J Hand Surg [Am].* 1994;19(5):720–727. https://doi.org/10.1016/0363-5023 (94)90174-0.

12. Katz MA, Beredjiklian PK, Bozentka DJ, Steinberg DR. Computed tomography scanning of intra-articular distal radius fractures: does it influence treatment? *J Hand Surg*

[Am]. 2001;26(3):415–421. https://doi.org/10.1053/jhsu.2001.22930a.

13. Nana AD, Joshi A, Lichtman DM. Plating of the distal radius. J Am Acad Orthop Surg. 2005;13(3):159–171.

14. Rhee PC, Medoff RJ, Shin AY. Complex distal radius fractures: an anatomic algorithm for surgical management. J Am Acad Orthop Surg. 2017;25(2):77–88. https://doi.org/10.5435/jaaos-d-15-00525.

15. Rozental TD, Blazar PE, Franko OI, Chacko AT, Earp BE, Day CS. Functional outcomes for unstable distal radial fractures treated with open reduction and internal fixation or closed reduction and percutaneous fixation. J Bone Joint Surg Am. 2009;91(8):1837–1846. https://doi.org/10.2106/jbjs.h.01478.

16. Rhee PC, Dennison DG, Kakar S. Avoiding and treating perioperative complications of distal radius fractures. Hand Clin. 2012;28(2):185–198. https://doi.org/10.1016/j.hcl.2012.03.004.

17. Lozano-Calderón SA, Doornberg J, Ring D. Fractures of the dorsal articular margin of the distal part of the radius with dorsal radiocarpal subluxation. J Bone Joint Surg Am. 2006;88(7):1486–1493. https://doi.org/10.2106/jbjs.e.00930.

18. Rikli DA, Rosenkranz J, Regazzoni P. Complex fractures of the distal radius. Eur J Trauma. 2003;29(4):199–207. https://doi.org/10.1007/s00068-003-1205-8.

19. Jakob M, Rikli DA, Regazzoni P. Fractures of the distal radius treated by internal fixation and early function. J Bone Joint Surg (Br). 2000;82(3):340–344. https://doi.org/10.1302/0301-620x.82b3.10099.

20. Williksen JH, Frihagen F, Hellund JC, Kvernmo HD, Husby T. Volar locking plates versus external fixation and adjuvant pin fixation in unstable distal radius fractures: a randomized, controlled study. J Hand Surg [Am]. 2013;38(8):1469–1476. https://doi.org/10.1016/j.jhsa.2013.04.039.

21. Gavaskar AS, Muthukumar S, Chowdary N. Fragment-specific fixation for complex intra-articular fractures of the distal radius: results of a prospective single-centre trial. J Hand Surg Eur Vol. 2012;37(8):765–771. https://doi.org/10.1177/1753193412439677.

22. Song J, Yu A-X, Li Z-H. Comparison of conservative and operative treatment for distal radius fracture: a meta-analysis of randomized controlled trials. Int J Clin Exp Med. 2015;8(10):17023–17035.

23. Knirk JL, Jupiter JB. Intra-articular fractures of the distal end of the radius in young adults. J Bone Joint Surg Am. 1986;68(5):647–659. https://doi.org/10.2106/00004623-198668050-00003.

24. Schneeberger AG, Ip WY, Poon TL, Chow SP. Open reduction and plate fixation of displaced AO type C3 fractures of the distal radius: restoration of articular congruity in eighteen cases. J Orthop Trauma. 2001;15(5):350–357. https://doi.org/10.1097/00005131-200106000-00008.

25. Bartl C, Stengel D, Bruckner T, Gebhard F. The Treatment of Displaced Intra-articular Distal Radius Fractures in Elderly Patients. Dtsch Arztebl Int. 2014. https://doi.org/10.3238/arztebl.2014.0779.

26. Martinez-Mendez D, Lizaur-Utrilla A, de Juan-Herrero J. Intra-articular distal radius fractures in elderly patients: a randomized prospective study of casting versus volar plating. J Hand Surg Eur Vol. 2017;43(2):142–147. https://doi.org/10.1177/1753193417727139.

27. Arora R, Lutz M, Deml C, Krappinger D, Haug L, Gabl M. A prospective randomized trial comparing nonoperative treatment with volar locking plate fixation for displaced and unstable distal radial fractures in patients sixty-five years of age and older. J Bone Joint Surg Am. 2011;93(23):2146–2153. https://doi.org/10.2106/jbjs.j.01597.

28. Zengin EC, Ozcan C, Aslan C, Bulut T, Sener M. Cast immobilization versus volar locking plate fixation of AO type C distal radial fractures in patients aged 60 years and older. Acta Orthop Traumatol Turc. 2018;53(1):15–18. https://doi.org/10.1016/j.aott.2018.10.005.

29. Toon DH, Premchand RAX, Sim J, Vaikunthan R. Outcomes and financial implications of intra-articular distal radius fractures: a comparative study of open reduction internal fixation (ORIF) with volar locking plates versus nonoperative management. J Orthop Traumatol. 2017;18(3):229–234. https://doi.org/10.1007/s10195-016-0441-8.

30. Arora R, Gabl M, Gschwentner M, Deml C, Krappinger D, Lutz M. A comparative study of clinical and radiologic outcomes of unstable colles type distal radius fractures in patients older than 70 years nonoperative treatment versus volar locking plating. J Orthop Trauma. 2009;23(4):237–242. https://doi.org/10.1097/bot.0b013e31819b24e9.

31. Mulders MAM, Walenkamp MMJ, Goslings JC, Schep NWL. Internal plate fixation versus plaster in displaced complete articular distal radius fractures, a randomised controlled trial. BMC Musculoskelet Disord. 2016;17(1):68. https://doi.org/10.1186/s12891-016-0925-y.

32. Walenkamp MMJ, Mulders MAM, van Hilst J, Goslings JC, Schep NWL. Prediction of distal radius fracture redisplacement. J Orthop Trauma. 2018;32(3):e92–e96. https://doi.org/10.1097/bot.0000000000001105.

33. Lutz M, Arora R, Krappinger D, Wambacher M, Rieger M, Pechlaner S. Arthritis predicting factors in distal intraarticular radius fractures. Arch Orthop Trauma Surg. 2010;131(8):1121–1126. https://doi.org/10.1007/s00402-010-1211-3.

34. Beumer A, McQueen MM. Fractures of the distal radius in low-demand elderly patients: closed reduction of no value in 53 of 60 wrists. Acta Orthop Scand. 2003;74(1):98–100. https://doi.org/10.1080/00016470310013743.

35. Trumble TE, Schmitt SR, Vedder NB. Factors affecting functional outcome of displaced intra-articular distal radius fractures. J Hand Surg [Am]. 1994;19(2):325–340. https://doi.org/10.1016/0363-5023(94)90028-0.

36. Synn AJ, Makhni EC, Makhni MC, Rozental TD, Day CS. Distal radius fractures in older patients: is anatomic reduction necessary? Clin Orthop Relat Res. 2008;467

(6):1612–1620. https://doi.org/10.1007/s11999-008-0660-2.

37. Strange-Vognsen HH. Intraarticular fractures of the distal end of the radius in young adults: a 16 (2–26) year follow-up of 42 patients. *Acta Orthop Scand*. 1991;62(6):527–530. https://doi.org/10.3109/17453679108994488.

38. Young BT, Rayan GM. Outcome following nonoperative treatment of displaced distal radius fractures in low-demand patients older than 60 years. *J Hand Surg [Am]*. 2000;25(1):19–28. https://doi.org/10.1053/jhsu.2000.jhsu025a0019.

39. Vakhshori V, Rounds AD, Heckmann N, et al. The declining use of wrist-spanning external fixators. *Hand N Y*. 2018;15(2). https://doi.org/10.1177/1558944718791185,15589447187 91185.

40. Wang D, Shan L, Zhou J-L. Locking plate versus external fixation for type C distal radius fractures: a meta-analysis of randomized controlled trials. *Chin J Traumatol*. 2017;21(2):113–117. https://doi.org/10.1016/j.cjtee.2017.11.002.

41. Wang J, Lu Y, Cui Y, Wei X, Sun J. Is volar locking plate superior to external fixation for distal radius fractures? A comprehensive meta-analysis. *Acta Orthop Traumatol Turc*. 2018;52(5):334–342. https://doi.org/10.1016/j.aott.2018.06.001.

42. Wei DH, Poolman RW, Bhandari M, Wolfe VM, Rosenwasser MP. External fixation versus internal fixation for unstable distal radius fractures. *J Orthop Trauma*. 2012;26(7):386–394. https://doi.org/10.1097/bot.0b013e318225f63c.

43. Han LR, Jin CX, Yan J, Han SZ, He XB, Yang XF. Effectiveness of external fixator combined with T-plate internal fixation for the treatment of comminuted distal radius fractures. *Genet Mol Res*. 2015;14(1):2912–2919. https://doi.org/10.4238/2015.march.31.22.

44. Navarro CM, Ahrengart L, Törnqvist H, Ponzer S. Volar locking plate or external fixation with optional addition of K-wires for dorsally displaced distal radius fractures: a randomized controlled study. *J Orthop Trauma*. 2016;30 (4):217–224. https://doi.org/10.1097/bot.000000000 0000519.

45. Shukla R, Jain RK, Sharma NK, Kumar R. External fixation versus volar locking plate for displaced intra-articular distal radius fractures: a prospective randomized comparative study of the functional outcomes. *J Orthop Traumatol*. 2014;15(4):265–270. https://doi.org/10.1007/s10195-014-0317-8.

46. Anderson JT, Lucas GL, Buhr BR. Complications of treating distal radius fractures with external fixation: a community experience. *Iowa Orthop J*. 2004;24:53–59.

47. Capo JT, Rossy W, Henry P, Maurer RJ, Naidu S, Chen L. External fixation of distal radius fractures: effect of distraction and duration. *J Hand Surg [Am]*. 2009;34 (9):1605–1611. https://doi.org/10.1016/j.jhsa.2009.07.010.

48. Ma C, Deng Q, Pu H, et al. External fixation is more suitable for intra-articular fractures of the distal radius in elderly patients. *Bone Res*. 2016;4(1):16017. https://doi.org/10.1038/boneres.2016.17.

49. Sanders RA, Keppel FL, Waldrop JI. External fixation of distal radial fractures: results and complications. *J Hand Surg [Am]*. 1991;16(3):385–391. https://doi.org/10.1016/0363-5023(91)90002-s.

50. Saving J, Enocson A, Ponzer S, Navarro CM. External fixation versus volar locking plate for unstable dorsally displaced distal radius fractures-a 3-year follow-up of a randomized controlled study. *J Hand Surg [Am]*. 2018;44 (1):18–26. https://doi.org/10.1016/j.jhsa.2018.09.015.

51. Szabo RM, Weber SC. Comminuted intraarticular fractures of the distal radius. *Clin Orthop Relat Res*. 1988. https://doi.org/10.1097/00003086-198805000-00005.

52. Weber SC, Szabo RM. Severely comminuted distal radial fracture as an unsolved problem: complications associated with external fixation and pins and plaster techniques. *J Hand Surg [Am]*. 1986;11(2):157–165. https://doi.org/10.1016/s0363-5023(86)80045-4.

53. van Dijk JP, Laudy FGJ. Dynamic external fixation versus non-operative treatment of severe distal radial fractures. *Injury*. 1996;27(1):57–61. https://doi.org/10.1016/0020-1383(95)00151-4.

54. Zanotti RM, Louis DS. Intra-articular fractures of the distal end of the radius treated with an adjustable fixator system. *J Hand Surg [Am]*. 1997;22(3):428–440. https://doi.org/10.1016/s0363-5023(97)80009-3.

55. Vidal J, Buscayret C, Paran M, Melka J. Ligamentotaxis. In: Mears DC, ed. *External Skeletal Fixation*. Baltimore: Williams & Wilkins; 1983:493–496.

56. Ochi R, Nakano T, Abe Y, Shimizu Y, Seike I, Iwamoto K. Clinical results of external fixation for distal radius fractures. *Orthop Traumatol*. 1999;48(3):966–969. https://doi.org/10.5035/nishiseisai.48.966.

57. Egol K, Walsh M, Tejwani N, McLaurin T, Wynn C, Paksima N. Bridging external fixation and supplementary Kirschner-wire fixation versus volar locked plating for unstable fractures of the distal radius: a randomised, prospective trial. *J Bone Joint Surg (Br)*. 2008;90(9):1214–1221. https://doi.org/10.1302/0301-620x.90b9.20521.

58. Comparison of external and percutaneous pin fixation with plate fixation for intra-articular distal radial fractures. A randomized study. In: *Cochrane Central Register Control Trials Central*. 2008(2); 2018. https://doi.org/10.1002/central/cn-00622070.

59. Pradhan R, Lakhey S, Pandey B, Manandhar R, Rijal K, Sharma S. External and internal fixation for comminuted intra-articular fractures of distal radius. *Kathmandu Univ Med J*. 1970;7(4):369–373. https://doi.org/10.3126/kumj.v7i4.2756.

60. Gouk C, Ng S-K, Knight M, Bindra R, Thomas M. Long term outcomes of open reduction internal fixation versus external fixation of distal radius fractures: a meta-analysis. *Orthop Rev*. 2019;11(3):7809. https://doi.org/10.4081/or.2019.7809.

61. Kumbaraci M, Kucuk L, Karapinar L, Kurt C, Coskunol E. Retrospective comparison of external fixation versus

volar locking plate in the treatment of unstable intra-articular distal radius fractures. *Eur J Orthop Surg Traumatol.* 2013;24(2):173–178. https://doi.org/10.1007/s00590-012-1155-0.

62. Diaz-Garcia RJ, Oda T, Shauver MJ, Chung KC. A systematic review of outcomes and complications of treating unstable distal radius fractures in the elderly. *J Hand Surg [Am].* 2011;36(5):824–835. e2 https://doi.org/10.1016/j.jhsa.2011.02.005.

63. Burke EF, Singer RM. Treatment of comminuted distal radius with the use of an internal distraction plate. *Tech Hand Up Extrem Surg.* 1998;2(4):248–252. https://doi.org/10.1097/00130911-199812000-00004.

64. Lauder A, Agnew S, Bakri K, Allan CH, Hanel DP, Huang JI. Functional outcomes following bridge plate fixation for distal radius fractures. *J Hand Surg [Am].* 2015;40(8):1554–1562. https://doi.org/10.1016/j.jhsa.2015.05.008.

65. Alluri RK, Hill JR, Ghiassi A. Distal radius fractures: approaches, indications, and techniques. *J Hand Surg [Am].* 2016;41(8):845–854. https://doi.org/10.1016/j.jhsa.2016.05.015.

66. Hanel DP, Ruhlman SD, Katolik LI, Allan CH. Complications associated with distraction plate fixation of wrist fractures. *Hand Clin.* 2010;26(2):237–243. https://doi.org/10.1016/j.hcl.2010.01.001.

67. Hanel DP, Lu TS, Weil WM. Bridge plating of distal radius fractures. *Clin Orthop Relat Res.* 2006;91–99. https://doi.org/10.1097/01.blo.0000205885.58458.f9.

68. Richard MJ, Katolik LI, Hanel DP, Wartinbee DA, Ruch DS. Distraction plating for the treatment of highly comminuted distal radius fractures in elderly patients. *J Hand Surg [Am].* 2012;37(5):948–956. https://doi.org/10.1016/j.jhsa.2012.02.034.

69. Ginn TA, Ruch DS, Yang CC, Hanel DP. Use of a distraction plate for distal radial fractures with metaphyseal and diaphyseal comminution. *J Bone Joint Surg Am.* 2006;88(1_suppl_1):29–36. https://doi.org/10.2106/00004623-200603001-00004.

70. Lewis S, Mostofi A, Stevanovic M, Ghiassi A. Risk of tendon entrapment under a dorsal bridge plate in a distal radius fracture model. *J Hand Surg [Am].* 2015;40(3):500–504. https://doi.org/10.1016/j.jhsa.2014.11.020.

71. Dahl J, Lee DJ, Elfar JC. Anatomic relationships in distal radius bridge plating: a cadaveric study. *Hand N Y.* 2015;10(4):657–662. https://doi.org/10.1007/s11552-015-9762-y.

72. Alluri RK, Bougioukli S, Stevanovic M, Ghiassi A. A biomechanical comparison of distal fixation for bridge plating in a distal radius fracture model. *J Hand Surg [Am].* 2017;42(9):748.e1–748.e8. https://doi.org/10.1016/j.jhsa.2017.05.010.

73. Wolf JC, Weil WM, Hanel DP, Trumble TE. A biomechanic comparison of an internal radiocarpal-spanning 2.4-mm locking plate and external fixation in a model of distal radius fractures. *J Hand Surg [Am].* 2006;31(10):1578–1586. https://doi.org/10.1016/j.jhsa.2006.09.014.

74. Dodds SD, Save AV, Yacob A. Dorsal spanning plate fixation for distal radius fractures. *Tech Hand Up Extrem Surg.* 2013;17(4):192–198. https://doi.org/10.1097/bth.0b013e3182a5cbf8.

75. Azad, et al. Wrist-spanning fixation of radiocarpal dislocation: a cadaveric assessment of ulnar translation. *Hand (N Y).* 2019. https://doi.org/10.1177/1558944719873148.

76. Guerrero EM, Lauder A, Federer AE, Glisson R, Richard MJ, Ruch DS. Metacarpal position and lunate facet screw fixation in dorsal wrist-spanning bridge plates for intra-articular distal radial fracture: a biomechanical analysis. *J Bone Joint Surg Am.* 2020;102(5):397–403. https://doi.org/10.2106/jbjs.19.00769.

77. Jain MJ, Mavani KJ. A comprehensive study of internal distraction plating, an alternative method for distal radius fractures. *J Clin Diagn Res.* 2016;10(12):RC14–RC17. https://doi.org/10.7860/jcdr/2016/21926.9036.

78. Benson LS, Minihane KP, Stern LD, Eller E, Seshadri R. The outcome of intra-articular distal radius fractures treated with fragment-specific fixation. *J Hand Surg [Am].* 2006;31(8):1333–1339. https://doi.org/10.1016/j.jhsa.2006.07.004.

79. Perlus R, Doyon J, Henry P. The use of dorsal distraction plating for severely comminuted distal radius fractures: a review and comparison to volar plate fixation. *Injury.* 2019;50(Suppl 1):S50–S55. https://doi.org/10.1016/j.injury.2019.03.052 [Bone Joint J 96-B 7 2014].

80. Chaudhry H, Kleinlugtenbelt YV, Mundi R, Ristevski B, Goslings JC, Bhandari M. Are volar locking plates superior to percutaneous K-wires for distal radius fractures? A meta-analysis. *Clin Orthop Relat Res.* 2015;473(9):3017–3027. https://doi.org/10.1007/s11999-015-4347-1.

81. del Piñal F. Technical tips for (dry) arthroscopic reduction and internal fixation of distal radius fractures. *J Hand Surg [Am].* 2011;36(10):1694–1705. https://doi.org/10.1016/j.jhsa.2011.07.021.

82. Piñal FD, Klausmeyer M, Moraleda E, de Piero GH, Rúas JS. Arthroscopic reduction of comminuted intra-articular distal radius fractures with diaphyseal-metaphyseal comminution. *J Hand Surg [Am].* 2014;39(5):835–843. https://doi.org/10.1016/j.jhsa.2014.02.013.

83. Burnier M, Riquier MLC, Herzberg G. Treatment of intra-articular fracture of distal radius fractures with fluoroscopic only or combined with arthroscopic control: a prospective tomodensitometric comparative study of 40 patients. *Orthop Traumatol Surg Res.* 2018;104(1):89–93. https://doi.org/10.1016/j.otsr.2017.08.021.

84. Freeland AE, Geissler WB. The arthroscopic management of intra-articular distal radius fractures. *Hand Surg.* 2000;05(02):93–102. https://doi.org/10.1142/s021881040000020x.

85. Chung KC, Shauver MJ, Birkmeyer JD. Trends in the United States in the treatment of distal radial fractures in the elderly. *J Bone Joint Surg Am.* 2009;91(8):1868–1873. https://doi.org/10.2106/jbjs.h.01297.

86. Chou Y-C, Chen AC-Y, Chen C-Y, Hsu Y-H, Wu C-C. Dorsal and volar 2.4-mm titanium locking plate fixation for AO Type C3 dorsally comminuted distal radius fractures. *J Hand Surg [Am]*. 2011;36(6):974–981. https://doi.org/10.1016/j.jhsa.2011.02.024.

87. Jakubietz RG, Gruenert JG, Kloss DF, Schindele S, Jakubietz MG. A randomised clinical study comparing palmar and dorsal fixed-angle plates for the internal fixation of AO C-type fractures of the distal radius in the elderly. *J Hand Surg Eur Vol*. 2008;33(5):600–604. https://doi.org/10.1177/1753193408094706.

88. Earp BE, Foster B, Blazar PE. The use of a single volar locking plate for AO C3-type distal radius fractures. *Hand N Y*. 2015;10(4):649–653. https://doi.org/10.1007/s11552-015-9757-8.

89. Arora R, Lutz M, Hennerbichler A, Krappinger D, Espen D, Gabl M. Complications following internal fixation of unstable distal radius fracture with a palmar locking-plate. *J Orthop Trauma*. 2007;21(5):316–322. https://doi.org/10.1097/bot.0b013e318059b993.

90. Sharma H, Khare GN, Singh S, Ramaswamy AG, Kumaraswamy V, Singh AK. Outcomes and complications of fractures of distal radius (AO type B and C): volar plating versus nonoperative treatment. *J Orthop Sci*. 2014;19(4):537–544. https://doi.org/10.1007/s00776-014-0560-0.

91. Marcheix P-S, Dotzis A, Benkö P-E, Siegler J, Arnaud J-P, Charissoux J-L. Extension fractures of the distal radius in patients older than 50: a prospective randomized study comparing fixation using mixed pins or a palmar fixed-angle plate. *J Hand Surg Eur Vol*. 2010;35(8):646–651. https://doi.org/10.1177/1753193410364179.

92. Karantana A, Downing ND, Forward DP, et al. Surgical treatment of distal radial fractures with a volar locking plate versus conventional percutaneous methods. *J Bone Joint Surg Am*. 2013;95(19):1737–1744. https://doi.org/10.2106/jbjs.l.00232.

93. Catalano LW, Cole RJ, Gelberman RH, Evanoff BA, Gilula LA, Borrelli J. Displaced intra-articular fractures of the distal aspect of the radius. *J Bone Joint Surg Am*. 1997;79(9):1290–1302. https://doi.org/10.2106/00004623-199709000-00003.

94. Fernandez JJ, Gruen GS, Herndon JH. Outcome of distal radius fractures using the short form 36 health survey. *Clin Orthop Relat Res*. 1997;341. https://doi.org/10.1097/00003086-199708000-00007.

95. Orbay JL, Badia A, Indriago IR, Infante A. The extended flexor carpi radialis approach: a new perspective for the distal radius fracture. *Tech Hand Up Extrem Surg*. 2001;5(4):204–211.

96. Orbay J. Volar plate fixation of distal radius fractures. *Hand Clin*. 2005;21(3):347–354. https://doi.org/10.1016/j.hcl.2005.02.003.

97. Gruber G, Gerald G, Gruber K, et al. Volar plate fixation of AO type C2 and C3 distal radius fractures, a single-center study of 55 patients. *J Orthop Trauma*. 2008;22(7):467–472. https://doi.org/10.1097/bot.0b013e318180db09.

98. Beck JD, Harness NG, Spencer HT. Volar plate fixation failure for volar shearing distal radius fractures with small lunate facet fragments. *J Hand Surg [Am]*. 2014;39(4):670–678. https://doi.org/10.1016/j.jhsa.2014.01.006.

99. Harness NG, Jupiter JB, Orbay JL, Raskin KB, Fernandez DL. Loss of fixation of the volar lunate facet fragment in fractures of the distal part of the radius. *J Bone Joint Surg Am*. 2004;86-A(9):1900–1908.

100. Apergis E, Darmanis S, Theodoratos G, Maris J. Beware of the Ulno-palmar distal radial fragment. *J Hand Surg [Am]*. 2002;27(2):139–145. https://doi.org/10.1054/jhsb.2001.0712.

101. Brink P, Rikli D. Four-corner concept: CT-based assessment of fracture patterns in distal radius. *J Wrist Surg*. 2016;05(02):147–151. https://doi.org/10.1055/s-0035-1570462.

102. O'Shaughnessy M, Shin A, Kakar S. Stabilization of volar ulnar rim fractures of the distal radius: current techniques and review of the literature. *J Wrist Surg*. 2016;05(02):113–119. https://doi.org/10.1055/s-0036-1579549.

103. Martineau PA, Berry GK, Harvey EJ. Plating for distal radius fractures. *Orthop Clin North Am*. 2007;38(2):193–201. https://doi.org/10.1016/j.ocl.2007.01.001.

104. O'Shaughnessy MA, Shin AY, Kakar S. Volar marginal rim fracture fixation with volar fragment-specific hook plate fixation. *J Hand Surg [Am]*. 2015;40(8):1563–1570. https://doi.org/10.1016/j.jhsa.2015.04.021.

105. Dodds SD, Cornelissen S, Jossan S, Wolfe SW. A biomechanical comparison of fragment-specific fixation and augmented external fixation for intra-articular distal radius fractures. *J Hand Surg [Am]*. 2002;27(6):953–964. https://doi.org/10.1053/jhsu.2002.35897.

106. Taylor KF, Parks BG, Segalman KA. Biomechanical stability of a fixed-angle volar plate versus fragment-specific fixation system: cyclic testing in a C2-type distal radius cadaver fracture model. *J Hand Surg [Am]*. 2006;31(3):373–381. https://doi.org/10.1016/j.jhsa.2005.12.017.

107. Swigart CR, Wolfe SW. Limited incision open techniques for distal radius fracture management. *Orthop Clin North Am*. 2001;32(2):317–327. https://doi.org/10.1016/s0030-5898(05)70252-2.

108. Lutsky K, Boyer M, Goldfarb C. Dorsal locked plate fixation of distal radius fractures. *J Hand Surg [Am]*. 2013;38(7):1414–1422. https://doi.org/10.1016/j.jhsa.2013.04.019.

109. Farhan M, Wong J, Sreedharan S, Yong F, Teoh L. Combined volar and dorsal plating for complex comminuted distal radial fractures. *J Orthop Surg (Hong Kong)*. 2015;23(1):19–23. https://doi.org/10.1177/230949901502300105.

110. Ring D, Prommersberger K, Jupiter JB. Combined dorsal and volar plate fixation of complex fractures of the distal part of the radius. *J Bone Joint Surg Am*. 2005;87(Suppl 1 (Pt 2)):195–212.

111. Konrath GA, Bahler S. Open reduction and internal fixation of unstable distal radius fractures: results using the trimed

fixation system. *J Orthop Trauma.* 2002;16(8):578–585. https://doi.org/10.1097/00005131-200209000-00007.

112. Bakker AJ, Shin AY. Fragment-specific volar hook plate for volar marginal rim fractures. *Tech Hand Up Extrem Surg.* 2014;18(1):56–60. https://doi.org/10.1097/bth.0000000000000038.

113. Spiteri M, Roberts D, Ng W, Matthews J, Power D. Distal radius volar rim plate: technical and radiographic considerations. *World J Orthop.* 2017;8(7):567–573. https://doi.org/10.5312/wjo.v8.i7.567.

114. Biondi M, Keller M, Merenghi L, Gabl M, Lauri G. Hook plate for volar rim fractures of the distal radius: review of the first 23 cases and focus on dorsal radiocarpal dislocation. *J Wrist Surg.* 2018;08(02):093–099. https://doi.org/10.1055/s-0038-1667306.

115. Marcano A, Taormina DP, Karia R, Paksima N, Posner M, Egol KA. Displaced intra-articular fractures involving the volar rim of the distal radius. *J Hand Surg [Am].* 2015;40(1):42–48. https://doi.org/10.1016/j.jhsa.2014.09.013.

116. Sammer DM, Fuller DS, Kim HM, Chung KC. A comparative study of fragment-specific versus volar plate fixation of distal radius fractures. *Plast Reconstr Surg.* 2008;122(5):1441–1450. https://doi.org/10.1097/prs.0b013e3181891677.

117. Lozano-Calderón SA, Souer S, Mudgal C, Jupiter JB, Ring D. Wrist mobilization following volar plate fixation of fractures of the distal part of the radius. *J Bone Joint Surg Am.* 2008;90(6):1297–1304. https://doi.org/10.2106/jbjs.g.01368.

118. Chung KC, Squitieri L, Kim HM. Comparative outcomes study using the volar locking plating system for distal radius fractures in both young adults and adults older than 60 years. *J Hand Surg [Am].* 2008;33(6):809–819. https://doi.org/10.1016/j.jhsa.2008.02.016.

119. Beck JD, Brothers JG, Maloney PJ, Deegan JH, Tang X, Klena JC. Predicting the outcome of revision carpal tunnel release. *J Hand Surg [Am].* 2012;37(2):282–287. https://doi.org/10.1016/j.jhsa.2011.10.040.

CHAPTER 13

Extra-Articular Distal Radius Fractures With Metaphyseal Comminution

C.C. DRIJFHOUT VAN HOOFF • NIELS W.L. SCHEP
Department of Trauma Surgery, Maasstad Hospital, Rotterdam, Netherlands

KEY POINTS

- The mainstay treatment for displaced extra-articular distal radius fractures with limited metaphyseal comminution is closed reduction and plaster immobilization. However, not all patients benefit.
- Carpal alignment and coronal plane translation are less familiar parameters to surgeons but important reduction criteria for these extra-articular distal radius fractures.
- Patients aged 18–75 years benefit from early open reduction and volar plate fixation, notably in more comminuted fractures.
- Optimal plate and screw positioning will decrease likelihood of tendinitis or tendon rupture.
- In case of more extensive metaphyseal comminution, (longer) volar plates, various methods of external fixation and intramedullary nailing result in comparable good outcomes.

Panel 1: Case Scenarios

A 55-year-old, right-handed female interior decorator visits the emergency department with a swollen and deformed right wrist after a fall from a horse on the outstretched hand. Radiographs show an extra-articular distal radius fracture with 20 degrees of dorsal angulation and dorsal metaphyseal comminution (Fig. 1). After closed reduction 15 degrees dorsal angulation persists (Fig. 2).

At the same time a 97-year-old lady comes in with a comminuted metaphyseal DRF as part of a distal forearm fracture and associated 2 cm-wound on the volar ulnar side (Fig. 3).

Which treatment is most effective for these comminuted extra-articular distal radius fractures?

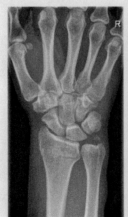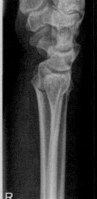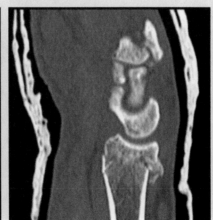

FIG. 1 Radiographs show an extra-articular distal radius fracture with 30 degrees of dorsal angulation and dorsal metaphyseal comminution.

Continued

Distal Radius Fractures. https://doi.org/10.1016/B978-0-323-75764-5.00009-3

Panel 1: Case Scenarios—cont'd

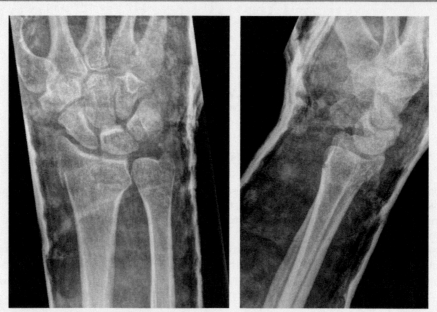

FIG. 2 After closed reduction 15 degrees dorsal angulation persists.

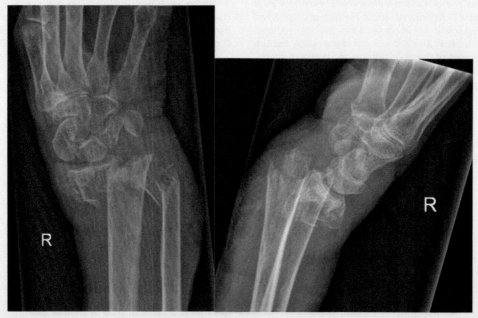

FIG. 3 Comminuted metaphyseal DRF as part of a distal forearm fracture and associated 2 cm-wound on the volar ulnar side.

IMPORTANCE OF THE PROBLEM

One in six fractures are distal radius fractures (DRFs).[1] Moreover, in the United States 600,000 DRFs are diagnosed every year[1] causing 480 million USD of direct cost of care.[2] As the population continues to age, the burden of distal radius fractures and the direct and indirect healthcare costs are expected to increase.

Overall incidence for DRFs in adults is 20 per 10,000 person-years. Extra-articular fractures are most common with an estimated incidence of 50%.[3] However, these figures are based on conventional radiographs. When using CT scans, the true incidence of AO type A fractures may be lower.

For displaced extra-articular distal radius fractures with limited comminution closed reduction and plaster immobilization is recommended as the treatment of choice. However, secondary dislocation is common and may result in poor patient-rated outcomes if left untreated.[4] Therefore, the question remains what the most effective therapeutic approach for comminuted extra-articular DRFs is?

Accurate assessment of standard radiographs is essential for appropriate treatment of extra-articular DRFs (Box 1, Fig. 4). Fracture anatomy and the degree of displacement may guide treatment.

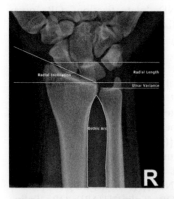

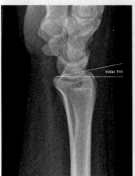 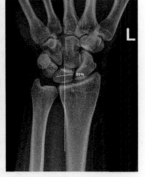

FIG. 4 Accurate assessment of standard radiographs is essential for appropriate treatment of extra-articular DRFs.

BOX 1
Radiographic Parameters

POSTERIOR ANTERIOR VIEW

– Radial inclination: Measures from the tip of radial styloid process (PSR) to the center point of the ulnar side of the distal radius. This center point (CRP) is located between the volar and dorsal rim which can easily be identified on the PA radiograph. Radial inclination is normally 20–25 degrees.[5]

– Ulnar Variance: The distance between the CRP and distal articular surface of the ulna. Normally +0.9 mm (range −4.2 to 2.3 mm).[6]

– Radial length: is defined by the length measured between the tip of the radial styloid and the distal articular surface of the ulna. Normally 10–13 mm.

– Coronal plane translation[7, 8]: is used to describe radial displacement of the distal fragment. Radial translation of the distal fragment might be associated with DRUJ instability due to lack of tension on the distal oblique bundle (the most distal part of the distal interosseous membrane) and the pronator quadratus. Coronal plane translation can be measured by drawing a line on the ulnar side of the radius which intersects the lunate. The point of intersection within the lunate is evaluated by drawing a second line along the transverse width of the lunate parallel with the distal joint. In a normal situation the lines should bisect at 50%.

– In a congruent DRUJ the ulnar side of the distal radius and radial side of the ulna should converge in the form of a Gothic arc. This arc should not be interrupted.

LATERAL VIEW

– On a pure lateral radiograph, the pisiform projects over the distal pole of the scaphoid, between the distal pole of the scaphoid and the capitate. Only then, can the surgeon assess volar or dorsal dislocation of the ulna.

– Volar tilt: Angle between a line drawn through the center of the radial shaft and a line drawn through the apices of the palmar and dorsal rims of the radius. The normal volar tilt is between 5 and 11 degrees[5]

– Carpal alignment: It is measured by drawing a line along the inner rim of the volar cortex of the radius (marginal line of Lewis) and determining the center of the capitate. (The center of the capitate is at the center of a circle drawn around the base of the capitate.) The carpus is aligned when the line along the inner rim transects the center of the capitate. By measuring the perpendicular distance to the center of the capitate, the degree of carpal malalignment can be quantified. Carpal malalignment is correlated with poor functional outcome.[9] Based on the study of Selles et al.,[10] a margin of 0.5 cm of dorsal and 0.5 cm of volar displacement would be within the range of normal alignment (Fig. 5).

Continued

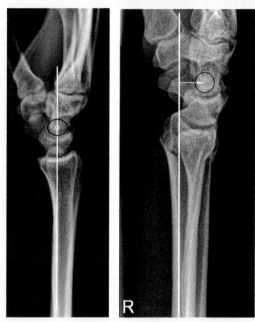

BOX 1
Radiographic Parameters—cont'd

R

FIG. 5 A margin of 0.5 cm of dorsal and 0.5 cm of volar displacement would be within the range of normal alignment.

The definition of a dislocated extra-articular fracture is when extra-articular radiologic parameters are not within the normal ranges as described in Box 1. In most situations, a closed reduction will be performed followed by a radiograph. However, what radiographic anatomy can we accept to continue nonoperative treatment? Historically, Lafontaine's criteria were used as the main guideline (See Chapter 9). Currently, the AAOS guidelines advise nonoperative treatment for fractures with post reduction radial shortening <3 mm and dorsal tilt of <10 degrees. On the contrary, the Dutch guidelines are more liberal: less than 10 degrees tilt in any direction and less than 5 mm radial shortening. If all of these are applicable, conservative treatment is advised.

In 2015, a systematic review was performed by Walenkamp et al.[11] to identify predictors of secondary displacement in DRFs. Female gender, age over 60 and dorsal comminution were significant predictors for secondary displacement. Associated ulnar styloid fractures, initial dorsal angulation >20 degrees or articular involvement were found to be nonsignificant.

MAIN QUESTION

What is the most effective therapeutic approach for comminuted extra-articular displaced DRFs?

CURRENT OPINION

The mainstay treatment of displaced extra-articular DRFs with limited comminution in adults is closed reduction and immobilization in a cast. However, even in case of adequate reduction, secondary dislocation of the fracture occurs in up to 60% of cases.[12] In recent years operative treatment of extra-articular DRFs with open reduction and fixation with a volar locking plate has become increasing popular. Open reduction and volar plate fixation allows for early mobilization and therefore may lead to improved functional outcome. In case of more extensive metaphyseal comminution, longer volar plates with optional bone grafting (Fig. 6) or alternative solid constructs such as bridging spanning plates, or external fixation are recommended.

FINDING THE EVIDENCE

Search algorithms used to retrieve evidence for the main question:

- Cochrane search: "distal radius fracture" OR "distal radial fracture" AND "plate fixation" OR "open reduction internal fixation"
- Pubmed (Medline): ((((("Radius Fractures"[Mesh] OR "distal radius fractures"[TIAB]) OR "distal radius"[TIAB]) OR Radius Fractures[TIAB]) AND ((((("Casts, Surgical"[Mesh] OR Casts[TIAB]) OR "Splint"[TIAB]) OR "Splinting"[TIAB]) OR casting [TIAB]) OR (((plate[TIAB] OR plating[TIAB]) OR orif[TIAB]) OR open reduction internal fixation [TIAB]))) OR ((((("Radius Fractures"[Mesh] OR "distal radius fractures"[TIAB]) OR "distal radius" [TIAB]) OR Radius Fractures[TIAB]) OR "forearm fractures"[TIAB]) AND ((((("Casts, Surgical"[Mesh] OR Casts[TIAB]) OR "Splint"[TIAB]) OR "Splinting"[TIAB]) OR casting[TIAB]) OR (((plate[TIAB] OR plating[TIAB]) OR orif[TIAB]) OR open reduction internal fixation[TIAB]))) AND ("Fracture Fixation, Intramedullary"[Mesh] OR "Fracture Fixation, Internal"[Mesh]))) AND (Dutch[lang] OR English [lang] OR German[lang])
- Only comparative studies were reviewed
- Only articles written in English, French or German were included
- Study protocols or abstracts of oral or poster presentations at congresses were excluded
- Article solely focusing on intra—or partial articular fractures were excluded

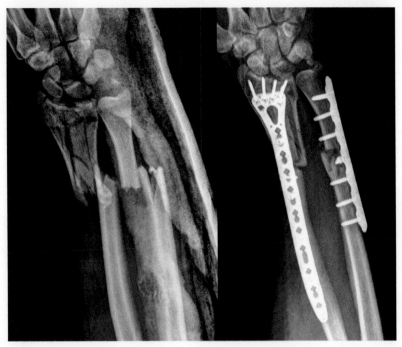

FIG. 6 Example of distal radius and ulna fractures with extensive metaphyseal comminution and intraarticular extension of the radius requiring long plating to achieve adequate stability. © Dr. Buijze 2020.

QUALITY OF THE EVIDENCE ON VLP VS CAST

Level I:
Randomized trials: 2
Level II:
Randomized trials with methodological limitations: 3
Level III:
Retrospective comparative studies: 3

QUALITY OF THE EVIDENCE ON OTHER TYPES OF SURGERY

Level I:
Randomized trials and systematic reviews: 6
Level II:
Randomized trials with methodological limitations: 5

FINDINGS

This chapter focuses on nonoperative treatment versus plate fixation in adult patients with extra-articular DRFs with a variable degree of comminution. A meta-analysis of Vannabouathong et al.[13] concluded that open reduction and plate fixation offers the best results for adult patients with a DRF, in terms of radiological and functional outcome and fracture healing. However, naturally other less invasive operative techniques have been described to treat DRFs such as closed reduction and Kirschner wire fixation, various methods of (non-) bridging external fixation, and intramedullary nailing. As ORIF with a volar locking plate (VLP) is the mainstay, it will be the primary focus of main part of this review, while alternative methods of fixation will be discussed at the end. Randomized controlled trials or comparative cohort studies evaluating plate fixation versus closed reduction and cast immobilization of displaced distal radius fractures in adults were included. Most studies included elderly with AO Type A and C DRFs.

Evidence From Level-1 VLP Studies

We have deemed the studies from Mulders et al.[12, 14] the only level-1 evidence available to the main question considering that the other articles either also included intra-articular fractures or focused on the elderly.

Mulders et al. randomized 92 patients (ages 18–75) with acceptably reduced extra-articular distal radius fractures between volar plate fixation (VLP) and cast immobilization (CI). At 6 weeks, 3 months, 6 months, and 12 months follow-up the VLP group had significant better DASH, PRWE scores and radiographic parameters (Fig. 7). However, at 12 months differences were below the MCID threshold. At 12 months VLP patients had significantly better flexion (80 degrees [70–86] vs 70 degrees [60–80]

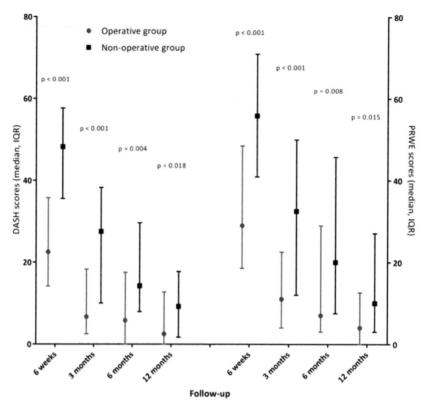

FIG. 7 At 6 weeks, 3 months, 6 months, and 12 months follow-up the VLP group had significant better DASH, PRWE scores, and radiographic parameters.

$P < .01$), extension (85 degrees [80–90] vs 80 degrees [70–90] $P < .01$), pronation (90 degrees [80–90] vs 85 degrees [75–90] $P < .01$), supination (85 degrees [75–90] vs 75 degrees [70–85] $P < .01$) and grip strength (26 kg [19–35] vs 20 kg [17–29] $P < .01$). Twenty eight percent of the CI patients had early fracture dislocation which was managed with VLP. Fourteen percent of the patients in the CI group developed a symptomatic malunion for which a correction osteotomy was performed.

Moreover, a cost-effectiveness analysis was performed in the same population.[14] The use of resources was prospectively documented for 12 months. This included direct medical, direct nonmedical and indirect nonmedical costs related to the DRF and treatment. The mean total costs were lower in the VLP group (mean difference −$299 [95% CI −$1880 to $1024]). Difference in costs per QALY also favored VLP (−$1838 [95% CI, −$12,604 to $9787]), this was even higher in subgroup analysis for patients with paid employment (−$7459 [95% CI, −$23,919 to $3233]).

Evidence From Level-2 VLP Studies

Saving et al. performed an RCT[15] ($n = 140$) comparing cast and VLP for treating DRF (type A and C) in the elderly (age 70+). After 3 months they found better PRWE (10.3 vs 35.5, $P = .002$) and DASH (14.4 vs 29.2, $P = .016$) in favor of the VLP group. After 12 months, the PRWE (7.5 vs 17.5 $P = .014$) and DASH (8.3 vs 19.9 $P = .028$) favored the VLP group.

At 12 months VLP patient had better flexion (51 degrees [SD 14] vs 63 degrees [SD 13], $P < .001$), grip strength vs contralateral hand (81% [SD 24] vs 96% [SD 24], $P = .001$) and ulnar deviation (28 degrees [SD 8] vs 30 degrees [SD 11], $P < .03$). Radiographic measurements were also better at 3 and 12 months follow-up. There was no significant difference in complications. Sixty three percent were extra-articular fractures, there was no subgroup analysis.

In 2011, Arora et al.[16] preformed an RCT where they randomized 73 patients (ages 65 and older) with DRF (type A and C) to VLP vs CI. They found no significant difference in ROM, pain, PRWE (12.8 vs 14.6 $P=.73$) or DASH (5.7 vs 8.0 $P=.34$) at 12 months follow-up. Grip strength was better in the VLP group in all follow-up moments. They found that an anatomical reconstruction did convey improved ROM. Results were not specified for type A or C fractures.

Sirnio et al.[17] performed an RCT randomizing 80 patients (ages 50 years and older) between VLP ($n=38$) and CI ($n=42$) after successful reduction. Delayed surgery was performed if there was early loss of alignment in the CI group ($n=16$, 38%). The mean DASH after 24 months was 7.9 vs 14 ($P=.05$) in favor of the surgical group. The mean DASH score in the delayed surgery group was 17 ($P=.02$).

Evidence From Level-3 VLP Studies

In 2009, Arora et al.[18] retrospectively analyzed 114 patients older than 70 years with a displaced distal radius fracture (type A and C). They let the patient choose between VLP and closed reduction and CI. They found better radiographical results after VLP than CI ($P<.05$). After a mean follow-up of 4 years and 7 months there was no difference in ROM, DASH or PWRE.

This study is potentially biased because of its retrospective nature. Patient selection bias is introduced by the fact that less demanding patients generally favor CI over VLP. After VLP fixation, the patients in this study were also treated with a cast for 2 weeks. Which could possibly further influence the results in favor of CI. Eighty-nine percent of the primarily reduced fractures in CI had a malunion. This study had no subgroup analysis for type A fractures.

Hung et al.[19] retrospectively analyzed VLP ($n=26$) vs CI ($n=31$) in the active Chinese elderly population (ages 61 and up) with "unstable" DRF. The DASH after a mean follow-up at 12 months was better in the VLP group (4.5 vs 13.6 $P=.04$) as well as grip strength ($P=.017$).

Chan et al.[20] retrospectively analyzed VLP ($n=40$) vs CI ($n=35$) in the active Chinese elderly population (ages 65 and up with an independent lifestyle) with DRF (type A and C) which redislocated after initial successful reduction. They found improved ROM and grip strength after 3 months but no difference in ROM, grip strength of DASH after 6 or 12 months.

Kirschner Wire Fixation

McFadyen et al.[21] randomized between closed reduction and Kirschner wire fixation (CRPP) and open reduction and VLP for extra-articular DRFs. They found better functional scores (DASH) at 3 months (18.3 vs 27.2, $P=.001$) and 6 months (15.9 vs 21.5, $P=.017$) postoperatively and no significant loss of fracture reduction in patients treated with a VLP.

A large RCT ($n=461$) performed in 2014 by Costa et al.[22] compared VLP and CRPP for both A and C type fractures but excluded severe intra-articular fractures which required open reduction. They found no difference in PWRE scores at any time point (3, 6 and 12 months) There was a marginally significant difference in DASH score at 12 months in favor of VLPs with a small effect size (-3.2 (95% CI -6.5 to 0.0) $P=.051$).

Their 5-year follow-up study showed comparable results. Interestingly, 75% of VLP patients in their study were treated with a cast not allowing for early mobilization for at least the first 2 weeks. This might explain why they found higher mean PWRE (13.9) and DASH (13) scores 12 months after plate fixation than reported in other studies[12, 15–17] (Table 1). A meta-analysis by Chaudhry et al.[23] found that patients treated with a VLP had lower DASH scores at 3 and 12 months. However, this difference was less than the 10-point threshold of the minimal clinical important difference (MCID). They found that superficial wound infection requiring antibiotics was more common in the CRPP group. This might also contribute to the difference found in other recent RCTs.

It is difficult to draw firm conclusion from these studies because most included extra- and intra-articular fractures. It seems that VLPs yields slightly better results than CRRP with lower infection rates. Moreover, VLPs allow for early functional rehabilitation and patients have better outcomes especially the first 6 months compared with CI. Additionally, operative treatment of type A fractures is cost-effective.

Intramedullary Nailing

The potential benefits of intramedullary (IM) fixation over locking plate fixation are the minimal invasive approach and consequent less soft tissue dissection. Theoretically, this may result in less stiffness and

TABLE 1
PWRE and DASH Scores 12 Months After Volar Plate Fixation.

	PWRE	DASH
Costa et al. (2014)	13.9	13.0
Mulders et al.[a] (2019)	4.0	2.5
Saving et al.[b] (2019)	7.5	8.3
Arora et al.[b] (2011)	12.8	5.7
Sirnio et al.[b] (2019)	–	7.9

[a]Only extra-articular fractures.
[b]Elderly population.

hardware related complications such as tendinitis and tendon ruptures. In 2016, Zhang et al.[24] published a systematic review comparing IM to locking plate fixation in adult patients with extra-articular or simple intraarticular DRFs. There were 221 participants in the IM group and 242 in the VLP group. The authors concluded that IM had better results than VLP regardless of which function scoring system was used at 6 weeks and 3 months. However, this was based on only one study. Moreover, all differences were below the MCID threshold (10 points) of the DASH score. Therefore, a clear benefit of IM nailing over other fixation methods is yet to be proven. Moreover, a systematic review of Hardman et al.[25] including 357 patients showed good functional results with a mean DASH score of 6 points at a mean follow up of 12.7 months. However, 11% of patients had a transient radial nerve irritation. At this moment IM devices are relatively new and there is a limitation of which fracture types can be treated.

External Fixation

Handoll et al. performed a Cochrane review[26] to evaluate the evidence from randomized controlled trials comparing different methods of external fixation. They found insufficient evidence to favor any of method including nonbridging versus bridging fixation, hydroxyapatite coated pins versus with standard uncoated pins, and dynamic versus static external fixation.

Several authors performed systematic reviews where they compared external fixation to VLP which yielded similar results.[27–29] These article showed better DASH scores after 3, 6 and 12 months postoperatively and an improved volar tilt. In 2017, Gouk et al.[30] conducted a metaanalysis including 780 patients reporting that VLP resulted in statistically better DASH scores at 3, 6, and 12 months. However, the difference between the two groups exceeded the MCID of 10 points for the DASH at 3 months only.

RECOMMENDATION

In patients with an extra-articular displaced distal radius fracture, evidence suggests:

Recommendation	Overall Quality
• Open reduction and volar plate fixation provides improved radiographic and functional outcome scores compared to closed reduction and cast immobilization in patients with extra-articular DRFs, especially the first 6 months	⊕⊕⊕⊕ HIGH
• In adults with displaced extra-articular DRFs, volar plate fixation is a cost-effective intervention, especially in patients who have paid employment	⊕⊕⊕⊕ HIGH
• Early open reduction and volar plate fixation provides better functional outcome scores compared to delayed (after redislocation <2 weeks)	⊕⊕○○ LOW
• In case of more extensive metaphyseal comminution, (longer) volar plates, various methods of external fixation and intramedullary nailing result in comparable good outcomes	⊕⊕⊕○ MODERATE

CONCLUSION

In adult patients aged between 18 and 75 years with displaced extra-articular distal radius fractures, early open reduction and volar plate fixation leads to improved functional outcome, range of motion and grip strength, even when initial closed reduction is adequate. Volar plate fixation is cost-effective in this patient group. In elderly patients, the evidence does not specify for extra-articular fractures but the combined results suggest the same. With limited metaphyseal comminution, closed reduction and K-wire fixation seems to provide similar results at the cost of higher infection rates. When metaphyseal comminution is more extensive, various methods of external fixation and intramedullary nailing can be considered effective alternatives. In elderly, frail osteoporotic patients, other options such as spanning plate fixation or arthrodesis of the radiocarpal joint with titanium elastic nails can be considered, for instance in open fractures or risk of skin perforation.

Panel 2: Authors' Preferred Technique

Due to carpal malalignment, the first patient in the case scenarios was scheduled for open reduction and volar plate fixation which corrected the dorsal angulation and carpal alignment (Fig. 8). At 3 months of follow-up, the PRWE was 11 and at 6 months 7 points.

General preferred technique:

The patient will preferably be operated under axillary nerve block, 2 g cefazoline prophylaxis and tourniquet after exsanguination. A modified Henry approach to the distal radius is used where we dissect radially from the flexor carpi radialis leaving the tendon sheath intact. The pronator quadratus (PQ) is incised (L-shaped) along the radial border of and below the watershed line avoiding injury to the volar ligaments exposing the distal radius. The brachioradialis insertion is released from the distal fracture fragment until we see the first extensor compartment. The fracture site is debrided. The fracture is reduced, dependent of the fracture pattern and temporarily fixed with K-wires. If reduction is unsuccessful, Orbay's maneuver is performed (described below). Once adequate reduction is reached the plate is positioned. In some cases it is preferable to fixate the plate distally first. This way final adjustments in reduction can be made when fixating the plate on the radial shaft. Reduction and plate position is checked under image intensifier using AP, PA, true lateral and sky line views (Fig. 8 image 3).

An image perpendicular to distal part of the plate and articular surface of the radius may help to asses screw length and to avoid penetration of the dorsal cortex and therefore protects the extensor tendons (Fig. 9). Occasionally, better visualization of the dorsal radial cortex is achieved with the wrist in flexion (skyline view) and sometimes in extension (carpal shoot through). A pitfall is to confuse the scaphoid and lunate for dorsal radial cortex in these images.

The PQ is not sutured. Only the skin is closed using an absorbable monofilament suture. Pressure bandage is applied (making sure the MCP joints are free) for 48 h. The patient will start nonweight bearing wrist motion exercises the same day. Weight bearing is allowed 6 weeks postoperatively.

In the second case scenario, the 97-year-old lady with the comminuted metaphyseal DRF as part of a grade-2 open distal forearm fracture was immediately scheduled for surgery. In these cases, we chose between two treatment options: spanning plate fixation (Fig. 10) or arthrodesis of the radiocarpal joint with titanium elastic nails. A modified Clayton-Mannerfelt technique in which we use the second and third distal MCPs as point of entrance. Due to the fragility of the patient, comorbidities and crepey skin, this minimal invasive approach was preferred. Following surgery the patient was treated with a plaster of Paris for 5 weeks (Fig. 11).

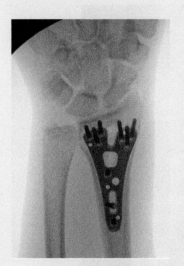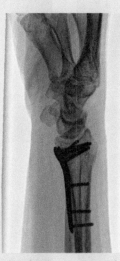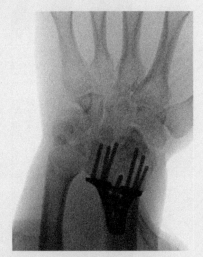

FIG. 8 Open reduction and volar plate fixation corrected the dorsal angulation and carpal alignment.

Continued

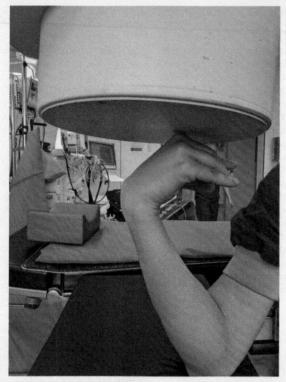

FIG. 9 Dorsal skyline view.

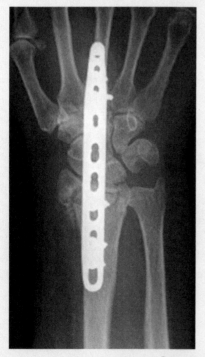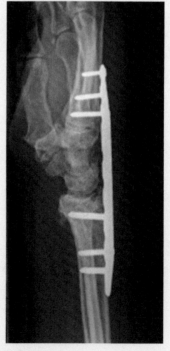

FIG. 10 Spanning plate fixation.

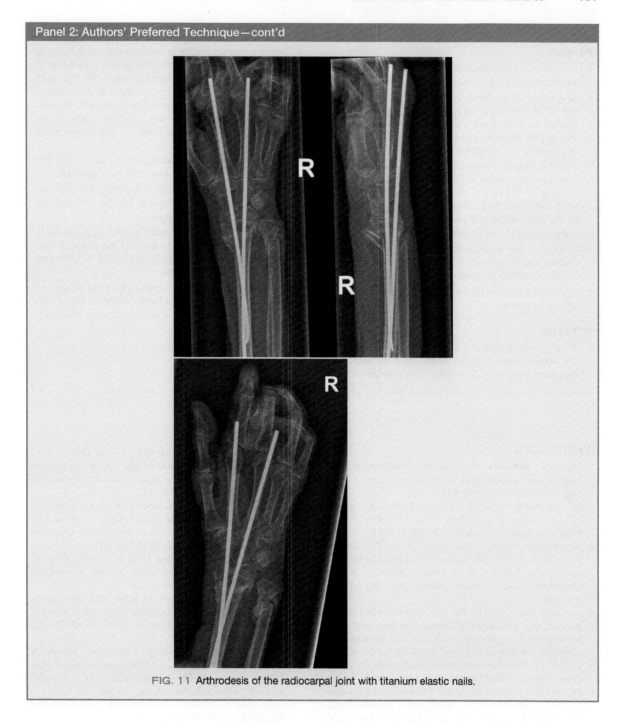

FIG. 11 Arthrodesis of the radiocarpal joint with titanium elastic nails.

Panel 3: Pearls and Pitfalls

PEARLS:

- Release of the brachioradialis insertion on the distal fracture fragment can aid in achieving anatomical reduction.
- One can avoid accidental injury to the palmar cutaneous branch of the median nerve by dissecting on the radial side of the FCR (flexor carpi radialis) instead of going through the tendon sheath when using a modified Henry approach to the distal radius.
- If the fracture is >2 weeks old. Getting adequate reduction, especially radial length, can be challenging. Performing an Orbay maneuver (pronating the proximal shaft with a reduction clamp, exposing the dorsal side of the distal radius and lifting off the extensor tendons subperiosteally) may enable reduction.
- In elderly, frail osteoporotic patients consider other options such as spanning plate fixation or arthrodesis of the radiocarpal joint with titanium elastic nails.
- When using a spanning plate consider plate removal as soon as 8 weeks.

PITFALLS:

- When using radial-sided (temporary) K-wires, protect the sensory branch of the radial nerve as neuromas can result from a (blind) percutaneous approach.

- Dorsal screw protrusion is common due to the irregular dorsal surface of the distal radius and can result in extensor tendinitis and rupture. Especially the most radial screw in the radial styloid process. Additionally, try to avoid penetrating the dorsal cortex with the drill. Skyline views are useful, although the scaphoid and lunate should not be confused for the dorsal radial cortex.
- When extending your incision proximally, mind the crossing of a radial artery branch to the medial side.
- There is no proven benefit in repairing the pronator quadratus muscle after volar plate fixation. It might actually reduce pronation strength.[31]
- Don't accept fracture translation as this can cause DRUJ instability due to lack of tension on the distal oblique bundle. Therefore, intraoperatively asses reduction of the radius at its ulnar border.
- Avoid positioning the plate distally from the watershed line. For it can cause flexor tendon irritation. Especially, the flexor pollicis longus is at risk and may eventually result in tendon rupture.

REFERENCES

1. Chung KC, Spilson SV. The frequency and epidemiology of hand and forearm fractures in the United States. *J Hand Surg [Am]*. 2001;26(5):908–915.
2. US Department of Health & Human Services Af, Quality HRa Welcome to H-CUPnet. Available from: http://hcupnet.ahrq.gov/. Accessed November 3, 2014.
3. Bentohami A, Bosma J, Akkersdijk GJ, van Dijkman B, Goslings JC, Schep NW. Incidence and characteristics of distal radial fractures in an urban population in The Netherlands. *Eur J Trauma Emerg Surg*. 2014;40(3): 357–361.
4. Grewal R, MacDermid JC. The risk of adverse outcomes in extra-articular distal radius fractures is increased with malalignment in patients of all ages but mitigated in older patients. *J Hand Surg [Am]*. 2007;32(7):962–970.
5. Medoff RJ. Essential radiographic evaluation for distal radius fractures. *Hand Clin*. 2005;21(3):279–288.
6. Schuind FA, Linscheid RL, An KN, Chao EY. A normal data base of posteroanterior roentgenographic measurements of the wrist. *J Bone Joint Surg Am*. 1992;74(9):1418–1429.
7. Ross M, Di Mascio L, Peters S, Cockfield A, Taylor F, Couzens G. Defining residual radial translation of distal radius fractures: a potential cause of distal radioulnar joint instability. *J Wrist Surg*. 2014;3(1):22–29.
8. Trehan SK, Orbay JL, Wolfe SW. Coronal shift of distal radius fractures: influence of the distal interosseous membrane on distal radioulnar joint instability. *J Hand Surg [Am]*. 2015;40(1):159–162.
9. McQueen MM, Hajducka C, Court-Brown CM. Redisplaced unstable fractures of the distal radius: a prospective randomised comparison of four methods of treatment. *J Bone Joint Surg (Br)*. 1996;78(3):404–409.
10. Selles CA, Ras L, Walenkamp MMJ, Maas M, Goslings JC, Schep NWL. Carpal alignment: a new method for assessment. *J Wrist Surg*. 2019;8(2):112–117.
11. Walenkamp MM, Aydin S, Mulders MA, Goslings JC, Schep NW. Predictors of unstable distal radius fractures: a systematic review and meta-analysis. *J Hand Surg Eur Vol*. 2016;41(5):501–515.
12. Mulders MAM, Walenkamp MMJ, van Dieren S, Goslings JC, Schep NWL, Collaborators VT. Volar plate fixation versus plaster immobilization in acceptably reduced extra-articular distal radial fractures: a multicenter randomized controlled trial. *J Bone Joint Surg Am*. 2019;101(9):787–796.
13. Vannabouathong C, Hussain N, Guerra-Farfan E, Bhandari M. Interventions for distal radius fractures: a network meta-analysis of randomized trials. *J Am Acad Orthop Surg*. 2019;27(13):e596–e605.

14. Mulders MAM, Walenkamp MMJ, van Dieren S, Goslings JC, Schep NWL, Collaborators VT. Volar plate fixation in adults with a displaced extra-articular distal radial fracture is cost-effective. *J Bone Joint Surg Am*. 2020;102(7):609–616. https://doi.org/10.2106/JBJS.19.00597.

15. Saving J, Severin Wahlgren S, Olsson K, et al. Nonoperative treatment compared with volar locking plate fixation for dorsally displaced distal radial fractures in the elderly: a randomized controlled trial. *J Bone Joint Surg Am*. 2019;101(11):961–969.

16. Arora R, Lutz M, Deml C, Krappinger D, Haug L, Gabl M. A prospective randomized trial comparing nonoperative treatment with volar locking plate fixation for displaced and unstable distal radial fractures in patients sixty-five years of age and older. *J Bone Joint Surg Am*. 2011;93 (23):2146–2153.

17. Sirnio K, Leppilahti J, Ohtonen P, Flinkkila T. Early palmar plate fixation of distal radius fractures may benefit patients aged 50 years or older: a randomized trial comparing 2 different treatment protocols. *Acta Orthop*. 2019;90(2): 123–128.

18. Arora R, Gabl M, Gschwentner M, Deml C, Krappinger D, Lutz M. A comparative study of clinical and radiologic outcomes of unstable colles type distal radius fractures in patients older than 70 years: nonoperative treatment versus volar locking plating. *J Orthop Trauma*. 2009;23 (4):237–242.

19. Hung LP, Leung YF, Ip WY, Lee YL. Is locking plate fixation a better option than casting for distal radius fracture in elderly people? *Hong Kong Med J*. 2015;21(5):407–410.

20. Chan YH, Foo TL, Yeo CJ, Chew WY. Comparison between cast immobilization versus volar locking plate fixation of distal radius fractures in active elderly patients, the Asian perspective. *Hand Surg*. 2014;19(1):19–23.

21. McFadyen I, Field J, McCann P, Ward J, Nicol S, Curwen C. Should unstable extra-articular distal radial fractures be treated with fixed-angle volar-locked plates or percutaneous Kirschner wires? A prospective randomised controlled trial. *Injury*. 2011;42(2):162–166.

22. Costa ML, Achten J, Parsons NR, et al. Percutaneous fixation with Kirschner wires versus volar locking plate fixation in adults with dorsally displaced fracture of distal radius: randomised controlled trial. *BMJ*. 2014;349:g4807.

23. Chaudhry H, Kleinlugtenbelt YV, Mundi R, Ristevski B, Goslings JC, Bhandari M. Are volar locking plates superior to percutaneous K-wires for distal radius fractures? A meta-analysis. *Clin Orthop Relat Res*. 2015;473(9):3017–3027.

24. Zhang B, Chang H, Yu K, et al. Intramedullary nail versus volar locking plate fixation for the treatment of extra-articular or simple intra-articular distal radius fractures: systematic review and meta-analysis. *Int Orthop*. 2017;41 (10):2161–2169.

25. Hardman J, Al-Hadithy N, Hester T, Anakwe R. Systematic review of outcomes following fixed angle intramedullary fixation of distal radius fractures. *Int Orthop*. 2015;39(12): 2381–2387.

26. Handoll HH, Huntley JS, Madhok R. Different methods of external fixation for treating distal radial fractures in adults. *Cochrane Database Syst Rev*. 2008;1:CD006522.

27. Wei DH, Poolman RW, Bhandari M, Wolfe VM, Rosenwasser MP. External fixation versus internal fixation for unstable distal radius fractures: a systematic review and meta-analysis of comparative clinical trials. *J Orthop Trauma*. 2012;26(7):386–394.

28. Walenkamp MM, Bentohami A, Beerekamp MS, et al. Functional outcome in patients with unstable distal radius fractures, volar locking plate versus external fixation: a meta-analysis. *Strategies Trauma Limb Reconstr*. 2013;8(2):67–75.

29. Li-hai Z, Ya-nan W, Zhi M, et al. Volar locking plate versus external fixation for the treatment of unstable distal radial fractures: a meta-analysis of randomized controlled trials. *J Surg Res*. 2015;193(1):324–333.

30. Gouk CJC, Bindra RR, Tarrant DJ, Thomas MJE. Volar locking plate fixation versus external fixation of distal radius fractures: a meta-analysis. *J Hand Surg Eur Vol*. 2018;43(9):954–960.

31. Sonntag J, Woythal L, Rasmussen P, et al. No effect on functional outcome after repair of pronator quadratus in volar plating of distal radial fractures: a randomized clinical trial. *Bone Joint J*. 2019;101-B(12):1498–1505.

CHAPTER 14

Bone Graft (Substitutes) in Distal Radius Fractures

PASCAL F.W. HANNEMANN[a] • TACO J. BLOKHUIS[a] •
JAN A. TEN BOSCH[a] • NIELS W.L. SCHEP[b]
[a]Department of Trauma Surgery, Maastricht University Medical Centre, Maastricht, Netherlands,
[b]Department of Trauma Surgery, Maasstad Hospital, Rotterdam, Netherlands

KEY POINTS

- The use of bone grafts or bone graft substitutes for treatment of comminuted distal radius fractures is dictated by tradition, training, and personal experience.
- The use of bone grafts (substitutes) for treatment of comminuted distal radius fractures does not improve outcome in elderly patients.
- The use of autologous bone graft is characterized by a significant number of complications related to the procedure of harvesting.

Panel 1: Case Scenario

A 50-year-old male presents with a grade 2 open comminuted distal radius and ulna fracture after a motor vehicle accident. Initial treatment consists of debridement of the wound, removal of devascularized bone and stabilization by means of joint-spanning external fixation. Postoperative radiographs show a comminuted extraarticular distal radius and ulna fracture with a significant segmental metaphyseal defect of 5 cm of the distal radius (Fig. 1).

What is the most effective approach for this metaphyseal defect in this patient?

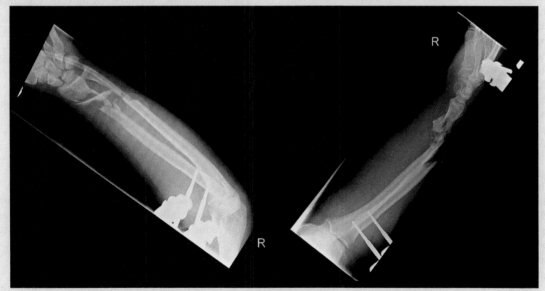

FIG. 1 Radiographs after initial stabilization in an external fixator. Comminuted extraarticular distal radius and ulna fracture with a significant segmental metaphyseal defect of 5 cm of the distal radius.

Distal Radius Fractures. https://doi.org/10.1016/B978-0-323-75764-5.00020-2

IMPORTANCE OF THE PROBLEM

Principles of treatment of distal radius fractures have changed in the last decades. While in the past, alignment of the bony fragments and maintenance of radial length were considered to be most important, nowadays meticulous reduction of the articular surface and adequate reconstruction of metaphyseal comminution along with reliable stabilization are key principles in most surgically treated distal radius fractures.

As more patients presenting with distal radius fractures are of older age, many clinicians are confronted with problems of osteoporosis when treating distal radius fractures. Osteoporotic fractures have an impaired ability to heal and often require more time to heal.[1] The degree of comminution is generally high and alignment is often lost, despite of some remaining healing potential of osteoporotic bone. As a result, metaphyseal comminution and impaction, especially in patients with osteoporotic bone, may result in a metaphyseal bony void with subsequent instability, loss of reduction, and malunion.[2] This may lead to serious functional impairment on short and long term.

Although healing of metaphyseal defects in distal radius fractures can be a slow process, the risk of non-union in distal radius fractures is minimal. As a consequence, bone grafts or bone graft substitutes are primarily used to provide structural stability and thereby support early return to function. By using bone grafts or bone graft substitutes for treatment of bony defects in the distal radius, the construct can be stabilized by providing mechanical support for the radiocarpal joint surface and a scaffold for ingrowth of new bone is provided.[3] The ideal implanted material is biocompatible, bio-resorbable and will lead to optimal structural stability by providing substantial initial compression strength while allowing rapid ingrowth of new bone with preservation of anatomical reduction of the joint surface.[3, 4]

Addressing bone defects as part of primary treatment of distal radius fractures is a challenge for the treating surgeon, since outcome of the fracture is dependent on how successful the defect is treated. Remodeling of metaphyseal defects in distal radius fractures that are fixated without additional bone graft or bone graft substitute does not lead to optimal bone quality after trabecular modeling.[5] Additionally, clinical evidence supports the hypothesis that the use of bone graft substitutes for treatment of metaphyseal defects may lead to faster healing.[6] On the other hand, structural stability is also directly influenced by the method of fixation.[4] As advances in plate design have led to the applicability of anatomically shaped and variable angle locking plates in recent years, perhaps bone graft substitutes are not essential in most situations.

MAIN QUESTION

- What is the role and additional value of bone graft substitutes in comminuted distal radius fractures?
- Which type of bone graft is most effective for treatment of bone defects in comminuted distal radius fractures? (autograft, allograft, or bone substitutes)

CURRENT OPINION

There are many surgical options for treatment of metaphyseal bone defects in distal radius fractures including autografts, allografts and bone substitutes, both biological and synthetic. However, the use of bone grafts or bone graft substitutes for treatment of comminuted distal radius fractures is dictated by tradition, training, and personal experience. In highly exceptional cases of bone defects larger than 6–8 cm, vascularized bone grafts are recommended. Strategies based on potential robust scientific evidence are very limited for treatment of bone defects in comminuted distal radius fractures.

FINDING THE EVIDENCE

We provide below a list of search algorithms used to retrieve evidence for the main question:

- Cochrane search: "distal radius fracture" OR "distal radial fracture" AND "bone substitutes"
- Pubmed (Medline): "Radius Fractures" [Mesh] OR "radius fracture" [tiab] OR "radial fracture" [tiab] OR "distal radius fracture" [tiab] OR "distal radial fracture" [tiab] AND "Bone Substitutes" [Mesh] OR "bone substitutes" [tiab]
- Only articles written in English, French or German were included.
- Study protocols or abstracts of oral or poster presentations at congresses were excluded.

QUALITY OF THE EVIDENCE

Overall, we found one cochrane systematic review and six prospective studies of relevance to the use of bone grafts or bone graft substitutes for treatment of distal radius fractures.[7–13] We also found one level 3 study and one level 4 case series.[2, 14]

Level I: Systematic review: 1[7]

Level II: Randomized trial with methodological limitations: 6[8–13]

LEVEL III: Case-controlled study: 1[14]

Level IV: Case series: 1[2]

FINDINGS

Evidence From Level-I Studies

A Cochrane systematic review from 2008 provided the only level-1 evidence available.[7]

For this review randomized or quasirandomized controlled clinical trials evaluating the use of bone grafts or bone graft substitutes for treatment of distal radius fractures in adults were included. Overall, 10 trials involving 874 adults with distal radius fractures were included in this review. All trials showed significant heterogeneity and no trial had proof of allocation concealment. For this reason, trials could be considered as level-2 evidence.

Overall, six comparisons regarding the use of bone grafts or bone graft substitutes could be made.

(1) Four trials with 239 participants compared the use of bone scaffolding with plaster cast immobilization for comminuted distal radius fractures.[11, 15–17] Improved anatomical outcomes were obtained when using bone grafts or bone graft substitutes. Differences between the intervention group and control group were significant with regards to dorsal angulation in favor of the intervention group (Fig. 2). The type of bone scaffolding used was quite different among studies. (Autogenous bone graft,[15] Norian SRS, a calcium phosphate bone cement[11, 16] or methylmetacrylate cement.[17]) Two studies showed that improved functional outcomes were obtained in the bone substitute group.[16, 17] Significantly more patients in the bone substitute group obtained excellent or good results (Fig. 3).

(2) One trial with 323 participants compared the use of percutaneous application of Norian SRS calcium phosphate cement to plaster cast or external fixation after closed reduction.[12] Subjects were followed clinically and radiographically up to 1 year. Initial functional recovery was faster in the Norian group, but no differences in functional outcome were seen at 1 year. No clinically relevant differences in anatomical outcomes were seen at 1 year. There were significantly more infections in the control group, always related to external fixator pins or Kirschner wires (16.7% vs 2.5%, $P<.001$). Subjects in the intervention group showed significantly more complications due to extraosseous Norian SRS deposits.

(3) One trial with 48 participants reported outcomes of autologous bone graft with surgical fixation by means of external fixation compared with surgical fixation alone.[18] All subjects had severely displaced and comminuted distal radius fractures. At 1-year follow up, there were no significant differences in functional outcome or anatomical measurements. There was no significant difference in numbers of malunions between both groups.

(4) One trial with 21 participants compared the use of hydroxyapatite cement with Kapandji's intrafocal pinning in 21 subjects with intraarticular distal radius fracture.[19] Grip strength was significantly worse in the bone substitute group (56% vs 73%). Furthermore, subjects in the bone substitute group showed significantly less palmar flexion at 6 months follow up (mean difference −10 degrees, 95% CI −18.89 to −1.11 degrees). No complications occurred in either group.

(5) Three trials with 180 participants with secondary displaced distal radius fractures compared the use of autogenous bone[15] or bone substitutes (Norian SRS[20] or methylmetacrylate cement[21]) with external fixation. No significant differences in functional outcome were seen between both groups. However, anatomical outcomes were somewhat superior in the groups using autogenous bone or bone substitutes when compared to external fixation only.

(6) One trial compared allogenic bone-graft substitutes with autologous bone graft for repair of comminuted distal radius fractures in 93 patients undergoing open reduction and dorsal plate fixation.[13] No clinically significant differences were seen regarding functional outcome between both groups. There was a significant number of complications in the autograft group due to the harvesting from the iliac crest. Half of these patients suffered postoperative pain and 13 patients still reported complaints of pain 1 year after iliac crest harvesting.

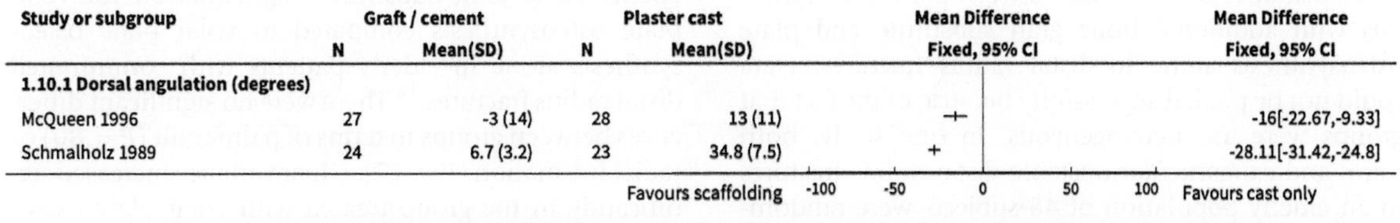

Study or subgroup	Graft / cement		Plaster cast		Mean Difference	Mean Difference
	N	Mean(SD)	N	Mean(SD)	Fixed, 95% CI	Fixed, 95% CI
1.10.1 Dorsal angulation (degrees)						
McQueen 1996	27	-3 (14)	28	13 (11)		-16[-22.67,-9.33]
Schmalholz 1989	24	6.7 (3.2)	23	34.8 (7.5)		-28.11[-31.42,-24.8]
					Favours scaffolding -100 -50 0 50 100 Favours cast only	

FIG. 2 Differences between the intervention group and control group regarding dorsal angulation.

Study or subgroup	Graft / substitute	Plaster cast	Risk Ratio	Risk Ratio
	n/N	n/N	M-H, Fixed, 95% CI	M-H, Fixed, 95% CI
1.1.1 Not excellent				
Sanchez-Sotelo 2000	25/55	38/55		0.66[0.47,0.92]
Schmalholz 1989	18/24	23/23		0.76[0.59,0.96]
1.1.2 Fair or poor				
Sanchez-Sotelo 2000	10/55	25/55		0.4[0.21,0.75]
Schmalholz 1989	1/24	21/23		0.05[0.01,0.31]

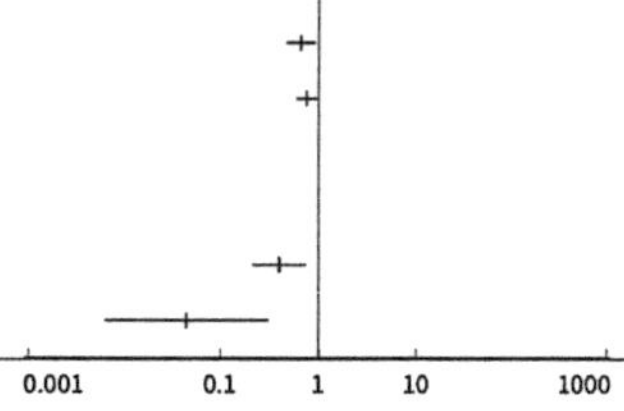

Favours scaffolding   0.001   0.1   1   10   1000   Favours cast only

FIG. 3 Differences between the intervention group and control group regarding functional outcome.

Overall, results from this review led to the conclusion that the use of bone grafts or bone graft substitutes for treatment of comminuted distal radius fractures may improve anatomical outcomes when compared to treatment with a cast alone, but there was insufficient evidence to draw any conclusions regarding other comparisons. No conclusions can be drawn with regards to functional outcome or safety.

Evidence From Level-II Studies

Two studies compared the use of bone graft substitutes with nonoperative treatment for comminuted distal radius fractures.[11, 12] Their data could not be pooled due to heterogeneous treatment groups.

Except for improved ulnar variance in favor of the calcium phosphate bone cement group in one study, no significant differences with regards to clinical, functional, and radiographical outcome were seen at final follow up.[12]

One study compared percutaneous pinning and cast immobilization with the use of injectable calcium phosphate bone cement with supplemented pin or screw fixation in 52 menopausal women with unstable intraarticular distal radius fractures.[9] Subjects were evaluated clinically and radiographically at 2 years.

Patients treated with injectable calcium phosphate had better DASH scores, better active range of motion in frontal and sagittal plane, better forearm rotation, and better grip strength ($P < .001$). Additionally, there was a significantly higher loss of reduction (radial length, radial inclination, and palmar tilt) in the control group ($P < .001$).

Two studies randomized between plate osteosynthesis with additional bone graft substitute and plate osteosynthesis alone in distal radius fractures. Data could not be pooled successfully because of the fact that groups were too heterogeneous. In one study, both intra- and extraarticular unstable distal radius fractures in an elderly population of 48 subjects were randomized between volar plate osteosynthesis alone and a combination of volar plate osteosynthesis and augmentation with calcium phosphate bone cement.[10] No statistic differences in clinical or radiographic outcome were seen between subjects at 1 year follow up.

In the other study, 39 patients with intraarticular fractures of the distal radius were randomized in 2 groups, one being treated with internal fixation by means of dorsal plating only while the second group received an additional bone graft substitute (compressed beta-tricalcium phosphate granules).[8] Subjects were followed clinically and radiographically up to 1 year. There was no statistically significant difference in functional or radiological outcome between groups at 12 months postoperatively, and complications were similar.

One study assessed clinical and radiological outcome of cancellous allograft compared to autologous bone grafting in comminuted distal radius fractures.[13] Ninety patients were randomized between allograft or autologous bone grafting. Subjects were followed for 12 months. Regarding range of motion, grip strength and radiological outcome parameters, no significant differences between groups were seen. Obviously, there were more complications related to the procedure of iliac crest bone graft harvesting. One year postoperatively, six patients (13%) still suffered from discomforting paresthesias of the upper lateral thigh. Operating time was significantly shorter in the allograft group ($P = .03$).

Evidence From Level-III Studies

One study assessed radiographic outcomes of hydroxyapatite bone graft substitute augmentation for volar plate osteosynthesis compared to volar plate osteosynthesis alone in elderly patients with comminuted distal radius fractures.[14] There were no significant differences between groups in terms of palmar tilt ($P = .80$) or radial inclination ($P = .17$). Ulnar variance increased significantly in the group treated with volar plate osteosynthesis alone ($P < .05$).

Evidence From Level-IV Studies

One study assessed functional, clinical, and radiological outcomes of synthetic hydroxyapatite bone graft substitute with closed reduction and Kirschner wire fixation for unstable distal radius fractures in elderly patients.[2] At 16 weeks postoperatively, subjects showed satisfactory clinical outcome without metaphyseal collapse in all fractures.

In recent literature, there are reports of successful reconstruction of large posttraumatic bone defects in distal radius fractures with free vascularized grafts, especially free vascularized fibular grafts.[22, 23] Although the majority of free vascularized fibular grafts are used for reconstructive option in patients with septic skeletal defects, they are also applied for indications of posttraumatic bony defects larger than 6–8 cm, often accompanied by poor vascularity of the surrounding soft tissues (Figs. 4–10). This technique offers the advantage of a 1-stage reconstruction, in which bony reconstruction and soft tissue coverage are addressed in a single procedure. However, experience in microsurgical techniques and careful postoperative surveillance is mandatory and satisfactory anatomical and functional outcomes have been achieved by the authors when addressing bone defects larger than 6–8 cm with nonvascularized techniques, such as the Masquelet technique, as well.[24]

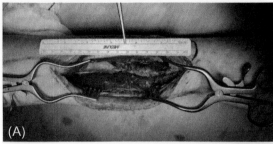
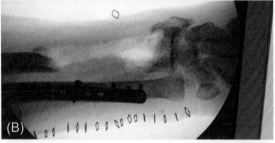

FIG. 5 (A) Intraoperative image after removal of unviable bone fragments and prior to regularization of the proximal bone segment, demonstrating a bone defect of approximately 7–8 cm. (B) Fluoroscopic view of the defect after ulna osteosynthesis was performed using a 2.7 mm plate. (Case courtesy Dr. Pérez Alba.)

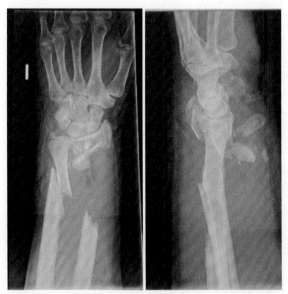

FIG. 4 Radiographs of a 32-year-old female patient after falling from the second floor (approximately 10 m) sustaining a Gustilo grade 2 open fracture of the distal radius and ulna with a large segmental bone defect of the metaphyseal radial shaft. (Case courtesy Dr. José Manuel Pérez Alba.)

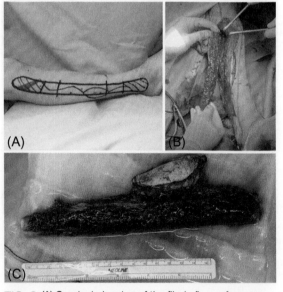

FIG. 6 (A) Surgical planning of the fibula flap, references, perforator marking and cutaneous island. (B) Adequate perfusion of the fibula flap is shown after removing the ischemia before cutting the pedicle. (C) Fibula flap with skin island before shortening for position within the radial bone segments. (Case courtesy Dr. Pérez Alba.)

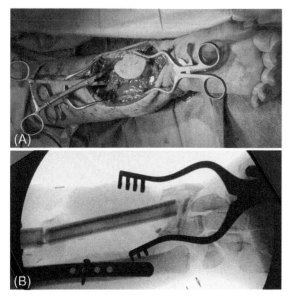

FIG. 7 (A) Intraoperative image after provisional placement of the fibula flap in the forearm. (B) Fluoroscopic image of the provisional placement of the flap. (Case courtesy Dr. Pérez Alba.)

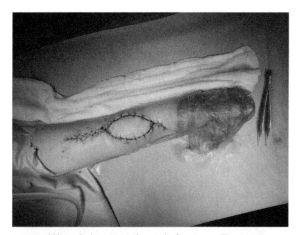

FIG. 8 Wound closure at the end of surgery. The proper closure and adequate color of the skin island are appreciated. (Case courtesy Dr. Pérez Alba.)

As a result, the latter technique may be the preferred technique in the majority of cases when addressing large metaphyseal bone defects in distal radius fractures.

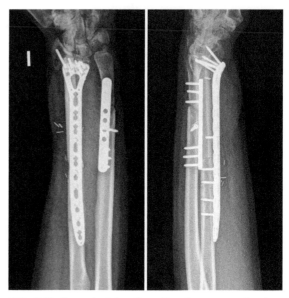

FIG. 9 Radiographs taken 3 months after surgery showing adequate reduction and osteosynthesis of both fractures with the contribution of the fibula flap for the reconstruction of the bone defect. (Case courtesy Dr. Pérez Alba.)

RECOMMENDATION

In patients with unstable, comminuted distal radius fracture, evidence suggests:

Recommendation	Overall Quality
• The use of bone grafts or bone graft substitutes for treatment of comminuted distal radius fractures in adult patients does not yield superior clinical outcomes.	⊕⊕⊕◯ MODERATE
• The use of bone grafts or bone graft substitutes for treatment of comminuted distal radius fractures in adult patients does not lead to superior functional outcomes.	⊕⊕⊕◯ MODERATE
• Bone grafts or bone graft substitutes may improve radiological or anatomical outcomes when compared to immobilization in a cast alone.	⊕⊕◯◯ LOW
• The use of autologous bone graft is characterized by a significant number of complications related to the procedure of harvesting.	⊕⊕⊕⊕ HIGH

CONCLUSION

Available level-I and level-II evidence has not demonstrated significant advantage from the use of bone grafts or bone graft substitutes to justify routine use in

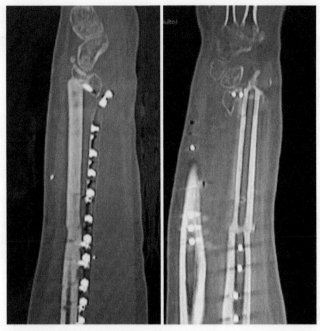

FIG. 10 CT images 4 months after surgery showing distal and proximal consolidation of the fibula flap with the radius. (Case courtesy Dr. Pérez Alba.)

comminuted distal radius fractures in elderly for purpose of improved functional or clinical outcomes. All available evidence regarding the use of bone grafts or bone graft substitutes for treatment of comminuted distal radius fractures however is targeted at elderly patients. There is no available level I, II, or III evidence regarding the use of bone grafts or bone graft substitutes for comminuted distal radius fractures or distal radius fractures with significant bone loss in younger patients. Due to the fact that bone graft substitutes may improve anatomical outcomes in selected populations, the use of bone graft substitutes for distal radius fractures in younger patients with significant metaphyseal bone loss could be considered. One should realize, however, that the use of autologous bone grafts is accompanied by a clinically important number of complications due to the harvesting from the donor site. This should be considered when treating a patient with comminuted distal radius fracture with significant metaphyseal bone loss, especially as satisfactory alternatives are available.

Panel 2: Author's Preferred Technique (Related to Case Scenario)

In the presented case, a significant metaphyseal defect after debridement of the open fracture is present, accompanied by a severe soft tissue defect. The bony defect is initially filled with a bone graft substitute—gentamicin-loaded polymethyl methacrylate (PMMA)—and an anterolateral thigh flap is used as soft tissue coverage (Fig. 11). Adequate soft tissue coverage at this stage is strongly recommended as it is a vital contribution to stimulate (bony) healing and prevent early stage infection. In addition, a primary Sauve Kapandji procedure was performed due to a severely damaged and irreconstructable distal radioulnar joint.

After 6 weeks, the cement is removed and autologous bone graft harvested from the ipsilateral femur by means of Reamed Irrigation Aspirator (RIA) grafting technique is used to fill the defect (Fig. 12). Due to necessary large volumes of bone graft, the RIA technique is preferred over iliac crest bone graft harvesting in case of large segmental bone defects.

At 1 year follow up, functional and clinical outcome is quite satisfactory and follow up radiographs show complete consolidation of the segmental metaphyseal defect in the distal radius as well as fusion of the distal radioulnar joint after Sauve Kapandji procedure (Fig. 13).

Continued

Panel 2: Author's Preferred Technique (Related to Case Scenario)—cont'd

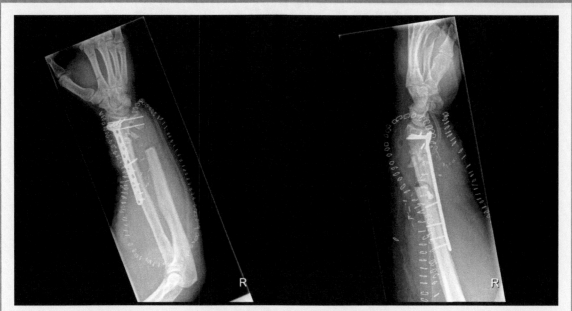

FIG. 11 Radiographs after second surgery (Case Scenario 1). The bony defect is initially filled with PMMA bone cement and an anterolateral thigh flap is used as soft tissue coverage.

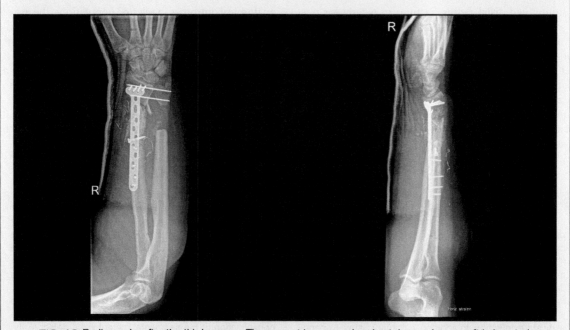

FIG. 12 Radiographs after the third surgery. The cement is removed and autologous bone graft is inserted.

Panel 2: Author's Preferred Technique (Related to Case Scenario)—cont'd

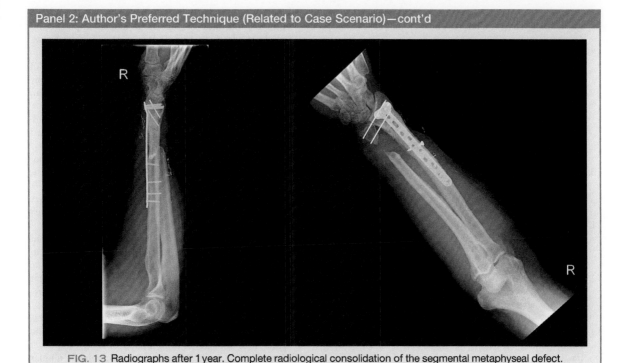

FIG. 13 Radiographs after 1 year. Complete radiological consolidation of the segmental metaphyseal defect.

Panel 3: Pearls and Pitfalls

PEARLS

- Antibiotic-loaded bone graft substitute such as gentamicin-loaded polymethyl methacrylate (PMMA) is particularly useful in open defects as it produces significant local antimicrobial activity.
- Consider the use of bone graft substitutes over autologous bone graft harvesting when possible as it prevents the occurrence of procedure related complications.

PITFALLS

- Bone graft substitutes are not an alternative for adequate osteosynthesis of comminuted distal radius fractures. Rigid and adequate fixation of all involved corners is paramount in treatment of comminuted distal radius fractures in order to prevent collapse, malunion or nonunion.

REFERENCES

1. Van Lieshout EM, Alt V. Bone graft substitutes and bone morphogenetic proteins for osteoporotic fractures: what is the evidence? *Injury*. 2016; 47(Suppl 1):S43–S46.
2. Hegde C, et al. Use of bone graft substitute in the treatment for distal radius fractures in elderly. *Eur J Orthop Surg Traumatol*. 2013;23(6):651–656.
3. Blokhuis TJ. Management of traumatic bone defects: metaphyseal versus diaphyseal defects. *Injury*. 2017; 48 (Suppl 1):S91–S93.
4. Ozer K, Chung KC. The use of bone grafts and substitutes in the treatment of distal radius fractures. *Hand Clin*. 2012; 28 (2):217–223.
5. Lutz M, et al. The metaphyseal bone defect in distal radius fractures and its implication on trabecular remodeling-a histomorphometric study (case series). *J Orthop Surg Res*. 2015;10:61.
6. Larsson S, Bauer TW. Use of injectable calcium phosphate cement for fracture fixation: a review. *Clin Orthop Relat Res*. 2002;395:23–32.

7. Handoll HH, Watts AC. Bone grafts and bone substitutes for treating distal radial fractures in adults. *Cochrane Database Syst Rev.* 2008;2:CD006836.

8. Jakubietz MG, Gruenert JG, Jakubietz RG. The use of beta-tricalcium phosphate bone graft substitute in dorsally plated, comminuted distal radius fractures. *J Orthop Surg Res.* 2011;6:24.

9. Zimmermann R, et al. Injectable calcium phosphate bone cement Norian SRS for the treatment of intra-articular compression fractures of the distal radius in osteoporotic women. *Arch Orthop Trauma Surg.* 2003; 123(1):22–27.

10. Kim JK, Koh YD, Kook SH. Effect of calcium phosphate bone cement augmentation on volar plate fixation of unstable distal radial fractures in the elderly. *J Bone Joint Surg Am.* 2011;93(7):609–614.

11. Kopylov P, et al. Norian SRS versus functional treatment in redisplaced distal radial fractures: a randomized study in 20 patients. *J Hand Surg (Br).* 2002;27 (6):538–541.

12. Cassidy C, et al. Norian SRS cement compared with conventional fixation in distal radial fractures. A randomized study. *J Bone Joint Surg Am.* 2003;85 (11):2127–2137.

13. Rajan GP, et al. Cancellous allograft versus autologous bone grafting for repair of comminuted distal radius fractures: a prospective, randomized trial. *J Trauma.* 2006;60(6):1322–1329.

14. Goto A, et al. Use of the volar fixed angle plate for comminuted distal radius fractures and augmentation with a hydroxyapatite bone graft substitute. *Hand Surg.* 2011;16(1):29–37.

15. McQueen MM, Hajducka C, Court-Brown CM. Redisplaced unstable fractures of the distal radius: a prospective randomised comparison of four methods of treatment. *J Bone Joint Surg (Br).* 1996;78(3):404–409.

16. Sanchez-Sotelo J, Munuera L, Madero R. Treatment of fractures of the distal radius with a remodellable bone cement: a prospective, randomised study using Norian SRS. *J Bone Joint Surg (Br).* 2000;82(6):856–863.

17. Schmalholz A. Bone cement for redislocated Colles' fracture. A prospective comparison with closed treatment. *Acta Orthop Scand.* 1989;60(2):212–217.

18. Widman J, Isacson J. Primary bone grafting does not improve the results in severely displaced distal radius fractures. *Int Orthop.* 2002;26(1):20–22.

19. Jeyam M, et al. Controlled trial of distal radial fractures treated with a resorbable bone mineral substitute. *J Hand Surg (Br).* 2002;27(2):146–149.

20. Kopylov P, et al. Norian SRS versus external fixation in redisplaced distal radial fractures. A randomized study in 40 patients. *Acta Orthop Scand.* 1999;70(1):1–5.

21. Schmalholz A. External skeletal fixation versus cement fixation in the treatment of redislocated Colles' fracture. *Clin Orthop Relat Res.* 1990;(254):236-41.

22. Noaman HH. Management of upper limb bone defects using free vascularized osteoseptocutaneous fibular bone graft. *Ann Plast Surg.* 2013;71(5):503–509.

23. Toros T, Ozaksar K. Reconstruction of traumatic tubular bone defects using vascularized fibular graft. *Injury.* 2019; https://doi.org/10.1016/j.injury.2019.08.013.

24. Giannoudis PV, et al. Restoration of long bone defects treated with the induced membrane technique: protocol and outcomes. *Injury.* 2016;47(Suppl 6):S53–S61.

CHAPTER 15

Arthroscopic-Assisted Treatment of Distal Radius Fractures

MARC SAAB[a] • CHRISTOPHE CHANTELOT[a] • MATTHIEU EHLINGER[b] • THOMAS BAUER[c]

[a]Orthopedic and Traumatology Department, Hôpital Roger Salengro, Lille University Hospital, Lille, France, [b]Orthopedic and Traumatology Department, Hôpital de Hautepierre, Strasbourg University Hospital, Strasbourg, France, [c]Orthopedic and Traumatology Department, Hôpital Ambroise Paré, Paris University Hospitals, Boulogne-Billancourt, France

KEY POINTS

- Arthroscopic assistance allows direct visualization and correction of the reduction of intraarticular distal articular radius fractures
- A high percentage of concomitant scapholunate interosseous ligament (SLIL) and triangular fibrocartilage complex (TFCC) lesions are diagnosed with this technique
- Arthroscopy allows same-stage treatment of SLIL and TFCC injuries after fracture fixation, although its clinical relevance remains debated due to the favorable natural course of the vast majority of these lesions.

Panel 1: Case Scenario

A 25-year-old, right-handed man fell on his outstretched right hand during professional basketball. He presented to the emergency department with a comminuted intraarticular distal radius fracture (Fig. 1). What is the most effective approach for management of this fracture and likely associated ligament injuries?

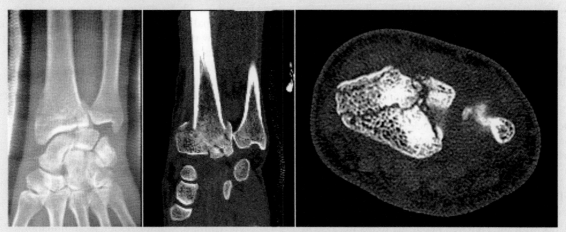

FIG. 1 Radiograph and CT scan in the coronal and axial planes showing an intraarticular distal radius fracture. Note the dorso-ulnar fragment.

Distal Radius Fractures. https://doi.org/10.1016/B978-0-323-75764-5.00005-6

IMPORTANCE OF THE PROBLEM

Arthroscopic-assisted treatment of distal radius fractures allows for potentially improved reduction through direct visualization. Moreover, it provides an accurate diagnosis of associated ligamentous injuries including SLIL or TFCC lesions that can otherwise be underdiagnosed. These injuries could be diagnosed at a state of advanced degenerative changes (such as SLAC wrist) that could lead to palliative surgery. For the TFCC, persistent ulnar-sided wrist pain could occur, as well as distal radio-ulnar joint (DRUJ) instability. Beyond 30 degrees of displacement of the radial epiphysis in the sagittal plane, associated TFCC injuries are very frequent and could be underdiagnosed without arthroscopy evaluation. The functional cost of these lesions makes early management important, especially in young adults.

MAIN QUESTION

- Can arthroscopic assistance improve the reduction of intraarticular distal radius fractures?
- How does arthroscopy contribute to the diagnosis and treatment of concomitant ligament injuries?
- Does arthroscopic assistance help to improve long-term functional outcome?

CURRENT OPINION

Arthroscopic assistance in the management of intraarticular distal radius fracture (IADRF) allows a better reduction of articular surface and could prevent degenerative arthritis of the wrist. It is also the only tool that allows control of intraoperative reduction of "Die punch" type impaction fractures and check for the absence of intraarticular protruding screws when aiming for the stable subchondral fixation. Furthermore, it allows to assess and manage associated ligament injuries at the same time. Nevertheless, enthusiasm is tempered by inconsistent evidence of its benefits and relevance in routine management of IADRF.

FINDING THE EVIDENCE

A systematic literature review was performed in accordance with the Preferred Reporting Items for Systematic Reviews and Meta-Analyses (PRISMA) guideline.[1] The PubMed, Ovid, and Cochrane databases were searched for articles published between January 1, 2006 and March 1, 2020, using the key indexing terms "distal radius fracture," "articular," and "wrist arthroscopy." Articles were potentially eligible if they compared internal IADRF fixation and/or the diagnosis and treatment of acute carpal injuries with versus without arthroscopic assistance or if they were case-series studies of patients managed with arthroscopic assistance. Only studies of adult patients were included. Fracture displacement and interfragmentary gap had to be among the criteria used to assess improvements in IADRF reduction. The diagnosis and treatment of carpal injuries had to be described. Finally, outcomes had to be reported based on the functional scores used for wrist surgery (range of motion, grip strength, visual analog scale [VAS] scores, Disabilities of the Arm, Shoulder, and Hand [DASH] score, Mayo Wrist score, and/or Patient-Rated Wrist Evaluation [PRWE]). The following article types were excluded: literature reviews, biomechanical and anatomical studies, technical notes, letters to editors, continuing medical education articles, and articles in languages other than French or English. The above-described inclusion criteria were assessed by reading the titles and abstracts or, if these were not available, the full-length article. Each abstract was read by two observers after the elimination of duplicates. Disagreements about eligibility for inclusion in the literature review were resolved by the senior author. Selected articles were read in their entirety. For each selected article, the data were categorized as follows: author information; year of publication; study design; level of evidence; number of patients; diagnostic and therapeutic methods that were used or compared; diagnosis and management of concomitant carpal injuries; assessment criteria, with the results; follow-up duration; and clinical and radiological outcomes at final follow-up.

Cochrane Search: "Distal radius fracture arthroscopy," from 2006 to 2020

Pubmed (Medline): "Distal Radius Fractures" AND "articular" AND "arthroscopy"; date 1/1/2006 to 03/01/2020

QUALITY OF THE EVIDENCE

Level I:
Randomized trials: 1
Level II:
Randomized trials with methodological limitations: 4
Level III:
Retrospective comparative studies: 1
Level IV:
Case series: 18

FINDINGS

Can Arthroscopy Improve the Reduction of Intraarticulardistal Radius Fractures (IADRFs)?

Seventeen articles were able to answer this question, with a total of 770 patients, a mean of 45 patients per article, and a mean follow-up of 14.8 months. Of the 17 studies, 11 were case series, 5 were prospective,[2-6] and 1 was retrospective.[7] The quality of reduction was compared using computed tomography (CT) measurements in two studies,[4, 7] whereas the other studies relied on radiographic parameters,[2, 3, 5, 8] arthroscopic findings,[6, 9-13] or both.[14-17] The system used to classify the fractures varied across studies, with the AO classification[18] being used most often and the classifications devised by Frikman[8, 19] and Castaing[9] less often. The internal fixation methods varied as well. Pinning was used alone in some studies[2, 9] and combined with external fixation in others.[3, 8] Several studies used an anterior locking plate[4-6, 10, 12, 13, 15-17] or several different fixation methods depending on the type of fracture.[7, 11, 19] In studies comparing two groups, the contribution of arthroscopy was chiefly assessed based on step-off and interfragmentary gap.[2-5, 7] These same criteria were also used in noncomparative studies. In one study, step-off was evaluated according to the Knirk and Jupiter grade.[8]

Of the 17 studies, 13 indicated a beneficial effect of arthroscopy for IADRF reduction. A beneficial effect was defined in comparative studies as statistically significant improvements in the assessment criteria compared to the group without arthroscopy and in noncomparative studies as improvements in step-off and interfragmentary gap with the use of arthroscopy. Table 1 recapitulates the main findings from these studies.

How Does Arthroscopy Contribute to the Diagnosis and Treatment of Concomitant Ligament Injuries?

Thirteen studies provided information on this topic, with a total of 517 patients and a mean follow-up of 21.4 months. Two studies reported data from the first described cohort of patients with IADRF that were evaluated arthroscopically by Lindau et al.[20] and were followed up for at least 13 years.[21, 22] In nine other studies, follow-up was 1 year or less.[6-9, 17, 23-27] Of the 13 studies, 2 were comparative[3, 7] and 10 noncomparative. The assessment criteria in these studies were the proportions of patients diagnosed with injuries to the scapholunate interosseous ligament (SLIL) and/or

triangular fibrocartilage complex (TFCC). The methods used to treat these injuries in the noncomparative studies were described. Some studies also analyzed clinical assessment criteria.[6, 9, 21-23, 26, 27] Arthroscopy was deemed beneficial when its use enabled the diagnosis and/or treatment of carpal injuries or when failure to treat carpal injuries resulted in poorer clinical and radiological outcomes.[23, 26] Arthroscopy was considered unhelpful when the diagnosis and/or treatment of concomitant carpal injuries failed to improve patient outcomes. Arthroscopy provided the diagnosis of SLIL injuries in 41.7% of cases with a total of 200 lesions. SLIL injuries were classified according to Geissler[28] in all but one study, which used the European Wrist Arthroscopy Society (EWAS) classification.[29] Of the 200 lesions, 147 (73.5%) were Geissler grade I or II (partial injuries) and 53 (26.5%) were Geissler grade III or IV (complete injuries). SLIL tears were managed by scapholunate pinning.[7, 8, 26, 27] In some studies, diagnosed SLIL injuries were left untreated,[6, 9, 21, 22] whereas in others pinning was performed routinely in patients with diagnosed injuries, with no concomitant arthroscopic procedure.[3, 11, 24] In one study, grade IV injuries were managed by open repair.[25] Arthroscopy showed TFCC injuries in 52.32% of cases. The 167 lesions were classified according to Palmer,[30] which showed the following distribution: Class 1A, $n = 47$ (28.14%); Class 1B, $n = 55$ (32.93%); Class 1C, $n = 19$ (11.3%); and Class 1D, $n = 37$ (22.16%); 3 injuries were not classified. In several studies, diagnosed TFCC injuries were left untreated.[6, 8, 9, 22, 23] Class 1B injuries were repaired by arthroscopic suture in all but one study,[3] which used open repair. Other lesion types were generally managed by arthroscopic debridement,[3, 7, 11, 24, 25] although splinting was used in one study for type 1D injuries.[25] In eight studies, the results supported a positive contribution of arthroscopy to the diagnosis and treatment of carpal injuries concomitant to IADRFs.[3, 7, 8, 11, 23-26] Only seven studies reported lunotriquetral lesions and classified them with the Geissler classification, with a mean of 25% of lesions.[3, 6, 8, 11, 23, 25, 26] Treatment were LT pinning for grade 3–4 lesions. Table 2 lists the data from the selected studies and the main conclusions.

Does Arthroscopy Help to Improve the Functional Scores at Long-Term Follow-Up?

The 13 studies that assessed functional scores at final follow-up had a total of 574 patients with a mean follow-up of 28.9 months, although follow-up was 12 months or less in half of the studies.[5, 6, 8, 9, 13, 17, 27] Four studies used a prospective comparative

TABLE 1
Main Data on Quality of Articular Surface Restoration.

Year/Study	Patients (Ascp)	Level of Evidence	Treatment	Mean Follow-Up, Months	Outcomes	Conclusion	Favorable to ARIF, Yes or No
2006 Hardy et al.	18 (18)	IV	ARIF	12	Mayo Wrist Score decreased with increasing Knirk-Jupiter (step-off) grade	Articular surface restoration is the most important prognostic criterion	Yes
2007 Battistella et al.	80 (40)	II	ORIF versus ARIF	38	With Ascp, better coronal inclination, ulnar variance, and joint surface restoration	ARIF is better than the conventional method	Yes
2007 Hattori et al.	28 (28)	IV	ARIF and volar plate or external fixation in patients >70years	24.9	Mayo Wrist Score 80.1 ± 0.5 23 returned to previous activities	ARIF is an effective option in older, physically active patients	Yes
2008 Varitimidis et al.	40 (20)	II	Open reduction external fixation versus ARIF	24	After 24months, smaller step-off with vs without Ascp (0.3 vs 0.8, $P < .01$)	ARIF improves articular surface restoration	Yes
2008 Lutsky et al.	16 (16)	IV	Ascp and Fscp to guide reduction compared using a subjective VAS	0	Fscp: 8.2/10 Ascp: 6.4/10	Fscp assessment underestimates residual displacement	Yes
2010 Ono et al.	31 (31)	IV	Ascp to assess step-off and interfragment gap after ORIF with volar locking plate	0	7 patients with displacement ≥2mm	ARIF if preoperative displacement	Yes
2011 Levy et al.	35 (35)	IV	ORIF with Ascp assessment after 6 weeks	12	Only 9 patients with interfragment gap >1mm and 2 with step-off >1mm	≥5.80 mm Reserve ARIF for young patients	No
2012 Ono et al.	70 (70)	IV	Ascp to assess step-off and interfragment gap after ORIF with volar locking plate	13	15 patients with step-off ≥1mm 40 patients with interfragment gap ≥1mm	ARIF is helpful when the preoperative sup of step-off and interfragment gap is >7.85mm	Yes
2013 Abe et al.	153 (153)	IV	ARIF and plate presetting arthroscopic reduction technique (PART)	30	35.2% of patients with displacement corrected with Ascp assistance	Plate presetting and ARIF provide effective reduction and decrease surgery invasiveness.	Yes

Study	Level of evidence	N	Intervention	Results	Conclusion	Ascp assessment
2013 Khanchandani et al.	IV	27 (27)	ARIF	In 5 patients intraoperative IF modification after Ascp evaluation	Ascp assessment allows correction of residual step-off	Yes
2014 Del Pinal et al.	IV	4 (4)	ARIF of comminuted diaphyseal-metaphyseal fractures	Step-off <1mm in 4 patients	ARIF allows the reduction of intraarticular fractures with diaphyseal-metaphyseal comminution	Yes
2014 Zemirline et al.	IV	20 (20)	ARIF via a 15-mm anterior approach	19 patients with step-off <1mm	Inconspicuous scar, anatomical reduction, diagnosis and treatment of concomitant ligament injuries	Yes
2015 Yamazaki et al.	II	74 (37)	ORIF versus ARIF	No significant difference in step-off or interfragment gap between the 2 groups after 6 or 48 weeks	ARIF does not improve articular surface restoration	No
2016 Thiart et al.	IV	44 (44)	ORIF then intraoperative Ascp assessment	Step-off: 0mm (33 patients) 0–1mm (3 patients) 1–2mm (8 patients) Interfragment gap: 0mm (37 patients) 0–2mm (6 patients) 3mm (1 patient)	Ascp showed acceptable step-off and interfragment gap with Fscp assistance. Limited role for Ascp assistance in reducing intraarticular fractures	No
2017 Christiaens et al.	III	40 (20)	ORIF vs ARIF	After 3 months, smaller step-off in the Ascp group	ARIF improves the reduction of IADRFs	Yes
2018 Burnier et al.	II	40 (20)	ORIF versus ARIF with CT after 3 months to compare step-off and interfragment gap	No Ascp: step-off reduction not significant ($P > .05$). With Ascp: significant step-off reduction ($P < .05$)	ARIF improves articular surface restoration	Yes
2019 Selles et al	I	50 (22) 770 (605)	Assess reduction in Ascp group after ORIF	No step off for 16 patients 1–2mm for 4 patients >2mm for 2 patients No gap for 16 patients 1–2mm for 5 patients >2mm for 1 patients	Anatomic reduction in 13 patients	No

Ascp, arthroscopy; *IF*, internal fixation; *Fscp*, fluoroscopy; *VAS*, visual analog scale; *CT*, computed tomography; *IADRF*, intraarticular distal radius fracture; *ARIF*, arthroscopic reduction internal fixation; *ORIF*, open reduction internal fixation.

TABLE 2

Main Data on the Diagnosis and Treatment of Carpal Cligamentous Injuries Concomitant to Intraarticular Distal Radius Fractures.

Year/Study	Patients (Ascp)	Mean FU (mo)	SLIL (%)	Geissler Grade 1	Geissler Grade 2	Geissler Grade 3	Geissler Grade 4	TFCC (%)	Palmer 1A	Palmer 1B	Palmer 1C	Palmer 1D	Treatment SLIL	Treatment TFCC	Conclusion	Favorable to Ascp, Yes or No
2006 Hardy et al.	18 (18)	12	28	4 "partial"		1 "complete"		17			1	2	SLIL pinning in 2 patients	None	ARIF allows the treatment of concomitant injuries	Yes
2007 Forward et al.	51 (51)	12	86	11	23	10							None	None	After 12 months, significant increase in the SL angle, SL pain and instability if Geissler 3	Yes
2008 Varitimidis et al.	40 (20)	24	45		7	2		60		6		6	SLIL pinning in 9 patients	Debridement of all lesions with Ascp repair in 1 case and open repair in 1 case	The treatment of concomitant lesions may have contributed to the better scores in the Ascp group	Yes
2011 Levy et al.[a]	35 (35)	12	28	3 grade 1 or 2		7 EWAS grade 3, 4 or 5		28		3[a]			None	None	No correlation between anatomical ligament injuries and functional scores after 1 year	No
2013 Araf et al.	30 (30)	0	36.6	2	6	2	1	76.7	4	7	14	2	Repair of all identified lesions		High incidence of carpal lesions in IADRFs	Yes
2013 Ogawa et al.	85 (85)	0	54.5	39		6	3	40	27	2		5	Grade 1–2: none; grade 3: SLIL pinning; grade 4: open repair	1A: debridement, 1B Ascp suture, 1D=above-elbow cast	High incidence of carpal injuries, independently from the fracture	Yes
2013 Khanchandani et al.	27 (27)	26	29	3	2	1	2	62		15		2	Grades 2–3–4: SLIL pinning 8 weeks	1B suture if large lesion, debridement for 1D and small 1B lesions	Ascp contributes to the diagnosis and treatment of concomitant injuries.	Yes

Study											SLIL injuries treatment	TFCC injuries treatment	Influence on outcome	Conclusion
2012–2015 Mrkonjic et al.	38 (38)	156	68.4	17 grade 1–2	9	7	2	7	9		None	None	No	SLIL injuries grades 1–3 and TFCC injuries do not influence the objective or subjective functional scores or the radiographic outcomes after a minimum follow-up of 13 years
2015 Kasapinova et al.	40 (40)	6	35	2	5	5	2	86.8	7		Grade 3–4: SLIL pinning	None	Yes	Lower functional scores at 3 and 6 months if SLIL injury ARIF useful for managing these lesions
2016 Thiart et al.	44 (44)	3	6.8	15	5		34.1				None	Repair of a single TFCC lesion	No	High incidence of carpal lesions in patients with IADRFs
2017 Swart et al.	42 (42)	12	45	11	7	1	50	7	6	8	Grade 3: SLIL pinning	Debridement	No	No difference in functional scores at 12 months between groups with vs without SLIL and/or TFCC injuries
2017 Christiaens et al.	40 (20)	3	30	3	1	2	30	2	1	2	Grade 3: SLIL pinning	1B Ascp suture, debridement for 1C and 1D	Yes	ARIF allows the management of these lesions.
2019 Selles et al	50 (22) / 517 (472)	12 / 50	21.38 (25) / 41.72 (25)	Partial lesions (grade 1 or 2): 147/200 (73.5%) / Complete lesions (>grade 3): 53/200 (26.5%)	5	1	3	91	52.32	2 — 47/167 (28.14%) / 10 — 55/167 (32.93%) / 1 — 19/167 (11.38%) / 1 — 37/167 (22.16%)	None	None	No	Most of soft-tissue Injuries do not Require treatment

FU, follow-up; *mo*, months; *SLIL*, scapho–lunate interosseous ligament; *TFCC*, triangular fibrocartilage complex; *SL*, scapholunate; *IADRF*, intraarticular distal radial fracture; *Ascp*, arthroscopy; *ARIF*, arthroscopic reduction internal fixation.

[a]1B, C, or D (not specified).

design.[2, 3, 5, 6] The most often used functional parameters were the MWS, DASH, VAS, and range of motion. Grip strength was measured in several studies[2, 3, 5, 10, 12, 13, 21, 22] and the PRWE score in two studies.[6, 12] Finally, the development of radiocarpal osteoarthritis was evaluated in two studies including one with a long-term follow-up.[8, 21] Of the 13 studies, 6 supported a beneficial effect of arthroscopy in improving the functional scores at final follow-up.[2, 3, 8, 10, 12, 13] One case-series study was inconclusive[11] and the six remaining studies were not in favor of arthroscopy,[5, 8, 16, 19, 25] including the randomized controlled trial study that did not find better outcomes after ORIF followed by arthroscopic removal of hematoma and debris compared to ORIF alone at 12 months follow-up.[6] Table 3 reports the main data on functional scores at final follow-up.

TABLE 3
Main Data on the Functional Scores at Final Follow-Up.

Year/ Study	Patients	Type	Outcome Measures	Mean FU (mo)	Outcomes	Conclusion	Favorable to Ascp, Yes or No
2006 Hardy et al.	18	IV	Mayo Wrist Score	12	Mayo Wrist Score decreases as Knirk-Jupiter grade (step-off) increases	Articular surface restoration is the most important prognostic criterion	Yes
2007 Battistella et al.	80	II	ROM, grip, VAS, DASH	38	ARIF group: better functional scores, greater motion range, greater grip strength ($P < .05$)	ARIF is better than the conventional method.	Yes
2008 Varitimidis et al.	40	II	ROM, grip, DASH, Mayo Wrist Score at 12 and 24 months	24	After 12 and 24 months: Mayo Wrist Score better in the Ascp group, DASH not significantly different At 12 months: flexion-extension, and supination better in the Ascp group	Functional scores and ROM better with Ascp	Yes
2011 Levy et al.	35	IV	ROM, DASH	12	Mean DASH 34.9 ± 21 VAS: 3	No correlation between anatomical reduction and functional scores	No
2013 Abe et al.	145	IV	ROM, grip, Mayo Wrist Score, DASH	30	Mean DASH: 4.1 Mayo: 112 excellent, 31 good, 2 fair	Plate presetting and ARIF provide effective reduction and decrease surgery invasiveness	Yes
2013 Khanchandani et al.	27	IV	Mayo Wrist Score	26	20 excellent, 3 good, 4 fair	No conclusion regarding the clinical score	

TABLE 3

Main Data on the Functional Scores at Final Follow-Up.—cont'd

Year/ Study	Patients	Type	Outcome Measures	Mean FU (mo)	Outcomes	Conclusion	Favorable to Ascp, Yes or No
2014 Del Pinal et al.	4	IV	ROM, grip, VAS, DASH, PRWE	36	Mean PRWE: 9 mean DASH: 10 Flexion 70% Extension 90% Grip 95% (vs normal side)	Clinical outcomes similar to those in other studies	Yes
2014 Zemirline et al.	17	IV	ROM, Quick DASH, grip, VAS	4	VAS 1.9 (0–7) Quick DASH 24.6 (0–70) ROM vs normal side, 71% to 86% Grip 67% of normal side	Inconspicuous scar, longer follow-up required	Yes
2015 Mrkonjic et al.	38	IV	DASH, VAS, grip, Gartland and Werley, osteoarthritis (if SLIL injury)	156	None of the subjective or objective criteria differed significantly between peripheral partial or central vs complete TFCC injury or between SLIL injury grade 0–1–2 vs 3	Grade 1–3 SLIL injuries and TFCC injuries did not influence the subjective or objective scores or the radiographic outcomes after a minimum of 13 years.	No
2015 Yamazaki et al.	74	II	ROM, grip, DASH	11	DASH, grip, ROM: no significant difference between groups	Functional scores at last follow-up not better with ARIF	No
2016 Thiart et al.	44	IV	ROM	3	Flexion 41 ± 10 degrees extension 51 ± 17 pronation 85 ± 5 degrees supination 74 ± 20 degrees	Good outcomes but longer-term data on functional scores needed	No
2017 Swart et al.	30	IV	DASH, VAS, ROM	12	DASH, VAS, ROM: no significant differences	No difference in functional scores at 12 months between the groups with vs without SLIL and/or TFCC injuries	No
2019 Selles et al.	22 574		VAS, DASH, PRWE	12 28.92	VAS 6 weeks no significant differences between the two groups PRWE and DASH 12 mo: no significant differences between the two groups	No benefits of arthroscopic removal of hematoma and debris after ORIF	No

Ascp, arthroscopy; *ROM*, range of motion; *VAS*, visual analog scale; *PRWE*, patient-rated wrist evaluation; *SLIL*, scapholunate interosseous ligament; *TFCC*, triangular fibrocartilage complex; *FU*, follow-up; *mo*, months; *ARIF*, arthroscopic reduction internal fixation.

RECOMMENDATION

In patients with an intraarticular distal radius fracture, evidence suggests:

Recommendation	Overall Quality
• Arthroscopic assistance may allow for a better intraarticular reduction than fluoroscopy	⊕⊕◯◯ LOW
• Arthroscopic assistance improves the diagnosis and classification of acute carpal ligament and TFCC injuries	⊕⊕⊕⊕ HIGH
• Although arthroscopy allows for direct treatment of severe SLIL injuries and of peripheral ulnar TFCC detachment, its benefit has not been consistently proven in comparative series	⊕⊕⊕◯ MODERATE
• Overall, arthroscopic assisted fixation has not proven consistent improved functional outcomes at long term follow-up	⊕⊕⊕◯ MODERATE

CONCLUSION

Studies on the contribution of arthroscopic assistance to control accurate articular surface restoration in patients with IADRFs have reported conflicting results. The available data provides convincing evidence that arthroscopy is valuable for diagnosing and classifying concomitant ligament injuries, although its clinical relevance remains speculative as treatment has not proven consistent benefit over neglect, which is likely due to the generally favorable natural course of these lesions. Finally, the retrospective design and short-term follow-up of most published studies preclude definitive conclusions about whether arthroscopy improves the functional scores on long-term follow-up.

Panel 2: Author's Preferred Technique

The authors prefer beginning by a provisional osteosynthesis with an anterior locking plate using a modified Henry's approach for stabilization and fluoroscopic control of metaphyseal and epiphyseal reduction. A first metaphyseal cortical screw is placed and if the plate height and epiphyseal reduction are satisfactory under fluoroscopic control, additional epiphyseal screws can be placed to fix well reduced fragments, notably the radial styloid fragment. Subsequently, standard arthroscopy is performed using a 2.7 mm arthroscope inclined at 30 degrees through the 3–4 portal with a probe of 1.5 mm diameter through the 6R portal. Haemarthrosis is removed by minimal irrigation and debridement in a "semidry" fashion. The probe is used to browse the cartilage for interfragmentary gaps and step-off and evaluate the scapholunate and lunotriquetral ligaments and TFCC.

If the reduction is unsatisfying, we correct it, if necessary, by removing an epiphyseal screw to re-allow fragment mobilization (Fig. 2) With the probe holding fragments in place, epiphyseal locking screws can be re positioned by an assistant. If necessary, additional pinning can help with the reduction. Pins could be left in place to stabilize osteosynthesis. Finally, we re-explore for any ligament injury including the TFCC by radiocarpal arthroscopy, and SLIL and LTIL by midcarpal arthroscopy. When a grade 3 or 4 SLIL injury is diagnosed, scapholunate pinning or arthroscopic capsulodesis is performed (Fig. 3). When a grade 3 or 4 LTIL injury is diagnosed, a lunotriquetral pinning is performed. Peripheral TFCC lesions are repaired by an inside-out suture. When a foveal lesion is diagnosed, it is repaired by performing a foveal reinsertion with an anchor inserted in the fovea of the ulna, which is prepared using an additional direct foveal portal.

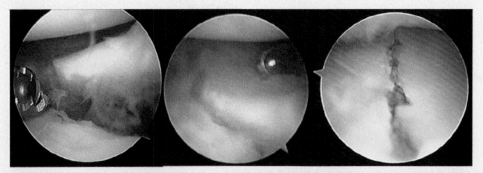

FIG. 2 Arthroscopic control and reduction. The step-off between fragments *(left image)* is greater than 1 mm. The probe is used to push on the fragment to align it *(center image)*. Arthroscopic view of the final reduction *(right image)*.

Panel 2: Author's Preferred Technique—cont'd

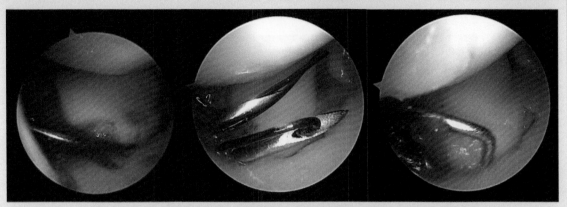

FIG. 3 Scapholunate lesion, stage 3C of the EWAS classification *(left)*: arthroscope in ulnar midcarpal portal, probe in radial midcarpal portal assessing the scapholunate interval. Note the passage of the probe in the dorsal portion of the scapholunate interval. Arthroscopic capsulodesis using two needles loaded with absorbable 3–0 sutures *(center)*. Final aspect of dorsal capsulodesis and testing with the probe unable to re-enter in the dorsal scapholunate interval *(right)*.

Panel 3: Pearls and Pitfalls

PEARLS

- A preoperative CT scan allows for better understanding of the fracture pattern
- Total procedure time should be aimed to remain within 1 h 30 min–2 h for multiple reasons such as the risk of compartment syndrome.
- Save time in the first stage of the procedure (modified Henry's approach and provisional osteosynthesis)
- Reactional synovitis of the radiocarpal joint can be shaved to allow better visualization; haemarthrosis should be evacuated as much as possible by utilizing the shaver aspiration while browsing the entire radio-carpal surface until obtaining a clear vision
- Follow the shaver with the scope in order to not commit iatrogenic injuries.

PITFALLS

- Be aware of the risk of nerve lesion (dorsal sensory branch of the ulnar nerve) and tendon injury while realizing arthroscopic portals
- Wrist arthroscopy can be challenging. Starting your learning curve with a noncomminuted IADRF such as a simple radial styloid is recommended.
- Be cautious about using irrigation during "wet arthroscopy" as increased forearm compartment pressure through leakage at the fracture site can result in a devastating complication. Pressure-pumps should be avoided.

Editor's Tips & Tricks: ARIF for Die Punch Fractures
Michael Bouyer and Geert Alexander Buijze

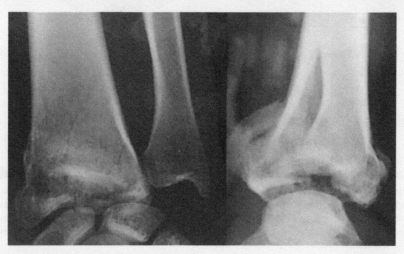

Fig. 1. Die punch fractures such as the one presented are arguably the best indication for ARIF as it offers live view of articular restoration while assuring absence of intraarticular screws having to be placed closely subchondral (see Video 1 from https://www.elsevier.com/books-and-journals/book-companion/9780323757645).

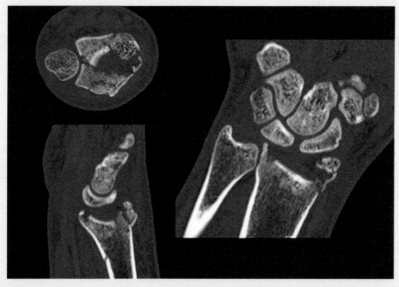

Fig. 2. CT scanning is necessary to appreciate true articular impaction. As central impaction cannot be restored by ligamentotaxis, either an extraarticular "push technique" under fluoroscopy or an intraarticular "pull technique" under arthroscopic control is mandatory.

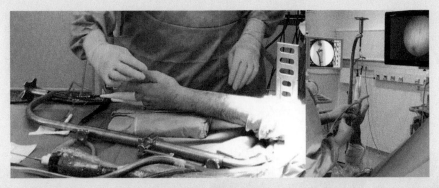

Fig. 3. An articulated axial traction tower allows for preoperative setup in horizontal position to provisionally apply a volar rim plate with a single adjustable metaphyseal screw. Next, the tower only needs to be verticalized to allow 360 degrees access to the distal radius while saving tourniquet time.

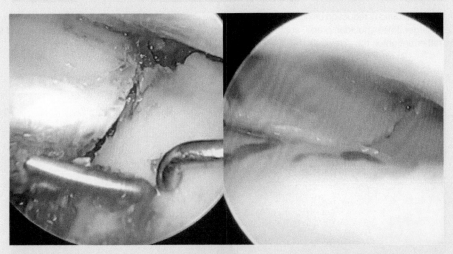

Fig. 4. Arthroscopy can guide both articular reduction and temporary K-wire fixation followed by screw fixation closely subchondral at the scaphoid and lunate fossae (see Video 1 from https://www.elsevier.com/books-and-journals/book-companion/9780323757645).

Continued

Editor's Tips & Tricks: ARIF for Die Punch Fractures—cont'd

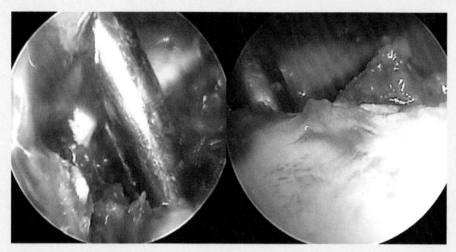

Fig. 5. In case of difficult reduction using a small 1.5 mm probe, consider more resistant blunt curved instruments such as a larger (knee/shoulder) probe, spatula or haemostat. Do not use excessive force on incarcerated fragments, rather untighten the screw.

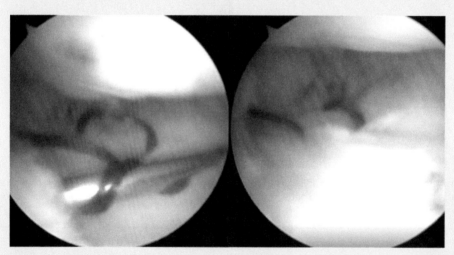

Fig. 6. To assess concomitant foveal TFCC disruption, we suggest combining the trampoline test with the hook test and "ghost sign" (see Video 2 from https://www.elsevier.com/books-and-journals/book-companion/9780323757645). Acute repair can generally be done by simple stitching techniques without anchors.

Editor's Tips & Tricks: ARIF for Die Punch Fractures—cont'd

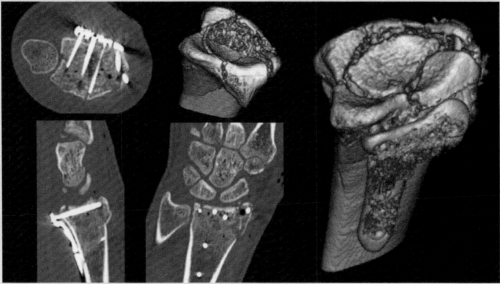

Fig. 7. Postoperative CT with 3D reconstruction of the distal radius (eliminating the segmented carpus and ulna) provides an accurate overview of the scapholunate facets and sigmoid notch.

REFERENCES

1. Shamseer L, Moher D, Clarke M, et al. Preferred reporting items for systematic review and meta-analysis protocols (PRISMA-P) 2015: elaboration and explanation. *BMJ*. 2015;350, g7647.

2. Battistella F, Verga M, Delaria G, Peri A. 2.3 Wrist arthroscopy in intra-articular distal radius fracture. *J Hand Surg Eur Vol*. 2006;31:7–8. https://doi.org/10.1016/j.jhsb.2006.03.177.

3. Varitimidis SE, Basdekis GK, Dailiana ZH, Hantes ME, Bargiotas K, Malizos K. Treatment of intra-articular fractures of the distal radius: fluoroscopic or arthroscopic reduction? *J Bone Joint Surg (Br)*. 2008;90(6):778–785. https://doi.org/10.1302/0301-620X.90B6.19809.

4. Burnier M, Le Chatelier Riquier M, Herzberg G. Treatment of intra-articular fracture of distal radius fractures with fluoroscopic only or combined with arthroscopic control: a prospective tomodensitometric comparative study of 40 patients. *Orthop Traumatol Surg Res*. 2018;104(1):89–93. https://doi.org/10.1016/j.otsr.2017.08.021.

5. Yamazaki H, Uchiyama S, Komatsu M, et al. Arthroscopic assistance does not improve the functional or radiographic outcome of unstable intra-articular distal radial fractures treated with a volar locking plate: a randomised

controlled trial. *Bone Joint J*. 2015;97-B(7):957–962. https://doi.org/10.1302/0301-620X.97B7.35354.

6. Selles CA, Mulders MAM, Colaris JW, van Heijl M, Cleffken BI, Schep NWL. Arthroscopic debridement does not enhance surgical treatment of intra-articular distal radius fractures: a randomized controlled trial. *J Hand Surg Eur Vol*. 2019. https://doi.org/10.1177/1753193419866128.

7. Christiaens N, Nedellec G, Guerre E, et al. Contribution of arthroscopy to the treatment of intraarticular fracture of the distal radius: retrospective study of 40 cases. *Hand Surg Rehabil*. 2017. https://doi.org/10.1016/j.hansur.2017.03.003.

8. Hardy P, Gomes N, Chebil M, Bauer T. Wrist arthroscopy and intra-articular fractures of the distal radius in young adults. *Knee Surg Sports Traumatol Arthrosc*. 2006;14 (11):1225–1230. https://doi.org/10.1007/s00167-006-0123-9.

9. Levy S, Saddiki R, Normand J, Dehoux E, Harisboure A. Arthroscopic assessment of articular fractures of distal radius osteosyntheses by percutaneous pins. *Chir Main*. 2011;30(3):218–223. https://doi.org/10.1016/j.main.2011.04.004.

10. Abe Y, Yoshida K, Tominaga Y. Less invasive surgery with wrist arthroscopy for distal radius fracture. *J Orthop Sci*.

2013;18(3):398–404. https://doi.org/10.1007/s00776-013-0371-8.

11. Khanchandani P, Badia A. Functional outcome of arthroscopic assisted fixation of distal radius fractures. *Indian J Orthop.* 2013;47(3):288–294. https://doi.org/10.4103/0019-5413.109872.

12. Del Piñal F, Klausmeyer M, Moraleda E, de Piero GH, Rúas JS. Arthroscopic reduction of comminuted intra-articular distal radius fractures with diaphyseal-metaphyseal comminution. *J Hand Surg [Am].* 2014;39(5):835–843. https://doi.org/10.1016/j.jhsa.2014.02.013.

13. Zemirline A, Taleb C, Facca S, Liverneaux P. Minimally invasive surgery of distal radius fractures: a series of 20 cases using a 15mm anterior approach and arthroscopy. *Chir Main.* 2014;33(4):263–271. https://doi.org/10.1016/j.main.2014.04.007.

14. Lutsky K, Boyer MI, Steffen JA, Goldfarb CA. Arthroscopic assessment of intra-articular distal radius fractures after open reduction and internal fixation from a volar approach. *J Hand Surg [Am].* 2008;33(4):476–484. https://doi.org/10.1016/j.jhsa.2007.12.009.

15. Ono H, Furuta K, Fujitani R, Katayama T, Akahane M. Distal radius fracture arthroscopic intraarticular displacement measurement after open reduction and internal fixation from a volar approach. *J Orthop Sci.* 2010;15(4):502–508. https://doi.org/10.1007/s00776-010-1484-y.

16. Ono H, Katayama T, Furuta K, Suzuki D, Fujitani R, Akahane M. Distal radial fracture arthroscopic intraarticular gap and step-off measurement after open reduction and internal fixation with a volar locked plate. *J Orthop Sci.* 2012;17(4):443–449. https://doi.org/10.1007/s00776-012-0226-8.

17. Thiart M, Ikram A, Lamberts RP. How well can step-off and gap distances be reduced when treating intra-articular distal radius fractures with fragment specific fixation when using fluoroscopy. *Orthop Traumatol Surg Res.* 2016;102(8):1001–1004. https://doi.org/10.1016/j.otsr.2016.09.005.

18. Müller ME, Nazarian S, Koch P. *Classification AO Des Fractures: Tome I: Les Os Longs.* 1st ed. Berlin: Springer-Verlag; 1987. Part 2.

19. Hattori Y, Doi K, Estrella EP, Chen G. Arthroscopically assisted reduction with volar plating or external fixation for displaced intra-articular fractures of the distal radius in the elderly patients. *Hand Surg.* 2007;12(01):1–12. https://doi.org/10.1142/S021881040700333X.

20. Lindau T, Arner M, Hagberg L. Intraarticular lesions in distal fractures of the radius in young adults. A descriptive arthroscopic study in 50 patients. *J Hand Surg (Br).* 1997;22(5):638–643.

21. Mrkonjic A, Lindau T, Geijer M, Tägil M. Arthroscopically diagnosed scapholunate ligament injuries associated with distal radial fractures: a 13- to 15-year follow-up. *J Hand Surg [Am].* 2015;40(6):1077–1082. https://doi.org/10.1016/j.jhsa.2015.03.017.

22. Mrkonjic A, Geijer M, Lindau T, Tägil M. The natural course of traumatic triangular fibrocartilage complex tears in distal radial fractures: a 13-15 year follow-up of arthroscopically diagnosed but untreated injuries. *J Hand Surg [Am].* 2012;37(8):1555–1560. https://doi.org/10.1016/j.jhsa.2012.05.032.

23. Forward DP, Lindau TR, Melsom DS. Intercarpal ligament injuries associated with fractures of the distal part of the radius. *J Bone Joint Surg Am.* 2007;89(11):2334–2340. https://doi.org/10.2106/JBJS.F.01537.

24. Araf M, Mattar Junior R. Arthroscopic study of injuries in articular fractures of distal radius extremity. *Acta Ortop Bras.* 2014;22(3):144–150. https://doi.org/10.1590/1413-78522014220300813.

25. Ogawa T, Tanaka T, Yanai T, Kumagai H, Ochiai N. Analysis of soft tissue injuries associated with distal radius fractures. *BMC Sports Sci Med Rehabil.* 2013;5(1):19. https://doi.org/10.1186/2052-1847-5-19.

26. Kasapinova K, Kamiloski V. Influence of associated lesions of the intrinsic ligaments on distal radius fractures outcome. *Arch Orthop Trauma Surg.* 2015;135(6):831–838. https://doi.org/10.1007/s00402-015-2203-0.

27. Swart E, Tang P. The effect of ligament injuries on outcomes of operatively treated distal radius fractures. *Am J Orthop.* 2017;46(1):E41–E46.

28. Geissler WB, Freeland AE, Savoie FH, McIntyre LW, Whipple TL. Intracarpal soft-tissue lesions associated with an intra-articular fracture of the distal end of the radius. *J Bone Joint Surg Am.* 1996;78(3):357–365.

29. Messina JC, Van Overstraeten L, Luchetti R, Fairplay T, Mathoulin CL. The EWAS classification of scapholunate tears: an anatomical arthroscopic study. *J Wrist Surg.* 2013;2(2):105–109. https://doi.org/10.1055/s-0033-1345265.

30. Palmer AK. Triangular fibrocartilage complex lesions: a classification. *J Hand Surg [Am].* 1989;14(4):594–606.

CHAPTER 16

Simultaneous Fractures of the Distal Radius and Scaphoid

NICK JOHNSON[a] • JULIA BLACKBURN[a] • SASA POCNETZ[a] •
TOMMY R. LINDAU[a,b]
[a]Pulvertaft Hand Centre, University Hospitals Derby and Burton, Derby, United Kingdom,
[b]University of Derby, Derby, United Kingdom

KEY POINTS

- Simultaneous distal radius and scaphoid fractures are rare. If diagnosed, rule out or confirm if they are part of a trans-styloid, trans-scaphoid perilunate fracture dislocation (greater arc) with CT or MRI.
- These injuries are most often caused by high-energy trauma, sometimes as part of polytrauma which will affect how to manage the fractures.
- There is low-grade evidence that they should be treated, operatively.

Panel 1: Case Scenario

A 36-year-old male sustains an isolated injury to his left dominant wrist after a motorcycle road traffic accident. There is an obvious deformity to the wrist. Radiographs reveal a comminuted volarly angulated distal radius fracture with a minimally displaced scaphoid waist fracture and an ulnar styloid fracture (Fig. 1). What are your options for further diagnosis and treatment?

Continued

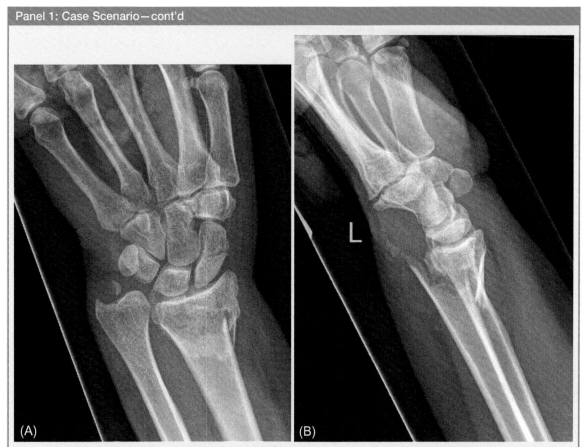

Panel 1: Case Scenario—cont'd

FIG. 1 Radiographs of simultaneous distal radius fracture and scaphoid fracture sustained with a high-energy mechanism. (A) PA view of the wrist demonstrating a radially and axially displaced radius fracture, a minimally displaced scaphoid fracture and an ulnar styloid fracture, which in this case is an avulsion fracture from the tip as opposed to a base of the styloid fracture potentially representing a destabilizing TFCC tear. (B) Lateral view showing palmar and axial displacement of the radius and an advanced carpal boss.

IMPORTANCE OF THE PROBLEM

In contrast to isolated distal radius fractures, simultaneous fractures of the distal radius and scaphoid are rare with studies reporting prevalence of 0.5%–5%.[1–10]

The second recognized pattern of injury is the fracture part (greater arc) of a perilunate (PL) dislocation with a distal radius fracture that most often is a radial styloid injury.[11] These two patterns of injury will be addressed as separate questions in this chapter.

Most of these injuries are due to high-energy trauma mechanisms.[8] That means that patients may have other fractures as part of polytrauma where lower limb or pelvis fractures may dictate how the upper limb injuries are managed.

Scaphoid fractures are less common than distal radius fractures, but account for 2%–7% of all fractures[12] and are the most frequently injured carpal bone. They usually affect young males. Nonunion rates of up to 50% are reported for displaced scaphoid fractures. Untreated nonunion often leads to early development of arthritis. As the scaphoid fracture seen with a distal radius fracture is often undisplaced,[3] it can commonly be missed.[5] Therefore, a high index of suspicion is necessary and a CT or MRI may be required to prevent nonunion of missed injuries.

MAIN QUESTIONS

1. What is the most effective treatment of simultaneous fractures of the distal radius and scaphoid?
2. What is the most effective treatment of simultaneous fractures of the distal radius and scaphoid in patients with a trans-styloid, trans-scaphoid perilunate (greater arc) dislocation?

CURRENT OPINION

Simultaneous fractures of the scaphoid and distal radius are most often diagnosed and treated as bony injuries although some surgeons argue that they can only co-exist with a trauma mechanism of a greater arc injury, like in complete perilunate dislocations, with a variable extent of partial or complete intercarpal ligament tears. Most surgeons will opt for an open reduction and internal fixation of a simultaneous distal radius and scaphoid fracture to allow early mobilization, which in turn may improve functional outcome. Although this is a common opinion, it is not clear if there is any evidence to support it.

FINDING THE EVIDENCE

We provide below our EMBASE search algorithm used to construct this chapter:

exp *"RADIUS FRACTURES"/ OR exp *"WRIST INJURIES"/ OR exp *"COLLES' FRACTURE"/ OR (exp *"SCAPHOID BONE"/ AND exp *"FRACTURES, BONE"/) OR (exp *"DISTAL RADIUS"/ AND exp *"FRACTURES, BONE"/) OR ((((radi*).ti,ab OR (wrist*).ti,ab OR (colles).ti,ab OR (scaphoid).ti,ab) AND (fractur*).ti,ab) AND (distal*).ti,ab)) AND (simultaneous OR concurrent OR coinciding OR together OR "same time" OR concomitant).ti,ab.

We did a systematic review of the literature and extracted appropriate papers for detailed analysis. Unfortunately, all papers did not present data in a coherent way, hence our results are presented with various numbers.

QUALITY OF THE EVIDENCE

We found 20 studies of simultaneous distal radius and scaphoid fractures. However, no studies were found that compared treatment. The evidence in relation to these is as follows:

Level IV:
Retrospective noncomparative studies: 14
Case reports: 6

We found 13 studies covering simultaneous fractures of the distal radius and scaphoid in patients with a trans-styloid, trans-scaphoid perilunate (greater arc) dislocation. However, no studies compared treatment. The evidence in relation to these is as follows:

Level IV:
Retrospective noncomparative studies: 6
Case reports: 7

FINDINGS

Diagnosis

Simultaneous fracture of the distal radius and the scaphoid are most often clear on normal wrist radiographs, although sometimes proper scaphoid views are needed. As these fractures can be part of a greater arc mechanism in young patients a high level of suspicion is needed and additional imaging with CT, to find further fractures, and/or MRI, to potentially find intercarpal ligament or TFCC tears, is useful. In specialized centers, arthroscopy is a useful adjunct to fully assess both bony and soft-tissue injuries.

As a bare minimum, patients who have been operated on should at the end of the procedure be re-examined with a C-arm regarding intercarpal ligament injuries, by radial and ulnar deviation of the wrist to rule out any gaps or steps. They should also have a clinical assessment of DRU-joint stability with a DRU-joint ballotment test.

Isolated Distal Radius and Scaphoid Fractures

As there were no comparative studies or prospective randomized trials of the treatment of simultaneous scaphoid and distal radius fractures, it is not possible to evaluate the most effective treatment.

In the 20 included studies, there were a total of 178 patients with 182 simultaneous fractures of the distal radius and scaphoid (Table 1). From those studies where it was possible to ascertain the mechanism of injury, most cases (134/155) were due to high-energy trauma mechanisms. Only 5/182 fractures were reported to be open.

High energy injuries did not only cause wrist injuries, but also other upper limb injuries (25/49) or lower limb injuries (24/49). It is likely that polytrauma patients are treated with operative management of their simultaneous distal radius and scaphoid fractures as part of operative management of other fractures, which will facilitate partial weightbearing for their lower limb injuries. However, great caution must be taken as the increased wrist forces involved in weightbearing on standard crutches can destabilize reduction and

TABLE 1
Summary of Findings From Included Studies of Patients Treated for Simultaneous Fractures of the Distal Radius and Scaphoid.

	No. of Patients	Fractures	Age (Range)	Gender (Male/Female)	Mechanism High Energy/Low Energy	Associated Injury Polytrauma/Upper Limb Only	Distal Radius Fractures Intra/Extra Articular	Distal Radius Fracture Treatment Open/Closed/Plaster	Scaphoid Displacement Displaced/Un displaced	Scaphoid Anatomy Proximal/Waist/Distal	Scaphoid Fracture Treatment Operative/Nonoperative	Union	Complications
Vukov (1988)	26	26	26 (16–61)	9M:17F	Unknown	–	8/18	0/0/26	0/26	0/26/0	0/26	100%	–
Oskam (1996)	23	23	39 (18–74)	13F:10M	23/0	–	8/15	1/4/18	4/19	0/21/2	4/19	100%	2/23
Fowler (2018)	23	23	37 (19–74)	19M:4F	19/4	–	17/6	18/5/0	1/22	4/17/2	23/0	95% scaphoid 100% distal radius	1/23
Gurbuz (2018)	21	22	34.9 (18–92)	17M:4F	22/0	1/10	22/0	14/8/0	–	0/22/0	22/0	100%	1/22
Rutgers (2008)	10	10	27 (19–41)	4M:6F	9/1	3/5	9/1	6/2/2	6/4	2/7/1	9/1	90% scaphoid 100% distal radius	4/10
Smith (1988)	9	9	34 (21–90)	7M:2F	6/3	2/1	0/9	1/4/4	0/9	0/9/0	0/9	100%	1/9
Hove (1994)[a]	9	9	38.6 (16–73)	5M:4F	7/2	1/3	5/4	0/0/9	–	0/7/2	0/9	100%	1/9
Moller (1983)	9	9	46.8 (27–69)	4M:5F	5/4	–	6/3	0/0/9	0/9	0/6/3	0/9	100%	–
Chang (2000)	8	8	55 (38–90)	5M:3F	4/4	3/0	7/1	2/5/1	1/7	0/8/0	5/3	100%	3/8
Komura (2012)	8	7	36.6 (19–68)	6M:1F	7/0	0/3	8/0	4/0/4	2/6	3/2/3	3/5	100%	–
Slade (2005)	7	7	30 (18–58)	5M:2F	5/2	0/1	4/3	7/0/0	7/0	1/6/0	7/0	100%	1/7

Tountas (1987)	7	7	30 (16–59)	7M	7/0	5/0	4/3/0	5/2	1/6	0/5/2	3/4	100%	4/7
Trumble (1993)	6	6	31.5 (14–49)	4M:2F	6/0	6/0	5/1/0	4/2	3/3	1/5/0	6/0	100%	4/6
Stother (1976)	3	4	41 (26–65)	3M	4/0	2/0	0/0/4	0/4	0/4	0/4/0	0/4	100%	1/4
Helm (1992)[a]	3	3	20.3 (20–21)	3M	3/0	0/0	3/0/0	3/0	–	–	3/0	100%	–
Proubasta (1991)	2	2	30 (28–32)	2M	2/0	0/1	0/2/0	2/0	0/2	0/2/0	2/0	100%	–
Richards (1992)	2	2	29 (20–38)	2M	2/0	0/0	1/1/0	2/0	0/2	0/2/0	2/0	100%	–
Oskan (2008)	1	1	28	M	2/0	1/0	2/0/0	2/0	2/0	0/2/0	2/0	100%	–
Jenkins (1986)	1	1	22	F	1/0	–	0/1/0	0/1	1/0	0/1/0	1/0	100%	–
Kristiansen (1982)	1	1	68	F	0/1	0/0	0/0/1	0/1	0/1	–	0/1	100%	–

Complications included: AVN (5), arthritis (5), malunion (4), nerve injury (2), metalwork problems (2), stiffness requiring capsulotomy (2), nonunion (2), tendon rupture (1), tenosynovitis (1).
[a]Excluding children or as part of perilunate dislocations/fracture dislocations.

fixation and potentially lead to nonunion. Forearm gutter crutches or axillary crutches are safe functional alternatives.

Most distal radius fractures were intraarticular (112/182) and most scaphoid fractures were undisplaced (120/148) involving the waist (152/178).

For both the distal radius fractures and the scaphoid fractures, roughly half were managed operatively (104/182 distal radius, 92/182 scaphoids). There was a tendency for earlier studies to use nonoperative management[6, 13, 14] while more recent studies used operative management for both these fractures[3, 8] although some fractures were still successfully managed nonoperatively in recent studies.[4, 15]

The union rate for both distal radius and scaphoid fractures was very high. Just two patients were reported to have scaphoid nonunion.[3, 15] Both these patients underwent internal fixation of their scaphoid.[15] Only three patients were reported to have malunion of their distal radius fracture[2, 16] and one with scaphoid malunion that was reportedly asymptomatic.[17]

Complications of treatment, and/or injury, included scaphoid avascular necrosis in 5 patients,[15, 18, 19] arthritis in 5 patients,[1, 16, 18] nerve injury in 2 patients[2, 8] and stiffness sufficient to require capsulotomy in 2 patients.[15] Wrist instability doesn't seem to be a great long-term concern.

It is very difficult to assess the outcome after these injuries due to the heterogeneity of the papers. Only one study used a validated patient-reported outcome measure.[8] In this study of 21 patients with 22 fractures, the results were excellent with an average Patient Rated Wrist Evaluation (PRWE) at 25 months (range 12–97 months) of 5.5 (range 0–8.5).[8]

Furthermore, range of movement outcomes at follow up[8, 15, 19–23] was reported in only seven studies, with variable results,[8, 15, 19–23] and only five studies reported grip strength[8, 19–21, 23]

Perilunate Fracture Dislocations

No comparative studies or prospective randomized trials were found regarding the treatment of simultaneous trans-styloid, trans-scaphoid fractures as part of perilunate fracture dislocations. Hence, it was not possible to evaluate the most effective treatment for these simultaneous fractures.

Patients with trans-radial styloid, trans-scaphoid perilunate fracture dislocations (PLFD) were identified

in eight out of the total of 13 studies.[24–31] In the 5 other studies,[11, 32–35] although some were large (with 166 patients,[36] 23 patients,[32] 20 patients[35] and 16 patients[34]), it was not possible to extract specific patients with trans-radial styloid and trans-scaphoid PLFD from the total.

No conclusions can be drawn regarding the management of these injuries as no included study had more than 10 patients with trans-styloid and trans-scaphoid PLFD. However, most cases found in our heterogenic systematic review were managed operatively.

RECOMMENDATION

In patients with a simultaneous fracture of the distal radius and scaphoid:

Recommendation	Overall Quality
• Perilunate (greater arc mechanism) injuries should always be suspected and may be diagnosed or excluded by MRI or wrist arthroscopy. In the absence of these diagnostic tools and as a bare minimum, patients who have been operated on should at the end of the procedure be re-examined with a C-arm regarding intercarpal ligament injuries, by radial and ulnar deviation of the wrist to rule out any gaps or steps. They should also have a clinical assessment of DRU-joint stability with a DRU-joint ballotment test.	⊕○○○ VERY LOW
• There is an increasing tendency toward recommending operative treatment.	⊕⊕○○ LOW
• The same recommendation of operative management applies to trans-styloid, trans-scaphoid PLFD.	⊕○○○ VERY LOW

CONCLUSION

Simultaneous fracture of the distal radius and scaphoid is a rare but serious injury. Patients are most often male with injury due to a high-energy trauma mechanism sometimes as part of serious polytrauma. The distal radius fracture is usually displaced whereas the scaphoid fracture is undisplaced. Union rate for both distal radius and scaphoid fractures is very high. Plate fixation of the distal radius and headless compression screw to the scaphoid is most surgeons' current preference with the aim to enable early mobilization.

Panel 2: Author's Preferred Technique

In simultaneous fractures of the distal radius and the scaphoid we routinely request for a CT to rule out other fractures as part of a greater arc injury. We don't have access to MRI arthrogram.

At the time of procedure, we aim to start with arthroscopy to assess intraarticular steps, remove lose bodies such as pieces of cartilage and/or fracture fragments and to fully assess intercarpal ligament and TFCC tears. If that is not possible we always end our procedure with re-examination with a C-arm as presented earlier.

We prefer internal fixation of both fractures to provide stability and allow early mobilization in relation to any intercarpal ligament injuries detected (Figs. 1 and 2). As in our described case the scaphoid fracture is most often minimally or undisplaced. We recommend a percutaneous fixation using a headless compression screw to the scaphoid first. Following this the displaced distal radius fracture can be reduced and fixed with a volar locking plate through an open approach without fear of displacing the scaphoid.

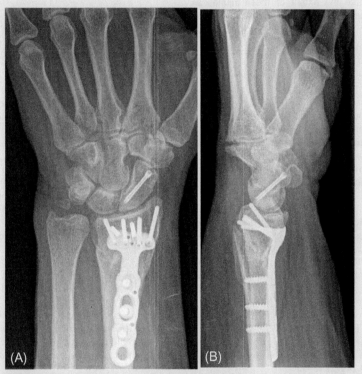

(A)   (B)

FIG. 2 (A and B) Postop PA and lateral views after initial percutaneous screw fixation of the scaphoid and subsequent ORIF of the distal radius fracture. Scaphoid fixation allows the surgeon to freely manipulate and reduce the radius fracture with a satisfactory outcome. At the end of the procedure we re-examined the wrist with a C-arm and ruled out intercarpal ligament injuries. We radially and ulnarly deviated the wrist and there were no gaps or steps. We also clinically assessed the DRU-joint stability with a DRU-joint ballotment test and found the joint stable.

Panel 3: Pearls and Pitfalls

PEARLS

- Scaphoid fixation requires compression whereas distal radius fixation usually needs traction to reduce the fracture.
- Stabilizing the scaphoid first with a percutaneous approach allows the surgeon to apply traction or any other reduction manoeuvers to reduce the displaced distal radius without causing displacement of the scaphoid fracture.

PITFALLS

- Don't underestimate the extent of these injuries as simultaneous distal radius and scaphoid fractures may represent part of a greater arc mechanism with a trans-styloid, trans-scaphoid injury with or without lunate dislocation (perilunate injury no dislocation; PLIND[37]).
- A high level of suspicion is needed and additional imaging with CT, to find further fractures, and/or MRI, to potentially find intercarpal ligament or TFCC tears, is useful. In specialized centers, arthroscopy is a useful adjunct to fully assess both bony and soft-tissue injuries.

REFERENCES

1. Hove L. Simultaneous scaphoid and distal radius fractures. *J Hand Surg (Br Eur Vol).* 1994;19B:384–388.
2. Chang C, Tsai Y, Sun J, Hou S. Ipsilateral distal radius and scaphoid fractures. *J Formos Med Assoc.* 2000;99:733–737.
3. Fowler TP, Fitzpatrick E. Simultaneous fractures of the ipsilateral scaphoid and distal radius. *J Wrist Surg.* 2018;7(4):303–311.
4. Komura S, Yokoi T, Nonomura H, Tanahashi H, Satake T, Watanabe N. Incidence and characteristics of carpal fractures occurring concurrently with distal radius fractures. *J Hand Surg Am.* 2012;37(3):469–476.
5. Vukov V, Ristic K, Stevanovic M, Bumbasirevic M. Simultaneous fractures of the distal end of the radius and the scaphoid bone. *J Orthop Trauma.* 1988;2(2):120–123.
6. Stother I. A report of 3 cases of simultaneous Colles' and scaphoid fractures. *Injury.* 1976;7(3):185–188.
7. Chrisman O, Shortell J. Fractures of the distal end of the radius complicated by fractures of the carpal scaphoid. *N Engl J Med.* 1949;241(2):58–59.
8. Gurbuz Y, Sugun TS, Kayalar M. Combined fractures of the scaphoid and distal radius: evaluation of early surgical fixation (21 patients with 22 wrists). *J Wrist Surg.* 2018;7(1):11–17.
9. Stober R, Wohlgensinger G. Karpale Begleitverletzungen bei Radiusfraktur. Art und Haufigkeit, Analyse der letzten 10 Jahre. *Z Unfallchir Versicherungsmed Berufskr.* 1989;82(1):63–65.
10. Gologan R, Ginter VM, Ising N, Kilian AK, Obertacke U, Schreiner U. Carpal lesions associated with dislocated fractures of the distal radius. A systematic screening of 104 fractures using preoperative CT and MRI. *Unfallchirurg.* 2014;117(1):48–53.
11. Herzberg G, Comtet J, Linscheid R, Amadio P, Cooney W, Stalder J. Perilunate dislocations and fracture-dislocations: a multicenter study. *J Hand Surg.* 1993;18A:768–779.
12. Hove L. Epidemiology of scaphoid fractures in Bergen, Norway. *Scand J Plast Reconstr Surg Hand Surg.* 1999;33(4):423–428.
13. Kristiansen A. Simultaneous Colles' fracture and fracture of the carpal scaphoid. *Ugeskr Laeger.* 1982;144:799.
14. Moller B. Simultaneous fracture of the carpal scaphoid and adjacent bones. *Hand.* 1983;15(3):258–261.
15. Rutgers M, Mudgal C, Shin R. Combined fractures of the distal radius and scaphoid. *J Hand Surg Eur Vol.* 2008;33E(4):478–483.
16. Oskam J, De Graaf J, Klasen H. Fractures of the distal radius and scaphoid. *J Hand Surg (Br Eur Vol).* 1996;21B(6):772–774.
17. Smith J, Keeve J, Bertin K, Mann R. Simultaneous fractures of the distal radius and scaphoid. *J Trauma.* 1988;28(5):676–679.
18. Tountas A, Waddell J. Simultaneous fractures of the distal radius and scaphoid. *J Orthop Trauma.* 1987;1(4):312–317.
19. Trumble T, Benirschke S, WVedder N. Ipsilateral fractures of the scaphoid and radius. *J Hand Surg Am.* 1993;18A(1):8–14.
20. Helm R, Tonkin M. The Chauffeur's fracture: simple of complex? *J Hand Surg.* 1992;17B:156–159.
21. Slade JF, 3rd, Taksali S, Safanda J. Combined fractures of the scaphoid and distal radius: a revised treatment rationale using percutaneous and arthroscopic techniques. *Hand Clin.* 2005;21(3):427–441.
22. Ozkan K, Ugutmen E, Unay K, Poyanli O, Guven M, Eren A. Fractures of the bilateral distal radius and scaphoid: a case report. *J Med Case Reports.* 2008;2:93.
23. Richards R, Ghose T, McBroom R. Ipsilateral fractures of the distal radius and scaphoid treated by Herbert screw and external skeletal fixation a report of two cases. *Clin Orthop Relat Res.* 1992;(282):219–220.
24. Dunn JC, Koehler LR, Kusnezov NA, et al. Perilunate dislocations and perilunate fracture dislocations in the U.S. Military. *J Wrist Surg.* 2018;7(1):57–65.

25. Banerjee A. Transstyloid perilunate carpal dislocation. *Acta Orthop Scand.* 1991;62(4):397–398.
26. Henault B, Duvernay A, Tchurukdichian A, Trouilloud P, Malka G, Trost O. Posterior perilunate carpal dislocation associated with a multifragmentary distal radius fracture. *J Plast Reconstr Aesthet Surg.* 2010;63(11):1926–1928.
27. Kohli S, Khanna V, Virani N, Chaturvedi H. Transradial, transscaphoid, transcapitate, perilunate dislocation; a case report and approach to the patient. *Bull Emerg Trauma.* 2016;4(1):54–57.
28. Morin ML, Becker GW. An unusual variant of perilunate fracture dislocations. *Case Reports Plast Surg Hand Surg.* 2016;3(1):7–10.
29. Russell T. Inter-carpal dislocations and fracture-dislocations a review of fifty-nine cases. *J Bone Joint Surg.* 1949;31B(4):524–531.
30. Schranz P, Fagg P. Trans-radial styloid, trans-scaphoid, trans-triquetral perilunate dislocation. *J R Army Med Corps.* 1991;137:146–148.
31. Yamaguchi H, Takahara M. Transradial styloid, transtriquetral perilunate dislocation of the carpus with an associated fracture of the ulnar border of the distal radius. *J Orthop Trauma.* 1994;8(5):434–436.
32. Brown KV, Tsekes D, Gorgoni CG, Di Mascio L. The treatment of perilunate ligament injuries in multiply injured patients. *Eur J Trauma Emerg Surg.* 2019;45(1):73–81.
33. Capo JT, Corti SJ, Shamian B, et al. Treatment of dorsal perilunate dislocations and fracture-dislocations using a standardized protocol. *Hand (N Y).* 2012;7(4):380–387.
34. Griffin M, Roushdi I, Osagie L, Cerovac S, Umarji S. Patient-reported outcomes following surgically managed perilunate dislocation: outcomes after perilunate dislocation. *Hand (N Y).* 2016;11(1):22–28.
35. Savvidou OD, Beltsios M, Sakellariou VI, Papagelopoulos PJ. Perilunate dislocations treated with external fixation and percutaneous pinning. *J Wrist Surg.* 2015;4(2):76–80.
36. Herzberg G, Comtet J, Linscheid R, Amadio P, Cooney WP, Perilunate Dislocations SJ. Fracture-dislocations: a multicenter study. *J Hand Surg Am.* 1993;18:768–779.
37. Herzberg G. Perilunate injuries, not dislocated (PLIND). *J Wrist Surg.* 2013;2(4):337–345.

CHAPTER 17

Galeazzi Fracture Dislocations

ANDREA CHAN • RYAN PAUL
University of Toronto—Toronto Western Hospital, Toronto, ON, Canada

KEY POINTS

- Recognition of a Galeazzi pattern of injury is essential, as failure to recognize the distal radioulnar joint (DRUJ) injury can lead to permanent impairment.
- The primary goal of management is to obtain anatomic restoration of the radius and subsequent alignment/stability of the DRUJ.
- Surgical reduction is indicated except in patients with comorbidities/conditions that preclude surgery.
- After open reduction and internal fixation of the radius in an anatomical position, stability of the DRUJ must be assessed through a full range of pronosupination.
- Treatment of the DRUJ is based on the extent of persistent instability and the arc of motion in which it occurs. Immobilization in a reduced position is preferred when instability persists only in one extreme of rotational motion (i.e., immobilization in supination when unstable only in full pronation).
- Cases of persistent instability that cannot be easily maintained or irreducible dislocations are best treated with reduction and ulnoradial Kirschner wire transfixation of the DRUJ, with consideration of repair of the ulnar styloid/triangular fibrocartilage complex (TFCC) to increase stability. Before this line of treatment is considered, it is assumed that the radius has been reduced anatomically.

Panel 1: Case Scenario

A 47-year-old, right hand dominant male accountant suffered an isolated injury to his right upper extremity after biking on his morning commute. He presented to the emergency department with a displaced distal third radial shaft fracture and dislocation of the distal radioulnar joint (Fig. 1). What is the most effective approach to management of this acute Galeazzi fracture dislocation?

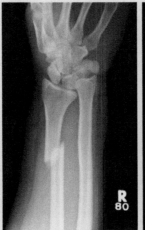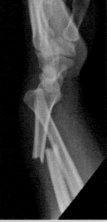

FIG. 1 Posteroanterior and lateral radiographs demonstrating a Galeazzi fracture dislocation.

Distal Radius Fractures. https://doi.org/10.1016/B978-0-323-75764-5.00003-2

IMPORTANCE OF THE PROBLEM

Recognition of the Galeazzi fracture pattern is critical to successful management of these injuries. While the majority of radial shaft fractures are isolated and do not have associated instability,[1] the DRUJ must be scrutinized for subluxation or dislocation, especially those occurring at the junction of the middle and distal third of the radius. Most true Galeazzi injuries will result in frank dislocation of the DRUJ, however, the ulnar head may demonstrate more subtle subluxation in about 20% of cases making diagnosis more difficult.[2] While Galeazzi fracture-dislocations comprise ≤7% of adult forearm fractures,[3] misidentification and inadequately treated injuries may result in ongoing DRUJ instability, restricted forearm rotational range of motion, and persistent ulnar sided wrist pain.[4] Patients may experience limited function as well as reduced strength as a result.[5] Additionally, the results of acute operative treatment are superior to that of nonoperative management or delayed reconstruction, particularly with regards to reduction and stability of the DRUJ.[2, 6, 7]

MAIN QUESTION

- In adult patients with acute Galeazzi fracture-dislocations, what is the most effective approach to management in order to restore stability and full range of motion to the distal radioulnar joint?

CURRENT OPINION

After anatomic reduction of the radius with rigid fixation, assessment of stability of the DRUJ should be performed through a full range of pronosupination. When the DRUJ may be safely reduced and easily maintained, immobilization in a stable position is recommended. For injuries where the reduction is difficult to maintain, or stable only through a short arc of motion, pin fixation of the DRUJ is indicated. Open reduction is performed when the joint is unable to be reduced by closed means.

FINDING THE EVIDENCE

We conducted a search of the Cochrane library, Medline and Embase via OVID, and the Cumulative Index of Nursing and Allied Health Literature (CINAHL). The search terms included using "Galeazzi" as a keyword and combining "radius" and "radius fracture" with "wrist injuries," "joint dislocations," "ulna," "ulna fractures." We excluded papers not published or translated into English. The reference list of included articles were also reviewed to identify additional papers not included in our initial search.

QUALITY OF THE EVIDENCE

No Level I, II, or III evidence exists regarding adult Galeazzi fracture-dislocation management. The best available evidence included in this review are Level IV:
- 13 Case Series, 2 Small Retrospective Cohort Studies and 1 Systematic Review (of case reports).

FINDINGS

We included comparative studies and any series reporting results in 10 or more adult patients. Sixteen studies were identified for inclusion (total 573 patients, range 10–95). Thirteen studies were case series (Level IV) of which a total of 448 patients were treated operatively and 108 patients were initially treated nonoperatively. Two of the studies included were retrospective cohort studies (Level IV) with a total of 17 patients with Galeazzi injuries. There was also one systematic review of case reports (Level IV) describing irreducible DRUJ dislocations.

Nonoperative Management

Closed reduction alone consistently results in poor outcomes as demonstrated by early case series.[2, 6–8] Ninety-two percent of nonoperative patients (38/41) in Hughston's case series demonstrated persistent DRUJ instability, nonunion, shortening or angulation.[6] Similarly, Mikic showed an 80% failure rate with nonoperative management.[2] Wong reported only 3 of 34 patients were able to maintain successful radial alignment and DRUJ stability after closed reduction, and 0 of 4 patients were successfully treated by immobilization without reduction.[8] Similarly, Reckling and Cordell only achieved fair or poor results (N=8) with reduction and immobilization. They noted that while all 8 of their nonoperative patients went on to achieve radial union, all had persistent ulnar head dislocation.[7] In fact, multiple studies report early conversion from nonoperative to operative management for persistent ulnar head dislocation and/or radial malreduction (N=39).[6–10] In those patients who did not receive surgery, persistent ulnar head dislocation was often associated with severe limitations in prosupination, ultimately requiring salvage procedures (most commonly Darrach/ulnar head resection). Hughston's early study recognized this issue with radial malreduction and advocated for early ulnar head resection, however, subsequent authors recommend such salvage procedures to be reserved for delayed presentations of refractory DRUJ instability.[6]

Fixation Type

The main consensus following review of the available evidence is that open reduction and rigid internal fixation of the radial shaft fracture is necessary.

In his landmark paper, Mikic described satisfactory results with both flexible intramedullary (Rush) rod and plate fixation. He went on to acknowledge that Rush rod fixation is most applicable in simple 2-part fractures and that plate fixation more readily provided rigid fixation in complex cases.[2] This combined with modern AO principles and inferior clinical results with Rush rod/intramedullary fixation reported by Reckling and Cordell (1 of 3 "poor"),[7] Macule Beneyto (3 of 3 "poor")[11] and Hughston (2 of 4 "unsatisfactory")[6] has led to plate fixation being the accepted standard of care for modern treatment.

Furthermore, plate and screw fixation has resulted in the most consistent satisfactory results in the literature. Mohan and colleagues performed open reduction and internal fixation (ORIF) on 50 patients (20 with square nail fixation, 30 with semitubular plate fixation). Despite overall 80% good results, they found that time to union occurred earlier with plate fixation and concluded that plate fixation is a better construct for this injury pattern.[10] Reckling and Cordell found that all patients treated with ORIF demonstrated good results when compared to fixation with Kirschner wires, screws or Rush rod alone.[7]

The most common, yet rare, complication following ORIF compared to nonoperative treatment is infection. In this review, 13 of 448 patients (3%) undergoing operative fixation were reported to have either superficial or deep infections.

Lastly, a 2010 paper by Gadegone et al. described the use of flexible intramedullary nails for adult patients with Galeazzi fracture dislocations.[12] They analyzed 22 cases in patients aged 20- to 56-year-old (mean 35), reporting excellent outcomes in 18 patients and fair outcomes in 4 by Mikic criteria (Table 1).[2] However, they did experience 4 cases (18%) of recurrent DRUJ instability—including 2 cases with loss of radial reduction. Given these results and the lack of other reported cases of flexible nailing, anatomic reduction, and rigid plate fixation is considered the standard of care.

DRUJ Management

Once internal fixation of the radius is performed, and the reduction deemed anatomic, assessment of the DRUJ is critical. We have elected to focus on evidence from contemporary studies (published in 2000 or later) which have a consistent means of plate fixation of the radius prior to management of the DRUJ.

Five studies were identified describing results in 178 patients all treated with plate fixation of the radius. In general, DRUJ stability was well restored, with only 2 patients demonstrating refractory instability requiring salvage procedure (Darrach). These results, however, may be overstated as 2 of the studies (N = 36) excluded

TABLE 1	
Mikic Outcome Criteria for Galeazzi Fracture-Dislocations.[2]	
Excellent	Union, perfect alignment, no loss of length, no subluxation of the distal radioulnar joint, no limitation of elbow or wrist function, and no limitation of supination or pronation.
Fair	One or more of the following: delayed union, minimum malalignment and shortening of the radius, subluxation of the ulnar head, excessive scar, limitation of pronation/supination up to 45 degrees, and some degree of restriction of motion of the elbow and wrist.
Poor	One or more of the following: nonunion, remarkable shortening or angulation of the radius, dislocation of the distal radioulnar joint, limitation of pronation/supination of more than 45 degrees, and excessive restriction of elbow and wrist function.

patients that required additional DRUJ procedures beyond immobilization in a reduced position.

The series by Korompilias et al. (N = 95), is the largest in the literature examining surgically treated Galeazzi fracture dislocations.[13] They had 72 male and 23 female patients with an average age of 41 (range 26–80) and a mean follow up of 81 months (range 18–132). They demonstrated that 54% of radial fractures occurring in the distal third shaft resulted in DRUJ instability, compared to 12% and 11% of those occurring in the proximal or middle third respectively. All patients were treated with plate fixation of the radius, and subsequent above elbow immobilization in supination for 6 weeks. Fifty-five patients were found to be stable after radius fixation alone, while 40 patients had ongoing instability and were thus treated with ulnoradial transfixation pinning of the DRUJ with a single Kirschner wire (N = 38) for 4 weeks or repair of the ulnar styloid (N = 2). The ulnar head was irreducible in 2 cases (2%) requiring open reduction and repair of the TFCC. Following this protocol, at medium-term follow up the authors report no incidence of persistent DRUJ instability or need for subsequent surgical procedures.

Rettig et al. used a similar protocol in their series (N = 40), with plate fixation of the radius and above elbow immobilization in supination for 6 weeks.[14] They found only 10 patients had persistent instability after radius fixation which were treated with ulnoradial transfixation pinning with two Kirschner wires. Three of these patients were irreducible by closed means, and thus open reduction and repair of the TFCC was performed in addition to pinning. This protocol was successful in the vast majority of patients, with 38 patients (95%) having excellent results by Mikic criteria and the remaining 2 patients having chronic instability treated with a Darrach procedure.

These studies provide the framework of the current approach to Galeazzi injuries. Two smaller studies are worth examining as they have challenged the duration and position of above elbow immobilization necessary to achieve satisfactory results (particularly in cases where the DRUJ is stable after radius fixation).

Park et al. performed a retrospective cohort study of 10 patients with Galeazzi injuries treated with radius fixation and found to be stable on examination postoperatively.[15] Five patients were immobilized above elbow in supination for 4 weeks, while 5 patients were immobilized above elbow in neutral rotation for 2 weeks. At an average of 68 months postoperative (range 26–124), all patients achieved an excellent outcome by Mikic criteria and there were no cases of residual DRUJ instability.

Gwinn et al. described an early motion protocol in 26 patients with Galeazzi injuries that were also found to be stable after radius fixation.[16] They immobilized patients in 30 degrees of supination with a Munster-type splint for the first 2 weeks, followed by 2 weeks of active and active-assisted range of motion from neutral to full supination, followed by 2 weeks of unrestricted active and active assisted motion. Short-term follow up at an average of 9 months (range 3–31 months) demonstrated all patients had a stable DRUJ on examination, although one patient continued to have pain localizing to the DRUJ. Additional complications included one hardware failure related to radius fixation, one ulnar nerve palsy and one case of extensor pollicis longus tendonitis.

Despite having few patients, the studies by Park and Gwinn demonstrate that acceptable results may be achieved with positioning in either supination or neutral, a shorter duration of immobilization, and earlier range of motion in cases which are stable after radius fixation. That said, no significant clinical benefit has been demonstrated aside from the potential anticipated benefits of reducing the period of immobilization. Position of fixation demonstrated equipoise between supinated and neutral positioning in Park's study (albeit with only five patients per group). Range of motion values were reported in both studies but insufficient evidence exists to make inferences based on the results or compare these to other treatment protocols.

Finally, Strehle and Gerber published a series of 19 patients in which radius open reduction and plate fixation was performed.[17] Their postoperative protocol was not well defined, however, no restriction of rotational motion was utilized. They found 4 out of 19 (21%) patients had ongoing DRUJ dysfunction; this was more common in patients with nonanatomic reduction of the radius ($N = 3$) than those with anatomic reduction ($N = 1$). Their findings demonstrate the importance of radius alignment on the distal radioulnar joint. Despite the increased rates of dysfunction being attributed to malreduction, this also raises concern about the potential for higher rates of instability with no DRUJ immobilization in the early postoperative period.

Associated Ulnar Styloid/Head Fracture

Mikic et al. reported 31.2% of Galeazzi injuries were associated with ulnar styloid fractures.[2] Two of the patients included in his case series went on to an acute ulnar head resection for ulnar head fracture. Mohan and colleagues demonstrated that there was no difference in outcome between those patients who did not have an associated styloid fracture and those who went on to fibrous/nonunion.[10] Only two patients amongst the included case series underwent an ulnar styloid ORIF for persistent instability after radial fixation,[13] however, the results in these patients were not separately reported. The authors of this study point out that fracture of the ulnar styloid was present in an additional 10 patients that did not require intervention.

TFCC Repair

No patients in the included case series underwent an open repair of the TFCC when the DRUJ was stable after radial fixation.

Irreducible Dislocations

When the distal radioulnar joint is not reducible by closed means, one must be particularly critical of the reduction of the radial shaft. Ensuring anatomic alignment will allow closed DRUJ reduction in the vast majority of cases. Yohe et al. performed a systematic review of case reports which document a total of 17 cases of irreducible Galeazzi fracture dislocations in the literature.[18] These primarily involved younger patients (mean age 26) and high-energy mechanisms. Dorsal dislocations were the most common, with 13 of 14 cases involving interposed extensor tendons (ECU and/or EDM). There were 3 volar dislocations which were blocked by fracture fragments or entrapment through the volar capsule. In their review, more than half of the irreducible dislocations were identified postoperatively requiring secondary interventions (between 1 day and 5 months after the index procedure). This underscores the need to have a high index of suspicion and to critically assess the DRUJ both clinically and radiographically. Despite these delays in diagnosis, only one case in this systematic review resulted in salvage ulnar head resection (after a 2-month missed dislocation).

When open reduction is required, one may consider concomitant repair of the TFCC or associated ulnar styloid fractures to increase stability.[13, 14]

RECOMMENDATIONS

Initial Management

In patients with an intraarticular displaced distal radius fracture, evidence suggests:

Recommendation	Overall Quality
• Anatomic reduction of the radius and rigid plate fixation is recommended.	⊕⊕⊕⊕ HIGH
• DRUJ stability must be tested intraoperatively after radial fixation is complete.	⊕⊕⊕⊕ HIGH

Stable DRUJ

When the DRUJ is stable after radius fixation:

Recommendation	Overall Quality
• When the DRUJ is stable after radius fixation, there is no difference in maintenance of DRUJ reduction between neutral or supinated position.	⊕◯◯◯ VERY LOW
• When the DRUJ is stable after radius fixation, associated ulnar styloid/TFCC injuries do not require surgical repair.	⊕⊕⊕◯ MODERATE

Reducible DRUJ

When the DRUJ is reducible but unstable after anatomic radius fixation:

Recommendation	Overall Quality
• Percutaneous ulnoradial Kirschner wire transfixation is recommended.	⊕⊕⊕⊕ HIGH

Irreducible DRUJ

When the DRUJ is irreducible after radius fixation:

Recommendation	Overall Quality
• Open reduction is recommended with removal of blocks to reduction.	⊕⊕⊕⊕ HIGH
• Acute ulnar head resection is not recommended as an initial treatment.	⊕⊕⊕◯ MODERATE

Postoperative Management

Recommendation	Overall Quality
• For cases in which pinning or open reduction of the DRUJ is necessary, postoperative above-elbow immobilization is recommended for a total 6 weeks.	⊕⊕⊕◯ MODERATE
• Transfixation wires may be removed at 3–4 weeks postoperatively.	⊕⊕◯◯ LOW

CONCLUSIONS

The Galeazzi fracture-dislocation is a fracture of necessity which demands anatomic fixation of the radius and maintained reduction of the DRUJ (possibly requiring ulnoradial transfixation pinning or open reduction). There is

---

Panel 2: Author's Preferred Technique

- The radial shaft fracture ORIF should be addressed first. Authors use a Henry approach to the volar forearm. Rigid fixation with a contoured 3.5 mm limited contact dynamic compression plate (LCDCP) is preferred. Anatomic reduction with restoration of the radial bow must be achieved.

- Once anatomic fixation of the radial shaft is obtained, DRUJ stability must be tested through a full range of pronosupination.

- If the DRUJ is reducible and can be easily maintained, then it is preferred to immobilize the patient in an above-elbow cast in the position of stability. The patient is immobilized for 4–6 weeks (based on intraoperative assessment of stability).

- If the DRUJ is reducible but unstable, then it is preferred to maintain reduction in the position of stability utilizing two percutaneously-placed 0.062″ ulnoradial transfixation K-wires. These should be placed approximately just proximal to the DRUJ and parallel to the articular surface of the distal ulna.

- If the DRUJ is irreducible, then it is preferred to perform a dorsal open reduction of the joint using an inverted "L" capsulotomy through the floor of the fifth extensor compartment. The authors prefer to perform a dorsal DRUJ capsular imbrication as well as a suture anchor repair of the TFCC if a deep foveal tear is present. Ulnoradial transfixation K-wires are also used to augment the soft tissue repair.

- Following pinning of the DRUJ, the authors will remove the wires at 4 weeks, and maintain above-elbow immobilization for a total 6 weeks. We recommend ensuring the pins are advanced slightly beyond the far cortex in order to allow retrieval from either side, should it inadvertently break while in situ.

CASE SCENARIO

- In the case provided, the patient initially underwent ORIF of the radius without postoperative above elbow immobilization of the DRUJ (Fig. 2).

Continued

Panel 2: Author's Preferred Technique—cont'd

- At 2 weeks postoperatively, the patient had a firm block to supination and imaging evidence of DRUJ subluxation/dislocation despite near anatomic alignment of the radius (Fig. 3).
- The patient subsequently underwent revision surgery to perform open reduction of the DRUJ with foveal TFCC

repair, dorsal capsular imbrication, and ulnoradial transfixation pinning (Fig. 4).

- At 4 months postoperatively, the patient demonstrates preserved stability of the DRUJ with excellent rotational range of motion and improving functional strength (Figs. 5 and 6).

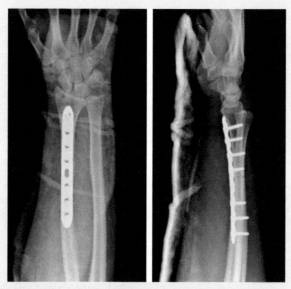

FIG. 2 Postoperative posteroanterior and lateral radiographs demonstrating plate fixation of the radius shaft. Note dorsal positioning of the ulna relative to the radius.

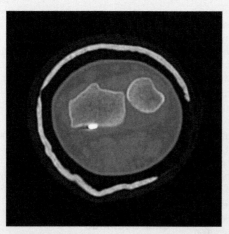 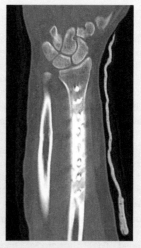

FIG. 3 Computed tomography scans showing malalignment of the DRUJ despite adequate reduction of the radius shaft (performed with patient in below elbow cast and repeated in full pronation, supination and neutral rotation for comparison).

Panel 2: Author's Preferred Technique—cont'd

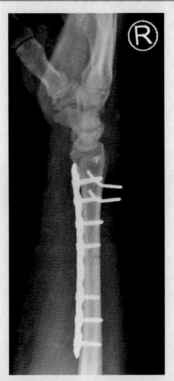

FIG. 4 Postoperative lateral radiograph demonstrating reduction of the DRUJ, ulnoradial transfixation pinning, and suture anchor repair of the TFCC.

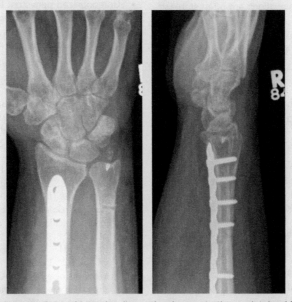

FIG. 5 Final posteroanterior and lateral radiographs demonstrating maintained DRUJ alignment.

Continued

Panel 2: Author's Preferred Technique—cont'd

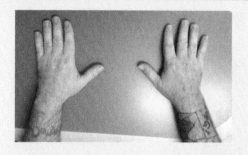
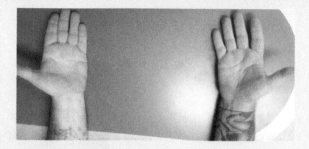
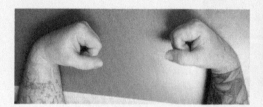
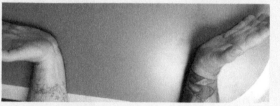

FIG. 6 Clinical photos demonstrating postoperative range of motion at 4 months.

Panel 3: Pearls and Pitfalls

PEARLS

- If the DRUJ is irreducible following radius fixation, recheck radial reduction to ensure anatomic alignment.
- Dorsal dislocations of the ulna are most commonly stable in supination; volar dislocations are often stable in pronation.
- If the DRUJ remains irreducible, consider potential blocks to reduction (including the extensor carpi ulnaris or extensor digitorum minimi tendons, fracture fragments, or joint capsule).

PITFALLS

- Unrecognized persistent DRUJ dislocation after radius fixation (>50% of cases in the literature).
- Applying rigid plates without contouring can result in malreduction of both the radius and DRUJ.

sufficient evidence to suggest that closed treatment of these injuries will result in an unacceptable outcome.

REFERENCES

1. Ring D, Rhim R, Carpenter C, Jupiter JB. Isolated radial shaft fractures are more common than Galeazzi fractures. *J Hand Surg Am.* 2006;31(1):17–21.
2. Mikić ZD. Galeazzi fracture-dislocations. *J Bone Joint Surg Am.* 1975;57(8):1071–1080.
3. Eberl R, Singer G, Schalamon J, Petnehazy T, Hoellwarth ME. Galeazzi lesions in children and adolescents: treatment and outcome. *Clin Orthop Relat Res.* 2008;466(7):1705–1709.
4. Atesok KI, Jupiter JB, Weiss AP. Galeazzi fracture. *J Am Acad Orthop Surg.* 2011;19(10):623–633.
5. Ploegmakers JJ, The B, Brutty M, Ackland TR, Wang AW. The effect of a Galeazzi fracture on the strength of pronation and supination two years after surgical treatment. *Bone Joint J.* 2013;95-B(11):1508–1513.
6. Hughston JC. Fracture of the distal radial shaft; mistakes in management. *J Bone Joint Surg Am.* 1957;39-A(2):249–264 [passim].
7. Reckling FW, Cordell LD. Unstable fracture-dislocations of the forearm. The Monteggia and Galeazzi lesions. *Arch Surg.* 1968;96(6):999–1007.
8. Wong PC. Galeazzi fracture—dislocations in Singapore 1960-64; incidence and results of treatment. *Singapore Med J.* 1967;8(3):186–193.
9. Mestdagh H, Duquennoy A, Letendart J, Sensey JJ, Fontaine C. Long-term results in the treatment of fracture-dislocations of Galeazzi in adults. Report on twenty-nine cases. *Ann Chir Main.* 1983;2(2):125–133.
10. Mohan K, Gupta AK, Sharma J, Singh AK, Jain AK. Internal fixation in 50 cases of Galeazzi fracture. *Acta Orthop Scand.* 1988;59(3):318–320.

11. Maculé Beneyto F, Arandes Renú JM, Ferreres Claramunt A, Ramón Soler R. Treatment of Galeazzi fracture-dislocations. *J Trauma*. 1994;36(3):352–355.

12. Gadegone WM, Salphale Y, Magarkar D. Percutaneous osteosynthesis of Galeazzi fracture-dislocation. *Indian J Orthop*. 2010;44(4):448–452.

13. Korompilias AV, Lykissas MG, Kostas-Agnantis IP, Beris AE, Soucacos PN. Distal radioulnar joint instability (Galeazzi type injury) after internal fixation in relation to the radius fracture pattern. *J Hand Surg Am*. 2011;36(5): 847–852.

14. Rettig ME, Raskin KB. Galeazzi fracture-dislocation: a new treatment-oriented classification. *J Hand Surg Am*. 2001;26 (2):228–235.

15. Park MJ, Pappas N, Steinberg DR, Bozentka DJ. Immobilization in supination versus neutral following surgical treatment of Galeazzi fracture-dislocations in adults: case series. *J Hand Surg Am*. 2012;37(3):528–531.

16. Gwinn DE, O'Toole RV, Eglseder WA. Early motion protocol for select Galeazzi fractures after radial shaft fixation. *J Surg Orthop Adv*. 2010;19(2):104–108.

17. Strehle J, Gerber C. Distal radioulnar joint function after Galeazzi fracture-dislocations treated by open reduction and internal plate fixation. *Clin Orthop Relat Res*. 1993;293:240–245.

18. Yohe NJ, De Tolla J, Kaye MB, Edelstein DM, Choueka J. Irreducible Galeazzi fracture-dislocations. *Hand (N Y)*. 2019;14(2):249–252.

CHAPTER 18

Diagnosis and Treatment of an Essex-Lopresti Injury

B.J.A. SCHOOLMEESTERS[a,b,c] • B. THE[c] • R.L. JAARSMA[a] •
JOB N. DOORNBERG[a,b,d]
[a]Department of Orthopaedic Surgery, Flinders Medical Centre and Flinders University, Adelaide, SA, Australia, [b]Department of Orthopaedic Surgery, Amsterdam University Medical Centre, Amsterdam, The Netherlands, [c]Department of Orthopaedic Surgery, Amphia Hospital, Breda, The Netherlands, [d]Department of Orthopaedic Surgery, University Medical Centre Groningen and Groningen University, Groningen, The Netherlands

---

KEY POINTS

- Essex-Lopresti injuries are frequently missed, therefore every proximal radius fracture requires at least a clinical and radiological examination of the elbow, forearm and wrist.
- In case of a clinical suspect Essex-Lopresti injury the recommended diagnostic tools to find or rule out an intraosseous membrane (IOM) rupture are either MRI or ultrasound (US).
- During proximal radius fracture surgery, forearm stability should always be examined by a combination of the radius push/pull test and Joystick test.
- An Essex-Lopresti injury should be preferably treated in the acute phase (<4 weeks).
- Treatment of a chronic Essex-Lopresti injury should be assessed on a case-to-case basis.

IMPORTANCE OF THE PROBLEM

An ELI is a pattern injury that consist of a fracture of the proximal radius, disruption of the distal radial ulnar joint, and a rupture of the interosseous membrane (IOM) of the forearm.[1] ELIs are rare and due to the predominant symptoms of a proximal radius fracture they are regularly missed or poorly treated. Most case series show a missed diagnosis frequency that exceeds 60%.[2] In some cases longitudinal forearm instability due to a rupture of the interosseous membrane can be diagnosed acutely (<4 weeks); however, it is more common that the interosseous membrane is partly ruptured causing progressing forearm instability over time.[3, 4]

A late treatment of an ELI is associated with a worse outcome for the patient.[2, 5] Patients who were treated in the acute phase showed an 80% success rate, well 80% of the patients treated for a chronic ELI demonstrated failure.[2, 5, 6] Therefore it is crucial to know how to diagnose and treat ELIs in the acute phase.

MAIN QUESTION

How can an Essex-Lopresti injury be diagnosed and what is the most effective management in the acute and chronic phase?

Current Opinion

ELI should be part of the differential diagnosis in every radial head fracture. Therefore, every radial head fracture requires a full radiological assessment of the elbow, forearm, and wrist. To diagnose subluxation or dislocation of the distal radioulnar joint (DRUJ) it is crucial to perform both a true posterior anterior as well as a true lateral view radiographs in neutral position. An additional radiograph of the wrist on the uninjured side enables assessment of the normal DRUJ variance. However, earlier studies found that radiographs alone are not reliable to either diagnose or rule out an ELI.[7, 8] Therefore, clinical examination is the most important indicator to decide if further investigation is required. A painful wrist and pain trough the forearm during

Distal Radius Fractures. https://doi.org/10.1016/B978-0-323-75764-5.00030-5

clinical examination is the most important reason to perform additional radiologic examination. In the acute phase it is possible to detect an IOM injury by ultrasound (US) or magnetic resonance imaging (MRI). Furthermore, intraoperative examination can be performed to diagnose an IOM injury.

The IOM is known for having a low healing potential.[9] Therefore, the golden standard treatment for acute or chronic ELIs has become surgical treatment. The treatment is focusing on restoring the radio-ulnar length and stabilizing the forearm. The acute treatment typically consists of either a replacement or fixation of the radial head in combination with pinning of the DRUJ. Depending on the grade of the distal instability, a TFCC repair could be considered. However, adding a TFCC repair to the procedure is more invasive and expensive compared to DRUJ pinning and should therefore be considered carefully. Chronic ELIs are treated by restoring the longitudinal stability between radius and ulna by reconstructive surgery. However, it is not clear what diagnostic tool and surgical technique is best to use to diagnose and treat an acute or chronic ELI.

Finding the Evidence

- Cochrane database: "Essex-Lopresti" 0; "Longitudinal forearm instability" 0; "Distal radio ulnar dislocation" 0; "Interosseous membrane" 0; "Interosseous ligament" 0.
- Pubmed (systematic review): "Essex-Lopresti" 1; "Longitudinal forearm instability" 0; "Distal radio

ulnar dislocation" 0, "Interosseous membrane" 1; "Interosseous ligament" 2.
- Pubmed: "Essex-Lopresti" 231; "Longitudinal forearm instability" 62; "Distal radio ulnar dislocation" 152; interosseous membrane 594; Interosseous ligament 842.
- Articles that were not in English, French, or German were excluded.

Quality of Evidence

Level III:
- Systematic reviews of case series: 2
- Cadaveric case-control studies: 8
- Cohort studies: 7

FINDINGS

Results for Diagnostic Tests

There were nine studies evaluating MRI, US, or intraoperative testing. Only two studies were comparative studies including one systematic review and one cadaveric study.[10, 11] Rodriguez-Martin and colleagues performed a systematic review of available publications and compared MRI with US. They concluded that, both US and MRI are equivalent in their capacity to diagnose IOM pathology.[10] This is in line with the remaining four cadaveric studies that are evaluating US or MRI. These studies indicate sensitivities from 87.5% to 100%, specificity from 89% to 100%, and accuracy from 94% to 100% (Table 1).[11–13] Furthermore, one study found that

---

TABLE 1
Diagnostic Performance Characteristics for Detecting an Essex-Lopresti Injury.

Author	Imaging Modility	Specimens	Examiners	Sensitivity	Specificity	Accuracy	PPV	NPV	IOA
Fester[11]	MRI	38	3	93	100	96	91	100	1.0–0.79
	US	19	3	100	89	94	89	91	NA
McGinley[12]	MRI	16	1	87.5	100	94	100	89	NA
Jaakkola[13]	US	18	3	NA	NA	95	NA	NA	NA
Soubeyrand[14]	US[a]	12	2	100	100	100	100	100	1.0
Smith[15]	Intraoperative[b]	13	NA	83	83	83	83	83	NA
Kachooei[16]	Intraoperative[c]	12	2	70	70	70	70	70	0.37
Soubeyrand[17]	Intraoperative[d]	20	2	100	88	94	90	100	0.97
Kachooei[18]	Intraoperative[d]	10	1	100	90	NA	NA	NA	NA

PPV, positive predictive value; *NPV*, negative predictive value; *IOA*, interobserver agreement.
[a]Ultrasound with muscle herniation as a predictor.
[b]Using the push/pull test with longitudinal displacement of more than 3 mm.
[c]Using the Joystick test with increased lateral displacement without a cut off value.
[d]Using the Joystick test with lateral displacement with lateral displacement of more than 5.5 mm.

a muscular herniation during dynamic US is a valuable predictor for a partial lesion of the IOM.[14] According to these studies both MRI and US are reliable techniques to identify an IOM injury. As these studies were all performed using the interpretation of experienced musculoskeletal specialized radiologists, an experience bias should be considered for the interpretation of the results. To our best knowledge, there are no studies published focusing on the less specialized and experienced radiologists.

Another technique that is used to identify a possible lesion of the IOM is the intraoperative radial push/pull test or the Joystick test. The radial push/pull test focuses on the longitudinal displacement of the radius and the Joystick test is focusing on the lateral displacement of the radius in reference to the ulna. Four cadaveric studies reported on the intraoperative proximal radius push/pulling test.[15–18] Most studies stated that a longitudinal displacement of the radius during the testing of >3 mm during the radial push/pull test and a lateral displacement of the radius of more than 5.5 mm during the Joystick test is suggestive for an IOM rupture. Kachooei and colleagues found that the most reliable way to perform the Joystick test is by flexion the elbow in 90 degrees and maximal supination.[18] However, the outcomes of these studies were varying a lot, possibly due to the difference in examining technique, examiner experience and cadaveric preparation (Table 2).

MRI and US both showed to be reliable to identify an ELI; however, in our opinion intraoperative testing of every radial head fracture that needs surgery might be the key assessment to reduce the chance of missing ELIs.

Results for Treatment

There are three studies concerning acute ELI treatment, two studies reporting on chronic ELI treatment, and two about both acute and chronic ELI treatment. Although eight studies illustrated the treatment of either an acute or chronic ELI, there were no comparative studies. Duckworth and colleagues reported on conservative treatment of acute diagnosed "stable" Essex-Lopresti injuries. They assessed all 237 patients with a radial head fracture and found that 60 patients had ipsilateral wrist pain. The wrist radiographs of 20 of these patients showed a proximalization of the radius ranged from 2 to 4 mm. The possible rupture of the IOM was not confirmed by either MRI or US. All of these patients were treated by collar and cuff immobilization for 1 week followed by supervised physiotherapy. All patients had an excellent or good Mayo Elbow Score at 6-month follow-up. They stated that patients with less than 4 mm proximalization of the radius on radiographs can be treated conservatively.[21] However, earlier research suggest that radiographs are not reliable to identify injuries of the IOM.[7] Therefore, the results of Duckworth's study should be interpreted with caution.

Treatment options that were reported in literature for acute ELI were as follows: radial head fixation or replacement, DRUJ pinning, IOM reconstruction, or a combination of these treatments. IOM reconstructions were described as "true" reconstructions with the use of an allograft or autograft as well as reconstructions using a synthetic graft according to the bracing principle to guide healing. All studies that reported on the acute treatment of an ELI showed a good clinical outcome (Table 2).[2, 5, 6, 20, 22] Chronic ELI was treated in literature with; radial head replacement, "true" IOM reconstruction, DRUJ reconstruction, and ulnar shortening or a combination of treatments. However, none of these treatments were superior and therefore a case-to-case treatment should always be considered (Table 3).[2, 6, 19, 23] Furthermore, two studies reported on the use of a fresh frozen radial head allografts. Both studies had a high complication and failure rate, and unsatisfying clinical outcomes.[24, 25]

Currently, there is still a lack of series that are truly comparable. The main problem is that ELIs vary significantly in complexity and are therefore hard to compare. However, general treatment for acute and chronic ELI consists of stabilizing the forearm and restoring the anatomy of the DRUJ. To establish this in an acute ELI it is recommended to repair or replace the radial head fracture in combination with pinning of the DRUJ, as this is easier, cheaper, and less invasive than an IOM reconstruction. If the DRUJ remains unstable after 6 weeks, a chronic ELI treatment should be considered. In case of a chronic ELI it is recommended to reconstruct the IOM, repair, or replace the radial head, and if required shorten the ulna.

TABLE 2
Clinical Outcomes of Acutely Treated Essex-Lopresti Injuries.

Author	Surgical Technique	Patients	Follow-Up (Months)	MEPS	MEWS	DASH	Morrey Score	Ext./Flex. (Wrist)	Ext./Flex. (Elbow)	Pron./Supin.	Complications
Grassmann[19]	RHP +DRUJ pinning	12	59	86.7	88.4	20.5	NA	50/50	8/138	75/81	4 × degeneration +heterotropic ossification
Trousdale[2]	RHF	1	120	NA	NA	NA	Excellent	60/60	30/125	40/80	None
	RHP +Darrach resection	1	50	NA	NA	NA	Good	60/50	10/135	45/30	None
Edwards[6]	RHF	2	17	NA	NA	NA	Excellent	NA	NA	NA	None
	RHE	1	30	NA	NA	NA	Poor	NA	NA	NA	None
	RHP	2	13	NA	NA	NA	Excellent/ good	NA	NA	NA	None
Schnetzke[5]	RHP +DRUJ pinning	15	64	91.3	81.3	12.5	NA	54/63	11/130	68/68	2 × nerve palsy
Fontana[20]	RHP	1	16	83	88	NA	NA	NA	NA	NA	Persistent wrist pain
	RHP +IOMR	1	15	95	95	NA	NA	NA	NA	NA	None
	RHP +TFCC	1	14	90	92	NA	NA	NA	NA	NA	None
	RHP +IOMR +TFCC	2	20	96	89.5	NA	NA	NA	NA	NA	None

RHF, radial head fixation; *RHP*, radial head prosthesis; *RHE*, radial head excision; *IOMR*, interosseous membrane reconstruction; *TFCC*, triangular fibrocartilage complex reinsertion; *MEPS*, Mayo Elbow Performance Score; *MEWS*, Modified Mayo Wrist Score; *DASH*, disability of the arm, shoulder and hand score.

TABLE 3
Clinical Outcomes of Treatment of Chronic Essex-Lopresti Injuries.

Author	Initial Treatment	Additional Treatment	Patients	Follow-Up (Months)	Morrey Score	Ext./Flex. (Wrist)	Ext./Flex. (Elbow)	Pron./ Supin.	Complications
Edwards[6]	Conservative	RHP+USO	2	10	Fair/Good	NA	NA	NA	None
Trousdale[2]	RHE/RHP	Darrach	1	115	Fair	60/30	20/110	80/50	Instability of elbow and wrist
		USO	1	43	Fair	45/45	30/90	30/10	Degeneration of elbow
		USO+IOMR	1	144	Fair	60/65	5/140	60/20	Nonunion of USO
		None	3	145	Fair	53/60	20/135	75/62	2 × subluxation of DRUJ
		USO+removal of RHP	1	96	Fair	60/60	10/150	75/75	Instability of elbow
Heijink[19]	Conservative/ RHE/RHF	RHP	8	49	NA	NA	16/135	69/66	NA
Venouziou[23]	RHE	RHP+USO	7	33	NA	56/57	12/132	53/66	None

RHP, radial head prothesis; *RHE*, radial head excision; *RHF*, radial head fixation; *IOMR*, interosseous membrane reconstruction; *USO*, ulnar shortening osteotomy.

RECOMMENDATION

In patients that have a suspected IOM injury, evidence suggest the following:

Recommendation	Overall Quality
• MRI or US are both reliable examinations to diagnose an ELI. Diagnostic of choice is best based on local availability and expertise.	⊕⊕◯◯ LOW
• Intraoperative testing should be done in every proximal radius fracture to avoid missing forearm instability.	⊕◯◯◯ VERY LOW
• Although all described techniques showed good results for the treatment of an acute ELI, DRUJ pinning seems to be the most cost-effective and less invasive option.	⊕◯◯◯ VERY LOW
• Chronic ELI should be assessed on a case-by-case basis, reconstruction seems indicated in case of a remaining longitudinal instability.	⊕◯◯◯ VERY LOW

CONCLUSION

A good clinical exam is crucial to diagnose an ELI in the acute phase. Based on these findings the physician can decide to perform either an MRI or US of the IOM, in addition to standard radiologic examination. Furthermore, it is recommended to check forearm stability during surgery in every proximal radius fracture case by using the radial push/pull test or the joystick test. Treatment is preferably done in the acute phase. However, an ELI is frequently missed and therefore chronic treatment is regularly necessary. As there is no consensus and a lack of literature concerning the best treatment of an acute or chronic ELI, the ideal treatment remains a subject of debate.

Panel 1: Case Scenario

A 35-year-old woman fell on her left dominant outstretched hand during a motorcycle ride. At the emergency department the woman especially complained about pain in her elbow. Radiographically, a complex fracture of the radial head was identified. The surgeons decided to treat her with a radial head arthroplasty. After 2 months, her wrist pain persistent. Wrist radiographs showed a DRUJ dislocation suspect for an Essex-Lopresti injury (Fig. 1). This raises the question: how can an Essex-Lopresti injury be diagnosed and what is the most effective management in the acute and chronic phase?

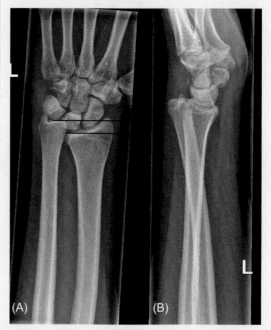

FIG. 1 Radiographs 2 months after trauma of the forearm, showing a proximalization of the distal radius of more than 4 mm (A) and a dorsal dislocation of the distal ulna (B).

Panel 2. Author's Preferred Treatment

AN ACUTE ESSEX-LOPRESTI INJURY

The patient is positioned in a supine position with the arm resting on an arm table. The radial head fracture is approached through an extensor digitorum communis splitting lateral approach. The forearm is pronated at this stage to keep the posterior interosseous nerve out of harms way. The alignment at the wrist is checked using an image intensifier. A temporary K-wire can be used to hold the corrected longitudinal alignment (in neutral forearm position to allow easier placement of the radial head/neck plate) after pushing the radius distally from the lateral exposure. The radial head fracture is stabilized using a low contour radial neck plate which is positioned to enable maximum rotational freedom without impingement, especially in supination.

If gross instability at the DRUJ is present an acute repair using a small bone anchor through an open dorsal approach is added to the procedure. The DRUJ is then pinned with two K wires that are positioned proximal the DRUJ joint and are removed after 6 weeks. The forearm should be supinated to minimize the tension on the distal radioulnar ligaments during this period.

A CHRONIC ESSEX-LOPRESTI INJURY

The DRUJ dislocation associated with a chronic Essex-Lopresti injury can be treated by specific surgical techniques depending on the finding at clinical examination, imaging, and intraoperative inspection. Regularly used techniques are: arthrolysis of the elbow joint including the proximal radioulnar joint, radial head removal/revision, radial head osteotomy, shortening or resection, ligamentous reconstructive surgery, and (ulnar) nerve surgery.

The stability of the forearm should be checked specifically focusing on correction of an ulnar plus configuration at the wrist. We use the push/pull test to check the longitudinal stability. An interosseous membrane (IOM) reconstruction is advised if the longitudinal movement of the radial head is more than 3 mm. If the correction—by manually pushing the radius distally—is only partial an additional ulnar shortening osteotomy will be added after reconstruction of the IOM.

The IOM reconstruction starts with an anterior partial Henry approach to access the proximal to mid diaphyseal part of the radius (Fig. 2). To create a force vector that is mostly in the longitudinal direction and as minimal as possible in the radio-ulnar direction we aim to create a ligament that originates proximal to the pronator teres insertion on the radius (Fig. 3). The insertion at the distal ulna is as distal as possible, but still allowing for an ulnar shortening osteotomy distal to that insertion if needed (Fig. 4).

Surgeons can choose to use an all synthetic reconstruction using—for example a LARS ligament—or to use an autograft or allograft. The distal (ulnar) insertion is typically approximately 6 cm proximal from the ulnar head. Depending on the preferred fixation technique drill tunnels are created in the proximal radius and distal ulna. When using a graft, it should be prestretched and reinforced with nonresorbable sutures that run from origin to insertion and are weaved through the graft itself.

We prefer fixation with endobuttons for maximum pull out strength. Finally, the longitudinal correction, the range of motion of elbow and forearm and stability of the DRUJ are checked.

Immediate movement is allowed but loading is not applied during the first 6 weeks. Normal daily activities should be possible at 12 weeks. More strenuous activities are not allowed until 26 weeks postsurgery

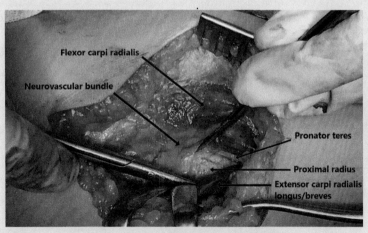

FIG. 2 Anterior partial Henry approach.

Continued

Panel 2. Author's Preferred Treatment—cont'd

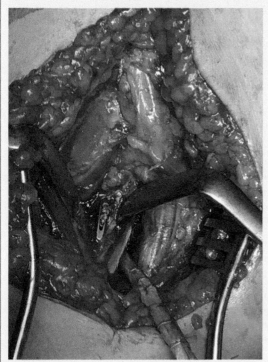

FIG. 3 Fixation of the allograft with endobuttons on the proximal radius.

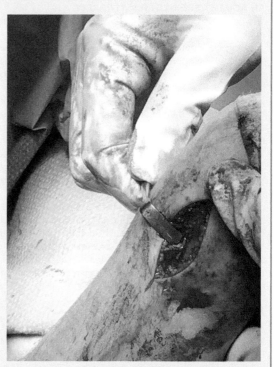

FIG. 4 Fixation of the allograft with endobuttons on the distal ulna.

Editor's Tips and Tricks: Acute Essex Lopresti and Unstable DRUJ
Geert Alexander Buijze

When ELI is suspected based on a comminuted/impacted radial head fracture, bilateral wrist radiographs and/or dynamic imaging are highly useful in diagnosing ELI. © Dr. Buijze 2020.

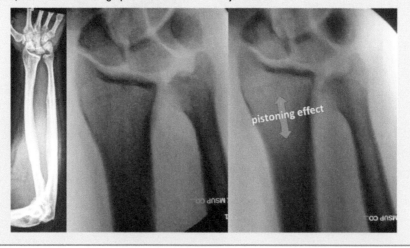

pistoning effect

Editor's Tips and Tricks: Acute Essex Lopresti and Unstable DRUJ—cont'd

When opting for an internal brace implant, I do not recommend a minimal-invasive approach as such "blind" techniques are reportedly at risk for the anterior and posterior interosseous nerves which should be protected when drilling. © Dr. Buijze 2020.

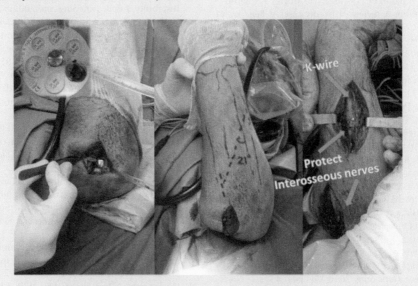

In case of an acute ELI with concomitant disrupted TFCC/unstable DRUJ, an internal brace implant stabilizing the IOM (traditionally recommended at 21 degrees) can be combined with one or two large K-wires stabilizing the DRUJ for 4–6 weeks in a neutral position to allow the TFCC to heal (superiority of anchor-repair has not been demonstrated). © Dr. Buijze 2020.

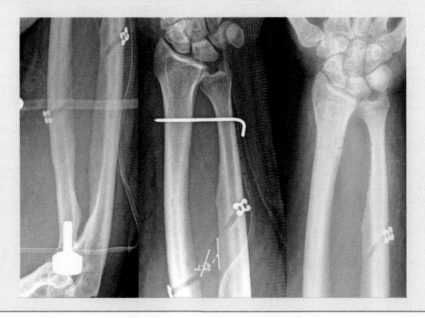

REFERENCES

1. Essex-Lopresti P. Fractures of the radial head with distal radio-ulnar dislocation; report of two cases. *J Bone Joint Surg Br.* 1951;33B(2):244–247.
2. Trousdale RT, Amadio PC, Cooney WP, Morrey BF. Radio-ulnar dissociation. A review of twenty cases. *J Bone Joint Surg Am.* 1992;74(10):1486–1497.
3. Dodds SD, Yeh PC, Slade 3rd JF. Essex-lopresti injuries. *Hand Clin.* 2008;24(1):125–137.
4. Adams JE, Culp RW, Osterman AL. Interosseous membrane reconstruction for the Essex-Lopresti injury. *J Hand Surg Am.* 2010;35(1):129–136.
5. Schnetzke M, Porschke F, Hoppe K, Studier-Fischer S, Gruetzner PA, Guehring T. Outcome of early and late diagnosed Essex-Lopresti injury. *J Bone Joint Surg Am.* 2017;99(12):1043–1050.
6. Edwards Jr GS, Jupiter JB. Radial head fractures with acute distal radioulnar dislocation. Essex-Lopresti revisited. *Clin Orthop Relat Res.* 1988;(234):61–69.
7. Sowa DT, Hotchkiss RN, Weiland AJ. Symptomatic proximal translation of the radius following radial head resection. *Clin Orthop Relat Res.* 1995;317:106–113.
8. Rodriguez-Martin J, Pretell-Mazzini J, Vidal-Bujanda C. Unusual pattern of Essex-Lopresti injury with negative plain radiographs of the wrist: a case report and literature review. *Hand Surg.* 2010;15(1):41–45.
9. Marcotte AL, Osterman AL. Longitudinal radioulnar dissociation: identification and treatment of acute and chronic injuries. *Hand Clin.* 2007;23(2):195–208 [vi].
10. Rodriguez-Martin J, Pretell-Mazzini J. The role of ultrasound and magnetic resonance imaging in the evaluation of the forearm interosseous membrane. A review. *Skeletal Radiol.* 2011;40(12):1515–1522.
11. Fester EW, Murray PM, Sanders TG, Ingari JV, Leyendecker J, Leis HL. The efficacy of magnetic resonance imaging and ultrasound in detecting disruptions of the forearm interosseous membrane: a cadaver study. *J Hand Surg Am.* 2002;27(3):418–424.
12. McGinley JC, Roach N, Hopgood BC, Limmer K, Kozin SH. Forearm interosseous membrane trauma: MRI diagnostic criteria and injury patterns. *Skeletal Radiol.* 2006;35(5):275–281.
13. Jaakkola JI, Riggans DH, Lourie GM, Lang CJ, Elhassan BT, Rosenthal SJ. Ultrasonography for the evaluation of forearm interosseous membrane disruption in a cadaver model. *J Hand Surg Am.* 2001;26(6):1053–1057.
14. Soubeyrand M, Lafont C, Oberlin C, France W, Maulat I, Degeorges R. The "muscular hernia sign": an original ultrasonographic sign to detect lesions of the forearm's interosseous membrane. *Surg Radiol Anat.* 2006;28(4):372–378.
15. Smith AM, Urbanosky LR, Castle JA, Rushing JT, Ruch DS. Radius pull test: predictor of longitudinal forearm instability. *J Bone Joint Surg Am.* 2002;84(11):1970–1976.
16. Kachooei AR, Rivlin M, Wu F, Faghfouri A, Eberlin KR, Ring D. Intraoperative physical examination for diagnosis of interosseous ligament rupture-cadaveric study. *J Hand Surg Am.* 2015;40(9):1785–1790. e1781.
17. Soubeyrand M, Ciais G, Wassermann V, et al. The intra-operative radius joystick test to diagnose complete disruption of the interosseous membrane. *J Bone Joint Surg Br.* 2011;93(10):1389–1394.
18. Kachooei AR, Rivlin M, Shojaie B, van Dijk CN, Mudgal C. Intraoperative technique for evaluation of the interosseous ligament of the forearm. *J Hand Surg Am.* 2015;40(12):2372–2376. e2371.
19. Heijink A, Morrey BF, van Riet RP, O'Driscoll SW, Cooney 3rd WP. Delayed treatment of elbow pain and dysfunction following Essex-Lopresti injury with metallic radial head replacement: a case series. *J Shoulder Elbow Surg.* 2010;19(6):929–936.
20. Grassmann JP, Hakimi M, Gehrmann SV, et al. The treatment of the acute Essex-Lopresti injury. *Bone Joint J.* 2014;96-B(10):1385–1391.
21. Duckworth AD, Watson BS, Will EM, et al. Radial shortening following a fracture of the proximal radius. *Acta Orthop.* 2011;82(3):356–359.
22. Fontana M, Cavallo M, Bettelli G, Rotini R. Diagnosis and treatment of acute Essex-Lopresti injury: focus on terminology and review of literature. *BMC Musculoskelet Disord.* 2018;19(1):312.
23. Venouziou AI, Papatheodorou LK, Weiser RW, Sotereanos DG. Chronic Essex-Lopresti injuries: an alternative treatment method. *J Shoulder Elbow Surg.* 2014;23(6):861–866.
24. Karlstad R, Morrey BF, Cooney WP. Failure of fresh-frozen radial head allografts in the treatment of Essex-Lopresti injury. A report of four cases. *J Bone Joint Surg Am.* 2005;87(8):1828–1833.
25. Szabo RM, Hotchkiss RN, Slater Jr RR. The use of frozen-allograft radial head replacement for treatment of established symptomatic proximal translation of the radius: preliminary experience in five cases. *J Hand Surg Am.* 1997;22(2):269–278.

CHAPTER 19

Acute Distal Radioulnar Joint Instability

RICK TOSTI[a,b]

[a]Philadelphia Hand to Shoulder Center, Philadelphia, PA, United States, [b]Orthopaedic Surgery, Thomas Jefferson University Hospital, Philadelphia, PA, United States

KEY POINTS

- All fractures of the distal radius should be evaluated with a physical exam to test for concurrent instability at the distal radioulnar joint.
- Radiographs that show excessive radial shortening, widening at the distal radioulnar joint, or a large ulnar styloid fracture should raise suspicion for instability.
- Most cases of instability can be managed with immobilization of the forearm in the position of stability.
- Cases in which stability cannot be maintained with immobilization are indicated for pinning of the forearm or repair of the ulnar structures.

Panel 1: Case Scenario

A 28-year-old man fell from a ladder at 14 ft and presented with a dorsally displaced and shortened distal radius fracture. The fracture was repaired with a volar plate and immobilized in a short arm splint. At the first follow up visit, the patient complains of a clunking sensation with rotation of the forearm. How can one diagnose acute instability of the forearm preoperatively or intraoperatively? How is acute distal radioulnar joint instability treated?

IMPORTANCE OF THE PROBLEM

Stability at the distal radioulnar joint (DRUJ) is imparted by the bony congruity of the sigmoid notch and the ulna and by the integrity of the soft tissue constraints of the triangular fibrocartilage complex (TFCC), radioulnar ligaments, and interosseous membrane (IOM).[1–3] Dynamic stabilizers such as the pronator quadratus and extensor carpi ulnaris play a minor role. Instability at the DRUJ may result from several causes:

(1) Simple dislocation from hyperpronation or hypersupination
(2) Essex-Lopresti dislocation from longitudinal rupture of the IOM
(3) Galeazzi fracture-dislocation from diaphyseal radial fracture

(4) Distal radius fracture and rupture of the soft tissue stabilizers

The aim of the following chapter will focus on those associated with distal radius fractures—a common fracture representing 16% of skeletal failures.[4] Fractures of the distal radius are often associated with an additional soft tissue injury. Studies reporting on wrist arthroscopy in distal radius fractures have estimated that concomitant TFCC injuries occur in 43%–84% of cases.[5, 6] Those with a complete TFCC rupture were more likely to develop instability at the DRUJ and experienced an inferior outcome.[7, 8] Significant morbidities associated with residual instability of the DRUJ include poor strength, reduction in range of motion, pain, and premature arthrosis.

MAIN QUESTION

What is the most effective diagnostic approach and treatment for acute DRUJ instability associated with DRF (including TFCC lesions)?

CURRENT OPINION

No consensus exists on the optimal method of diagnosis or treatment. Most surgeons would likely agree that an anatomic reduction of the distal radius is critical. Generally, intraoperative clinical exam is performed after fixation using rotation or translation maneuvers.

Radiographs may suggest instability if the radial articular segment is severely shortened, if the DRUJ is seen to be wide on the posteroanterior view, or if the radius is grossly dislocated from the ulna on the lateral view (Figs. 1 and 2). If instability is discovered treatment

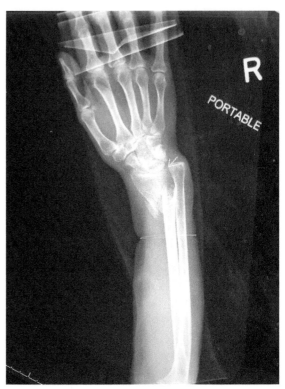

FIG. 2 AP radiograph showing a distal radial fracture with shortening and widening at the DRUJ. Intraoperative physical exam after fixation revealed laxity. The patient was placed into a long arm sugar tong splint in supination for 4 weeks.

options include immobilization in the position of stability, radioulnar pinning, or repair of the TFCC/ulnar styloid.

FINDING THE EVIDENCE

Pubmed (Medline) search was performed using keywords "distal radius" and "distal radioulnar joint" and "dislocation" or "instability."

Bibliography of eligible articles.

Articles not in English, French, or German were excluded.

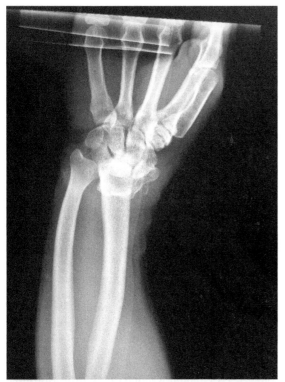

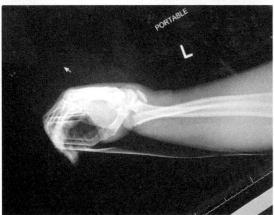

FIG. 1 AP and lateral radiographs showing excessive shortening and fragmentation of the sigmoid notch. Intraoperative physical exam of the DRUJ after fixation noted gross instability.

QUALITY OF THE EVIDENCE

Level I: 2 studies

Level II: 1 study

Level IV: 4 studies

FINDINGS

Despite not being a commonly studied lesion, a few high-quality evaluations have reported on the prognosis and treatment of acute instability of the DRUJ associated with distal radius fracture. However, diagnosis was most commonly performed with the ballottement test, which is a subjective evaluation; thus making the long-term consequences of a positive test difficult to interpret. The following studies are summarized in Table 1 with more recent studies described in detail below.

Lindau et al. evaluated 51 distal radial fractures with wrist arthroscopy in order to correlate findings with presence of DRUJ instability.[8] Distal radius fractures were treated with external fixation, closed reduction, and open reduction internal fixation. If a TFCC tear was present, it was classified by Palmer's criteria[9] but not treated. Their method of diagnosis of instability was postoperative physical exam using ballottement

(translation) of the ulna in the posterior and anterior direction with the forearm in neutral (Fig. 3). The examiner was blinded to the intraoperative findings and rated the joint as unstable if it had increased translation compared to the contralateral side. They classified 19 of 51 fractures as unstable and noted that instability of the DRUJ was associated with significantly lower Gartland and Werley scores. Neither preoperative nor postoperative radiographic measures correlated with instability. Ulnar styloid nonunion did not correlate with instability. DRUJ instability correlated only with rupture of the TFCC; in fact 10/11 cases of instability had a complete peripheral rupture. However, TFCC injury didn't necessarily result in instability, as 2/3 of TFCC tears were discovered in stable forearms.

Lee et al. performed a prospective study comparing operative and nonoperative treatment for DRUJ instability following distal radius fracture in 157 patients.[10]

TABLE 1
Selected Studies Evaluating Distal Radioulnar Joint Instability With Distal Radius Fractures.

LoE	Author	Study Aim	Number of Patients	Method of Diagnosis	Conclusion
I	Kim et al.	Determine if intraoperative laxity was associated with adverse outcome after distal radius fracture	84	Ballottement test	Laxity did not affect outcome at 1 year, but groups were treated differently
I	Lee et al.	Compare conservative vs operative treatment for laxity of DRUJ	157	Ballottement test. CT scan	No difference in outcome at 1 year
II	May et al.	Determine if ulna styloid size or displacement was associated with DRUJ instability	166	Ballottement test. Radiographs. CT scan	Size and displacement were associated with instability
IV	Stoffelen et al.	Determine the effect of instability on outcome score	272	Ballottement test, forearm rotation and compression test	Instability had a worse outcome
IV	Lindau et al.	Determine if TFCC tear was associated with DRUJ instability	51	Ballottement test	Unstable DRUJs often had peripheral TFCC tear
IV	Solgaard	Describe prognosis of distal radius fractures	154	Ballottement test	DRUJ pain and or instability was the most frequent problem at 3.5 years
IV	Frykman	Gross description of outcomes of distal radius fractures	430	Ballottement test	19% of all fractures complained of pain or instability at DRUJ. Ulnar styloid fracture has worse outcome

LoE, level of evidence.

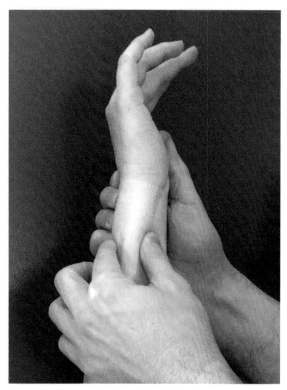

FIG. 3 Ballottement test indicates instability by observing increased translation of the ulna with force in an anterior and posterior direction.

At the time of injury the patients were assigned into three groups based on the ulna fracture morphology: (A) no fracture, (B) tip, and (C) Base. Classification of these groups was based on X-ray and MRI obtained in each patient. Each group was then randomized into three treatment arms: (1) sugar tong splint, (2) pinning of the DRUJ, or (3) fixation of TFCC or styloid fracture. All patients were initially immobilized for 4 weeks. The conservative group had the option of longer duration of immobilization if persistent laxity was discovered. Pins were all removed at 4 weeks. The patients were followed 12 months with exams and CT scan performed in all patients. The primary outcome measures were presence of instability, range of motion, grip strength, and functional scores (DASH and Modified Mayo). Instability was defined by either physical exam using anteroposterior translation with the forearm in neutral or by subluxation noted on CT scan using the epicenter method. No significant differences were noted between the groups in any of the outcome measures except the operative groups had a better range of motion at 3 months.

Kim et al. prospectively followed 84 patients with distal radius fractures to compare whether or not intraoperative laxity in the DRUJ affected the ultimate outcome after volar plating.[11] Although wrist arthroscopy was also performed in all patients to record the morphology of the tear, no ulnar sided lesions were treated surgically. DRUJ laxity was defined by the ballottement test intraoperatively. Stable fractures were treated with a short arm splint for 4 weeks while unstable fractures were treated with a sugar tong splint in supination for 4 weeks. Outcome measures were defined as DASH score, range of motion, pain, and grip strength. They deemed that 19 of 84 were unstable. All of the unstable patients had a TFCC tear, and most tears were described as peripheral ruptures (Palmer class 1B). However, TFCC tear was noted in 50% of the stable group as well. No differences in outcome measures were noted at 12 months.

May et al. prospectively evaluated 166 patients with distal radius fractures to determine the effect of ulna styloid fracture on instability.[12] Patients sorted to the instability group had any of the following: laxity determined by ballottement test intraoperatively, radiographs with gross instability, and subluxation on CT scan. Ulnar styloid fracture size was graded as a percentage of the styloid. Displacement was defined as: nondisplaced, minimally displaced (less than 2 mm) or displaced (greater than 2 mm). They noted that 55% of fractures had an ulnar styloid fracture. DRUJ laxity was noted in 11% of cases and appeared to positively correlate with displacement and size of ulnar styloid fracture.

Stoffelen et al. prospectively followed 272 patients with distal radius fracture to investigate the functional outcome as a function of DRUJ stability.[13] Patient were treated with cast immobilization, pinning, open reduction internal fixation or external fixation. Assessment for instability was done by physical exam at 6 weeks and 1-year posttreatment; none of the patients were treated specifically for the instability. Instability was defined by several physical exam maneuvers: ballottement test, forearm rotation test, and forearm rotation-compression test (Fig. 4). Fractures were classified by Frykman's criteria.[7] Strength, range of motion, and Cooney score were outcome measures. Outcomes appeared to be worse for those with instability and with ulnar styloid fracture.

Solgaard[14] and Frykman[7] each published descriptive case series of distal radius fractures. Included in their findings were that persistent complaints about the DRUJ were present in 27% and 19% of all fractures, respectively.

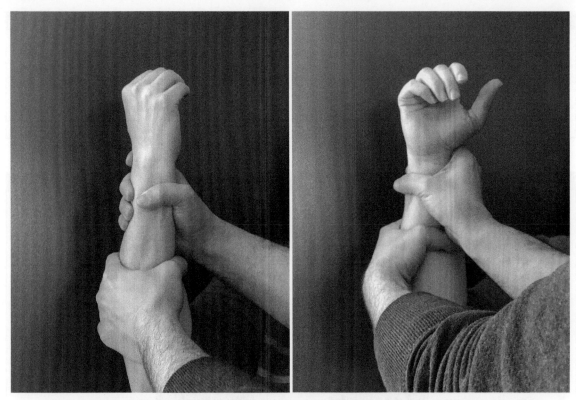

FIG. 4 Forearm rotation test indicates instability if the examiner perceives a clunk with rotating the forearm from supination to pronation. Forearm compression test is the same maneuver but the examiner compresses the ulna and radius while rotating them.

RECOMMENDATION

In patients with concomitant acute DRUJ laxity, evidence suggests the following:

Recommendation	Overall Quality
• Restoring articular congruity at the distal radioulnar joint is critical in preventing instability.	⊕⊕⊕○ MODERATE
• All distal radius fractures should have a physical exam to test for instability at the DRUJ.	⊕⊕⊕○ MODERATE
• Splinting in the position of stability (supination or pronation) for 4 weeks, radioulnar pinning and ulnar styloid/TFCC fixation have shown equivalent outcomes.	⊕⊕⊕○ MODERATE

CONCLUSION

Restoring articular congruity at the distal radioulnar joint is critical in preventing instability. Despite the method chosen, it is recommended it all fractures undergo a physical exam. Diagnosis of DRUJ laxity or instability may be determined intraoperatively by using a simple ballottement test. Preoperative radiographs should also be obtained, as instability may be evident from them. The presence of an ulnar styloid fracture may not necessarily affect stability or outcome, but larger fractures and displaced fractures should raise suspicion that instability might be discovered intraoperatively. Peripheral TFCC tears are associated with DRUJ laxity but have not been shown to be solely causative. Several studies have noted the presence of peripheral TFCC tear in stable fractures, thus the routine use of arthroscopy or MRI to identify these lesions is not necessary.

Untreated laxity or instability have been shown to result in inferior outcomes. If DRUJ laxity is discovered intraoperatively, then splinting in the position of stability (supination or pronation) for 4 weeks has been shown to produce a stable joint with equivalent outcome to operative techniques. K wire pinning of the forearm can be considered if the splint is unable to hold the reduction. Operative fixation of the ulna styloid or the TFCC can be considered if early motion is desired, as outcome studies have only shown superior range of motion in the short term.

Panel 2: Author's Preferred Treatment

Routinely, I perform an intraoperative ballottement test to determine stability of the joint. I usually rotate the forearm with and without compression of the radius against the ulna maintaining it through the full passive rotation to feel for a clunk or crepitus, which may indicate instability, malreduction, or intraarticular screw projection. Additionally, I perform the ballottement test in neutral, pronation, and supination to gain a full appreciation of the mechanics of the forearm. If these maneuvers are performed diligently, I believe the situation described in the case would be prevented. However, if I discovered instability intraoperatively or at a recent follow up visit, I would place the limb in an above elbow splint in the position of stability (supination or pronation) for 4 weeks.

Panel 3: Pearls and Pitfalls

PEARLS

- If the reduction cannot be held with splinting, 2 or 3 K wires can be placed across the forearm.
- It's easier to place the wires from ulna to radius because the ulnar doesn't rotate and the radius is larger.

PITFALLS

- Large or obese arms may be difficult to control with splinting.
- Use larger diameter wires (0.62 mm) to prevent breakage.
- Advance the wire out of the skin on both sides, so that if the wire breaks it can be retrieved on either end. (Fig. 5).

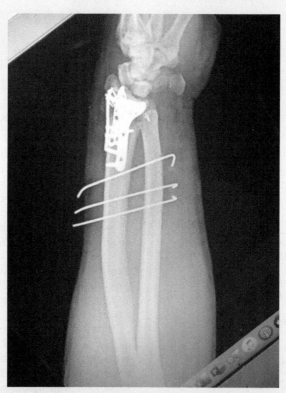

FIG. 5 This man had a comminuted distal radius fracture with an unstable DRUJ and compartment syndrome. The reduction could not be held with the splint. Note the pins emerge from the skin on both sides to ease retrieval if they broke.

REFERENCES

1. Stuart PR, Berger RA, Linscheid RL, et al. The dorsopalmar stability of the distal radioulnar joint. *J Hand Surg Am.* 2000;25(4):689–699.
2. Carlsen BT, Dennison DG, Moran SL. Acute dislocations of the distal radioulnar joint and distal ulna fractures. *Hand Clin.* 2010;26(4):503–516.
3. Sammer DM, Chung KC. Management of the distal radioulnar joint and ulnar styloid fracture. *Hand Clin.* 2012;28(2):199–206.
4. Owen RA, Melton 3rd LJ, Johnson KA, Ilstrup DM, Riggs BL. Incidence of Colles' fracture in a North American community. *Am J Public Health.* 1982;72(6):605–607.
5. Geissler WB, Freeland AE, Savoie FH, et al. Intra-carpal soft-tissue lesions associated with an intra-articular fracture of the distal end of the radius. *J Bone Joint Surg Am.* 1996;78(3):357–365.
6. Lindau T, Arner M, Hagberg L. Intraarticular lesions in distal fractures of the radius in young adults. A descriptive arthroscopic study in 50 patients. *J Hand Surg (Br).* 1997;22(5):638–643.
7. Frykman G. Fracture of the distal radius including sequelae—shoulder-hand-finger syndrome, disturbance in the distal radio-ulnar joint and impairment of nerve function. A clinical and experimental study. *Acta Orthop Scand.* 1967;108(Suppl.):1–124.
8. Lindau T, Adlercreutz C, Aspenberg P. Peripheral tears of the triangular fibrocartilage complex cause distal radioulnar joint instability after distal radial fractures. *J Hand Surg.* 2000;25A:464–468.
9. Palmer AK. Triangular fibrocartilage complex lesions: a classification. *J Hand Surg Am.* 1989;14:594–606.
10. Lee SK, Kim KJ, Cha YH, Choy WS. Conservative treatment is sufficient for acute distal radioulnar joint instability with distal radius fracture. *Ann Plast Surg.* 2016;77(3):297–304.
11. Kim JK, Yi JW, Jeon SH. The effect of acute distal radioulnar joint laxity on outcome after volar plate fixation of distal radius fractures. *J Orthop Trauma.* 2013;27(12):735–739.
12. May MM, Lawton JN, Blazar PE. Ulnar styloid fractures associated with distal radius fractures: incidence and implications for distal radioulnar joint instability. *J Hand Surg Am.* 2002;27:965–971.
13. Stoffelen D, de Smet L, Broos P. The importance of the distal radioulnar joint in distal radial fractures. *J Hand Surg.* 1998;23B:507–511.
14. Solgaard S. Function after distal radius fracture. *Acta Orthop Scand.* 1988;59:39–42.

CHAPTER 20

Distal Ulnar Fractures Concomitant With Distal Radius Fractures

C.L.E. LAANE[a] • JOB N. DOORNBERG[b] • D. RING[c] • M.M.E. WIJFFELS[a]

[a]Trauma Research Unit, Department of Surgery, Erasmus MC, University Medical Center Rotterdam, Rotterdam, The Netherlands, [b]Department of Orthopaedics and Trauma, Flinders Medical Centre, Adelaide, Australia, [c]Department of Psychiatry and Perioperative Care, Dell Medical School, University of Texas at Austin, Austin, TX, United States

KEY POINTS

- Database studies and case series suggest most ulnar fractures associated with distal radius fracture do not benefit from specific treatment. In particular, there is no advantage to fixation of the ulna if it lines up reasonably after the radius fracture is satisfactorily aligned and stabilized.

- In the absence of data, and in our opinion, fractures of the ulnar styloid base, head, neck, or shaft of the ulna that remain widely displaced after the radius is reduced and secured likely benefit from reduction and fixation.

- Primary distal ulna resection in elderly patients with distal radius fractures concomitant with distal ulna fractures is an acceptable treatment with less complications and reoperations compared to distal ulna fixation.

Panel 1: Case Scenarios

Case 1: A 45-year-old man fell from a height and fractured his distal radius and the ulnar styloid base (USB) (Fig. 1A and B).

Case 2: A 55-year-old right hand dominant woman fell off her bike resulting in a distal radius fracture on the right side with a concomitant dislocated USB fracture.

CT-scan showed a simple articular distal radius fracture (AO type 23C1.3) (Fig. 2A–C).

Open reduction and internal radial fixation was opted for in both cases. However, for which case would additional reduction and internal fixation of the fractured distal ulna be indicated?

Continued

Distal Radius Fractures. https://doi.org/10.1016/B978-0-323-75764-5.00018-4

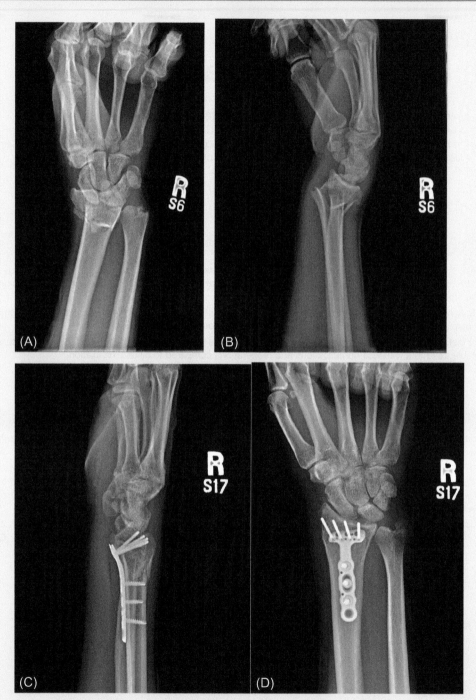

FIG. 1 (A, B) Radiographs showing a displaced distal radius fracture with concomitant, displaced ulnar styloid base fracture. (C, D) Postoperative radiographs showing volar plate fixation. The USB lined up well and was not repaired.

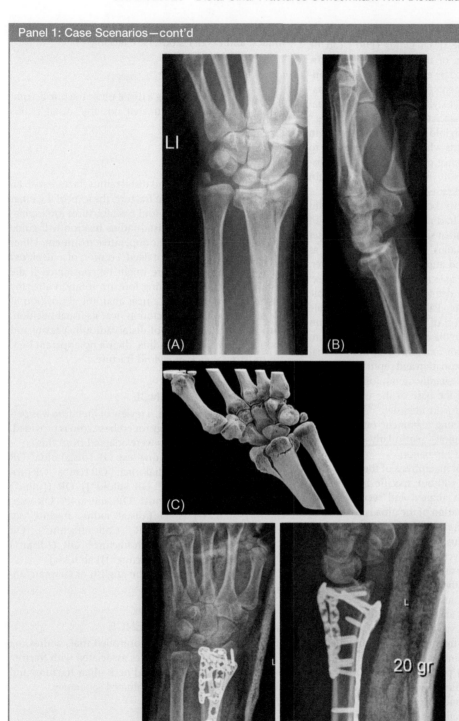

FIG. 2 (A–C) Radiographs and 3D-CT showing an unstable distal radius fracture with a concomitant displaced ulnar styloid base fracture. (D, E) The USB lined up well and was not repaired.

Continued

IMPORTANCE OF THE PROBLEM

Displaced fractures of the distal radius (DRF) can be expected to have rupture of the linkage between the radius and the ulna, caused by either avulsion of the origin of the radioulnar ligaments from the base of the ulnar styloid, or fracture of ulnar styloid base.[1–5] Of all distal ulnar fractures, 77% are associated with radial fractures.[6]

Fracture of the ulnar styloid base disrupts the origin of the radioulnar ligaments which remains attached to the fragment. In the absence of fracture, similarly displaced fractures likely result in avulsion of the origin from the base without fracture.

Surgeons express concern about distal radioulnar joint (DRUJ) "instability" after fracture of the distal radius. In our opinion, pain in the ulnar side of the wrist pain after fracture of the distal radius is often diagnosed as "instability" for unclear and imprecise reasons. However, the term "instability" is vague and nonspecific because: (1) There is no consensus definition and (2) no reliable and accurate measurement. Palpable and reproducible subluxation and dislocation of the DRUJ with forearm rotation are uncommon in the absence of malalignment of the radius. There is both rotational and translational motion at the DRUJ with pronation and supination. Moreover, evidence shows radiographic nonunion and malalignment of a fracture of the base of the ulnar styloid does not correspond with pain intensity.[7–9] This results in the risk of misinterpreting alignment on computed tomography as pathological, particularly at relative extremes of pronation and supination.

Fractures of the head or metaphysis of the distal ulna often line up and heal without specific intervention when the distal radius is aligned and secured. Open reduction and internal fixation of the ulna is considered when head, neck, and diaphyseal fractures remain notably malaligned after radius fixation. The degree of displacement that might affect symptoms and limitations is still a matter of debate and needs more evidence.

Fixation of fractures of the ulnar styloid and distal ulna is not straightforward, because of the need to avoid articular surfaces and tendons and because the bone is small and often osteoporotic. A variety of techniques are used. For ulnar styloid fixation frequently used techniques are (1) open reduction and internal fixation (ORIF) using tension band wiring; (2) plate and screw fixation; (3) screw fixation (either headless or headed); and K-wire fixation, sometimes percutaneous. For the ulnar head or metaphyseal fractures fixation is usually accomplished with a plate and screws. Loss of fixation, restriction of DRUJ motion, and iatrogenic injury of the dorsal branch of the ulnar nerve are potential harms of fixation.

Previous database studies and case series addressing fixation of distal ulnar fractures concomitant with distal radius fractures are heterogeneous in fixation techniques, and Level-1 studies are lacking.

MAIN QUESTION

Is there a benefit repairing a distal ulnar fracture accompanying an operatively treated unstable distal radius fracture?

CURRENT OPINION

In patients with a displaced distal radius fracture with an accompanying distal ulnar fracture, the level of the ulnar fracture and in case of styloid base fractures intraoperative stability tests after distal radius fixation will guide you to ulnar fixation or nonoperative treatment. Ulnar styloid tip fractures are not fixed. Fixation of a displaced ulnar styloid base fracture might be considered if the distal ulna dislocates during forearm rotation after the radial fracture is fixed in a near anatomical position. If the ulnar styloid base fracture is near its usual position, with an expected degree of distal radioulnar laxity and good alignment of the radius, there's no apparent benefit to fixing the ulnar styloid fracture.

FINDING THE EVIDENCE

To evaluate available data, a review of literature was performed. The search strategy for embase.com is provided. All other search strategies were adapted from this.

Embase.com: ('distal ulna'/exp OR (distal-ulna* OR ulna-distal* OR distal-radial-ulnar* OR ((ulna* OR process*) NEAR/1 (styloid* OR stiloid*)) OR ((ulna*) NEAR/3 (head* OR caput* OR subcapit* OR subcapit*))):ab,ti,kw AND ('distal radius fracture'/exp OR (Barton-fracture* OR Colles-fracture* OR Galeazzi-fracture* OR Smith-fracture* OR ((distal*) NEAR/3 (radi*) NEAR/3 (fracture*))):ab,ti,kw)

Articles that were not in the English or German language were excluded.

QUALITY OF THE EVIDENCE

There were no randomized controlled trials addressing fixation of distal ulna fractures associated with fracture of the distal radius. Head and neck ulnar fractures and ulnar styloid fractures are evaluated separately.
Ulnar styloid:
Level II: 1[10]
Level III: 3[11–14]
Distal ulna:
Level II: 1[15]
Level III: 1[16]
Level IV: 3[17–19]

Ulna resection:
Level III: 1[20]
Level IV: 2[21,22]

FINDINGS

Ulnar Styloid Base Fractures

One study[10] was designed to prospectively compare fixation with no fixation of ulnar styloid fractures prospectively randomized based on timepoint. When not repairing the ulnar styloid base fracture, they found better grip strength up to 12 weeks in the early postoperative period and regarding range of motion up to three weeks for dorsal flexion and supination, up to 2 weeks for pronation and in the third and fourth week for extension.

Four of 5 cohort studies[11–14] with a total of 735 patients (range 134–319 patients per study) found no difference in outcomes when a displaced fracture of the distal radius treated with volar locked plating has an associated base of ulnar styloid fracture treated nonoperative or no ulnar styloid fracture. Three studies tested motion,[10–12] two studies examined pain,[10,12] all studies reported on PROMs[10–14] (e.g., DASH, MHQ), and two studies administered physician-based scales[11,12] (e.g., Gartland and Werley or Mayo).

Nonstyloid Distal Ulna Fractures

One study[15] was designed to prospectively compare fixation with no fixation of ulnar neck fractures prospectively randomized based on timepoint. They found no significant differences between fixed and nonfixed distal ulnar fractures regarding range of motion, grip strength, pain, Gartland and Werley score and radiographic outcomes.[15]

One study retrospectively compared the treatment of ulnar neck fractures to no ulnar fixation. The authors found more complications and more operations in fixed distal ulna fractures.[16]

One study analyzing nonoperative treatment of ulnar head fractures associated with distal radius fractures found that satisfactory results regarding function and pain can be achieved when the distal radius is fixed rigidly. However, radiographic images showed early degenerative arthritis of the DRUJ in not fixed distal ulna fractures.[19]

As for fixation strategies, two cohort studies with a total of 49 patients (24 and 25, respectively) achieved alignment, good function and an acceptable amount of secondary surgery when fixing the ulnar neck and head fractures with distal ulnar hook plate fixation[17] and condylar blade plate fixation.[18]

Ulna Resection

Two cohort studies of patients treated with acute distal ulnar resection for distal ulna fractures in combination with unstable distal radius fractures with a total of 34 patients (11 and 23, respectively) achieved satisfactory outcomes after distal ulnar resection in older patients[21] and was considered to help avoid secondary surgeries and prevent DRUJ arthrosis.[22]

One study compared distal ulnar resection to fixation of distal ulna fractures in elder patients. They found acceptable results in the ulnar resection group, as no significant changes were found in range of motion, grip strength, pain, patient reported outcomes and radiographic outcomes in comparison to fixed distal ulna fractures. Moreover, the ulnar resection group showed less complications (7 vs 2, $P = 0.03$) and reoperations (6 vs 1, no P-value given) in comparison to fixed distal ulna fractures.[20]

RECOMMENDATION

In patients with an intraarticular displaced distal radius fracture, evidence suggests:

Recommendation	Overall Quality
• There is no good quality evidence to guide surgical decision making whether or not to fix a concomitant ulnar fracture.	⊕⊕⊕○ MODERATE
• Current database studies and case series do not suggest any benefit of fixation of distal ulnar fractures associated with fixed distal radius fractures.	⊕⊕○○ LOW
• Primary distal ulna resection in elderly patients with distal radius fractures concomitant with distal ulna fractures is an acceptable treatment with less complications and reoperations compared to distal ulna fixation.	⊕⊕○○ LOW

CONCLUSION

On average fixation of a fracture of the distal ulna associated with fracture of the distal radius does not improve motion, strength, pain intensity, or radiographic alignment. However, it should be acknowledged that research is limited to database studies and case series on operatively versus nonoperatively treated ulnar fractures and quality of evidence for included studies were very low. It's possible that prospective studies of selected fractures felt to be at greater risk of DRUJ problems would support fixation. Future studies might also address fixation options for distal ulna fractures after the radius is aligned and fixed.

Panel 2: Author's Preferred Technique

The authors' rationale for fixing a concomitant USB might be considered if the distal ulna dislocates during forearm rotation after the radial fracture is fixed in a near anatomical position. If the ulnar styloid base fracture is near its usual position, with an expected degree of distal radio-ulnar laxity and good alignment of the radius, there's no apparent benefit to fixing the ulnar styloid fracture. Hence in both cases, only open reduction and internal fixation of the radius was performed. (Figs. 1C,D and 2D,E)

If USB fracture fixation is needed, anatomical reduction and stable fixation are the main goals. A small straight ulnar incision should be made, preventing iatrogenic injury to the dorsal branch of the ulnar nerve. Anatomical reduction should be performed and we recommend tension band wiring with trans-osseous fixation using nonabsorbent wire (Fig. 3), since plate fixation in this area might result in soft tissue irritation. A more volar or dorsal position of the plate is prevented by the flexor and extensor carpi ulnaris, respectively.

For ulnar head or metaphyseal fractures the authors recommend angular stable plate fixation, by preference using anatomical precontoured plates to enable direct postoperative movement.

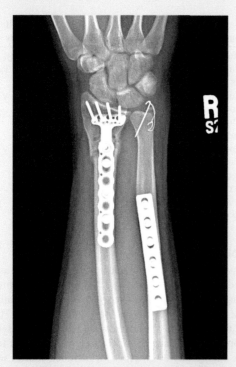

FIG. 3 Additional tension band wiring of a USB fracture after volar plate fixation of a fracture of the distal radius. The diaphyseal fracture of the ulna is from a prior injury.

Panel 3: Pearls and Pitfalls

PEARLS

- In case of a distal radius fracture with concomitant distal ulnar fracture, the ulnar fracture is an indicator for the radial reduction quality. If the ulnar fragment is still dislocated the distal radius might not be reduced properly.

PITFALLS

- When using an ulnar approach for ORIF of a distal ulnar fracture, protect the dorsal branch of the ulnar nerve.
- In distal metaphyseal or ulnar head fractures, screws that are too long protrude in the DRUJ and result in compromised function.

REFERENCES

1. Frykman G. Fracture of the distal radius including sequelae—shoulder-hand-finger syndrome, disturbance in the distal radio-ulnar joint and impairment of nerve function. A clinical and experimental study. *Acta Orthop Scand.* 1967; https://doi.org/10.3109/ort.1967.38.suppl-108.01.
2. Lindau T, Arner M, Hagberg L. Intraarticular lesions in distal fractures of the radius in young adults: a descriptive arthroscopic study in 50 patients. *J Hand Surg Eur.* 1997; 22(5):638–643. https://doi.org/10.1016/S0266-7681(97)80364-6.
3. Oskarsson GV, Aaser P, Hjall A. Do we underestimate the predictive value of the ulnar styloid affection in Colles fractures? *Arch Orthop Trauma Surg.* 1997; 116(6–7):341–344. https://doi.org/10.1007/BF00433986.
4. Richards RS, Bennett JD, Roth JH, Milne KJ. Arthroscopic diagnosis of intra-articular soft tissue injuries associated with distal radial fractures. *J Hand Surg Am.* 1997; 22(5):772–776. https://doi.org/10.1016/S0363-5023(97)80068-8.
5. Geissler WB, Fernandez DL, Lamey DM. Distal radioulnar joint injuries associated with fractures of the distal radius. In: *Clinical Orthopaedics and Related Research.* In: Springer New York LLC; 1996:135–146. https://doi.org/10.1097/00003086-199606000-00018.
6. Moloney M, Farnebo S, Adolfsson L. Incidence of distal ulna fractures in a Swedish county: 74/100,000 person-years, most of them treated non-operatively. *Acta Orthop.* 2020; 91(1):104–108. https://doi.org/10.1080/17453674.2019.1686570.
7. Yuan C, Zhang H, Liu H, Gu J. Does concomitant ulnar styloid fracture and distal radius fracture portend poorer outcomes? A meta-analysis of comparative studies. *Injury.* 2017; 48(11):2575–2581. https://doi.org/10.1016/j.injury.2017.08.061.

8. Mulders MAM, Fuhri Snethlage LJ, de Muinck Keizer RJO, Goslings JC, Schep NWL. Functional outcomes of distal radius fractures with and without ulnar styloid fractures: a meta-analysis. *J Hand Surg Eur Vol.* 2018; 43(2):150–157. https://doi.org/10.1177/1753193417730323.

9. Wijffels MME, Keizer J, Buijze GA, et al. Ulnar styloid process nonunion and outcome in patients with a distal radius fracture: a meta-analysis of comparative clinical trials. *Injury.* 2014; 45(12):1889–1895. https://doi.org/10.1016/j.injury.2014.08.007.

10. Zenke Y, Sakai A, Oshige T, Moritani S, Nakamura T. Treatment with or without internal fixation for ulnar styloid base fractures accompanied by distal radius fractures fixed with volar locking plate. *Hand Surg.* 2012; 17(2):181–190. https://doi.org/10.1142/S0218810412500177.

11. Kim JK, Do KY, Do NH. Should an ulnar styloid fracture be fixed following volar plate fixation of a distal radial fracture? *J Bone Jt Surg Ser A.* 2010; 92(1):1–6. https://doi.org/10.2106/JBJS.H.01738.

12. Souer JS, Ring D, Matschke S, et al. Effect of an unrepaired fracture of the ulnar styloid base on outcome after plate-and-screw fixation of a distal radial fracture. *J Bone Jt Surg Ser A.* 2009; 91(4):830–838. https://doi.org/10.2106/JBJS.H.00345.

13. Okoli M, Silverman M, Abboudi J, et al. Radiographic healing and functional outcomes of untreated ulnar styloid fractures following volar plate fixation of distal radius fractures: a prospective analysis. *Hand.* 2019; https://doi.org/10.1177/1558944719855445.

14. Sammer DM, Shah HM, Shauver MJ, Chung KC. The effect of ulnar styloid fractures on patient-rated outcomes after volar locking plating of distal radius fractures. *J Hand Surg Am.* 2009; 34(9):1595–1602. https://doi.org/10.1016/j.jhsa.2009.05.017.

15. Cha SM, Shin HD, Kim KC, Park E. Treatment of unstable distal ulna fractures associated with distal radius fractures in patients 65 years and older. *J Hand Surg Am.* 2012; 37(12):2481–2487. https://doi.org/10.1016/j.jhsa.2012.07.031.

16. Özkan S, Fischerauer S, Kootstra T, Claessen F, Ring D. Ulnar neck fractures associated with distal radius fractures. *J Wrist Surg.* 2018; 07(01):071–076. https://doi.org/10.1055/s-0037-1605382.

17. Lee SK, Kim KJ, Park JS, Choy WS. Distal ulna hook plate fixation for unstable distal ulna fracture associated with distal radius fracture. *Orthopedics.* 2012; 35(9):1358–1364. https://doi.org/10.3928/01477447-20120822-22.

18. Ring D, McCarty LP, Campbell D, Jupiter JB. Condylar blade plate fixation of unstable fractures of the distal ulna associated with fracture of the distal radius. *J Hand Surg Am.* 2004; 29(1):103–109. https://doi.org/10.1016/j.jhsa.2003.10.019.

19. Namba J, Fujiwara T, Murase T, Kyo T, Satoh I, Tsuda T. Intra-articular distal ulnar fractures associated with distal radial fractures in older adults: early experience in fixation of the radius and leaving the ulna unfixed. *J Hand Surg Eur Vol.* 2009; 34(5):592–597. https://doi.org/10.1177/1753193409103728.

20. Boretto JG, Zaidenberg EE, Gallucci GL, Sarme A, De Carli P. Comparative study of internal fixation of the ulna and distal ulna resection in patients older than 70 years with distal radius and distal metaphyseal ulna fractures. *Hand.* 2018; https://doi.org/10.1177/1558944718760000.

21. Yoneda H, Watanabe K. Primary excision of the ulnar head for fractures of the distal ulna associated with fractures of the distal radius in severe osteoporotic patients. *J Hand Surg Eur Vol.* 2014; 39(3):293–299. https://doi.org/10.1177/1753193413504160.

22. Ruchelsman DE, Raskin KB, Rettig ME. Outcome following acute primary distal ulna resection for comminuted distal ulna fractures at the time of operative fixation of unstable fractures of the distal radius. *Hand.* 2009; 4(4):391–396. https://doi.org/10.1007/s11552-009-9175-x.

CHAPTER 21

Persistent Ulnar-Sided Wrist Pain After Distal Radius Fracture

YUKIO ABE • YOUHEI TAKAHASHI
Department of Orthopaedic Surgery, Saiseikai Shimonoseki General Hospital, Shimonoseki City, Yamaguchi, Japan

KEY POINTS

- The development of palmar locking plate fixation for surgical treatment for distal radius fracture (DRF) provides successful outcome. However, persistent ulnar-sided wrist pain (USWP) after healed DRF is often encountered.
- USWP is common after DRF and can improve for a year or more, so patience is warranted.
- The main causes of persistent USWP after healed DRF are malunion of the distal radius, triangular fibrocartilage complex (TFCC) injury, and nonunion of ulnar styloid.
- TFCC injury is frequently associated to DRF and has a good healing potential. The type of TFCC tear that is most troublesome would be a foveal tear causing distal radioulnar joint instability.
- When conservative treatment fails, correction osteotomy for malunion, arthroscopic management for TFCC injury, and fixation or resection for nonunion of ulnar styloid seem to be the best solutions.

Panel 1: Case Scenarios

CASE 1: PALMARLY ANGULATED MALUNION

A 76-year-old, right-handed female suffered a left DRF. She underwent cast immobilization for 4 weeks. She visited our clinic with a swollen and deformed left wrist 3 months after removing the cast. She complained of persistent USWP. Range of motion (ROM) was restricted: extension (ex) 50 degrees (deg), flexion (flex) 60 deg, pronation (pro) 80 deg, supination (sup) 65 deg, grip strength was 60% of the contralateral side. Radiographs showed radial shortening with an ulnar variance (UV) which was +3.5 mm, radial inclination (RI) was 5 deg, and palmar tilt (PT) was 35 deg (Fig. 1). What is the most effective approach for management of USWP for this patient?

CASE 2: DORSALLY ANGULATED MALUNION

A 56-year-old, right-handed male injured his wrist by falling, was diagnosed with a DRF and treated with cast immobilization. He visited our clinic 3 months after injury with USWP. His radiographs showed a dorsally angulated malunion of the distal radius (RI: 23.5 deg, UV: 5.5 mm, PT: −27 deg) and an ulnar styloid nonunion (Fig. 2). This nonunion was already diagnosed before the DRF and seemed an old injury.

He often felt mild USWP before his DRF. How do you consider the best plan to resolve his USWP?

CASE 3: TFCC DISC TEAR

A 56-year-old, right-handed female sustained a right DRF, treated with cast fixation for 4 weeks. The DRF healed within normal range alignment (RI: 27 deg, PT: 10 deg, UV: +1.5 mm) (Fig. 3), however she complained of USWP for 10 months and therefore visited our clinic. Grip strength was 62% of the contralateral side. A TFCC slit tear was suspected on MRI. How would this be best managed?

CASE 4: TFCC FOVEAL TEAR

A 54-year-old, right-handed female suffered left DRF, classified as A3 in the AO classification. She underwent palmar plate fixation (Fig. 4A and B) with arthroscopic radiocarpal inspection, showing a normal appearing TFCC. The postoperative course was uneventful, plate removal was performed 6 months after surgery (Fig. 4C). Around 9 months after surgery, she gradually complained of USWP with instability of the ulnar head and grip weakness of 75% of the contralateral side. Radiographs showed widening of the DRUJ

Continued

Panel 1: Case Scenarios—cont'd

(Fig. 4D). How could this finding best be explained and managed?

CASE 5: ULNAR STYLOID NONUNION

A 28-year-old, right-handed male visited our clinic for USWP that appeared after slightly twisting the wrist several days earlier. His medical history revealed a left DRF that uneventfully healed with cast immobilization for 4 weeks at the age of 13 years. He complained not only of USWP but also of a slack sensation of the ulnar head during forearm rotation. Radiographs and MRI showed an ulnar styloid nonunion probably due to the old injury (Fig. 5). It is unclear if the foveal origin of the TFCC was still attached to the fragment or not. A removable wrist splint was applied for 4 months, but failed, USWP continued. How would this best be managed?

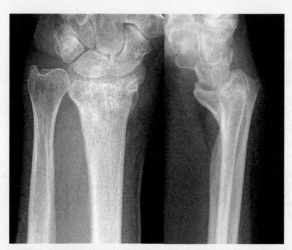

FIG. 1 Preoperative radiographs showed malunion with radial shortening and palmar angulation.

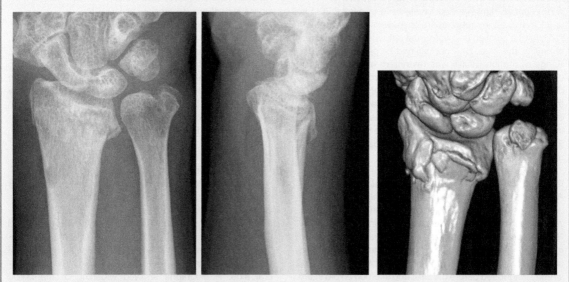

FIG. 2 Preoperative radiographs and CT showed a shortened and dorsally angulated malunion of the distal radius, and an ulnar styloid nonunion.

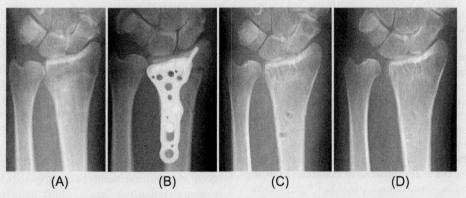

FIG. 3 Alignment of the distal radius was almost normal. On MRI, a TFCC slit tear was suspected *(red arrow)*.

(A)   (B)   (C)   (D)

FIG. 4 Extraarticular DRF was fixed with a volar plate (A and B). At 6 months after surgery, the plate was removed (C). At 9 months after surgery, the DRUJ was distended (D).

Continued

IMPORTANCE OF THE PROBLEM

USWP is a common complaint that contains a diagnostic challenge for hand surgeons because of the small and complex anatomic structures involved. The history and physical examination findings for a wide range of pathologies often overlap. Pain may derive from injured forearm and carpal bones, TFCC, ligament tears, tendinitis, vascular pathology, osteoarthritis and systemic arthritis, and ulnar nerve compression. DRF is the most common fracture in the upper extremity,

Panel 1: Case Scenarios—cont'd

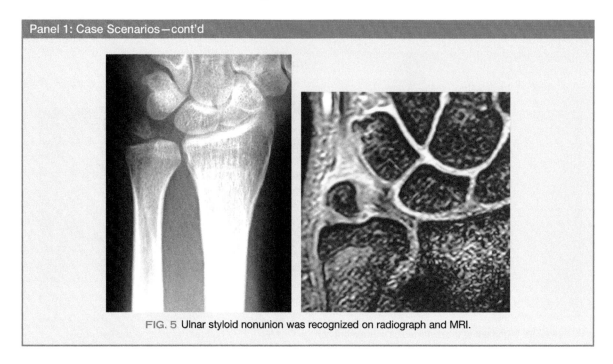

FIG. 5 Ulnar styloid nonunion was recognized on radiograph and MRI.

and is frequently associated with injury of the ulnar wrist structures such as the ulnar styloid, TFCC, lunotriquetral (LT) ligament, etc. The development of palmar locking plate fixation for surgical treatment for DRF provides rigid fixation, maintains accurate reduction acquired when the surgery was carried out, results successful outcome. However, USWP after DRF healed is often encountered, though only some of these patients have persistent moderate to severe pain that persists even a few years after, limiting proper function of the hand.[1–8] The causes of pain are often difficult to diagnose and resolve. A comprehensive examination of the wrist such as inspection, palpation, provocative maneuvers, radiography, computed tomography (CT), magnetic resonance imaging (MRI), and wrist arthroscopy are required.[9–12] Wrist arthroscopy plays an increasingly important role in the diagnosis and management of persistent USWP.[13] It is considered the benchmark for the diagnosis and management of TFCC injuries and other pathologies including carpal ligament injuries.

MAIN QUESTION

What are the main causes of persistent USWP after healed DRF and how is it best managed?

Current Opinion

USWP is common after DRF and can improve for a year or more, so patience and exhausting conservative trial outs are generally warranted. Acute injury of the TFCC and ulnar styloid fractures are common, and treatment remains controversial as routine repair is not indicated. As the natural course is mostly benign and self-limiting, persistent USWP is much less common and necessities a careful diagnostic work-up before surgical treatment.

What Are the Elements of USWP After DRF?

USWP after DRF has mainly been attributed to malunion, creating an imbalance distally, which might lead to ulnocarpal abutment, incongruency, and osteoarthrosis of the distal radioulnar joint (DRUJ). Although malunion is a three-dimensional deformity, extraarticular malunited DRF are often categorized on radiographs as palmarly angulated, dorsally angulated, loss of radial inclination, and/or radial shortening.[14, 15]

TFCC injuries are the most common associated intraarticular injuries with DRF, and may cause USWP.[5, 6, 16–18] TFCC injury can be divided into disc tear and peripheral tear.[18] "Disc" refers to the articular disc that acts as a shock absorber, while "peripheral" indicates the attachment of the disc to the surrounding tissue and the surrounding tissue itself. The surrounding tissue include both palmar and dorsal radioulnar ligaments, the ulnocarpal ligament, the sigmoid notch of the radius, the ulnar styloid and fovea. A disc tear may be treated by resection, on the other hand, peripheral tear should be repaired as it could lead to DRUJ or carpal instability.[6] Wrist arthroscopy is the best procedure to clearly recognize the associated TFCC tear.

Ulnar styloid fracture is often accompanied with DRF, and nonunion of this fracture is also common. However, the relationship between ulnar styloid nonunion and persistent USWP remains unclear.[1, 8, 19] It is considered that whether nonunion of ulnar styloid is symptomatic or not depends on the stability of DRUJ.

LT ligament tear could become the source of USWP after a healed DRF. However, the detail is still unclear.[5]

Finding the Evidence

* Cochrane search: Distal Radius Fracture, Ulnar-Sided Wrist Pain
* PubMed (Medline): Distal Radius Fracture, Ulnar-Sided Wrist Pain, Distal Radius Fracture AND Ulnar-Sided Wrist Pain, Distal Radius Fracture AND Distal Radius Malunion, Distal Radius Fracture AND Triangular Fibrocartilage Complex injury, Distal Radius Fracture AND Ulnar Styloid Nonunion
* Bibliography of eligible articles
* Articles that were not in English were excluded

Quality of the Evidence

Level II: Prospective case series: 2
Level III: Retrospective comparative studies: 6
Level IV: Case series: 2

FINDINGS

Although there were many high-level studies on DRF, there were no randomized controlled trials, systematic reviews, or metaanalyses about USWP after healed DRF. We only found 10 relevant articles with evidence levels II to IV (Table 1).

Kim et al. performed a retrospective study of longitudinal changes in the incidence of USWP after DRF treated by plate fixation, and factors associated with pain in 140 patients.[4] The incidence of USWP decreased significantly with time after surgery: 22 patients at 3 months, 11 patients at 6 months, and 3 patients at 12 months. The mean age, sex, the presence of an ulnar styloid fracture, and the classification of the DRF were not factors that were associated with an incidence of USWP, but

there was an association between higher patient-rated wrist evaluation scores and the presence of USWP (*Level III*).

Cheng et al. conducted a retrospective study analyzing 22 patients with chronic wrist pain after DRFs that were healed.[1] There were 17 males and 5 females with an average age of 40 years. They identified four patterns of pathoanatomy: (1) ulnar impaction syndrome caused by radial malunion and shortening; (2) ulnar styloid nonunion; (3) TFCC tear with or without DRUJ instability; (4) carpal instability or chondral lesions. Surgical treatment directed toward each identified abnormality gave satisfactory outcome. At 6 months after surgery, their wrist functional score improved on average by 36%, their mean pain score decreased by 50%, mean grip strength improved by 25%, and 64% of patients were able to return to work (*Level III*).

Prommersberger et al. reported a retrospective study that evaluated the outcome of corrective osteotomy for malunited DRF and investigated the influence of the radiological result on the clinical outcome.[14] Twenty nine patients underwent corrective osteotomy for dorsally angulated malunion, and 20 underwent corrective osteotomy for palmarly angulated malunion. Postoperative PT, RI, and UV were significantly improved, and radiological results correlated with the functional outcome (*Level III*).

Malunion is a common complication of DRF and can cause persistent USWP. Wada et al. retrospectively compared the clinical and radiographic results of opening-wedge with closing-wedge osteotomy.[15] Postoperative PT and UV improved significantly compared with the preoperative status in each procedure, however restoration of UV to within defined criteria (−2.5 to 0.5 mm) was significantly more frequent in the closing-wedge group than in the opening wedge osteotomy group. The postoperative mean extension-flexion arc of the wrist and Mayo Wrist Score were significantly better in the closing-wedge osteotomy group. They concluded that the closing-wedge osteotomy is an effective reconstructive procedure for the treatment of extraarticular distal radial malunion (*Level III*).

Deniz et al. performed a prospective study including 47 DRF patients who were treated with closed reduction and casting.[2] All patients underwent wrist MRI and 24 patients had associated traumatic TFCC tear according to Palmer's classification, the remaining 23 patients had no TFCC tear. In the mean follow-up period of about 39 months, TFCC tears did not affect the functional results. They concluded that further diagnostic tests and treatment of TFCC tears in patients with stable

TABLE 1
FINDINGS

Author	LoE	Study Design	Objective	Number of Patients	Content	Comments
Kim	IIIB	Retrospective	Longitudinal observation of the incidence of USWP after DRF treated by plate fixation	140	Number of cases of USWP. PO 3M: 22, PO 6M: 11, PO12M: 3	The incidence of USWP decreased significantly with time after surgery.
Cheng	IIIB	Retrospective	Analysis of 22 cases who complained of chronic wrist pain after DRF	22	Four patterns identified: (1) ulnar impaction due to malunion, (2) ulnar styloid nonunion, (3) TFCC injury with/without DRUJ instability, (4) intercarpal ligament and chondral lesion	Reconstruction for each abnormality gave satisfactory outcome
Prommersberger	IIIB	Retrospective	The outcome of corrective osteotomy for malunited DRF	Dorsally tilted: 29 Palmarly angulated: 20	Changes of XP index Dorsally tilted RI: 14 to 24, PT: −22 to 0, UV: 4 to 0 Palmarly angulated RI: 18 to 30, PT: 32 to 13, UV: 8 to 0	Postoperative XP index significantly improved and radiological results correlated with the functional outcome.
Wada	IIIB	Retrospective	Compared the clinical and radiographic results of opening and closing wedge osteotomy	Radial opening: 22 Radial closing and ulnar shortening: 20	Restoration of UV was significantly better in closing. exflex arc, Mayo wrist score: significantly better in closing	Closing osteotomy was significantly better than opening in terms of UV, exflex arc, and Mayo wrist score
Deniz	IIC	Prospective	Investigated the effect of untreated TFCC tear on the outcome of conservatively treated DRF	Total 47 Detect TFCC tear using MRI: 24 Undetected: 23	In the mean follow-up period of about 39months, TFCC tears did not affect the functional results	Further diagnostic tests and treatment of TFCC tears in patients with stable DRF may be unnecessary
Mrkonjic	IIC	Prospective	13–15years, longitudinal outcome study of the natural course of TFCC tears associated with DRF	38	Only 1 patient needed a stabilizing procedure because of painful instability of the DRUJ. The results did not provide evidence that a TFCC injury would influence the long-term outcome	Larger and preferably randomized studies needed
Abe	IV	Retrospective	The incidence of traumatic TFCC tear associated with DRF	456 intra- and extraarticular DRF	48.6%	
Wijffels	IIIB	Retrospective	The influence of nonunion of the ulnar styloid base fracture on the outcome of DRF is debated	Nonunion: 18 Union: 16	In the mean follow-up period of about 30months, There were no significant differences in both groups	Ulnar styloid nonunion is not associated with pain, instability or diminished function after DRF
Hauck	IIIB	Retrospective	Investigation for 20 cases of USWP associated with nonunion of the ulnar styloid	Type 1: with a stable DRUJ: 11 Type II: with subluxation of DRUJ: 9	Type 1: all excision and pain relief Type 2: ORIF 3 complete relief, excision 6 excellent 4, good 1, fair 1	DRUJ was stable or its stability was restored, long-term pain relief was achieved by treatment of the nonunion

LoE, level of evidence.

DRF may be unnecessary. However, they suggested that it should be borne in mind as a reason for continuing wrist pain and instability after DRF despite proper radiologic recovery (*Level II*).

In a prospective, longitudinal outcome study over 13–15 years of the natural course of TFCC tears associated with DRF in 38 patients. Mrkonjic et al. reported only one patient needed a stabilizing procedure because of painful instability of the DRUJ.[7] The subjective and objective results did not provide evidence that a TFCC injury would influence the long-term outcome. They concluded that there was no support for aggressive surgical management when TFCC tears are diagnosed in association with DRF, however they suggested larger and preferably randomized studies were needed (*Level II*).

TFCC injury associated DRF is considered one of the main causes of persistent USWP. Regarding the incidence of associated TFCC injury, Lindau summarized several articles and reported the incidence was 35%–78%.[5] Abe et al. previously reported that traumatic TFCC tear was arthroscopically diagnosed in 102 of 248 intraarticular DRF (41.1%), and 222 of 456 extra- and intraarticular DRF (48.6%).[16, 17] Our current investigation of 518 DRFs including both intra- and extraarticular fractures, TFCC traumatic injury was diagnosed in 250 wrists (48.3%). The type of injury classified according to our original classification are shown in Fig. 6 (*Level IV*).

Wijffels et al. reported a retrospective study of 34 adult DRF including 18 patients with an ulnar styloid base nonunion compared to 16 patients with union of an ulnar styloid base fracture with a mean postoperative follow-up of 30 months.[8] There were no significant differences in pain, complications, or function, and patients with nonunion had significantly greater grip strength. None of the patients had DRUJ instability. They concluded that ulnar styloid nonunion is not associated with pain, instability, or diminished function after DRF (*Level III*).

Hauck et al. classified symptomatic nonunion of ulnar styloid fractures dependent on stability of the DRUJ.[19] Type 1 is defined as a nonunion associated with a stable DRUJ. Type 2 is defined as a nonunion associated with subluxation of the DRUJ. Eleven type 1 were treated with excision of the fragments, and all patients had satisfactory pain relief. Nine type 2 required restoration of the TFCC anatomy. Three of these had large fragments that were treated by open reduction and internal fixation. All three patients experienced relief of discomfort. Six other patients underwent excision of the fragment and repair of the TFCC, and achieved four excellent, one good, and one fair results. They concluded that if the DRUJ is stable on presentation or if its stability is restored, then long-term relief of pain from ulnar styloid nonunion is achieved by treatment of the nonunion (*Level III*).

According to Lindau, LT ligament injuries occur in about one out of six DRFs, and to date there is no evidence that LT tears lead to long-term problems when associated with DRF.[5] He suggested that complete LT tear may need arthroscopic debridement of the tear and percutaneous pinning of the joint (*Level IV*) (Table 1).

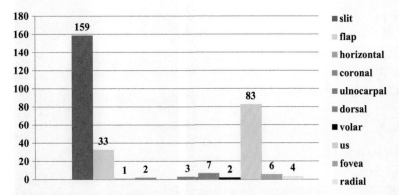

FIG. 6 The number of TFCC injuries associated with 518 DRFs, classified according to the Abe classification. A traumatic tear was recognized in 48.3% of cases (US: tear from ulnar styloid).

Panel 2: Case Scenarios; Author's Treatment Option and Results

CASE 1

Open-wedge osteotomy was carried out from the palmar side and fixed with a palmar plate; bone defect was filled with artificial bone graft (Fig. 7A and B). Intraarticular debridement for fibrous tissue proliferation and TFCC flap tear were performed simultaneously using arthroscopy (Fig. 7C and D). ROM exercise was introduced 2 days after surgery. Two and a half months after surgery, radiographs showed complete bone union. Sixteen months after surgery (Fig. 8), she did not complaint of any USWP, ROM was almost normal (ex: 75 deg, flex: 70 deg. pro: 85 deg, sup: 90 deg), grip strength was 105% of contralateral side

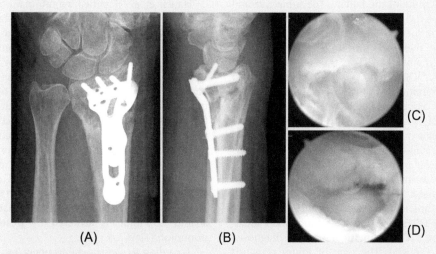

(A) (B) (C)

(D)

FIG. 7 Postoperative radiographs after correction osteotomy (A and B). Arthroscopy showed a flap tear of the TFCC disc (C) for which debridement was carried out (D).

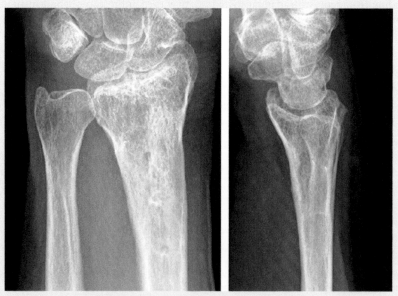

FIG. 8 Radiographs at 16 months after osteotomy, and hardware removal.

CASE 2

Open-wedge osteotomy was performed from dorsal side with a small (1 cm) skin incision and fixed from the palmar side with a locking plate. The bone defect was filled with artificial bone graft (Fig. 9). The ulnar styloid nonunion fragment was resected. Debridement of the TFCC degenerative tear was carried out under arthroscopy. Rehabilitation was started 2 days after surgery. One year after surgery, ROM recovered normal (ex: 85, flex: 70, pro: 85, sup: 90), grip strength was 92% of the contralateral side and pain free (Fig. 10).

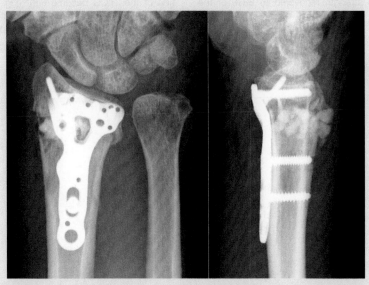

FIG. 9 Postoperative radiographs following open wedge osteotomy, wrist arthroscopy and resection of the ulnar styloid fragment.

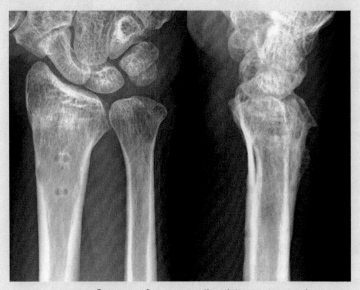

FIG. 10 One year after surgery, the plate was removed.

Continued

Panel 2: Case Scenarios; Author's Treatment Option and Results—cont'd

CASE 3

Wrist arthroscopy revealed a slit tear of TFCC disc (Fig. 11A) and synovitis around the TFCC. Debridement was carried out for these pathological lesions (Fig. 11B). Thereafter, she underwent ipsilateral thumb carpometacarpal arthroplasty. Nineteen months after TFCC debridement, there was no USWP, grip strength recovered to 88% of the contralateral side.

CASE 4

The TFCC at the fovea might be injured when the fracture occurred, and gradually peeled off during the postoperative

course. On MRI, a TFCC foveal tear was suspected (Fig. 12A). Twenty months after initial surgery, reconstructive surgery was carried out. DRUJ arthroscopy showed fibrous tissue continuation at the fovea but elongated (Fig. 12B), then arthroscopic transosseous repair[20, 21] for TFCC foveal tear was performed (Fig. 12C). The foveal portion of the TFCC became tight (Fig. 12D). After 3 years, USWP was not present, grip strength recovered to 93% of the contralateral side. Radiographs showed normal appearance of the DRUJ (Fig. 12E).

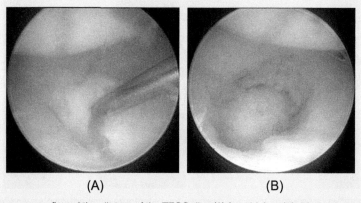

(A)   (B)

FIG. 11 Arthroscopy confirmed the slit tear of the TFCC disc (A) for which a debridement was carried out (B).

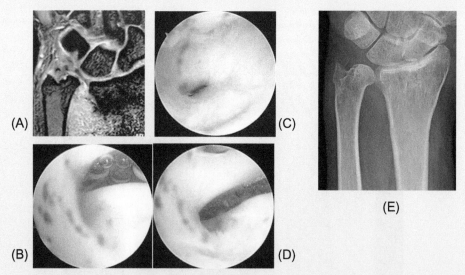

(A)   (C)

(B)   (D)   (E)

FIG. 12 TFCC foveal injury was suspected on MRI (A). Scar tissue was recognized at the fovea during DRUJ arthroscopy (B). Transosseous repair was carried out under arthroscopy (C: radiocarpal view, D: DRUJ view). At 3 years after repair, radiographs showed a normal appearance of the DRUJ (E).

Panel 2: Case Scenarios; Author's Treatment Option and Results—cont'd

CASE 5

Ulnar head instability was obvious under general anesthesia at surgery. Osteosynthesis for ulnar styloid nonunion was performed under direct vision. The nonunion site was refreshed and fixed with tension band wiring. A bone peg harvested at the olecranon was inserted into the hole created using 1.5mm Kirschner wire between the fragments (Fig. 13A). The ulnar head instability disappeared. DRUJ arthroscopy showed that TFCC foveal lesion was elongated before fixation (Fig. 13B), and subsequently became tight after fixation (Fig. 13C). The wrist was immobilized with a cast for 2 weeks and rehabilitation was started. Bone union was confirmed 3 months after surgery (Fig. 13D). One year after surgery, ROM and function of the wrist was normal and USWP had resolved.

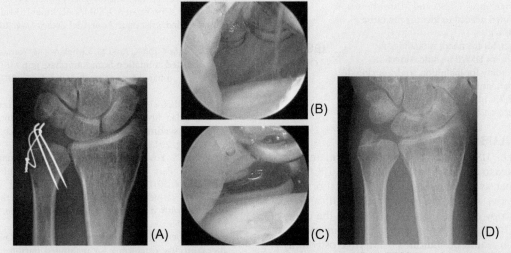

FIG. 13 The nonunion was fixed with tension band wiring and a bone peg graft (A). TFCC fovea became tight. (B: fovea before fixation, C: fovea after fixation.) Three months after surgery, there were signs of early union (D).

Panel 3: Pearls and Pitfalls

PEARLS

- The incidence of USWP after healed DRF significantly decreases with time after surgery, hence patience will yield high and predictable rates of improvement.
- Distal radius malunion: open-wedge osteotomy from both palmar and dorsal could achieve predictable good results if postoperative alignments on radiographs are restored to near anatomic. Closing wedge osteotomy can be expected to provide the same effect. During malunion surgery, wrist arthroscopy may be indicated for concern of associated intercarpal ligament injury or TFCC disruptions.
- TFCC injury associated with DRF might be the cause of persistent USWP after fracture healed. If USWP is encountered, MRI and wrist arthroscopy are strongly helpful to analyze and treat USWP.
- Ulnar styloid nonunion might become one of the causes of USWP. Nonunion with DRUJ instability should be considered for fixation, whereas nonunion without DRUJ instability could be treated with resection.

PITFALLS

- The indication of corrective osteotomy for malunion of the distal radius is based on the clinical findings, not merely on radiographs.
- Concomitant TFCC injury and/or ulnar styloid fracture without DRUJ instability do not need to be routinely repaired with distal radius osteosynthesis.

RECOMMENDATION

In patients with an intraarticular displaced distal radius fracture, evidence suggests:

Recommendation	Overall Quality
• USWP is common after DRF and can improve for a year or more, so patience is generally warranted	⊕⊕○○ LOW
• Careful evaluation such as inspection, palpation, provocative maneuvers, radiography, CT, MRI, and wrist arthroscopy are often needed to identify the cause of USWP	⊕⊕○○ LOW
• Successful treatment modalities for persistent USWP include correction osteotomy for malunion (open or closed wedge), arthroscopic or open management for TFCC injury, and fixation or resection for nonunion of ulnar styloid	⊕⊕○○ LOW

CONCLUSIONS

Persistent USWP after healed DRF has mainly been attributed to malunion of the distal radius, TFCC injury, and ulnar styloid nonunion. Careful evaluation such as provocative maneuvers, radiography, MRI, and wrist arthroscopy are often needed to identify the cause of USWP. If conservative treatment fails, surgical reconstruction would be indicated. Corrective osteotomy is a reliable treatment, DRUJ instability is the critical point to determine the surgical indication for TFCC injury and ulnar styloid nonunion. Wrist arthroscopy is helpful in dealing with persistent USWP.

REFERENCES

1. Cheng HS, Hung LK, Ho PC, Wong J. An analysis of causes and treatment outcome of chronic wrist pain after distal radial fractures. *Hand Surg.* 2008;13:1–10.
2. Deniz G, Kose O, Yanik S, Colakoglu T, Tugay A. Effect of untreated triangular fibrocartilage complex (TFCC) tears on the clinical outcome of conservatively treated distal radius fractures. *Eur J Orthop Surg Traumatol.* 2014;24: 1155–1159.
3. Diaz-Garcia RJ, Oda T, Shauver MJ, Chung KC. A systematic review of outcomes and complications of treating unstable distal radius fractures in the elderly. *J Hand Surg.* 2011;36A:824–835.
4. Kim JK, Kim DJ, Yun Y. Natural history and factors associated with ulnar-sided wrist pain in distal radial fractures treated by plate fixation. *J Hand Surg.* 2016; 41E:727–731.
5. Lindau T. Arthroscopic evaluation of associated soft tissue injuries in distal radius fractures. *Hand Clin.* 2017; 33:651–658.
6. Lindau T, Hagberg L, Adlercreutz C, Jonsson K, Aspenberg P. Distal radioulnar instability is an independent worsening factor in distal radial fractures. *Clin Orthop.* 2000;376:229–235.
7. Mrkonjic A, Geijer M, Lindau T, Tägil M. The natural course of traumatic triangular fibrocartilage complex tears in distal radial fractures: a 13-15-year follow-up of arthroscopically diagnosed but untreated injuries. *J Hand Surg.* 2012;37A:1555–1560.
8. Wijffels M, Ring D. The influence of non-union of the ulnar styloid on pain, wrist function and instability after distal radius fracture. *J Hand Microsurg.* 2011;3:11–14.
9. DaSilva MF, Goodman AD, Gil JA, Akelman E. Evaluation of ulnar-sided wrist pain. *J Am Acad Orthop Surg.* 2017;25: e150–e156.
10. Oda T, Wada T, Iba K, Aoki M, Tamakawa M, Yamashita T. Reconstructed animation from four-phase grip MRI of the wrist with ulnar-sided pain. *J Hand Surg.* 2013;38E: 746–750.
11. Sachar K. Ulnar-sided wrist pain: evaluation and treatment of triangular fibrocartilage complex tears, ulnocarpal impaction syndrome, and lunotriquetral ligament tears. *J Hand Surg.* 2012;37A:1489–1500.
12. Vezeridis PS, Yoshioka H, Han R, Blazar P. Ulnar-sided wrist pain. Part I: anatomy and physical examination. *Skelet Radiol.* 2010;39:733–745.
13. Lindau T. Treatment of injuries to the ulnar side of the wrist occurring with distal radial fractures. *Hand Clin.* 2005; 21:417–425.
14. Prommersberger KJ, Schoonhoven JV, Lanz UB. Outcome after corrective osteotomy for malunited fractures of the distal end of the radius. *J Hand Surg.* 2002;27B:55–60.
15. Wada T, Tatebe M, Ozasa Y, et al. Clinical outcomes of corrective osteotomy for distal radial malunion. A review of opening and closing-wedge techniques. *J Bone Joint Surg Am.* 2011;93:1619–1626.
16. Abe Y. Arthroscopic management. Distal radius fractures and carpal instabilities. In: Del Pinal F, ed. *FESSH IFSSH 2019 Instructional Book.* Stuttgart: Thieme; 2019:95–103.
17. Abe Y, Fujii K. Arthroscopic-assisted reduction of intraarticular distal radius fracture. *Hand Clin.* 2017; 33:659–668.
18. Abe Y, Tominaga Y, Yoshida K. Various patterns of traumatic triangular fibrocartilage complex tear. *Hand Surg.* 2012;17(2):191–198.
19. Hauck RM, Skahen III J, Palmer AK. Classification and treatment of ulnar styloid non-union. *J Hand Surg.* 1996;21A:418–422.
20. Nakamura T, Sato K, Okazaki M, Toyama Y, Ikegami H. Repair of foveal detachment of the triangular fibrocartilage complex: open and arthroscopic transosseous techniques. *Hand Clin.* 2011;27:281–290.
21. Abe Y, Fujii K, Fujisawa T. Midterm results after open versus arthroscopic transosseous repair for foveal tears of the triangular fibrocartilage complex. *J Wrist Surg.* 2018; 7:292–297.

CHAPTER 22

Association Between Radiological and Patient-Reported Outcomes

ANDREW MILLER
Philadelphia Hand to Shoulder Center, Thomas Jefferson University Hospital, Philadelphia, PA, United States

KEY POINTS

- Restoration of the main radiographic distal radial parameters has long been a focus of treatment in closed versus open management of distal radial fractures (DRFs).
- Commonly used radiographic predictors for assessing adequate anatomic restoration include radial inclination, sagittal tilt (dorsal and volar), radial shortening, as well as intraarticular incongruity.
- In review of the literature, radial height and articular incongruity have the most significant effect on patient-reported outcome measures (PROMs).
- In particular, radial height loss of greater than 5–6 mm and articular incongruity >2 mm is predictive of worse PROMs.
- Radial inclination and sagittal tilt, while important to restore do not impact PROMs as significantly.

Panel 1: Case Scenario

A 63-year-old active female physiotherapist falls from standing and presents to the emergency department with a moderately displaced extra-articular distal radius fracture. On postreduction radiographs, the dorsal tilt is neutral, radial inclination is 15 degrees and the distal radius is 5 mm shortened (Fig. 1). She strongly requests "anatomic reduction" and fixation as she fears the slightest malunion may jeopardize her function. Opting for shared decision-making, the main question arises: What radiographic parameters are most predictive of patient-reported outcomes?

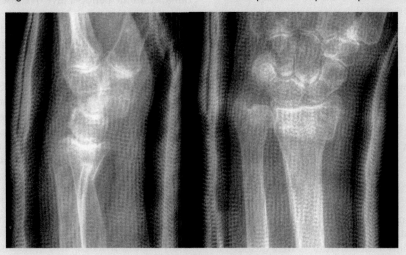

FIG. 1 Postreduction radiographs.

Distal Radius Fractures. https://doi.org/10.1016/B978-0-323-75764-5.00024-X

IMPORTANCE OF THE PROBLEM

Distal radius fractures (DRFs) are one of the more common musculoskeletal injuries that present to the emergency department or urgent care.[1] Deciding how to manage a DRF therefore has implications with respect to patient function. Displaced, comminuted intraarticular DRFs are challenging injuries to treat with closed management, prone to collapse or re-displacement, and are often indicated for open reduction and internal fixation.[2]

One of the first attempts to evaluate the functional outcomes of dorsally displaced DRFs was by Gartland and Werley in 1951.[3] They concluded that the degree of comminution was directly proportional to the development of posttraumatic arthritis. However, despite incomplete reduction, satisfactory functional results were obtained in 68.3% of the series over 1 year of follow-up.

Since this study, predicting the successful return to function and elimination of pain has been studied in the literature by several papers. Commonly used radiographic predictors for assessing adequate anatomic restoration radial inclination, sagittal tilt (dorsal and volar), radial shortening, as well as intraarticular incongruity.

MAIN QUESTION

To what extent do radiographic parameters of radial inclination, radial height, dorsal tilt, and articular incongruity predict patient-reported outcome measures (PROMs)?

CURRENT OPINION

Despite the fact that radiographic parameters influence treatment paradigms to a large extent and are widely used as core evaluation tool, there remains lacking consensus on which radiographic parameters have the greatest impact on PROMs.

FINDING THE EVIDENCE

Pubmed searches using keywords such as "distal radius patient-reported outcomes," "outcomes after distal radius fracture," "postoperative outcomes after distal radius fractures," "radiographic parameters of distal radius fractures," "volar tilt and distal radius fractures," "radial inclination and distal radius fractures," "articular incongruity and distal radius fractures," "radial shortening and distal radius fractures." Articles were excluded if not written in English.

QUALITY OF THE EVIDENCE

Level I: 1
Level II: 5
Level III: 31
Level IV: 3

FINDINGS

PROMs are tools that have been developed to identify and objectify patient satisfaction and function with respect to a particular injury. Patient outcomes include visual analog scale pain scores (VAS), patient satisfaction scores, return to work, and functional outcomes.

The most reliable and valid outcome measures reported for hand and wrist trauma are the disabilities of the arm, shoulder, and hand outcome (DASH) as well as the patient-rated wrist evaluation (PRWE).[4] The DASH was designed for patients to briefly define symptoms and functional status.[5] The PRWE was first published in 1998 by J.C. MacDermid as a result of the study of the International Wrist Investigators Group and was designed to measure pain and disability experienced by patients.[6]

Several variables have been cited as important to restore functional and painless range of motion and grip strength. If radiologic parameters are predictive with respect to patient-reported outcomes, then restoration of all radiologic parameters as close to anatomically possible would ensure optimal patient outcomes.

In order to objectively measure the key radiologic parameters of a distal radius, standardized radiographs (including posterior-anterior and lateral views) must be obtained in the perioperative or conservative treatment setting (Box 1).

Predicting outcomes from DRF radiographic assessment (Box 2) can be done in two segments: evaluating the injury and prereduction films versus evaluating the posttreatment films (closed or open).

This chapter is largely focused on radiographic assessment posttreatment but it is worth noting that Lafontaine's criteria of dorsal displacement greater than 20 degrees, dorsal comminution, intraarticular fracture, associated ulnar styloid fracture as well as age greater than 60 years suggest worse anatomic and radiographic results with an increasing number of these factors present.[2] However, Lafontaine's series did not evaluate functional or subjective outcomes, only the anatomic parameters.

Evaluating prereduction parameters associated with patient outcomes, radial shortening, and severity of injury were associated with 6 month PRWE scores.[10] When evaluating the 1 year PRWE scores, Grewal et al.

BOX 1
Standardized Radiographs.

1. Posterior-anterior
2. Lateral and lateral 10 degree projection
3. Distal radial ulnar joint (DRUJ) view

    In order to accurately measure the radiologic parameters, standardized radiographs must be performed. The posteroanterior requires the shoulder in 90 degrees of abduction, the elbow in 90 degrees of flexion and the wrist and forearm in neutral. For a lateral radiograph, the shoulder is fully adducted and the hand must be turned to lie in the same plane as the humerus. The pisiform should overlap the distal pole of the scaphoid. To obtain the tilted view, the forearm can be tilted 10 degrees to obtain a better view of the joint. For a DRUJ view, the wrist is in similar position as the PA view but the volar and dorsal cortex of the sigmoid notch should overlap.

BOX 2
Radiographic Parameters.

1. Radial inclination
2. Radial height
3. Dorsal tilt
4. Articular incongruity

    The normal radiographic parameters for the distal radius include an average volar tilt of 10–12 degrees, a radial inclination of 23 degrees, and a radial length of 12 mm.[7–9] The tear drop angle measures approximately 70 degrees on the lateral radiograph of the distal radius.[7]

did not identify any correlation with prereduction radiographic measurements: dorsal angulation (average 11 ± 17.5), ulnar variance (1.1 ± 2.3) or radial inclination (18.9 ± 7.1).[11]

RADIAL INCLINATION

The radial inclination parameter has been evaluated by several authors going back to Mason's fracture investigation in 1953.[12] Mason found that in a subset of patients with both clinical dysfunction and pain, patients demonstrated loss of radial inclination. The loss of radial inclination of the distal radial fragment can lead to altered DRUJ kinematics and noticeable arthritic changes.

Gartland et al. noted in their seminal series of 60 DRFs treated with closed reduction that radial inclination was markedly varied after immobilization from 13 to 30 degrees.[3] Despite reduction of the deviated radial fragment, there was a tendency to re-displace by follow-up examination. The authors do make note of the fact that radial inclination changes are associated with a rotation of the distal radial fragment into supination which can challenge the tension of the TFCC. However, little effect on functional outcome was noted overall.

Wilcke et al. found in series of 78 DRFs treated with closed reduction and immobilization, radial inclination greater than 10 degrees of the uninjured sided was associated with poorer DASH score and worse patient satisfaction.[13]

Perugia et al. found in 51 patients treated with volar locking plates for DRFs, approximately 75% had restoration of radial inclination. They suggested that small variations do not effect final outcome at 3 years.[14] Porter and Stockley found in their series of 115 patients with DRFs that when the radial inclination fell below 10 degrees, the grip strength was significantly reduced at 6 months and 2 years with a deficit measured at 33% and 30%, respectively.[15]

Jenkins and Mintowt reviewed 58 patients and found a significant negative correlation between flattening of the radial inclination and patient grip strength.[16] Further in agreement, Rubinovich concluded that a radial angle of less than 10 degrees resulted in a grip strength reduction. Additionally, patients with radial inclinations that exceeded normal values (16–28 degrees) led to unsatisfactory results in 50% of cases.[17, 18]

In 2005, Karnezis et al. demonstrated no correlation between loss of radial inclination and the PRWE score although the mean radial inclination was found to be 16 degrees and within a small variation to the normal range.[19] In 2007, Kumar et al. found that patient outcomes, as measured by the MHQ and DASH were satisfactory even if the radiologic parameters including radial inclination were not. There was also a stronger inverse correlation in older age groups than younger age groups in their study.[20]

Despite the variation in reported outcomes with altered radial inclination, subjective outcomes do not seem to be affected greatly by radial inclination. Of note, many patients that had worse functional or subjective outcomes with significant changes in radial inclination also had additional radiographic parameters that fell outside the normal range. Thus, in isolation, the impact of radial inclination is difficult to predict.

RADIAL SHORTENING

Loss of radial height, and by extension increased ulnar height and variance, is a well-studied radiographic parameter following DRFs treated by both closed and open techniques. One of the components of Gartland and Werley's study, radial shortening is an often-examined radiographic metric to evaluate for successful management of a DRF by closed or open means.[3] For patients with significant radial shortening during injury, regardless of postreduction improvements, there is a tendency toward re-shortening. Gartland and Werley found that significant shortening resulted in decreased ulnar deviation and that excellent functional results were obtained with average of 2.2 mm of shortening. On the contrary, Short et al. found that shortening of the radius altered force transmission and radiocarpal kinematics.[21]

There is also concern that radial shortening will lead to altered DRUJ mechanics and ulnocarpal impingement. Consequently, ulnar-sided wrist pain after closed and open management of DRFs with incomplete restoration of radial height has been studied.[22, 23]

The degree to which shortening impairs function has been found to be proportionate to the amount of shortening. Fujii et al. found in their review of 22 elderly patients treated with closed reduction or open reduction and percutaneous pinning, functional outcome was affected when shortening was greater than 6 mm. However, 4 mm or less of shortening did not affect patient outcomes especially over 60 years of age.[24]

However, Aro and Koivunen found that even minor shortening of the radius in patients 55 years and older could lead to unsatisfactory outcomes. Patients that had between 3 and 5 mm of shortening had significant disability according to the demerit score which evaluated functional as well as subjective outcomes. They also noted that there was no increased disability for patients that also had concomitant malalignment of the radial inclination or tilt in addition suggesting that radial shortening was the most important parameter to correct.[25]

Wilcke et al. found that there was a distinction between 2 mm of shortening and significant changes in the DASH. For patients with greater than 2 mm of shortening, the DASH score averaged 10 points higher and the VAS satisfaction score was lower.[13] Jenkins et al. found a significant increase in wrist pain for patients that had approximately 4.7 mm or greater of shortening compared to patients who were wrist pain-free with an average shortening of 2.3 mm or less.[16]

In older patients, Karnezis found that radial shortening up to 5 mm can be tolerated.[19] However, permanent shortening was strongly associated with persistent wrist pain and higher PRWE pain subscores. On the other hand, Barton et al. in a review of 60 patients treated with closed reduction and pinning found and average shortening of 2.6 mm [0–8 mm] and that no association between PRWE score was found suggesting that patients, especially older individuals, with moderate shortening would not have worse subjective outcomes.[26]

SAGITTAL TILT

One of the most commonly assessed radiologic parameters for DRFs is the dorsal tilt. The parameter is often utilized to justify open reduction internal fixation for significant variations in the parameter as well as the success of closed or open management in the posttreatment period. For fractures with greater degrees of dorsal tilt, especially with dorsal comminution, there is a high risk of re-displacement with closed reduction.[9]

Dorsal angulation has been shown to alter the radiocarpal pressure concentrations as well as DRUJ kinematics.[27] Acceptable ranges for dorsal angulation vary but largely include a range of 0–20 degrees.

In Gartland's study of patients managed non-operatively with immobilization, patients that had excellent functional outcome had final follow up dorsal tilt of 0 degrees. However, there is no significant mention of patient reported outcome or satisfaction based on the degree of dorsal tilting. While greater than 10 degrees of dorsal tilting was associated with reduction in palmar flexion by 20 degrees, this does not seem to correlate with patient satisfaction. Tsukazaki et al. also found that dorsal tilt was the most important factor associated with loss of palmar flexion several years later in follow-up.[28] Conversely, postreduction or intervention volar tilt that was increased beyond the average or contralateral seemed to lead to a decrease in wrist extension.[29]

A few studies have evaluated the patient-reported outcomes.[13, 19, 20, 30] Wilcke et al. found that dorsal tilt that exceeded 15 degrees was associated with a poorer DASH score by approximately 10 points. Similarly, excessive dorsal tilt was found to correlate with worse VAS patient satisfaction scores. Kumar et al. found that there was a significant correlation between volar tilt and functional outcomes in younger individuals but not in older individuals.[20] Despite many patients with poor radiologic results, there was a high proportion of patients with acceptable DASH and Michigan Hand Outcomes Questionnaire (MHQ) scores.

In 30 DRFs treated with closed reduction and percutaneous pinning and final volar tilt of 4.5 degrees

[−25 to 23 degrees], Karnezis et al. found that a permanent loss of volar tilt was associated with persisting wrist pain on the PRWE pain subscore which includes level of pain at rest as well as with various activities.[19] They did not find a correlation with the functional outcome in the PRWE. Anzarut et al. reviewed 74 patients older than 50 years of age with non-operatively managed DRFs and divided the radiographic criteria as acceptable or unacceptable.[30] Acceptable tilt was volar tilt <20 degrees and dorsal tilt <10 degrees, whereas unacceptable ranges were volar tilt >20 degrees and dorsal tilting greater than 10 degrees. Forty-seven patients had acceptable radiographic parameters compared to 27. The authors found that radiographic reduction was not significantly associated with improved patient reported outcomes as measured by the DASH, SF-12, and patient satisfaction survey. They did demonstrate that 44% of patients with acceptable reductions were satisfied compared to 26% of patients with unacceptable outcomes.

Dorsal tilt does not appear to significant impact patient reported disability despite alteration in functional outcome. Functionally, dorsal tilt does appear to affect wrist arc of motion. Excessive volar tilt reduces wrist extension while excessive dorsal tilt reduces palmar flexion. Overall, abnormal values appear to be well tolerated unless they alter the distal radial ulnar joint mechanics.

ARTICULAR STEP-OFF AND INCONGRUITY

Articular step-off following closed or open treatment of DRFs has recently garnered significant attention following Jupiter's classic article on measuring incongruity.[31] The implications of articular incongruity include radiocarpal arthrosis and long-term arthritis. In their series, only 43% of patients had an excellent or good result with development of posttraumatic arthritis. No development of secondary arthritic changes were discovered when articular step-off was less than 1 mm in a separate study by Fernandez and Geissler.[32]

While the degree of acceptable articular step-off has been challenged, as implant fixation improves and adjunct treatments such as arthroscopic-assisted reductions evolved, anatomic reduction of the articular surface remains an important goal and radiographic parameter.

Synn et al. evaluated four subjective assessment measures including the DASH and PRWE and found no relationship between subjective outcome and radiographic displacement with respect to articular step-off or articular gapping in patients older than 55 years of age.[33]

In a retrospective study, Perugia et al. found that articular step-off was present in over 1/3 of patients with DRFs treated with a volar plate.[14] The step-off was recorded as

either greater than or less than 2 mm on a standard radiographs. However, they did not find correlation with articular step-off and worsening DASH scores.

Karnezis et al. found in their prospective study of 30 consecutive DRFs treated with closed reduction and percutaneous pinning, the presence of >1 mm of articular step-off correlated with loss of dorsiflexion as well as worsening PRWE scores at 1 year.[19]

Mehta et al. found in arthroscopic-assisted reductions and pinning of DRFs that there was a direct correlation between the size of the step-off and the development of wrist pain postoperatively.[34] For patients with no step-off, VAS pain scores greater than 2 were found in 18% versus 38% with greater than 1 mm of step-off and 100% with >2 mm.

Forward et al. published their results on younger patients (less than 40 years old at time of injury) with malunited DRFs with a mean follow-up time of 38 years.[35] Nearly 70% had evidence of posttraumatic arthritis. However, their DASH scores were not dissimilar from population norms and overall pain was not significantly different to the contralateral wrist.

Similarly, Goldfarb et al. found that while radiocarpal arthrosis worsened over time after intraarticular fractures of the distal radius, patients maintained high function as longer term follow-up. No correlation between degree of arthrosis and the upper extremity function at average of 15 years.[36]

One challenge with articular incongruity and step-off is accurate measurement. Because of poor inter and intraobserver agreement for measuring the degree of step-off on plain films, CT scans are recommended for more accurate measurement compared to standard radiographic assessment.[37]

An important subparameter of the articular evaluation is the tear drop angle. On the lateral 10 degree projection, this parameter is easier to measure than articular incongruity. These parameters should be restored as variations in congruity.

The tear drop angle, which normally measures around 70 degrees, is the outline of the volar rim of the lunate face. The lunate facet is a major weight-bearing column of the distal radius and can determine articular incongruity and the direction of carpal instability.[7]

Loss of the tear drop angle between the fractured and uninjured wrist was seen to lead to significant reduction in grip strength and worse DASH scores.[38]

RECOMMENDATION

In patients with an intraarticular displaced distal radius fracture, evidence suggests:

Recommendation	Overall Quality
• Variations in the radiographic parameters do affect PROMs. However, there is a large degree of tolerance for abnormal radiographic parameters.	⊕⊕⊕◯ MODERATE
• Radial inclination affects mainly grip strength, but its effect on PROMS is difficult to quantify in isolation.	⊕⊕◯◯ LOW
• Radial shortening, particularly beyond 5–6 mm, has an effect on patient outcome, especially younger patients.	⊕⊕⊕◯ MODERATE
• Failure of restoration of the radial height appears to affect DRUJ mechanics and imparts the risk of ulnar sided wrist pain, ulnar wrist impaction, and loss of rotation.	⊕⊕⊕◯ MODERATE
• While articular incongruity is important to restore anatomic function, patients do seem to tolerate radiocarpal arthrosis as well as minor incongruities of less than 2 mm.	⊕⊕⊕◯ MODERATE
• Loss of the tear drop angle less than 70 degrees may impact long-term outcomes especially in younger and higher demand individuals.	⊕⊕◯◯ LOW
• As long as DRUJ mechanics are not altered, volar/dorsal tilt does not affect PROMs but may reduce wrist extension or flexion, respectively.	⊕⊕⊕◯ MODERATE

CONCLUSION

Patient satisfaction and pain relief are paramount in closed or open management of DRFs. While it is important to restore the native anatomy and approximate normal radiographic parameters, patients do tolerate incomplete restoration of these parameters and loss of some functionality without compromising satisfaction, especially in the elderly.

Assigning significance and causality to any one particular parameter is challenging. When viewed in combination, dorsal angulation, radial height, and radial inclination only accounted for 11% of the variability of clinical outcomes for displaced DRFs managed non-operatively as measured by VAS Pain, Q-DASH, PRWE, and Global Wrist Outcome Score (GWOS).[39] Thus, less tangible factors such as psychosocial determinants play a far greater role in PROMs than restoration of radiographic parameters.[40, 41]

Panel 2: Author's Preferred Treatment

For younger patients and manual laborers especially, I try to restore all anatomic parameters of the distal radius. For elderly patients, I prioritize radial shortening as the literature seems to demonstrate higher rates of ulnar sided wrist pain and DRUJ dysfunction. In the highlighted case above, I would opt to treat the patient with open reduction and internal fixation utilizing a volar plate with variable or fixed angle locking features in order to anatomically fix the distal radius and restore the radial height.

REFERENCES

1. Azad A, Kang HP, Alluri RK, Vakhshori V, Kay HF, Ghiassi A. Epidemiological and treatment trends of distal radius fractures across multiple age groups. *J Wrist Surg.* 2019;8(4):305–311.
2. Lafontaine M, Hardy D, Delince PH. Stability assessment of distal radius fractures. *Injury.* 1989;20(4):208–210.
3. Gartland Jr. JJ, Werley CW. Evaluation of healed Colles' fractures. *J Bone Joint Surg.* 1951;33(4):895–907.
4. Dacombe PJ, Amirfeyz R, Davis T. Patient-reported outcome measures for hand and wrist trauma: is there sufficient evidence of reliability, validity, and responsiveness? *Hand.* 2016;11(1):11–21.
5. Hudak PL, Amadio PC, Bombardier C, et al. Development of an upper extremity outcome measure: the DASH (disabilities of the arm, shoulder, and head). *Am J Ind Med.* 1996;29(6):602–608.
6. MacDermid JC, Turgeon T, Richards RS, et al. Patient rating of wrist pain and disability: a reliable and valid measurement tool. *J Orthop Trauma.* 1998; 12(8):577–586.
7. Medoff RJ. Essential radiographic evaluation for distal radius fractures. *Hand Clin.* 2005;21(3):279–288.
8. Friberg S, Lundström B. Radiographic measurements of the radio-carpal joint in normal adults. *Acta Radiol Diagn.* 1976;17(2):249–256.
9. Feipel V, Rinnen D, Rooze M. Postero-anterior radiography of the wrist normal database of carpal measurements. *Surg Radiol Anat.* 1998; 20(3):221–226.
10. MacDermid JC, Donner A, Richards RS, Roth JH. Patient versus injury factors as predictors of pain and disability six months after a distal radius fracture. *J Clin Epidemiol.* 2002;55(9):849–854.
11. Grewal R, MacDermid JC, Pope J, Chesworth BM. Baseline predictors of pain and disability one year following extra-articular distal radius fractures. *Hand.* 2007;2(3):104–111.
12. Mason ML. Colles's fracture a survey of end-results. *Br J Surg.* 1953;40(162):340–346.

13. Wilcke MK, Abbaszadegan H, Adolphson PY. Patient-perceived outcome after displaced distal radius fractures: a comparison between radiological parameters, objective physical variables, and the DASH score. *J Hand Ther.* 2007;20(4):290–299.

14. Perugia D, Guzzini M, Civitenga C, et al. Is it really necessary to restore radial anatomic parameters after distal radius fractures? *Injury.* 2014;45:S21–S26.

15. Porter M, Stockley I. Fractures of the distal radius. Intermediate and end results in relation to radiologic parameters. *Clin Orthop Relat Res.* 1987;220:241–252.

16. Jenkins NH, Mintowt-Czyz WJ. Mal-union and dysfunction in Colles' fracture. *J Hand Surg.* 1988;13(3):291–293.

17. Rubinovich RM, Rennie WR. Colles' fracture: end results in relation to radiologic parameters. *Can J Surg.* 1983;26(4):361–363.

18. Altissimi M, Antenucci RE, Fiacca CL, Mancini GB. Long-term results of conservative treatment of fractures of the distal radius. *Clin Orthop Relat Res.* 1986;206:202–210.

19. Karnezis IA, Panagiotopoulos E, Tyllianakis M, Megas P, Lambiris E. Correlation between radiological parameters and patient-rated wrist dysfunction following fractures of the distal radius. *Injury.* 2005;36(12):1435–1439.

20. Kumar S, Penematsa S, Sadri M, Deshmukh SC. Can radiological results be surrogate markers of functional outcome in distal radial extra-articular fractures? *Int Orthop.* 2008;32(4):505–509.

21. Short WH, Palmer AK, Werner FW, Murphy DJ. A biomechanical study of distal radial fractures. *J Hand Surg Am.* 1987;12(4):529–534.

22. Hollevoet N, Verdonk R. The functional importance of malunion in distal radius fractures. *Acta Orthop Belg.* 2003;69(3):239–245.

23. Geissler WB, Fernandez DL, Lamey DM. Distal radioulnar joint injuries associated with fractures of the distal radius. *Clin Orthop Relat Res.* 1996;327:135–146.

24. Fujii K, Henmi T, Kanematsu Y, Mishiro T, Sakai T, Terai T. Fractures of the distal end of radius in elderly patients: a comparative study of anatomical and functional results. *J Orthop Surg.* 2002;10(1):9–15.

25. Aro HT, Koivunen T. Minor axial shortening of the radius affects outcome of Colles' fracture treatment. *J Hand Surg Am.* 1991;16(3):392–398.

26. Barton T, Chambers C, Bannister G. A comparison between subjective outcome score and moderate radial shortening following a fractured distal radius in patients of mean age 69 years. *J Hand Surg Eur Vol.* 2007;32(2):165–169.

27. Pogue DJ, Viegas SF, Patterson RM, et al. Effects of distal radius fracture malunion on wrist joint mechanics. *J Hand Surg Am.* 1990;15(5):721–727.

28. Tsukazaki T, Takagi K, Iwasaki K. Poor correlation between functional results and radiographic findings in Colles' fracture. *J Hand Surg Br Eur Vol.* 1993;18(5):588–591.

29. Batra S, Gupta A. The effect of fracture-related factors on the functional outcome at 1 year in distal radius fractures. *Injury.* 2002;33(6):499–502.

30. Anzarut A, Johnson JA, Rowe BH, Lambert RG, Blitz S, Majumdar SR. Radiologic and patient-reported functional outcomes in an elderly cohort with conservatively treated distal radius fractures. *J Hand Surg Am.* 2004;29(6):1121–1127.

31. Knirk JL, Jupiter JB. Intra-articular fractures of the distal end of the radius in young adults. *J Bone Joint Surg Am.* 1986;68(5):647–659.

32. Fernandez DL, Geissler WB. Treatment of displaced articular fractures of the radius. *J Hand Surg Am.* 1991;16(3):375–384.

33. Synn AJ, Makhni EC, Makhni MC, Rozental TD, Day CS. Distal radius fractures in older patients: is anatomic reduction necessary? *Clin Orthop Relat Res.* 2009; 467(6):1612–1620.

34. Mehta JA, Bain GI, Heptinstall RJ. Anatomical reduction of intra-articular fractures of the distal radius: an arthroscopically-assisted approach. *J Bone Joint Surg.* 2000; 82(1):79–86.

35. Forward DP, Davis TR, Sithole JS. Do young patients with malunited fractures of the distal radius inevitably develop symptomatic post-traumatic osteoarthritis? *J Bone Joint Surg.* 2008;90(5):629–637.

36. Goldfarb CA, Rudzki JR, Catalano LW, Hughes M, Borrelli Jr. J. Fifteen-year outcome of displaced intra-articular fractures of the distal radius. *J Hand Surg Am.* 2006;31(4):633–639.

37. Katz MA, Beredjiklian PK, Bozentka DJ, Steinberg DR. Computed tomography scanning of intra-articular distal radius fractures: does it influence treatment? *J Hand Surg Am.* 2001;26(3):415–421.

38. Forward D, Davis T. The teardrop angle and AP distance in fractures of the distal radius. In: *Orthopaedic Proceedings.* The British Editorial Society of Bone & Joint Surgery; 2011:6vol. 93(Suppl_I).

39. Finsen V, Rod O, Rød K, Rajabi B, Alm-Paulsen PS, Russwurm H. The relationship between displacement and clinical outcome after distal radius (Colles') fracture. *J Hand Surg Eur Vol.* 2013;38(2):116–126.

40. Bot AG, Mulders MA, Fostvedt S, Ring D. Determinants of grip strength in healthy subjects compared to that in patients recovering from a distal radius fracture. *J Hand Surg Am.* 2012;37(9):1874–1880.

41. Jayakumar P, Teunis T, Vranceanu AM, Lamb S, Ring D, Gwilym S. Early psychological and social factors explain the recovery trajectory after distal radial fracture. *J Bone Joint Surg Am.* 2020;102(9):788–795.

CHAPTER 23

Rehabilitation Protocols After Distal Radius Fracture

HYUN IL LEE[a] • JONG PIL KIM[b]

[a]Department of Orthopedic Surgery, Ilsan Paik Hospital, Inje University, Goyang, South Korea,
[b]Department of Orthopedic Surgery, Dankook University College of Medicine, Cheonan, South Korea

KEY POINTS

- Current evidences show no significant difference of clinical outcomes between patients treated with versus without additional physiotherapeutic intervention, but high-quality studies are lacking.
- Patient education and exercise (so-called home exercise program) seems sufficient after distal radius fracture (DRF) based on current evidence, suggesting that there is no need to prescribe a routine supervised physiotherapy session for all patients.
- The subgroup who would obtain significant benefit from supervised physiotherapy session has not yet been identified. Future studies should aim to identify for whom this costly intervention is needed.
- Earlier rehabilitation after surgery leads to early recovery and return to work at short-term follow-up.

Panel 1

CASE 1

A 56-year-old homemaker presented to the emergency department with a displaced extra-articular distal radius fracture (DRF). Closed reduction and immobilization with a sugar-tong splint was achieved. Reduction was subsequently maintained via 5-week cast immobilization (Fig. 1). Is exercise prescribed by a therapist required for this patient during cast immobilization or after cast removal?

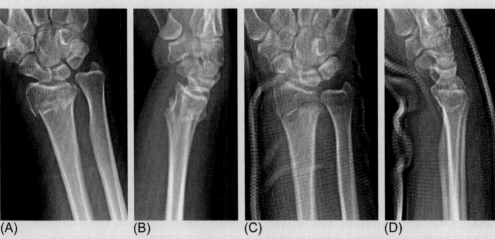

(A) (B) (C) (D)

FIG. 1 (A) Anteroposterior (AP) and (B) lateral wrist radiograph of Case 1, a 56-year-old woman with a displaced mainly extra-articular distal radius fracture. (C) AP and (D) lateral wrist radiograph after successful closed reduction and immobilization with sugar-tong splint.

Continued

Panel 1—cont'd

CASE 2

An 86-year-old woman presented to emergency department with DRF. An orthopedic resident attempted closed reduction and applied a sugar-tong splint, but loss of reduction was observed at the first outpatient visit. Thus, we decided to perform open reduction and internal fixation because of her high activity before injury, which appeared to achieve acceptable reduction and stable fixation of the fracture fragments (Fig. 2). Would there be any benefit of early start of mobilization and physiotherapy in this patient?

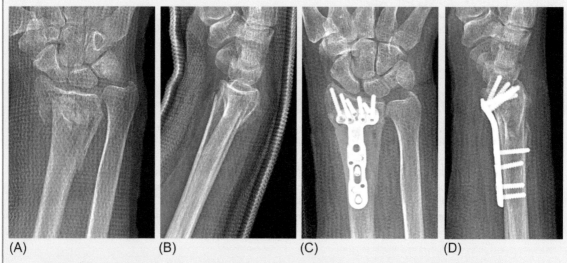

(A)   (B)   (C)   (D)

FIG. 2 (A) Anteroposterior (AP) and (B) lateral wrist radiograph of Case 2, an 86-year-old woman with a displaced distal radius fracture whose initial reduction was not maintained within a sugar-tong splint applied in the emergency department. (C) AP and (D) lateral wrist radiograph after successful operation with a volar locking plate. Reduction was satisfactory and fixation strength seemed stable.

IMPORTANCE OF THE PROBLEM

DRF is a very common injury. Nonoperative treatment with a cast remains the most popular treatment for stable fracture.[1] However, surgical treatment has been increasingly adopted as a reliable modality since the volar locking plate (VLP) was introduced as a robust implant.[2] Although many studies have focused on immobilization methods or surgical approaches, little attention has been given to rehabilitation protocols during or after those definitive treatments. However, achieving successful outcomes requires both sound definitive treatment and timely appropriate rehabilitation. Rehabilitation prevents fracture-related complications and optimizes functional recovery to maintain activities of daily living. Despite rehabilitation being critical to the final prognosis of DRF, sufficient evidence of its application and efficacy is lacking. This issue will become increasingly important because of the predicted increase in the number of affected patients and demand for cost-effective healthcare.

MAIN QUESTION

What is the effect of rehabilitation protocols (home exercise program [HEP] versus supervised physiotherapy session [SPS]) on functional outcome after DRF, and when should they be initiated?

Current Opinion

HEP and SPS are the two most frequently prescribed forms of rehabilitation. HEP consists of basic education and advice including fracture protection, cast care, and edema control as well as instructions to engage in progressive exercise at home. This is the simplest and most cost-effective form of rehabilitation after DRF. This measure is the minimal intervention usually provided to patients during or after immobilization, and many randomized controlled trials (RCTs) adopted HEP to the control group. In contrast, SPS consists of exercises performed in specific places, such as a hospital under the supervision of a physiotherapist or other medical personnel, for a certain period. Although it is assumed that patients who receive early structured physiotherapy achieve a faster recovery, it is unclear whether SPS is truly beneficial over natural recovery or HEP.

Finding the Evidence

- Cochrane search: "distal radius fracture"
- Pubmed (Medline): ("radius fractures" [Mesh] OR distal radius fracture*[tiab]) AND ("rehabilitation" OR "exercise" OR "physiotherapy" OR "occupational therapy" OR "mobilization" OR "training" OR "edema" OR "glove" OR "PEMF" OR "mirror")
- Manual review of eligible articles (especially systematic reviews and metaanalyses)
- Articles (at least abstracts) not published in English, French, or German were excluded.

Quality of Evidence

Level I:
Systematic reviews/metaanalyses: 5
Randomized trials: 28
Level II:
Randomized trials with methodological limitations: 1
Level III or IV: 2

FINDINGS

After a certain immobilization period, limited range of motion (ROM), weak grip strength, pain, and swelling or edema are typical indications for rehabilitation. Extensive rehabilitation intervention is frequently required to reduce pain, restore ROM, and improve muscle strength and function. According to Waljee et al.,[3] 20.6% of patients received either physical or occupational therapy (OT) after DRF. Patients who underwent open reduction and internal fixation (ORIF) were more likely to receive formal physiotherapy than patients who received nonoperative treatment. Furthermore, patients who undergo ORIF were referred to a physiotherapist sooner than those who receive other management are. Bruder et al.,[4] who performed an observational study of 14 physiotherapists, reported that most common interventions prescribed by surgeons were exercise (97%), advice (90%), passive joint mobilization (55%), and massage (38%).

Role of HEP

HEP can be the minimum requirement for effective rehabilitation; however, there is a paucity of evidence of its true effectiveness. Just one RCT by Kay et al.[5] compared an HEP group with a group received no instruction or intervention after cast or pin fixation. No significant intergroup difference was found regarding wrist ROM at 6 weeks. However, in terms of a decrease in pain visual analog scale score and increase in functional activity (Patient Rated Wrist Evaluation [PRWE] score), the HEP group showed superior outcomes at 3 and 6 weeks. In addition, patient satisfaction was higher in the HEP group. The authors concluded that HEP with advice provides some benefit over natural recovery without formal intervention.

Role of SPS

The need for additional SPS has been under debate for DRF rehabilitation. In at least three RCTs, SPS showed more favorable outcomes than HEP. Watt et al.[6] compared the effect of SPS and HEP after cast removal in 18 patients, and those treated with SPS showed significant increases in wrist extension and grip strength at 6 weeks. Accordingly, a recent study by Gutiérrez-Espinoza et al.[7] demonstrated that SPS was more effective than HEP in patients older than 60 years; in fact, the SPS group showed better results in terms of PRWE score at 6 weeks and 6 months. Gronlund et al.[8] studied the effect of early OT in 40 patients treated with a cast for stable Colle's fracture. A better functional score according to Gartland classification was found in OT group at 5 weeks but not at 9 weeks or 3 months. In terms of wrist ROM and complication rate, the two groups were similar at 3 months. Based on these findings, they concluded that early OT during immobilization has a favorable short-term effect on the recovery of hand function.

However, a larger number of studies including nine RCTs do not support those favorable effects of SPS.[9-19] Pasila et al.[16] investigated the effect of early SPS started during cast immobilization in 96 patients. At 3 months' follow-up, there were no significant differences in hand strength or ROM between the SPS and HEP groups. These findings were repeated in several RCTs comparing the effects of HEP and SPS in patients given nonoperative treatment (Table 1). The same conclusion was drawn from studies including RCTs of patients treated with a VLP (Table 1). Fig. 3 shows representative forest plots that demonstrate no difference in PRWE scores between the SPS and HEP groups at 6 weeks and 6 months. However, the data in each study are not reliable because of extreme study heterogeneity such as wide variations in interventions, timing, and measurement tools.

Systematic Reviews: HEP vs SPS

Five systematic reviews on this issue were retrieved in our literature search. Among them, two focused on DRF, while the other three included other upper limb conditions. Valdes et al.[20] published a systematic review

TABLE 1
Summary of Randomized Controlled Trials Comparing SPS and HEP After Nonoperative or Operative Treatment.

Author	Year	Number of Patients	Treatment Method	Time of Evaluation	Outcome Measured
Studies showing superior effect of SPS over HEP					
Watt	2010	18	Cast	6 weeks	Extension, grip strength
Gutiérrez-Espinoza	2017	74	Cast	6 weeks and 6 months	ROM, grip strength, pain, PRWE
Gronlund	1990	40	Cast	5 weeks, 9 weeks, and 5 months	Modified functional score
Studies showing similar effects of SPS and HEP					
Kay	2000	40	Cast or pin	6 weeks	ROM, grip strength, pain
Wakefield	2000	66	Cast	3 months and 6 months	ROM, grip strength, pain
Christensen	2001	30	Cast	5 weeks, 3 months, and 9 months	ROM, grip strength, pain, DASH
Maciel	2005	41	Cast	6 weeks and 6 months	ROM, grip strength, pain, PRWE
Bruder	2016	33	Cast	7 weeks and 6 months	PRWE, DASH
Valdes	2015	50	VLP	3 months	ROM, grip strength, pain, PRWE
Studies showing superior effect of HEP over SPS					
Krischak	2009	48	VLP	6 weeks	ROM, grip strength, PRWE
Souer	2011	94	VLP	3 months and 6 months	ROM, grip strength, pain, Mayo wrist score, DASH

DASH, disabilities of the arm, shoulder, and hand; *HEP*, home exercise program; *PRWE*, patient-rated wrist evaluation; *ROM*, range of motion; *SPS*, supervised physiotherapy session; *VLP*, volar locking plate.

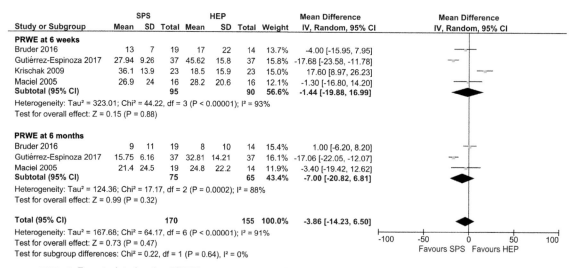

FIG. 3 Forest plot showing PRWE score measure at 6 weeks and 6 months. Mean difference (95% CI) of effect of SPS compared HEP after distal radius fracture. *HEP*, home exercise program; *PRWE*, patient-rated wrist evaluation; *SPS*, structured physiotherapy session.

of SPS versus HEP for patients with DRF in 2014 and observed that five of the seven RCTs found no intergroup differences in outcomes, especially when analyzing the patients who had no complications such as median nerve symptoms or chronic regional pain syndrome. However, they concluded that there was insufficient evidence to prove which method is superior as reliable physiotherapy. Handoll et al.[21] published a Cochrane systematic review about DRF rehabilitation in adults. In brief, they reviewed a total of 26 trials including 1269 patients who were mainly older women treated with SPS or HEP and reported no intergroup differences in clinical outcomes. However, the majority of the trials had methodological shortcomings (lack of blinding) and a high risk of bias. Despite poor-quality evidence, previous studies reported that early exercise consisting of either SPS or HEP have equal benefits for the early recovery of hand function.

Three other systematic reviews evaluated the role of physiotherapy in upper limb conditions including fracture. Bruder et al. conducted two consecutive systematic reviews of the effect of exercise on upper limb fractures including DRF.[22, 23] They concluded that current exercise regimens are ineffective at reducing impairment following upper limb fracture. They suggested that "early exercise combined with a shorter immobilization duration may be effective strategy." Otherwise, Roll and Hardison[24] systematically analyzed the role of OT for the treatment of hand, wrist, and forearm conditions and reported that it was difficult to identify the clinical effect of any one of specific intervention because of wide heterogeneity among the studies. Nevertheless, they suggested that there was no evidence to support the long-term effects of any OT versus no intervention on functional outcomes except for short-term effects on pain decrease.

Overall, the review of previous studies suggested that there was preliminary evidence that the addition of SPS to HEP provides no extra benefit on functional outcomes. Based on these studies, HEP is considered a sufficient rehabilitation protocol after DRF, which indicates that routine referral to SPS is not recommended. The important factors for early functional recovery and pain decreases might be mobilization period duration and early instruction to exercise rather than SPS. The role of SPS in patients at high risk of poor outcomes (e.g., malunion, poor preinjury function, comorbidities, older age) should be investigated in future.[19]

Otherwise, Chung KC et al.[11] reported an interesting case series study (level IV) in which patients who did not receive physiotherapy recovered more powerful grip strength and those who engaged in physiotherapy for a shorter time showed greater functional recovery and

satisfaction. The authors suggested that physiotherapy may not be required in older patients with DRF and that simply encouraging participants to resume their daily activities as soon as possible may be sufficient.

Timing of Rehabilitation After Surgery
Early mobilization could be adopted in patients with VLP because it provides immediate stability to the fracture construct. The optimum immobilization period following ORIF is closely related with the timing of the start of exercise, but it has not been established precisely. In one retrospective study with level 4 evidence, the mean number of days to visiting a therapist was 7 in the ORIF group that started ROM exercise early and 17 days in the cast immobilization group that started ROM exercise late, which may indicate a benefit of an early start of ROM exercise.[25]

Several RCTs mainly compared early start timing of exercise (0–3 weeks after surgery) with late starting (beyond 5–6 weeks after surgery) after VLP fixation. The results of these studies showed consistent short-term benefits, but the long-term benefits were unclear. Watson et al.,[26] who investigated the effect of immobilization period after internal fixation using VLP, reported that immobilization periods of 3 weeks or less showed superior short-term outcomes (2 months after surgery) than those of 6 weeks or longer in terms of functional ROM recovery and pain decrease. There were no significant adverse events in shorter versus longer periods of immobilization. However, the differences were not significant at 3 or 6 months of follow-up. Similar findings were reported in two more RCTs (Fig. 4).[27, 28] Lozano-Calderon et al.,[28] who compared the initiation time of wrist stretches at 2 weeks and those at 6 weeks after VLP placement in 60 patients, found no differences in pain, functional score, or ROM at 3 or 6 months of follow-up. Brehmer et al.[27] investigated the starting timing of rehabilitation after VLP placement in 81 patients and reported that patients in the accelerated group who started rehabilitation at 2 weeks had better mobility, strength, and DASH scores at 2 months than those in the standard rehabilitation group who started rehabilitation at 6 weeks. Quadlbauer et al.,[29] who compared immediate mobilization with 5 weeks of immobilization after VLP, demonstrated even longer persistence of the favorable effect of immediate mobilization. Early mobilization leads to better ROM and grip strength up to 6 months after surgery and better Quick-DASH score and PRWE scores up to 6 weeks, with no difference in loss of reduction. In another study, Duprat et al.[30] compared splinting for 2 weeks versus immediate mobilization after VLP fixation. At 3 months, the

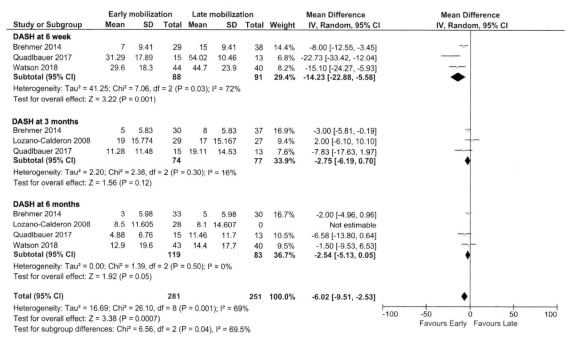

Study or Subgroup	Early mobilization			Late mobilization			Weight	Mean Difference IV, Random, 95% CI
	Mean	SD	Total	Mean	SD	Total		
DASH at 6 week								
Brehmer 2014	7	9.41	29	15	9.41	38	14.4%	-8.00 [-12.55, -3.45]
Quadlbauer 2017	31.29	17.89	15	54.02	10.46	13	6.8%	-22.73 [-33.42, -12.04]
Watson 2018	29.6	18.3	44	44.7	23.9	40	8.2%	-15.10 [-24.27, -5.93]
Subtotal (95% CI)			88			91	29.4%	-14.23 [-22.88, -5.58]
Heterogeneity: Tau² = 41.25; Chi² = 7.06, df = 2 (P = 0.03); I² = 72%								
Test for overall effect: Z = 3.22 (P = 0.001)								
DASH at 3 months								
Brehmer 2014	5	5.83	30	8	5.83	37	16.9%	-3.00 [-5.81, -0.19]
Lozano-Calderon 2008	19	15.774	29	17	15.167	27	9.4%	2.00 [-6.10, 10.10]
Quadlbauer 2017	11.28	11.48	15	19.11	14.53	13	7.6%	-7.83 [-17.63, 1.97]
Subtotal (95% CI)			74			77	33.9%	-2.75 [-6.19, 0.70]
Heterogeneity: Tau² = 2.20; Chi² = 2.38, df = 2 (P = 0.30); I² = 16%								
Test for overall effect: Z = 1.56 (P = 0.12)								
DASH at 6 months								
Brehmer 2014	3	5.98	33	5	5.98	30	16.7%	-2.00 [-4.96, 0.96]
Lozano-Calderon 2008	8.5	11.605	28	8.1	14.607	0		Not estimable
Quadlbauer 2017	4.88	6.76	15	11.46	11.7	13	10.5%	-6.58 [-13.80, 0.64]
Watson 2018	12.9	19.6	43	14.4	17.7	40	9.5%	-1.50 [-9.53, 6.53]
Subtotal (95% CI)			119			83	36.7%	-2.54 [-5.13, 0.05]
Heterogeneity: Tau² = 0.00; Chi² = 1.39, df = 2 (P = 0.50); I² = 0%								
Test for overall effect: Z = 1.92 (P = 0.05)								
Total (95% CI)			281			251	100.0%	-6.02 [-9.51, -2.53]
Heterogeneity: Tau² = 16.69; Chi² = 26.10, df = 8 (P = 0.001); I² = 69%								
Test for overall effect: Z = 3.38 (P = 0.0007)								
Test for subgroup differences: Chi² = 6.56, df = 2 (P = 0.04), I² = 69.5%								

FIG. 4 Forest plot showing DASH score measure at 6 weeks, 3 months, and 6 months. Mean difference (95% CI) of the effect of early and accelerated mobilization compared delayed mobilization up to 5–6 weeks after VLP fixation of a distal radius fracture. *DASH*, disabilities of the arm, shoulder, and hand; *VLP*, volar locking plate.

averages of all variables including ROM, pain visual analog scale score, QuickDASH, PRWE, and grip strength were better in the early mobilization group. These two studies[29, 30] indicated that even immediate mobilization is safe and effective in the treatment of DRF. However, immediate mobilization could cause additional pain without any benefit compared to 2 weeks of immobilization.[31]

Other Rehabilitation Programs With Some Beneficial Evidence

The following rehabilitation protocols are not frequently used but have shown some evidence of a positive effect:

1. **Hand strength-focused exercise**
   Nguyen et al.[32] studied whether an exercise program that focused to hand strength improves grip strength in older patients who were treated nonoperatively. The intervention group that received a home hand strength focused exercise program at 2–6 weeks after surgery showed a significant improvement in grip strength at 6 weeks and 3 months of follow-up.

2. **Contralateral strengthening exercise**
   There was preliminary evidence of improvement in hand strength and ROM of the injured wrist via strength training of the unaffected contralateral side during splint or cast immobilization of the affected side. Magnus et al.[33] evaluated the effect of "cross-education (strengthening exercise of the opposite hand)" intervention in an RCT of 51 patients. The patients who received cross-education achieved a restored grip strength and ROM of the injured side at 12 weeks, whereas patients who did not receive the education did not.

3. **Blood flow restriction therapy**
   In an RCT of 13 patients, Cancio et al.[32] demonstrated that blood flow restriction (BFR) therapy enables patients to increase their hand strength. The BFR group also showed significantly greater effect on pain reduction after 8 weeks of therapy than controls. Although the addition of BFR therapy is safe and well tolerated by patients, this is a new strategy based on a pilot study with limited evidence.

4. **Shoulder exercise**
   Shoulder problems are commonly associated with immobilization duration or methods such as long arm, short arm cast, or cast weight and may affect overall upper extremity function.[34] An RCT of 40 patients investigated whether postoperative rehabilitation extended to the shoulder girdle showed

favorable effects in patients with ORIF.[35] The study demonstrated that rehabilitation extending to the shoulder showed a greater and faster improvement in the physical function of the injured hand, which supports the importance of shoulder rehabilitation protocol.

5. **Compression glove**

Although the role of passive treatments including compression glove or wrapping remains debatable, its main effect is reducing edema of the affected side. Two RCTs[36, 37] also demonstrated a quicker reduction of swelling and faster restoration of ROM as well as a quicker restoration of function (according to DASH or PRWE scores) and decrease pain in patients who wore the fitted compression device.

6. **Mirror therapy**

Motor-cognitive approaches are new strategies using neuroscience or behavioral approaches. Although this approach is less familiar for orthopedic surgeons, it was first started with severe and disproportionate pain such as chronic regional pain syndrome,[38] and its use has now been extended to the treatment of simple fracture. Mirror therapy is a simple rehabilitation technique in which a mirror is positioned between the unaffected and affected limbs.[39] This blocks the patient's view of the affected limb, and when the patient performs exercises using both limbs, the reflection of the unaffected limb movement in the mirror creates some visual illusion of enhanced movement in the affected limb. An RCT of 36 patients reported that the graded motor imagery, a subset of mirror therapy appeared to provide beneficial effects to reduce pain, improved ROM, and thus increased function in patients with ORIF.[40] However, the results have not been promising until now.[41]

RECOMMENDATION

For the rehabilitation of patients with DRF, whether they were treated nonoperatively with a cast or operatively, the evidence suggests the following:

Recommendation	Overall Quality
• Advice and instruction for HEP is sufficient and SPS is not routinely required	⊕⊕⊕⊕ HIGH

Recommendation	Overall Quality
• Hand strength-focused exercise, contralateral strengthening, or compressive glove use can provide additional benefits, but concrete evidence is lacking	⊕⊕◯◯ LOW

Concerning patients at high risk of a poor outcome, the evidence suggests the following:

Recommendation	Overall Quality
• Older patients, those with co-morbidities, and those with early stiffness might benefit from SPS, but evidence is lacking	⊕⊕◯◯ LOW

For patients who underwent surgery (especially ORIF with VLP), the evidence suggests the following:

Recommendation	Overall Quality
• Shorter immobilization and accelerated rehabilitation will hasten recovery and return to work and provide better short-term functional outcomes, but this effect will not persist in the long term. The group with longer immobilization and delayed rehabilitation showed similar results to those with shorter immobilization and accelerated rehabilitation	⊕⊕⊕◯ MODERATE

CONCLUSION

Available evidence from RCTs remains insufficient to establish the relative effectiveness of the various interventions used in the rehabilitation of adults with DRF. Based on multiple RCTs, advice and general instructions for a HEP should be provided to all patients with DRF, while SPS may not effectively decrease impairment or increase functional activity and can be reserved to selected patients. Commencing an accelerated rehabilitation program following short immobilization for patients treated surgically may be beneficial at short-term follow-up, but it remains uncertain whether the benefit is because of the shorter duration of immobilization or the early vigorous exercise. However, few studies have shown significant differences in long-term outcomes.

Panel 2: Author's Preferred Technique

With or without surgery, the following is recommended for all patients to alleviate swelling and secondary stiffness:

(1) Elevation of the injured arm for the first few days.

(2) ROM exercise for nonimmobilized joints including the finger, elbow, and shoulder. The easiest finger exercise for patients to perform might be a composite fist with self-assist using the un-injured hand.

(3) Compression glove or handgrip strengthening and contralateral strengthening exercises can be used, but the demonstrated functional gain was not consistent because of the small number of trials. At a minimum, edema control will be effective with a compression glove and hand grip exercise.

CASE 1

For patients treated with cast immobilization, HEP for the wrist can be started after cast removal. Currently, a single instruction session regarding the HEP provided by a physiotherapist or orthopedic surgeon is the minimum requirement for patients. It seems reasonable that only patients

who have significant stiffness and those who cannot execute their self-training program for any reason would benefit from SPS. Routine referral to a structured physiotherapy session is not recommended if a low cost-benefit ratio is predicted.

CASE 2

For patients treated surgically, particularly ORIF with a VLP, we usually advise an early start of ROM exercises for all joints including the wrist if the fracture is sufficiently stable. This helps reduce the likelihood of a recurring pain cycle and swelling that may thicken into scar tissue around the joints. However, if joint instability because of a concomitant ligament injury were suspected, a late start to rehabilitation would be better. We can expect the same long-term outcome even with delayed exercise starting 6 weeks after surgery. In case 2, we delayed the exercise until 1 month after surgery and offered HEP only because of the patient's older age and severe osteoporosis. Active self-assisted exercises will be the mainstay for recovery in most patients.

Panel 3: Pearls and Pitfalls

PEARLS

• The incidence of physiotherapy-related complications is very low.

• Whether cast immobilization or surgery is performed, advice and instruction about fracture or HEP is the minimum requirement for rehabilitation of DRF. Stretching exercises for the wrist as well as the fingers, elbow, and shoulder—usually performed by the patients themselves—are an important part of recovery.

• Rehabilitation could start as soon as possible after surgery, especially after VLP fixation, to aid in early restoration of function and a faster return to previous activity.

PITFALLS

• Because of the significant heterogeneity across the reviewed studies, it is not possible to elucidate the effects of the variations such as dosage, provider experience, patient demographics, fracture severity, and

specific characteristics of individual interventions (e.g., exercise type).

• Consensus has not yet been established regarding whether HEP or SPS is most effective.

• HEP education has not yet been established, and it is unclear which delivery method is superior. Currently, educational booklets or flyers are commonly provided, but in the future, videos delivered via YouTube may be commonly used.

• SPS will place a transportation burden on patients and are costly on patients and the government or insurance companies.

• Not all patients receive physical therapy as instructed. Sex, distance from therapy, and driving status are factors that are significantly related to adherence.[42] Because home exercise adherence was an important predictor of short-term outcomes, it is important to monitor each patient's adherence to rehabilitation.[43]

REFERENCES

1. Chung KC, Shauver MJ, Birkmeyer JD. Trends in the United States in the treatment of distal radial fractures in the elderly. *J Bone Joint Surg Am.* 2009;91(8):1868–1873.

2. Orbay JL, Fernandez DL. Volar fixed-angle plate fixation for unstable distal radius fractures in the elderly patient. *J Hand Surg Am.* 2004;29(1):96–102.

3. Waljee JF, Zhong L, Shauver M, Chung KC. Variation in the use of therapy following distal radius fractures in the United States. *Plast Reconstr Surg Glob Open.* 2014;2(4):e130.

4. Bruder AM, Taylor NF, Dodd KJ, Shields N. Physiotherapy intervention practice patterns used in rehabilitation after distal radial fracture. *Physiotherapy.* 2013;99(3):233–240.

5. Kay S, McMahon M, Stiller K. An advice and exercise program has some benefits over natural recovery after distal radius fracture: a randomised trial. *Aust J Physiother.* 2008;54(4):253–259.

6. Watt CF, Taylor NF, Baskus K. Do Colles' fracture patients benefit from routine referral to physiotherapy following cast removal? *Arch Orthop Trauma Surg.* 2000;120(7–8): 413–415.

7. Gutierrez-Espinoza H, Rubio-Oyarzun D, Olguin-Huerta C, Gutierrez-Monclus R, Pinto-Concha S, Gana-Hervias G. Supervised physical therapy vs. home exercise program for patients with distal radius fracture: a single-blind randomized clinical study. *J Hand Ther.* 2017;30(3): 242–252.

8. Gronlund B, Harreby MS, Kofoed R, Rasmussen L. The importance of early exercise therapy in the treatment of Colles' fracture. A clinically controlled study. *Ugeskr Laeger.* 1990;152(35):2491–2493.

9. Bruder AM, Shields N, Dodd KJ, Hau R, Taylor NF. A progressive exercise and structured advice program does not improve activity more than structured advice alone following a distal radial fracture: a multi-centre, randomised trial. *J Physiother.* 2016;62(3):145–152.

10. Christensen OM, Kunov A, Hansen FF, Christiansen TC, Krasheninnikoff M. Occupational therapy and Colles' fractures. *Int Orthop.* 2001;25(1):43–45.

11. Chung KC, Malay S, Shauver MJ, Wrist and Radius Injury Surgical Trial Group. The relationship between hand therapy and long-term outcomes after distal radius fracture in older adults: evidence from the randomized wrist and radius injury surgical trial. *Plast Reconstr Surg.* 2019;144(2):230e–237e.

12. Kay S, Haensel N, Stiller K. The effect of passive mobilisation following fractures involving the distal radius: a randomised study. *Aust J Physiother.* 2000;46(2):93–101.

13. Krischak GD, Krasteva A, Schneider F, Gulkin D, Gebhard F, Kramer M. Physiotherapy after volar plating of wrist fractures is effective using a home exercise program. *Arch Phys Med Rehabil.* 2009;90(4):537–544.

14. Maciel JS, Taylor NF, McIlveen C. A randomised clinical trial of activity-focussed physiotherapy on patients with distal radius fractures. *Arch Orthop Trauma Surg.* 2005;125(8):515–520.

15. Oskarsson GV, Hjall A, Aaser P. Physiotherapy: an overestimated factor in after-treatment of fractures in the distal radius? *Arch Orthop Trauma Surg.* 1997;116(6–7): 373–375.

16. Pasila M, Karaharju EO, Lepisto PV. Role of physical therapy in recovery of function after Colles' fracture. *Arch Phys Med Rehabil.* 1974;55(3):130–134.

17. Souer JS, Buijze G, Ring D. A prospective randomized controlled trial comparing occupational therapy with independent exercises after volar plate fixation of a fracture of the distal part of the radius. *J Bone Joint Surg Am.* 2011;93(19):1761–1766.

18. Valdes K, Naughton N, Burke CJ. Therapist-supervised hand therapy versus home therapy with therapist instruction following distal radius fracture. *J Hand Surg Am.* 2015;40(6):1110–1116. e1111.

19. Wakefield AE, McQueen MM. The role of physiotherapy and clinical predictors of outcome after fracture of the distal radius. *J Bone Joint Surg Br.* 2000;82(7):972–976.

20. Valdes K, Naughton N, Michlovitz S. Therapist supervised clinic-based therapy versus instruction in a home program following distal radius fracture: a systematic review. *J Hand Ther.* 2014;27(3):165–173 [quiz 174].

21. Handoll HH, Elliott J. Rehabilitation for distal radial fractures in adults. *Cochrane Database Syst Rev.* 2015;9, CD003324.

22. Bruder AM, Shields N, Dodd KJ, Taylor NF. Prescribed exercise programs may not be effective in reducing impairments and improving activity during upper limb fracture rehabilitation: a systematic review. *J Physiother.* 2017;63(4):205–220.

23. Bruder A, Taylor NF, Dodd KJ, Shields N. Exercise reduces impairment and improves activity in people after some upper limb fractures: a systematic review. *J Physiother.* 2011;57(2):71–82.

24. Roll SC, Hardison ME. Effectiveness of occupational therapy interventions for adults with musculoskeletal conditions of the forearm, wrist, and hand: a systematic review. *Am J Occup Ther.* 2017;71(1). 7101180010p7101180011–7101180010p7101180012.

25. Valdes K. A retrospective pilot study comparing the number of therapy visits required to regain functional wrist and forearm range of motion following volar plating of a distal radius fracture. *J Hand Ther.* 2009; 22(4):312–318 [quiz 319].

26. Watson N, Haines T, Tran P, Keating JL. A comparison of the effect of one, three, or six weeks of immobilization on function and pain after open reduction and internal fixation of distal radial fractures in adults: a randomized controlled trial. *J Bone Joint Surg Am.* 2018;100(13):1118–1125.

27. Brehmer JL, Husband JB. Accelerated rehabilitation compared with a standard protocol after distal radial fractures treated with volar open reduction and internal fixation: a prospective, randomized, controlled study. *J Bone Joint Surg Am.* 2014;96(19):1621–1630.

28. Lozano-Calderon SA, Souer S, Mudgal C, Jupiter JB, Ring D. Wrist mobilization following volar plate fixation of fractures of the distal part of the radius. *J Bone Joint Surg Am.* 2008;90(6):1297–1304.

29. Quadlbauer S, Pezzei C, Jurkowitsch J, et al. Early rehabilitation of distal radius fractures stabilized by volar locking plate: a prospective randomized pilot study. *J Wrist Surg.* 2017;6(2):102–112.

30. Duprat A, Diaz JJH, Vernet P, et al. Volar locking plate fixation of distal radius fractures: splint versus immediate mobilization. *J Wrist Surg.* 2018;7(3):237–242.

31. Andrade-Silva FB, Rocha JP, Carvalho A, Kojima KE, Silva JS. Influence of postoperative immobilization on pain control of patients with distal radius fracture treated with volar locked plating: a prospective, randomized clinical trial. *Injury.* 2019;50(2):386–391.

32. Nguyen A, Vather M, Bal G, et al. Does a hand strength focused exercise program improve grip strength in older patients with wrist fractures managed non-operatively? A randomized controlled trial. *Am J Phys Med Rehabil.* 2019.

33. Magnus CR, Arnold CM, Johnston G, et al. Cross-education for improving strength and mobility after distal radius fractures: a randomized controlled trial. *Arch Phys Med Rehabil.* 2013;94(7):1247–1255.

34. Cantero-Tellez R, Orza SG, Bishop MD, Berjano P, Villafane JH. Duration of wrist immobilization is associated with shoulder pain in patients with after wrist immobilization: an observational study. *J Exerc Rehabil.* 2018;14(4):694–698.

35. Jancikova V, Opavsky J, Drac P, Krobot A, Cizmar I. The effect of activation of the shoulder girdle muscles on functional outcomes of rehabilitation in patients with surgically treated distal radius fractures. *Acta Chir Orthop Traumatol Cech.* 2017;84(2):114–119.

36. Schmidt J, Tessmann UJ, Schmidt I. Compression glove has advantages in the functional aftercare of distal radius fractures. *Z Orthop Unfall.* 2013;151(1):80–84.

37. Miller-Shahabar I, Schreuer N, Katsevman H, et al. Efficacy of compression gloves in the rehabilitation of distal radius fractures: randomized controlled study. *Am J Phys Med Rehabil.* 2018;97(12):904–910.

38. Cacchio A, De Blasis E, Necozione S, di Orio F, Santilli V. Mirror therapy for chronic complex regional pain syndrome type 1 and stroke. *N Engl J Med.* 2009;361(6):634–636.

39. Altschuler EL, Wisdom SB, Stone L, et al. Rehabilitation of hemiparesis after stroke with a mirror. *Lancet.* 1999;353(9169):2035–2036.

40. Dilek B, Ayhan C, Yagci G, Yakut Y. Effectiveness of the graded motor imagery to improve hand function in patients with distal radius fracture: a randomized controlled trial. *J Hand Ther.* 2018;31(1):2–9. e1.

41. Bayon-Calatayud M, Benavente-Valdepenas AM, Del Prado Vazquez-Munoz M. Mirror therapy for distal radial fractures: a pilot randomized controlled study. *J Rehabil Med.* 2016;48(9):829–832.

42. Hickey S, Rodgers J, Wollstein R. Barriers to adherence with post-operative hand therapy following surgery for fracture of the distal radius. *J Hand Microsurg.* 2015;7(1):55–60.

43. Lyngcoln A, Taylor N, Pizzari T, Baskus K. The relationship between adherence to hand therapy and short-term outcome after distal radius fracture. *J Hand Ther.* 2005;18(1):2–8 [quiz 9].

CHAPTER 24

Complex Regional Pain Syndrome in Distal Radius Fractures

ASSAF KADAR[a,b] • NINA SUH[a,b]

[a]Roth|McFarlane Hand and Upper Limb Centre, St. Joseph's Health Care London, London, ON, Canada,
[b]Department of Surgery, Division of Orthopaedic Surgery, Schulich School of Medicine & Dentistry, Western University, London, ON, Canada

KEY POINTS

- Diagnosis of complex regional pain syndrome (CRPS) is challenging and remains a hot topic of debate as despite decades of research, the etiology remains entirely unclear.
- Recent randomized controlled trials have questioned the role of vitamin C as a prophylactic treatment of CRPS in patients with distal radius fractures (DRFs).
- The risk of CRPS following DRFs is independent of the fixation technique. However, tight casts and over distraction of the wrist joint using a spanning external fixator should be avoided.
- Early detection and identification of a peripheral nerve compression that can be approached surgically is crucial to avoiding possible negative consequences such as drug dependency and long-term disability.
- Physiotherapy with behavioral therapy components may be effective in ameliorating symptoms of CRPS and help the patient build coping mechanisms to regain functionality.

Panel 1: Case Scenario

A 67-year-old women with a history of fibromyalgia fell on her right wrist and suffered a DRF. The fracture was reduced to an acceptable position and treatment consisted of short arm casting. She presents to clinic 2 weeks after the fracture with disproportionate pain and finger stiffness. Swelling appears within normal limits and she is not showing signs of acute carpal tunnel syndrome or compartment syndrome. What are the best methods to prevent, diagnose, and eventually treat CRPS type 1 in this patient?

IMPORTANCE OF THE PROBLEM

Complex regional pain syndrome (CRPS) type I is defined as chronic pain without an identifiable nerve injury[1] and is one of the principal causes of long-term disability following distal radius fractures.[2] Pain is accompanied by trophic changes, impaired function, and finger stiffness as well as autonomic dysfunction (Fig. 1). Patients with fibromyalgia,[3] women,[4] and smokers[5] have a higher likelihood of developing this condition. Incidence of DRFs complicated by CRPS varies and is reported to affect 1%–37% of patients[6]; however, the etiology of this complication is not well understood. It has been correlated to tight casts and over distraction of the wrist joint with spanning external fixators (Fig. 2), but these scenarios only account for a small fraction of the known clinical scenarios. Surgical decompression, particularly of the median nerve, has been shown to be effective in modulating the sequelae of CRPS associated with a DRF.[7, 8]

Diagnosis of CRPS is challenging as it is based on clinical criteria[9] (Box 1) with mainly subjective components. Several diagnosis algorithms have been published over the years and currently, the most validated and internationally accepted is the Budapest Criteria

Distal Radius Fractures. https://doi.org/10.1016/B978-0-323-75764-5.00029-9

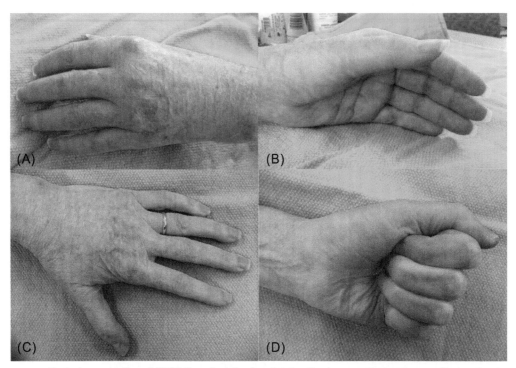

FIG. 1 Typical presentation of CRPS 8 weeks following distal radius fracture. Patient has swelling and peri-articular and palmar fibrosis with flexed posture as well as disproportional pain to light touch (A,B). Patient regained functional use of the hand following 4 months of intensive physical therapy (twice weekly sessions for greater than 90 min per session for 3 months then weekly until discharged) that also included use of edema gloves, continuous passive motion device, contrast bath for desensitization, and use of topical cream for pain relief (C,D). (Courtesy of Shrikant J. Chinchalkar, OTR, CHT.)

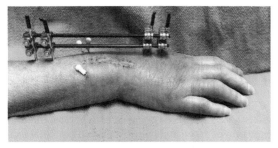

FIG. 2 External fixator for distal radius fracture without features of CRPS. (Courtesy of William Aibinder MD.)

(Box 1).[9] Radiographs may show disuse osteoporosis and peri-articular demineralization.[8] Bone scan may show increased uptake, especially in phase 3 of the scan, but has low sensitivity.[10] In general, imaging studies should be interpreted in light of the clinical findings and are usually not essential to diagnose CRPS. Early diagnosis is possible even 2 weeks after the injury and is associated with recovery in 80%–90% of cases.[6] Late diagnosis of CRPS and inappropriate treatment can lead to chronic CRPS with residual pain and long-term disability up to 10 years after the injury[2] with significant sociomedical and welfare consequences.[11] Conversely, some prominent hand surgeons claim that CRPS does not exist and the symptoms can be explained by another pathology that was overlooked such as subclinical nerve compression, undetected nonunion, or fracture malreduction.[12, 13] Certainly, imaging and other advanced studies should be performed to rule out any pathology that may cause disproportional pain that may have been overlooked.

The purpose of treatment of CRPS in DRFs is to restore the affected upper extremity within the acceptable mobility and durability requirements.[14] There are many treatment modalities to treat CRPS, most with poor supporting evidence. Treatments such as bisphosphonates, *N*-acetylcysteine, glucocorticoids, calcitonin, pregabalin, gabapentin, antidepressant, antiepileptic

---

BOX 1
Budapest Criteria for CRPS.[9]

1. Continuing pain, which is disproportionate to any inciting event
2. At least one symptom in three of the four following categories:
   - Sensory: hyperesthesia/allodynia
   - Vasomotor: temperature/color change or asymmetry
   - Sudomotor/edema: edema/sweating change or asymmetry
   - Motor/trophic: decreased range of motion, motor dysfunction, or trophic changes

3. At least one sign in two or more of the following categories:
   - Sensory: hyperalgesia (to pinprick) and/or allodynia (to light touch)
   - Vasomotor: temperature/color asymmetry
   - Sudomotor: edema/sweating change or asymmetry
   - Motor/Trophic: decreased range of motion, motor dysfunction and/or trophic changes
4. There is no other diagnosis that better explains the signs and symptoms

---

drugs, clonidine, epidural infusion systems, and neurostimulation have all been reported yet limited studies exist.[6] However, there has been extensive research regarding the role of vitamin C in the treatment of CRPS in patients with DRFs as well as literature regarding the role of physical therapy and cognitive behavioral therapy.[15] These latter treatment modalities will be the focus of this chapter.

MAIN QUESTION

How can CRPS type-1 be effectively prevented, diagnosed, and/or treated in patients with DRF?

CURRENT OPINION

The diagnosis of CRPS remains challenged and debated because of its lacking objectifiable character and etiologic understanding. Several treatment modalities have been offered over the years to treat CRPS following DRF, most with poor supporting evidence. There is an ongoing debate, accompanied by high quality evidence, about the role of Vitamin C in the prevention of CRPS. Other areas of controversy relate to the role of physical therapy with behavioral components in the treatment of CRPS and if there is an association between the distal radius fixation method to the occurrence of CRPS. Additionally, in recent years, a paradigm shift among surgeons has developed to find the culprit of the pain and offer surgical treatment. This paradigm shift is currently supported mainly by expert opinion and case series.

FINDING THE EVIDENCE

The search was conducted in MEDLINE via PubMed and the Cochrane library. The search terms were broad and included the intervention ("vitamin C,"

"physiotherapy," "physical therapy," "psychotherapy," "cognitive behavioral therapy," "nerve block," "cast," "external fixation," "open reduction internal fixation"), population ("wrist fracture," "distal radius fracture"), and disease of interest ["complex regional pain syndrome (or CRPS)," "reflex sympathetic dystrophy (or RSD)," "Sudeck's atrophy"]. Additionally, we searched for review articles of CRPS in DRF using the general terms "distal radius fracture" and "CRPS." No time limits were set. The reference list of the review articles and metanalyses retrieved were additionally reviewed to identify other papers not included in our other broader search.

QUALITY OF EVIDENCE

We attempted to limit our examination to level I or II prospective randomized trials and metanalyses. However, to better define the role of surgery in the treatment of CRPS, we included several case series.

Level I—4 randomized controlled trials, 5 systematic review and metanalysis.

Level II—3 randomized controlled trials with methodological limitations.

Level III—5 case series.

FINDINGS

Prevention of CRPS in Patients With DRFs With Prophylactic Vitamin C Treatment

Vitamin C, a free radical scavenger, was proposed as a treatment to address the prevailing theory that CRPS was caused by free oxygen radicals released at the time of injury. Zollinger et al. performed two level I randomized controlled trials touting the beneficial effects of vitamin C in the prevention of CRPS[16, 17] and in fact, their studies contributed to the 2009 AAOS recommendation supporting its routine use in DRFs.[18]

In their first study in 1999,[17] 115 patients with DRFs treated with cast immobilization were randomized to receive either 500 mg of vitamin C daily or placebo for 50 days starting on the first day of fracture. CRPS was defined by clinical symptoms (Table 1). The authors reported a statistically significant advantage for vitamin C at 1-year follow-up with 22% of patients treated with the placebo being diagnosed with CRPS as compared to 7% in the vitamin C treatment group. Other statistically significant factors associated with CRPS in the study were fracture comminution (odds ratio 0.09, $P=0.0037$) and compliance with the plaster immobilization (odds ratio 0.1, $P=0.0002$).

Subsequently, Zollinger et al.[16] sought to examine the dose-response of vitamin C on patients with DRFs. Three hundred and seventeen patients were equally randomized to receive 200, 500, or 1500 mg of vitamin C per day while 99 patients received pacebo. The prevalence of CRPS in the placebo group was 10.1% as compared to 2.4% in the vitamin C groups ($P=0.0002$). In the sub-analysis of vitamin C dosage, the prevalence of CRPS was 4.2% in the 200 mg group (NS), 2% in the 500 mg group ($P=0.007$) and 2% in the 1500 mg group ($P=0.005$). Patients receiving 200 mg of vitamin C did not differ significantly from the placebo group. Other factors associated with higher rates of CRPS were female gender and older age. In conclusion, the authors reported that a vitamin C dose of 500 mg for 50 days after the fracture was sufficient for the prevention of CRPS.

However, two further randomized prospective trials performed by other groups could not reproduce these beneficial effects[19, 20] (Table 1). In 2014, Ekrol et al.[19] published their randomized controlled trial examining the effects of vitamin C by allocating 167 patients to the placebo group and 169 patients to the vitamin C group. Study design was similar to the protocol described by Zollinger et al.[12] original paper with 500 mg of vitamin C or placebo for 50 days after the day of fracture with follow-up of 1 year. The primary outcome of interest was DASH (Disability of the Arm, Shoulder and Hand) score and secondary outcomes were complications, wrist and finger motion, grip strength, pain, and CRPS score. CRPS was defined using Atkins[21] Criteria (Table 1) requiring three positive symptoms of five: (1) neuropathic pain; (2) vasomotor instability and abnormalities of sweating; (3) swelling; (4) loss of joint mobility; and (5) joint and soft-tissue contractures.

The authors found no effect of vitamin C on the DASH score throughout the study period and the prevalence of CRPS was significantly higher at 6 weeks for patients treated with vitamin C. Additionally, at 26 weeks, the vitamin C group had significantly more complications and greater pain with wrist use. The authors concluded that there was no difference in functional outcome or any other objective measurement between patients treated with vitamin C or placebo. Interestingly, the authors reported a strong correlation between the functional outcome after distal radius fracture to the patient baseline level of anxiety (measured with the Hospital Anxiety and Depression Score).

The most recent study demonstrating discrepancy with initial positive reports was published in 2019 by Özkan et al.[20] The authors measured finger stiffness as a surrogate for CRPS as well as Patient-Reported Outcomes Measurement Information System (PROMIS) and pain scores with the numeric rating scale (NRS-pain) rather than dichotomizing the outcome of CRPS-based on subjective criteria. One hundred and thirty-four patients were equally randomized to receive 500 mg of vitamin C or placebo within 2 weeks of the fracture. At 6 weeks follow-up, patients were assessed for finger stiffness using the finger pulp to palmar crease distance and assessed for pain and function with NRS and PROMIS questionnaires, respectively. At 6 months follow-up, patients were assessed with the NRS and PROMIS questionnaires. They found that the administration of vitamin C was not associated with improved finger stiffness, range of motion, pain or function at 6 weeks or 6 months. Based on their findings and the paper by Ekrol et al.,[19] the authors concluded that vitamin C had no clinically important effect on pain intensity and upper extremity limitations.

A metanalysis of these conflicting studies, excluding the most recent paper by Özkan et al. which only considered a surrogate of CRPS, finger stiffness, and not CRPS scores, was published in 2017.[22] The authors found that the relative risk of CRPS after a DRF was not significantly diminished in the group given vitamin C with any dosage. However, when the analysis was confined to a dose of 500 mg of vitamin C, the relative risk for CRPS was 0.54 (0.33–0.91; $P=0.02$). As a result, the authors concluded that vitamin C supplementation at a dose of 500 mg for 50 days may halve the risk of CRPS within the first year after fracture but recommended that further research is necessary to establish the effectiveness of the treatment. Another metaanalysis of the same three studies[23] concluded that the evidences are conflicting and did not demonstrate a significant effect of vitamin C. The authors recommended that the decision to treat with vitamin C should be guided by patient preference and clinical expertise.

TABLE 1

Vitamin C in the Treatment of CRPS in Distal Radius Fractures.

Author	Study Design and Number of Participants	Intervention	Definition of CRPS	Occurrence of CRPS at 1 Year Follow Up, n (%)	Other Outcome Measures	Authors Recommendation for Use of Vitamin C in Prevention of CRPS
Zollinger (1999)[17]	Prospective RCT, n = 123	500 mg of Vit C vs placebo on fracture occurrence for 50 days with 1 year follow up	4/6 Symptoms: unexplained diffuse pain; difference in skin temperature relative to the other arm; difference in skin color; diffuse edema; limited range of motion; increase of these symptoms after activity.	Placebo: 14 (22%) 500 mg Vit C: 4 (7%), $P < 0.05$		Yes—Vitamin C is effective in CRPS prevention
Zollinger (2007)[16]	Prospective RCT, n = 416	200, 500, or 1500 mg of Vit C vs placebo on fracture occurrence for 50 days with 1 year follow up	4/5 Symptoms: unexplained diffuse pain; difference in skin temperature; difference in skin color; diffuse edema; limited range of motion; increase of these symptoms after activity.	Placebo: 10 (10.1%) 200 mg Vit C: 4 (4.2%), NS 500 mg Vit C: 2 (1.8%), $P = 0.007$ 1500 mg Vit C: 2 (1.7%), $P = 0.005$		Yes—Vitamin C is effective in CRPS prevention
Ekrol (2014)[19]	Prospective RCT, n = 336	500 mg of Vit C vs placebo on fracture occurrence for 50 days with 1 year follow up	Atkins criteria, 3/5 symptoms: neuropathic pain, vasomotor instability and abnormalities of sweating, swelling, loss of joint mobility, and joint and soft-tissue contractures.	Placebo: 14 (8.3%) 500 mg Vit C: 14 (8.2%), $P = 1$	*Placebo:* DASH: 11.8 Grip deficit: 13.9% Pain at use (VAS): 1.1 *500 mg Vit C:* DASH: 13 Grip deficit: 16.9% Pain at use (VAS): 1.8 *All NS*	No—Vitamin C has no effect in CRPS prevention
Özkan (2019)[20]	Prospective RCT, n = 134	500 mg of Vit C vs placebo within 2 weeks of fracture occurrence for 50 days with 6 months follow up	Objective measurements only: Distance of fingers to palmar crease (DTPC); function (PROMIS); pain (NRS)	N/A	At 6 weeks no association of Vit C to DTPC (RC -0.23, $P = 0.7$) at 6 months no association to PROMIS (RC, -0.21, $P = 0.9$) or NRS (RC, 0.31, $P = 0.5$)	No—Vitamin C does not facilitate recovery from distal radius fracture

RCT, randomized controlled trial; *CRPS*, complex regional pain syndrome; *PROMIS*, patient-reported; outcomes measurement information system; *DASH*, disability of the arm shoulder and hand score; *DTPC*, distance of fingers to palmar crease; *NR*, numeric rating scale; *VAS*, visual analog scale; *NS*, nonsignificant; *RC*, regression coefficient.

Is There a Correlation of CRPS to the DRF Fixation Technique?

Several fixation methods have been implicated as contributors to the development of CRPS in patients with DRFs. A poorly applied plaster cast may facilitate compartment syndrome, pressure ulcers, joint contracture, nerve damage, and chronic pain.[24] Similarly, wrist spanning external fixation has been suggested to cause nerve damage because of proximal pin malposition while chronic pain and joint stiffness may result in cases of wrist joint overdistraction secondary to wrist spanning external fixators.[25]

Wang et al.[24] performed a network metaanalysis to compare 7 different treatment methods of fixation for DRFs and their effect on the development of CRPS. He included 17 RCTs in his metaanalysis with 1658 DRF patients treated with wrist spanning external fixation, nonspanning external fixation, K-wire fixation, plaster fixation, dorsal plating, volar plating, or dorsal and volar plating. They found no marked difference in CRPS risk between all treatment options. This network metaanalysis also ranked the association of the seven treatment methods to CRPS as follows: plaster fixation, nonspanning external fixation, spanning external fixation, dorsal plating, volar plating, dorsal and volar plating and K-wire fixation. Consequently, they reported that plaster fixation and nonspanning external fixation were most effective in reducing the risk of CRPS in DRF patients.

What Is the Role of Surgery for Treatment of CRPS

Many hand surgeons are reluctant to operate on patients that develop disproportionate pain following injury or surgery as they doubt surgery can improve the pain and even more worrisome is the concern of worsening the pain. However, in recent years, a paradigm shift in the surgical approach for CRPS is being led by prominent hand surgeons who believe that most cases classified as CRPS are actually caused by an underlying pathology that was overlooked. Under this premise, proper surgical treatment is advocated as a method to improve the disproportionate pain experienced by patients with CRPS,[7] rather than rendering a suffering patient to prolonged and, at times, futile treatment in the pain clinic.

Such overlooked diagnoses that may induce severe pain were categorized by Del Piñal as unstable fractures, malreduced fractures, occult painful tumors (such as glomus tumors), and dysvascular states.[12] However, the most overlooked diagnosis that may be surgically treated is subclinical nerve compression and injury. These irritative nerve injuries will present differently than classical carpal tunnel or cubital tunnel syndrome and in 66% of cases, negative findings will be present on nerve conduction studies. However, large case series demonstrated significant pain reduction in 99% of patients who received nerve decompression surgeries, mainly carpal tunnel release, yet were previously diagnosed with CRPS.[7] Dellon et al. reported on 100 patients diagnosed with CRPS for whom 80% had an underlying nerve injury or compression that responded to surgery.[26] Dellon recommended that the initial step to determine treatment success was the presence of pain reduction following a nerve block of the suspected compressed or injured nerve. Treatment is dependent on nerve injury and ranges from simple decompression, neuroma resection, nerve graft or joint denervation.[13] Jupiter et al. also advocated for coverage of the injured nerve with vascular tissue in the form of a local vascular flap.[8]

The Role of Local Anesthetic Sympathetic Blockade for Treatment of CRPS

Local and intravenous anesthetic has been used for the treatment of CRPS in patients with DRFs. Early results from small case series appeared promising. Paraskevas et al.[27] reported treating 17 patients with CRPS with intravenous regional sympathetic block (Bier's block) sessions with guanethidine and lidocaine. All of the patients had complete disappearance of pain and return to normal function and movement of the extremity.

However, Livingstone et al.[28] performed a randomized control trial of 57 patients with CRPS 9 weeks following DRF. Patients received either intravenous regional blockade with 15 mg of guanethidine, a local anesthetic, or intravenous saline. They found no significant difference in finger tenderness, stiffness, or grip strength between the two groups. However, the guanethidine group experienced more pain in the affected hand ($P = 0.025$) and at 6 months, had more vasomotor instability ($P < 0.0001$). The authors concluded that intravenous regional blockade with guanethidine is not effective and may even delay the resolution of vasomotor instability.

Livingstone et al. finding are further supported by a recent Cochrane review of CRPS treatment with local anesthetic.[29] Twelve studies with 461 patients with CRPS, not confined to DRF patients, were reviewed. The authors found no evidence to support the effectiveness of local anesthetic blockade in the treatment of CRPS and therefore, did not endorse its use.

What Is the Role of Physical Therapy and Behavioral Therapy for Treatment of CRPS in Patients With DRFs?

There is a large variety of physiotherapy interventions recommended as part of the multimodal treatment of CRPS; however, very little evidence exists to support their use. The following interventions have been described for the treatment of CRPS and may be used as stand-alone treatments or in combination: manual therapy (e.g., mobilization, manipulation, massage, desensitization), therapeutic exercise and progressive loading regimens (including hydrotherapy), adjunctive modalities [e.g., contrast baths, transcutaneous electrical nerve stimulation (TENS), therapeutic ultrasound, shortwave diathermy, laser], physiotherapist-administered education (e.g., pain neuroscience education), as well as cortically directed sensory-motor rehabilitation strategies [e.g., graded motor imagery (GMI), mirror therapy (MT), sensory motor retuning, tactile discrimination training].[30]

Mirror therapy is based on the mirror image of the healthy extremity being seen in place of the affected extremity while exercises are performed in both extremities. Graded motor imagery (GMI) is a multidimension movement representation technique that includes three interventional phases: (1) Limb laterality recognition; (2) Explicit motor imagery; and (3) Mirror therapy[31] (Fig. 3). These physical therapy approaches are the only approaches supported by prospective controlled studies. Moseley et al. published two small prospective trials on treatment of CRPS following DRF with GMI. In his 2004 paper,[32] Moseley et al. randomized 13 patients with chronic CRPS following DRF to receive either 6 weeks of GMI or 12 weeks or physiotherapy. He reported statistically significant improvement in pain at 6 weeks follow-up with three patients needed to treat to obtain a 50% reduction in pain (NNT=3).

Subsequently, Moseley et al.[33] randomized 20 patients with CRPS following DRF to receive GMI with its three components delivered in the correct order or in an different order. The authors found a statistically significant improvement in pain and function in the correctly ordered GMI group at 12 weeks posttreatment compared to both comparison groups. Their conclusion was that the effect of the GMI is dependent on the order of components. This in turn is suggestive that the beneficial effects of GMI is not because of the sustained attention to the affected limb but rather is consistent with sequential activation of cortical motor networks.

A recent Cochrane review of the role of physiotherapy for CRPS, not confined to CRPS following DRF, reached similar conclusions.[30] Eighteen RCTs were reviewed with 739 patients treated with a broad range

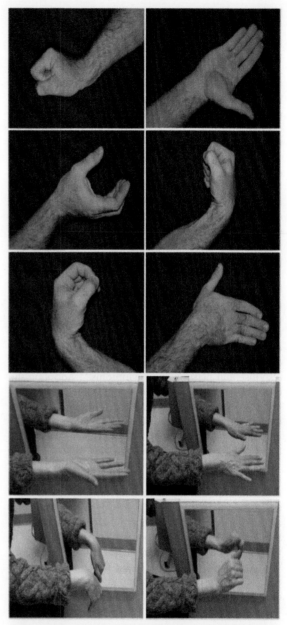

FIG. 3 Graded motor imagery. Photos for Phases 1 (limb laterality recognition) and 2 (explicit motor imagery) are represented in the top six panels. Phase 3 (mirror therapy) is represented in the bottom 4 panels.[31] (Courtesy of Corey McGee, PhD, MS, OTR/L, CHT.)

of physiotherapy interventions. GMI and mirror therapy[34] were found as the only treatment options with clinically meaningful improvement in pain and function. Of note, this recommendation is supported by low quality evidence, though prospective and randomized. Authors were unable to find evidence to support the effectiveness of any other physical therapy modality (including multi model PT, electrotherapy,[35] and lymphatic massage). GMI and MT as a treatment for CRPS was also supported by other systematic reviews but all concluded that the quality of evidence was poor.[36, 37] Future clinical randomized control studies are pending and may shed light on the effectiveness of this treatment.[31]

Patient education should focus on the negative effects of disuse and the importance of using the painful limb. The merits of preventing disuse-related pain was recently shown in a group of 127 patients treated non-surgically for DRF who were instructed to use their wrist early after cast removal despite pain. None of the patients developed CRPS. This approach is also termed pain exposure in physical therapy (PEPT).[38]

There is a growing awareness of the psychosocial factors affecting CRPS. While it has been confirmed in many studies that anxiety, depression, and personality are not predictors of the development of CRPS, experts agree that, similar to other chronic pain conditions such as chronic headache, back pain etc., there is an influence of psychosocial factors especially on the treatment response and persistence of symptoms.[11] Adopting the biopsychosocial approach is essential for the correct treatment of CRPS and also the reason why physical therapeutic modalities with behavioral therapy components, such as mirror therapy and graded motor therapy, has been proven to be more successful than other therapy.

There are no controlled studies of cognitive behavioral therapy (CBT) in the treatment of CRPS,[11] yet there is strong empirical support for CBT for the treatment of somatoform disorders, ineffective coping mechanism, and distress. Behavioral therapy, despite its stigma, may have merits and can be partially implemented in the office by educating the patient about the condition. The clinician should be empathic to the patient's pain and offer techniques to focus on thoughts that can decrease pain intensity.[15, 39]

RECOMMENDATION

In patients with a DRF, the evidence suggests the following:

Recommendation	Overall Quality
• The role of prophylactic treatment with vitamin C to prevent the development of CRPS is controversial. Consequently, patient preference and clinician judgment should be utilized to guide use of this treatment modality.	⊕⊕⊕⊕ HIGH
• CRPS may occur after DRF regardless of the fixation method chosen, including cast and spanning external fixation.	⊕⊕⊕⊕ HIGH
• Physiotherapy with behavioral modification components such as graded motor imagery, mirror therapy, and early active motion may be beneficial for the treatment of CRPS following DRF.	⊕⊕⊕○ MODERATE
• CRPS cases should be scrutinized for underlying pathology, such as nerve compression or injury that may benefit from an operative intervention.	⊕⊕○○ LOW

CONCLUSIONS

Despite early promising evidence that CPRS can be prevented and treated with the biomedical approach (e.g., vitamin C, intravenous anesthetics), it is now apparent that this multifactorial condition requires a multimodal tactic based on the biopsychosocial approach. Physical therapy combined with behavioral therapy components may provide some relief of pain. Yet, more importantly, clinician awareness and early detection of potential CRPS symptomology postwrist fracture is imperative in preventing long-term complications. The clinician must listen and show empathy to the patient condition and educate them on coping mechanisms to allow early use of the extremity despite the pain. Clinicians should be cognizant of potentially overlooked generators of pain and offer surgical intervention when appropriate.

Panel 2: Authors Preferred Technique

Signs and symptoms of CRPS following DRF can be detected as early as 2 weeks following the fracture with disproportional pain and finger stiffness. Early detection and counseling are imperative in preventing chronic pain. In the case presented, after diligently assuring the patient that the pain was not due to another treatable cause (e.g., tight cast, compartment syndrome, or acute carpal tunnel syndrome), the authors counselled the patient that she may be developing disproportional pain and educated her about the condition. The patient was empathically encouraged to range her fingers, elbow, and shoulder while in cast. Subsequently, after cast removal at 6 weeks, the wrist was encouraged to be ranged despite the pain and a removable

brace was provided for comfort and use in crowded places. The clinician also conveyed that pain and stiffness are normal aspects of recovery and coping with the pain was imperative for regaining future hand and wrist functionality.

Despite early promise and recommendations from the AAOS, subsequent conflicting reports make definitive endorsement of the routine use of vitamin C in the prevention of CRPS unclear. Rather, patient preference and clinician judgment should guide treatment with this supplement. Physical therapy such as graded motor imagery and mirror imagery may provide relief of pain, in the author's opinion, primarily because they include components of cognitive behavioral therapy.

Panel 3: Pearls and Pitfalls

PEARLS

- Awareness of the symptoms of CRPS and early detection in clinic will facilitate discussion about the condition and coping mechanisms to potentially avoid long term consequences.
- When discussing the condition with the patient, the clinician should be empathetic to the patient's pain and not imply that CRPS is a pathology with a known etiology that can be effectively treated by drugs or surgery.
- Refer the patient to physical therapy to focus on motor imagery and behavioral component therapy. Alternatively, refer to a mental health clinician in situations whereby the patient shows interest in building coping mechanisms to deal with disproportional pain.

PITFALLS

- Before diagnosing CRPS, be sure to rule out other, treatable conditions that inflict disproportional pain in distal radius fractures (e.g., tight cast, over distracted wrist spanning plates/fixators, infection, hardware malpositioning, articular malreduction, nerve injury, compartment syndrome or acute carpal tunnel syndrome).
- Focusing on psychosocial aspects and not looking for an underlying cause such as nerve injury/compression can be misleading and cause erroneous withholding of care.
- The "label" of CRPS may lead to misconception, anxiety, more testing, and invasive treatment.

FINANCIAL DISCLOSURE

The author has nothing to disclose.

Eminence-Based Medicine
Francisco del Piñal

DEMYSTIFYING CRPS: SURGICAL TREATMENT FOR CRPS AFTER DRF

Complex regional pain syndrome (CRPS) of the upper limb (a.k.a. reflex sympathetic dystrophy, Sudeck, or algodystrophy) is a poorly understood clinical condition that typically presents after surgery or trauma. The authors of the chapter correctly point to distal radius fractures as being the main cause of the condition in the upper limb.

CRPS is an elusive condition that has little strong scientific support, yet at the same time an abundance of clinical lore. Denying its existence[40–43] provokes passionate arguments in any meeting, but even with today's medical

advances,[44, 45] this "condition" has no clear-cut clinical picture, no specific diagnostic tests, an unknown pathophysiology, and lacks curative treatment.[46–48] The current body of evidence discourages surgery in all,[11, 45, 49] or under very exceptional,[50–52] circumstances.

Saying all this, which is universally held to be "THE EVIDENCE," I must add that I am totally skeptical about the existence of CRPS itself.[42, 43] In addition, there is the overwhelming abuse of the diagnosis that stems from the nonspecificity of the criteria used to label CRPS (the so-called Budapest criteria),[9] whose signs and symptoms can be mimicked by genuine diseases.[13, 53] Furthermore, some

Continued

Eminence-Based Medicine—cont'd

authorities on the matter, consider that the Budapest criteria to be too stringent, and recommend lowering the threshold in order to avoid missing any case which could progress to the chronic stage.[11, 45, 50, 51, 54] Yet, nobody has proved that early treatment is of any benefit or improves the prognosis. This misconception precipitates a hasty diagnosis that may well have major consequences on the patient's well-being: i.e., catastrophic thoughts, medicalization, and nocebo effect.[15, 55–58] Many patients are sent to the Pain Clinic without a proper diagnosis and once there, there is no way out. The mission of the Pain Doctor is to ease pain, not to know what the etiology of the pain is—this is the responsibility to the referral orthopedist! This nonsensical sequence of events makes the number of CRPS cases soar to 50,000 a year in the USA alone.[59]

My utter bewildering at this condition started more than 25 years ago, when I was confronted with cases that having been diagnosed with CRPS (with their attached label of "no cure"), I was able to identify what was causing the pain and subsequently solve it. Since June 2018 I have prospectively gathered 159 patients who had come to the office diagnosed with CRPS. Of those, 56 developed the condition after a distal radius fracture. They fall into three groups:

- *Bad doctoring*. This represents 40% in my series, and particularly this is high in DRF. In other words, voluntarily or not, CRPS is being used as a shelter for sloppy treatment (Fig. 1).

- *Flare reactions*. For years it has been known that some patients develop a hyperresponse to trauma. The vast majority self-heal in some weeks with PT, NSAID, and support. Occasionally, low doses of pregabaline (an antiseizure) can be added for short periods. It is a major mistake to label them with CRPS1 as there is a high risk of catastrophic thinking and medicalization.[15, 55–58] Clinically, they are similar to the next group below, but have less pain, and tolerable sleep. In this series of 159 patients there were 4 who had stellate ganglion blocks and were given neuropathic drugs despite never having had severe pain, albeit presenting swelling, redness, and stiffness. (The case the authors show in Fig. 1 of their chapter is an excellent example of a flare reaction).

- *Irritative carpal tunnel syndrome*. When the pain is unbearable and/or disturbs sleep, then, there is a high likelihood of an *irritation* of the median nerve in the carpal canal. I named this condition "Irritative Carpal Tunnel type II" (ICTS-II) (see Discussion). I do not use the term "compression," as in approximately 60% of patients, their electrophysiological studies were negative. This is not surprising as standard electrophysiologic studies do not detect the activity of the small fibers (A∂ and C fibers) that are afferent for pain, temperature, and vasomotor changes. All patients with an ICTS had a carpal tunnel release (CTR) under local anesthesia.

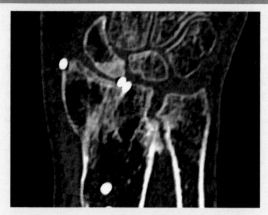

Fig. 1 This 48-y-o had limited and painful motion in the radiocarpal and distal radioulnar joints, as well as difficulty clenching his fingers. He was diagnosed with CRPS and had had several invasive treatments in the Pain Clinic for more than 1 year with little improvement. A CT scan was ordered at his first visit demonstrating poor extraarticular reduction, and intraarticular screw penetration. (© Dr. Piñal 2020.)

It is difficult to give exact figures, as some patients had a flare reaction in the midst of a malunion, and some had a malunion combined with an ICTS-II. Most important is that the care was below the standard in 40%. Globally, I have operated only 36 cases diagnosed with CRPS secondary to a DRF in different stages of the evolution of the "CRPS." I include 5 cases who were operated on by our team with a volar locking plate, and who develop CRPS-like symptoms, and the progression was aborted by CTR. The rest, including some overt cases of bad-doctoring, dismissed the recommendation of having surgery on advice from their surgeons such as: "the literature is against surgery," "that doctor [the author of this paper] only wants to get your money." This is quite unfortunate, as it has deprived them of the benefit of surgery.

Of the whole group of CRPS secondary to DRF operated on the response was immediate and curative (Fig. 2). There were 2 patients (1 in the acute stage and 1 in the chronic stage of CRPS) who did not respond to surgery as expected, although both improved in pain and range of motion. It is not clear to me why this may have happened, but my colleague and friend Carlos Heras-Palou (Derby, UK) has warned me that perhaps behind some of the failures there is an entrapment of the posterior interosseus nerve secondary to the fracture.[60] As a matter of fact, he systematically carries out an infiltration with 2 cc of lidocaine in the interosseous membrane to rule out its involvement. This makes a lot of sense as irritation of the posterior interosseous nerve is responsible for neuropathic pain.[61] The corollary is that any nerve (injury) may be behind failed surgery, i.e., anything other than using CRPS as an easy scapegoat.

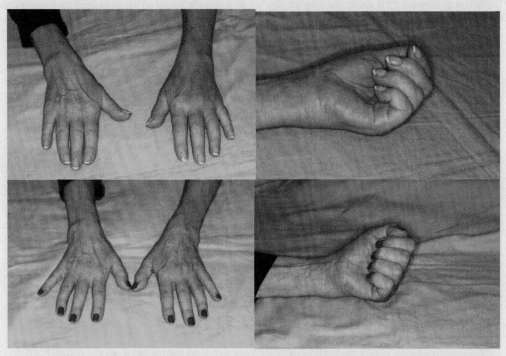

FIG. 2 This 68-y-o sustained bilateral distal radius fractures that were anatomically reduced and treated in a cast (by his brother, himself an orthopaedic surgeon). While the right side had a normal evolution, the left developed all the signs and symptoms of severe acute CRPS. (A) and (B) Swelling and attempting to clench her fist 11 weeks post fracture. Pain 9.5/10; EMG normal. (C) and (D) Range-of-motion and swelling at the time of stitch removal 2 weeks after the operation. Her pain fell to 0. (© Dr. Piñal 2020.)

DISCUSSION

I am aware that all the literature is against surgery, though one of the co-authors of this book achieved excellent results in CRPS patients with a nerve injury.[8] Some reluctantly concede that if there is an identifiable nociceptive focus, demonstrable with neurophysiologic tests, and which responds to a sympathetic block, surgery can be warranted with the protective umbrella of intra and postoperative sympathetic blocks.[50–52] Several authors have recommend releasing the median nerve if it is demonstrated to be compressed in the carpal tunnel.[62–66] However, this restrictive policy would leave the majority of my patients without the benefit of surgery and consequently in pain, perhaps, forever.

The rationale of this against-the-flow approach is based on **observation**—presently reviled by the scientific methodology—that a subset of patients diagnosed with carpal tunnel syndrome (CTS) shared a similar clinical picture to CRPS patients. Said CTS patients had: poorly localized pain with dysesthesias in the hand, inability to make a full fist, and

worsening of the symptoms at night.[43, 67] None had a precipitating injury, most of them had bilateral involvement, were aged 60+, and responded immediately to CTR. I named this group Irritative Carpal Tunnel Syndrome type I (ICTS-1). The clinical picture of ICTS-1 patients was indistinguishable from some of the features displayed by CRPS patients, though this group were all unilateral, younger individuals, and the pain fared much worse. It seemed logical to offer them the same operative approach taking into account their no-hope status. Offering unproven surgery may be considered unethical, but if unsuccessful, surgery has minimal morbidity. On the other hand, aggressive-invasive medical approaches are accepted at the rallying cries that "it is better do something than nothing," or "the absence of evidence is not the same as the evidence of absence"[11, 44, 45, 50–52, 54]; despite the lack of scientific evidence validating this,[46–48] and the risks incurred.[15, 55–58] Yet this is the gold standard.

In light of our results, and considering the innocuity of the procedure, I recommend CTR to all patients with

Continued

CRPS-like symptoms, provided other sources of pain have been ruled out. I stress again the obvious: sloppy surgery skyrockets the number of patients with pain— *not of CRPS*—and, likewise, *CTR would not cure a badly treated distal radius fracture* (see flowchart).

Flowchart summarizing the author's policy for any patient whose signs and symptoms may fit into the CRPS constellation: Note that the decision to wait or to proceed to surgery is based on the severity of the pain: interference with sleep indicates severe pain. (*Some patients are too sore as to accept having any sort of nonvital painful test).

PAIN DISTURBS SLEEP

NO

YES *

FLARE REACTION

EMG

P.T.
NSAID
(Pregabalin)

\+

\-

1 criteria

2 criteria

RESISTANT

ICTS

RESPONDS

CTR

CRITERIA FOR ICTS.

INABILITY TO MAKE A FULL FIST
DISTURBING PAIN AT NIGHT
SIGNS OR SYMPTOMS OF CTS
PASSIVE FINGER FLEXION PAINFUL
WRIST/ELBOW EXTENSION PAINFUL
ALLODYNIA /BURNING PAIN
MULTIPLE TRIGGER POINTS
CRUMPLING WHEN ABDUCTING ARM
STRING SIGN.

REFERENCES

1. Li Z, Smith BP, Tuohy C, Smith TL, Koman LA. Complex regional pain syndrome after hand surgery. *Hand Clin.* 2010; 26(2):281–289.
2. Field J, Warwick D, Bannister G. Features of algodystrophy ten years after Colles' fracture. *J Hand Surg Br Eur Vol.* 1992; 17(3):318–320.
3. Crijns TJ, Van Der Gronde BA, Ring D, Leung N. Complex regional pain syndrome after distal radius fracture is uncommon and is often associated with fibromyalgia. *Clin Orthop Relat Res.* 2018; 476(4):744.
4. Roh YH, Lee BK, Noh JH, et al. Factors associated with complex regional pain syndrome type I in patients with surgically treated distal radius fracture. *Arch Orthop Trauma Surg.* 2014; 134(12):1775–1781.
5. An HS, Hawthorne KB, Jackson WT. Reflex sympathetic dystrophy and cigarette smoking. *J Hand Surg Am.* 1988; 13(3):458–460.
6. Mathews AL, Chung KC. Management of complications of distal radius fractures. *Hand Clin.* 2015; 31(2): 205–215.
7. Del Piñal F. Reflex sympathetic dystrophy (RSD)/CRPS/SUDECK does not exist. *Ezine IFSSH.* 2019; 9(3):23–33.
8. Jupiter JB, Seiler 3rd JG, Zienowicz R. Sympathetic maintained pain (causalgia) associated with a demonstrable peripheral-nerve lesion. Operative treatment. *JBoneJointSurg(AmVol).* 1994;76(9):1376–1384.
9. Harden RN, Bruehl S, Perez RS, et al. Validation of proposed diagnostic criteria (the "Budapest Criteria") for complex regional pain syndrome. *Pain.* 2010; 150 (2):268–274.
10. Holder L, Mackinnon S. Reflex sympathetic dystrophy in the hands: clinical and scintigraphic criteria. *Radiology.* 1984; 152(2):517–522.
11. Birklein F, O'Neill D, Schlereth T. Complex regional pain syndrome: an optimistic perspective. *Neurology.* 2015; 84 (1):89–96.
12. Del Piñal F. *I Have a Dream... Reflex Sympathetic Dystrophy (RSD or Complex Regional Pain Syndrome-CRPS I) Does Not Exist.* London, England: Sage Publications Sage UK; 2013.
13. Dellon AL. Surgical treatment of upper extremity pain. *Hand Clin.* 2016; 32(1):71–80.
14. Schneppendahl J, Windolf J, Kaufmann RA. Distal radius fractures: current concepts. *J Hand Surg Am.* 2012; 37 (8):1718–1725.
15. Ring D, Barth R, Barsky A. Evidence-based medicine: disproportionate pain and disability. *J Hand Surg Am.* 2010; 35(8):1345–1347.
16. Zollinger PE, Tuinebreijer W, Breederveld R, Kreis R. Can vitamin C prevent complex regional pain syndrome in patients with wrist fractures?: a randomized, controlled, multicenter dose-response study. *J Bone Joint Surg.* 2007; 89(7):1424–1431.
17. Zollinger PE, Tuinebreijer WE, Kreis RW, Breederveld RS. Effect of vitamin C on frequency of reflex sympathetic dystrophy in wrist fractures: a randomised trial. *Lancet.* 1999; 354(9195):2025–2028.
18. Surgeons AAoO. *The treatment of distal radius fractures: guideline and evidence report.* [Adopted by the American AcademyofOrthopaedicSurgeonsBoardofDirectors2013].
19. Ekrol I, Duckworth AD, Ralston SH, McQueen MM. The influence of vitamin C on the outcome of distal radial fractures: a double-blind, randomized controlled trial. *J Bone Joint Surg.* 2014; 96(17):1451–1459.
20. Özkan S, Teunis T, Ring DC, Chen NC. What is the effect of vitamin C on finger stiffness after distal radius fracture? A double-blind, placebo-controlled randomized trial. *Clin Orthop Relat Res.* 2019; 477(10):2278–2286.
21. Atkins R, Duckworth T, Kanis J. Features of algodystrophy after Colles' fracture. *J Bone Joint Surg Br Vol.* 1990; 72 (1):105–110.
22. Aim F, Klouche S, Frison A, Bauer T, Hardy P. Efficacy of vitamin C in preventing complex regional pain syndrome after wrist fracture: a systematic review and meta-analysis. *Orthop Traumatol Surg Res.* 2017; 103 (3):465–470.
23. Evaniew N, McCarthy C, Kleinlugtenbelt YV, Ghert M, Bhandari M. Vitamin C to prevent complex regional pain syndrome in patients with distal radius fractures: a meta-analysis of randomized controlled trials. *J Orthop Trauma.* 2015; 29(8):e235–e241.
24. Wang J-H, Sun T. Comparison of effects of seven treatment methods for distal radius fracture on minimizing complex regional pain syndrome. *Arch Med Sci.* 2017; 13(1):163.
25. Zollinger PE, Kreis RW, van der Meulen HG, van der Elst M, Breederveld RS, Tuinebreijer WE. No higher risk of CRPS after external fixation of distal radial fractures—subgroup analysis under randomised vitamin C prophylaxis. *Open Orthop J.* 2010; 4:71.
26. Dellon AL, Andonian E, Rosson GD. CRPS of the upper or lower extremity: surgical treatment outcomes. *J Brachial Plex Peripher Nerve Inj.* 2009; 4(1):e7–e12.
27. Paraskevas KI, Michaloglou AA, Briana DD, Samara M. Treatment of complex regional pain syndrome type I of the hand with a series of intravenous regional sympathetic blocks with guanethidine and lidocaine. *Clin Rheumatol.* 2006; 25(5):687–693.
28. Livingstone J, Atkins R. Intravenous regional guanethidine blockade in the treatment of post-traumatic complex regional pain syndrome type 1 (algodystrophy) of the hand. *J Bone Joint Surg Br Vol.* 2002; 84(3):380–386.
29. O'Connell NE, Wand BM, Gibson W, Carr DB, Birklein F, Stanton TR. Local anaesthetic sympathetic blockade for complex regional pain syndrome. *Cochrane Database Syst Rev.* 2016; 7.
30. Smart KM, Wand BM, O'Connell NE. Physiotherapy for pain and disability in adults with complex regional pain syndrome (CRPS) types I and II. *Cochrane Database Syst Rev.* 2016; 2:CD010853.
31. McGee C, Skye J, Van Heest A. Graded motor imagery for women at risk for developing type I CRPS following closed treatment of distal radius fractures: a randomized comparative effectiveness trial protocol. *BMC Musculoskelet Disord.* 2018; 19(1):202.

32. Moseley G. Graded motor imagery is effective for long-standing complex regional pain syndrome: a randomised controlled trial. *Pain*. 2004; 108(1–2):192–198.

33. Moseley GL. Is successful rehabilitation of complex regional pain syndrome due to sustained attention to the affected limb? A randomised clinical trial. *Pain*. 2005; 114(1–2):54–61.

34. McCabe C, Haigh R, Ring E, Halligan P, Wall P, Blake D. A controlled pilot study of the utility of mirror visual feedback in the treatment of complex regional pain syndrome (type 1). *Rheumatology*. 2003; 42(1):97–101.

35. Durmus A, Cakmak A, Disci R, Muslumanoglu L. The efficiency of electromagnetic field treatment in complex regional pain syndrome type I. *Disabil Rehabil*. 2004; 26 (9):537–545.

36. Méndez-Rebolledo G, Gatica-Rojas V, Torres-Cueco R, Albornoz-Verdugo M, Guzmán-Muñoz E. Update on the effects of graded motor imagery and mirror therapy on complex regional pain syndrome type 1: a systematic review. *J Back Musculoskelet Rehabil*. 2017; 30(3):441–449.

37. Daly AE, Bialocerkowski AE. Does evidence support physiotherapy management of adult complex regional pain syndrome type one? A systematic review. *Eur J Pain*. 2009; 13(4):339–353.

38. Boersma EZ, Meent HV, Klomp FP, Frölke JM, Nijhuis-van der Sanden MW, Edwards MJ. Treatment of distal radius fracture: does early activity postinjury lead to a lower incidence of complex regional pain syndrome? *Hand*. 2020; :1558944719895782.

39. Bruehl S, Chung OY. Psychological and behavioral aspects of complex regional pain syndrome management. *Clin J Pain*. 2006; 22(5):430–437.

40. Ochoa JL. Truths, errors, and lies around "reflex sympathetic dystrophy" and "complex regional pain syndrome". *J Neurol*. 1999; 246:875–879.

41. Dellon AL, Andonian E, Rosson GD. CRPS of the upper or lower extremity: surgical treatment outcomes. *J Brachial Plex Peripher Nerve Inj*. 2009; 4:1.

42. del Piñal F. Editorial. I have a dream … Reflex sympathetic dystrophy (RSD or complex regional pain syndrome—CRPS I) does not exist. *J Hand Surg Eur Vol*. 2013; 38 (6):595–597.

43. del Piñal F. Reflex sympathetic dystrophy (RSD)/CRPS/Sudeck does not exist. *Ezine (IFSSH)*. 2019; 9(3):22–31.

44. Marinus J, Moseley GL, Birklein F, et al. Clinical features and pathophysiology of complex regional pain syndrome. *Lancet Neurol*. 2011; 10(7):637–648.

45. Bruehl S. Complex regional pain syndrome. *BMJ*. 2015; 351:h2730.

46. Schott GD. Interrupting the sympathetic outflow in causalgia and reflex sympathetic dystrophy. *BMJ*. 1998; 316(7134):792–793.

47. O'Connell NE, Wand BM, McAuley J, et al. Interventions for treating pain and disability in adults with complex regional pain syndrome. *Cochrane Database Syst Rev*. 2013; 4:CD009416.

48. Straube S, Derry S, Moore RA, Cole P. Cervico-thoracic or lumbar sympathectomy for neuropathic pain and complex regional pain syndrome. *Cochrane Database Syst Rev*. 2013; 2013(9):CD002918.

49. Noordenbos W, Wall PD. Implications of the failure of nerve resection and graft to cure chronic pain produced by nerve lesions. *J Neurol Neurosurg Psychiatry*. 1981; 44 (12):1068–1073.

50. Patterson RW, Li Z, Smith BP, Smith TL, Koman LA. Complex regional pain syndrome of the upper extremity. *J Hand Surg Am*. 2011; 36(9):1553–1562.

51. Koman AL, Smith BP, SmithTL. A practical guide for complex regional pain syndrome in the acute stage and late stage. In: Wolfe SW, Hotchkiss RN, Pederson WC, et al. *Green's Operative Hand Surgery*. 7th ed. Philadelphia: Churchill Livingstone; 2017:1797–1827.

52. Goebel A, Barker CH, Turner-Stokes L, et al. *Complex Regional Pain Syndrome in Adults: UK Guidelines for Diagnosis, Referral and Management in Primary and Secondary Care*. London: Royal College of Physicians; 2018.

53. Thimineur MA, Saberski L. Complex regional pain syndrome type I (RSD) or peripheral mononeuropathy? A discussion of three cases. *Clin J Pain*. 1996; 12:145–150.

54. Øyluk A, Puchalski P. Complex regional pain syndrome: observations on diagnosis, treatment and definition of a new subgroup. *J Hand Surg Eur Vol*. 2013; 38(6):599–606.

55. Gupta A, Silman AJ, Ray D, et al. The role of psychosocial factors in predicting the onset of chronic widespread pain: results from a prospective population-based study. *Rheumatology (Oxford)*. 2007; 46(4):666–671.

56. Munglani R. Does a diagnosis in pain medicine promote disability? *Pain News*. 2012; 10:16–18.

57. Hayes PJ, Louis DS, Kasdan ML. Additional considerations in complex regional pain syndrome. *J Hand Surg Am*. 2012; 37(3):625.

58. Bass C. Complex regional pain syndrome medicalises limb pain. *BMJ*. 2014; 348:g2631.

59. Bruehl S, Chung OY. How common is complex regional pain syndrome—type I? *Pain*. 2007; 129(1–2):1–2.

60. Heras-Palou C. *Personal Communication*. .

61. Lluch A. Treatment of radial neuromata and dysesthesia. *Tech Hand Up Extrem Surg*. 2001; 5(4):188–195.

62. Stein Jr. AH. The relation of median nerve compression to Sudeck's syndrome. *Surg Gynecol Obstet*. 1962; 115:713–720.

63. Grundberg AB, Reagan DS. Compression syndromes in reflex sympathetic dystrophy. *J Hand Surg Am*. 1991; 16 (4):731–736.

64. Monsivais JJ, Baker J, Monsivais D. The association of peripheral nerve compression and reflex sympathetic dystrophy. *J Hand Surg Br*. 1993; 18(3):337–338.

65. Placzek JD, Boyer MI, Gelberman RH, Sopp B, Goldfarb CA. Nerve decompression for complex regional pain syndrome type II following upper extremity surgery. *J Hand Surg Am*. 2005; 30(1):69–74.

66. Koh SM, Moate F, Grinsell D. Co-existing carpal tunnel syndrome in complex regional pain syndrome after hand trauma. *J Hand Surg Eur Vol*. 2010; 35(3):228–231.

67. del Piñal F. *The Irritative Carpal Tunnel Syndrome. A New Entity*; n.d. [in preparation].

CHAPTER 25

Pediatric Distal Radius Fractures

A.R. POUBLON[a] • A.E. VAN DER WINDT[b] • J.J.W. PLOEGMAKERS[c] •
JOOST W. COLARIS[d]

[a]Department of Orthopedics, ETZ, Tilburg, The Netherlands, [b]Department of Orthopedics, Maxima MC, Utrecht, The Netherlands, [c]Department of Orthopedics, UMCG, Groningen, The Netherlands, [d]Department of Orthopedics, Erasmus MC, Rotterdam, The Netherlands

KEY POINTS

- Treatment of pediatric distal radius fractures (DRFs) is challenging because of possible involvement of the physis and the remodeling capacity by growth.
- Young children with a fracture close to the most active distal physis angulated in the sagittal plane have the highest remodeling capacity.
- Predictors for secondary fracture displacement in cast are initial complete displacement and inadequate reduction. Cast index is not a predictor for failure.
- Additional K-wire fixation of displaced distal radius fractures reduces re-displacement rates but does not improve functional outcome.

Panel 1: Case Scenario

A 12-year-old, right-handed boy with a painful and swollen right wrist visits the emergency department after a fall from his bike. Radiographs show a Salter Harris type II (SH II) distal radius fracture (Fig. 1). What is the most effective treatment of his fracture?

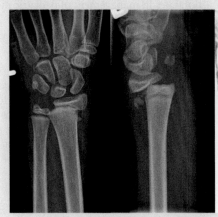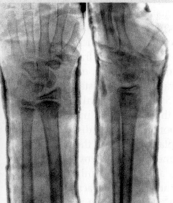

FIG. 1 Radiographs of a 12-year-old child with a SH II fracture before and after reduction.

Continued

Panel 1: Case Scenario—cont'd

After a week, the boy visits your outpatient clinic for follow-up and the radiographs show secondary displacement of the fracture (Fig. 2). What is the most effective treatment of his secondary displaced fracture?

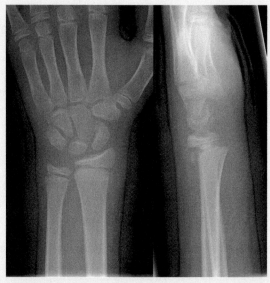

FIG. 2 Radiographs of a 12-year-old child with a SH II fracture with secondary fracture displacement in cast.

IMPORTANCE OF THE PROBLEM

Distal forearm fractures are one of the most common fractures accounting for about 40% of all long bone fractures in children.[1, 2] A peak incidence is seen in girls between 10 and 12 years and in boys between 12 and 14 years. The key difference between the child's bone and that of an adult is the physis that needs to be taken into account for the treatment of these fractures. Physeal injuries are very common in children, making up 15% of all distal forearm fractures.[3] The distal physis of the radius accounts for 75% of the growth of the radius and 40% of the growth of the entire upper extremity, thereby remodeling potential in the distal forearm is highest in the sagittal plane because of the highest range of motion in this plane (flexion-extension). Multiple attempts at reduction, and late re-manipulation more than 7 days post injury are known risk factors for physeal growth arrest (Fig. 3).[4, 5] Remodeling potential[6, 7] of pediatric distal radius fractures (DRFs) makes the choice between nonoperative treatment and operative treatment more complex than in the adult population.

MAIN QUESTION

What is the relative effect of additional K-wire fixation in closed reduction on functional outcome and complication rates in management of pediatric metaphyseal and physeal DRFs?

CURRENT OPINION

Relatively stable buckle/torus or greenstick DRFs with minimal angulation do not require closed reduction and can be treated with cast or pressure bandage treatment. Current opinion is divided with regard to more unstable displaced greenstick fractures, SH Type I–IV fractures, complete DRFs, or both-bone distal forearm fractures.[8, 9]

FINDING THE EVIDENCE

- Cochrane search: Pediatric DRF
- Pubmed (Medline):

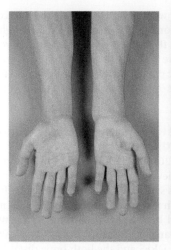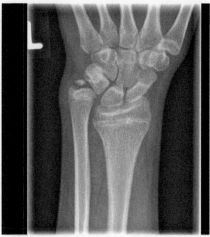

FIG. 3 Physeal arrest of the distal radius after physeal fracture.

- Embase ("forearm fracture"/de OR "radius fracture"/exp. OR "ulna fracture"/exp. OR "wrist fracture"/de OR "distal radius fracture"/exp. OR (((forearm* OR fore-arm OR radius* OR ulna OR wrist* OR antebrach* OR both-bone* OR colles* OR monteggia*) NEAR/3 (fracture*)) OR ((salter-harris* OR epiphys*-plate* OR growth-plate* OR intra-articul* OR intraarticul*) AND (wrist* OR radius* OR ulna))):ab,ti,kw) **AND** ("fracture treatment"/exp. OR "closed reduction (procedure)"/exp. OR "open reduction (procedure)"/exp. OR "bone resection"/de OR "orthopedic surgery"/de OR (ORIF OR CRIF OR plaster* OR cast* OR K-wire* OR plate* OR nail* OR reduction* OR fixat* OR osteosynth* OR ilizarov* OR splint* OR ((therapy OR therapies OR treat* OR immobili*) NEAR/3 (fracture*)) OR ((orthoped*) NEAR/3 (surgic* OR surger* OR procedur*))):ab,ti,kw) **AND** ("Controlled clinical trial"/exp. OR "Crossover procedure"/de OR "Double-blind procedure"/de OR "Single-blind procedure"/de OR "review"/exp. OR "meta analysis"/de OR (meta-analys* OR metaanalys* OR review* OR random* OR factorial* OR crossover* OR (cross NEXT/1 over*) OR placebo* OR ((doubl* OR singl*) NEXT/1 blind*) OR assign* OR allocat* OR volunteer* OR trial OR groups):ab,ti,kw) **AND** (child/exp. OR adolescent/exp. OR adolescence/exp. OR pediatrics/exp. OR childhood/exp. OR "child welfare"/de OR "child development"/de OR "child growth"/de OR "child health"/de OR "child health care"/exp. OR "child care"/exp. OR "childhood disease"/exp. OR "pediatric ward"/de OR "pediatric hospital"/de OR "pediatric anesthesia"/de OR (adolescen* OR preadolescen* OR infan* OR child* OR kid OR kids OR toddler* OR teen* OR boy* OR girl* OR minors OR underag* OR (under NEXT/1 (age* OR aging OR ageing)) OR juvenil* OR youth* OR kindergar* OR puber* OR pubescen* OR prepubescen* OR prepubert* OR pediatric* OR paediatric* OR school* OR preschool* OR highschool* OR suckling* OR PICU OR NICU OR PICUs OR NICUs):ab,ti,kw) **NOT** ((animal/exp. OR animal*:de OR nonhuman/de) **NOT** ("human"/exp)) NOT ([Conference Abstract]/lim)
- Bibliography of eligible articles
- Articles that were not in the English, French, or German language were excluded.

QUALITY OF THE EVIDENCE

Level I:
Systematic Reviews/Metaanalyses: 9
Randomized trials: 9
Level II:
Randomized trials with methodological limitations: 1
Prospective studies: 3
Level III:
Retrospective comparative studies: 12
Level IV:
Case series: 2

FINDINGS

For pediatric DRFs, we divided the evidence into fractures with and without involvement of the physis. The fractures without involvement of the physis were further divided into non-/minimally displaced fractures and displaced fractures.

For the fractures with involvement of the physis, we wanted to answer the question:

1. Can the fracture be treated with a closed reduction and cast alone or is additional K-wire fixation required?

For the fractures without involvement of the physis with minimal displacement, we wanted to answer the question:

1. Is a splint or swim cast as effective as a rigid below-elbow cast for nonoperative treatment?
2. Is a below-elbow cast as effective as an above-elbow cast for nonoperative treatment?

For the fractures without involvement of the physis with displacement, we wanted to answer the question:

1. What is the relative effect of additional K-wire fixation in closed reduction on the functional outcome and complication rate in management of displaced fractures without involvement of the physis?

Distal Forearm Fractures With Involvement of the Physis

There is a paucity of evidence on physeal fractures of the distal radius in children. The best evidence is on SH II fractures. We therefore discuss one systematic review[3] and four retrospective case series.[4, 10–12]

Larsen et al.[3] in 2016 performed a systematic review of the literature. They included 7 retrospective studies[4, 10, 13–17] with a total of 434 SH II fractures. In this review, there were no studies directly comparing operative versus nonoperative treatment. Two studies reported long-term outcomes after treatment of SH II fractures. Out of 224 patients, 213 had good results. Eleven patients had moderate to poor results varying from nonspecific wrist pain with sports to radial shortening requiring additional intervention. The studies also showed a 22% re-displacement rate. The retrospective study of Houshian et al.[4] concluded that although some remodeling occurred in all ages, complete remodeling only occurred in children below age 10. Nietosvaara et al.[10] showed that 2 out of 109 patients had a high residual angular deformity and wrist symptoms. Both fractures occurred 6 months prior to skeletal maturity. There have been two case series on volar buttress plating of volarly displaced physeal fractures of the distal radius. Cha et al.[12] presented nine cases in which a SH II fracture was treated with a volar buttress plate. In this case series, there was a minor impairment of flexion and extension of

the wrist (140 vs 146 degrees). No complications were reported. Shah et al.[11] presented eight cases in which a SH III fracture was treated with a volar plate. Patients were between 11 and 16 years of age. After 8 weeks, only one patient had mild wrist pain and the range of motion was 90%–100% compared to the contralateral side.

Distal Forearm Fractures Without Involvement of the Physis

In 2018, Handoll et al.[18] did an extensive systematic review on pediatric DRFs. For this part of the chapter, this study will serve as a main guideline complemented with a number of newer studies. In most studies, DRFs and both-bone distal forearm fractures are not clearly separated. Therefore, in this section, we will discuss both the DRFS and the both-bone distal forearm fractures.

Because of the variation in treatment, metaphyseal fractures can be divided into two groups: Non-/minimally displaced distal radius and both-bone metaphyseal fractures, displaced distal radius, and both-bone metaphyseal fractures.

Non-/Minimally Displaced Fractures

While non- and minimally displaced fractures do not need fracture reduction, the threshold for reduction depends on several factors. Young children with a fracture close to the most active distal physis angulated in the sagittal plane have the highest remodeling capacity.[19–22] Ploegmakers et al.[23] performed a metaanalysis of acceptable angulation in the literature and combined this with expert opinions. The acceptable angulation for distal physeal-, torus-, greenstick-, distal radius-, and both-bone distal forearm fractures varies with age (Graph 1A–E).

In the review of Handoll, multiple studies[19, 24–30] compared removable splints/soft cast/bandages to rigid casts. In a study by Pountos et al.,[19] the removable splint group showed excellent functional outcome. The other studies also favored the splint when it comes to return to normal activities, pain, patient and parent satisfaction and complications. Only one study by Karimi[24] showed more edema in patients with removable splints. Treatment duration in most studies was 2–4 weeks.

Both the reviews of Handoll et al.[18] (Cochrane review) and Schreck et al.[31] describe four trials comparing below-elbow versus above-elbow casts in the treatment of distal forearm fractures without involvement of the physis. In three trials (333 children), casts were applied after closed reduction of displaced distal radius or both radius and ulna fractures,[32–34] whereas Colaris et al.[30] is the only study in which all 66 children had minimally displaced metaphyseal fractures of both the radius and ulna.

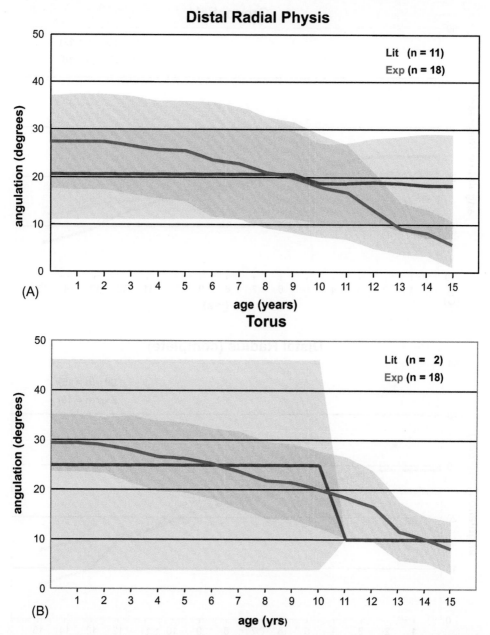

GRAPH 1 Graphs showing age (years) plotted against angulation (degrees): (A) distal radial physis, (B) torus, *(Continued)*

Greenstick

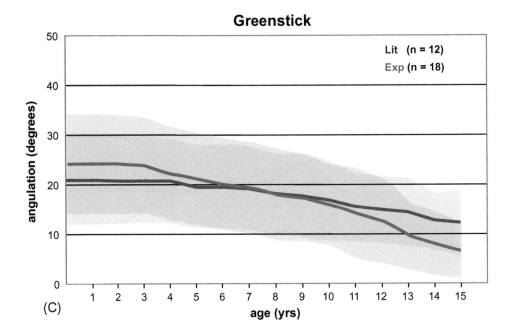

Distal Radius (complete)

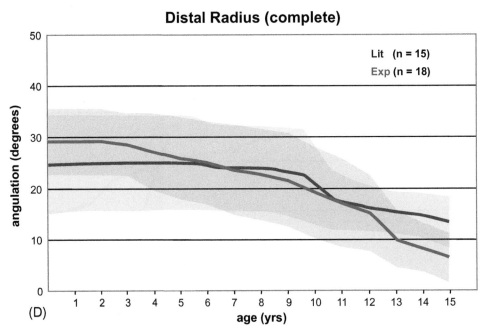

GRAPH 1, CONT'D   (C) greenstick, (D) distal radius (complete),

Both Bone Forearm (distal 1/3)

GRAPH 1, CONT'D   (E) both-bone forearm (distal 1/3). The lines represent the limit of acceptance of deformity for each age. Pooled data from literature (Lit, *blue line*) and experts' opinion (Exp, *red line*) with one standard deviation.

The primarily applied casts were circumferential in the three trials but noncircumferential in the trial of Colaris et al. A below-elbow cast reduces the risk for secondary fracture displacement by 44% (21/133 vs 42/146; RR 0.56, 95% CI 0.36–0.87; 279 children, 3 studies) and the risk for secondary reduction by 73% (2/177 vs 9/189; RR 0.27, 95% CI 0.07–1.06; 366 children; 4 studies) compared to an above-elbow cast. Only Paneru et al.[33] reported on pain, and found that in children who were treated with below-elbow cast the mean VAS score was reduced by 1.91 points after 1 week (MD −1.91, 95% CI −2.55 to −1.27; 85 children).

Displaced Fractures

Sengab et al.[35] performed a metaanalysis on risk factors for re-displacement during cast treatment. Anatomical reduction reduced the risk of re-displacement by 82% when compared to nonanatomical reduction (RR 0.18 95% CI 0.1–0.32). Also, a complete displacement of the distal radius gave a 3.3 times higher risk of re-displacement (RR 3.3 95% CI 2.4–4.5). A cast index of lower than 0.8 was not found to be a significant factor, however, the studies were statistically very heterogeneous

on this matter. Ploegmakers et al.[36] also performed a study on the predictors of losing reduction during cast treatment. They found that persistent fracture displacement after reduction increased the risk of re-displacement (RR 1.99 overall) with a relative risk of 1.42 for residual displacement in the frontal plane and an RR of 1.01 for residual displacement in the sagittal plane. A residual displacement of >20% gave a RR of 1.41. They also found no correlation between re-displacement and cast index.

Colaris et al.[37] showed that in a subgroup of 67 stable reduced distal metaphyseal both bone fractures 30 re-displaced, 19 of which in the first week of follow-up. It is therefore paramount that seemingly stable fractures receive regular radiographic follow-up at the outpatient clinic.

The Cochrane review by Handoll et al.[18] described five trials comparing percutaneous K-wire fixation and cast immobilization versus cast alone for displaced metaphyseal fractures of the distal forearm. Only Colaris et al.[37] and McLauchlan et al.[38] had exclusively or mainly both-bone fractures. Children who were included in the study of Gibbons et al. had isolated displaced DRFs and the other two trials did not mention ulna involvement. The authors stated that there is low-quality evidence that additional percutaneous K-wire fixation reduces the risk of fracture re-displacement (6/159 vs 69/164; RR 0.11, 95% CI 0.05–0.23; 323 children, 5 studies) and treatment (typically re-manipulation) for loss of fracture position (1/124 vs 40/129; RR 0.06, 95% CI 0.02–0.22; 253 children; 4 studies) This means 1.8 patient needs to be treated with additional K-wires to prevent one secondary fracture displacement. And 1.7 patient need to be treated with additional K-wires to prevent re-manipulation. Colaris et al. described less limitation of pronation and supination (mean limitation 6.9 ($\pm$9.4) degrees vs 14.3 ($\pm$13.6) degrees) but more complications (14 vs 1), including subcutaneously migrated K-wires, re-fractures, superficial infections, and failed insertion of K-wires in the surgery group.

Sengab et al.[39] included six studies[6, 37, 38, 40–42] in a metaanalysis which analyzed treatment of displaced DRFs with cast alone versus cast plus K-wire fixation. In this study, additional K-wire fixation gave less re-displacement after primary and secondary reduction. However, there was no statistically significant difference between cast alone and additional K-wires with regards to range of motion and functional outcome. However, there was significant statistical heterogeneity between the studies for flexion/extension and pronation/supination. Colaris et al.[37] did however find a statistically significant worse outcome with regard to pronation and supination in the largest RCT in this metaanalysis. Khandekar et al.[43] found in their systematic review that K-wire fixation of displaced distal radius fractures gave a re-displacement rate ranging from 0% to 43%, with a 43% re-displacement rate only found in one study. Thereby, they reported only minor complications (0%–38%) without any nonunion, growth arrest, compartment syndrome, or permanent nerve injury.

In addition to the trials in the Cochrane review, we found one retrospective study by Egmond et al.[42] In this study, 42% of the patients with a complete metaphyseal both-bone fracture required secondary reduction after treatment with closed reduction and cast alone. None of the patients in the K-wire group required secondary reduction.

Furthermore, van Egmond et al.[44] performed a retrospective cohort study on the outcome after volar plating of unstable DRFs in children with a median age of 12.5 years (IQR 9–15). In 26 consecutive children, no statistically significant difference in radiographic outcome was seen between the treated and untreated forearm. Two children complained of wrist stiffness.

RECOMMENDATION

In pediatric distal forearm fractures with involvement of the physis:

Recommendation	Overall Quality
• Closed/open reduction and cast immobilization provide excellent functional outcome.	⊕⊕⊕○ MODERATE
• If closed reduction does not result in an anatomical alignment, open reduction and additional K-wire fixation is recommended, especially in older children	⊕⊕⊕○ MODERATE
• In displaced SH II/III fractures a volar buttress plate can be used in selected cases of volar displacement	⊕⊕○○ LOW
• Closed reduction of a SH II fracture after 7 days should only be performed if the fracture does not have enough remodeling potential	⊕⊕○○ LOW

In pediatric distal forearm fractures without involvement of the physis:

Recommendation	Overall Quality
• In a minimally displaced torus/greenstick fracture a splint or swim cast can be applied for 2–4 weeks	⊕⊕⊕○ MODERATE
• Minimally displaced fractures of the distal forearm are most effectively treated with a below-elbow cast.	⊕⊕⊕⊕ HIGH
• Follow-up at 1-week interval is paramount because even seemingly stable fractures can displace during treatment (Fig. 4).	⊕⊕⊕○ MODERATE
• Additional percutaneous K-wire fixation after reduction of displaced metaphyseal forearm fractures reduces the risk of fracture re-displacement and secondary reduction.	⊕⊕⊕○ MODERATE
• Additional K-wire fixation after reduction of displaced metaphyseal forearm fractures does not improve functional outcome when compared to cast alone	⊕⊕⊕○ MODERATE
• Unstable distal radius fractures can be treated with volar plating	⊕⊕○○ LOW

CONCLUSION

Fractures With Involvement of the Physis

Regarding physeal fractures of the DRFs, nonoperative treatment seems to be the treatment of choice with a high rate of success. Multiple attempts at reduction, and late re-manipulation at more than 7 days post injury are known risk factors for physeal arrest. Especially in older children with a persistent fracture displacement after

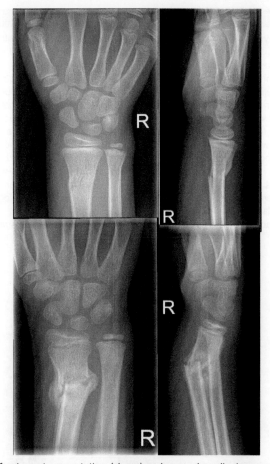

FIG. 4 Greenstick fracture at presentation *(above)* and secondary displacement at 6 weeks *(below)*.

closed reduction, open reduction and fixation with a K-wire is recommended. With regards to volar plating, the quality of evidence is too low to recommend its' routine use.

Fractures Without Involvement of the Physis

In non- or minimally displaced fractures of the distal radius in children a splint or swim cast gives similar results with regards to outcome and complications as a full rigid cast, with better patient and parent satisfaction. Minimally displaced fractures of the distal forearm in children are

recommended to treat nonoperatively with a below-elbow cast. In displaced fractures of the distal forearm, additional percutaneous K-wire fixation reduces the risk of fracture re-displacement and secondary reduction. The frequently seen complications of pinning might be reduced by a proper surgical technique, especially not cutting the K-wires too short to prevent subcutaneous migration. Treatment of DRFs with volar plating is reported in the literature but comparison with other treatment modalities is lacking. Therefore, better evidence for the use volar plating in pediatric distal radius fractures is needed.

Panel 2: Author's Preferred Technique

Displaced DRFs involving the physis, such as the one presented in the case scenario (Fig. 1), are generally reduced and treated in cast. If an acceptable reduction cannot be achieved additional K-wire fixation should be performed.

In case of secondary displacement after 1 week (Fig. 2), re-reduction should not be performed because of the chance of physeal damage with growth disturbance.

The boy was asked to return to the outpatient clinic at 2 years follow-up to exclude growth abnormalities. Radiographs show complete remodeling (Fig. 5).

PERCUTANEOUS ADDITIONAL K-WIRE FIXATION

The fracture is reduced in the operating room under general anesthesia with fluoroscopic guidance (Fig. 6). After optimal reduction by closed means, the fracture is tested for stability.

A fracture is defined as unstable if full range of pronation and supination of the proximal forearm causes re-displacement of the fracture.

A small skin incision is made over the radial styloid and blunt dissection of soft tissue is carried out down to the bone. A K-wire is directed proximally and ulnarly across the fracture site, engaging the opposite cortex. A second K wire is inserted from dorsal to volar across the fracture site through a small incision over the interval between the fourth and fifth dorsal compartments after blunt dissection down to the bone. Care is taken not to cross the K-wires at the level of the fracture.

Injury to the sensory branch of the radial nerve and the extensor tendons is avoided. The K-wires are bent, cut and left outside the skin.

A below-elbow cast is applied.

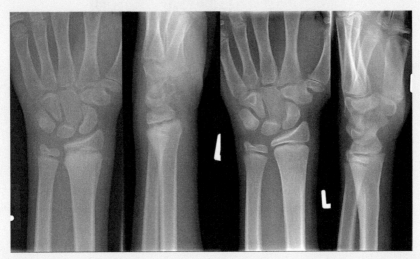

FIG. 5 Radiographs of a 14 year-old child with a SH II fracture with secondary fracture displacement in cast after 2 years of remodeling.

Continued

Panel 2: Author's Preferred Technique—cont'd

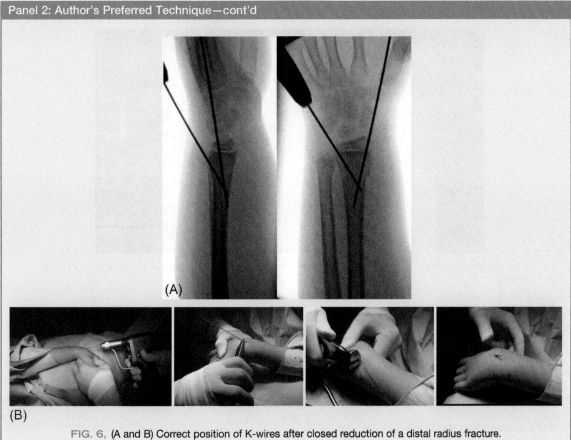

FIG. 6, (A and B) Correct position of K-wires after closed reduction of a distal radius fracture.

Panel 3: Pearls and Pitfalls

PEARLS:

- In case of a nonreducible SH II fracture, be mindful that interposition of a periosteal flap or the pronator quadratus muscle can prevent reduction.
- Proper blunt dissection prevents injury to the superficial branch of the radial nerve when performing K-wire fixation.[45]
- Fractures involving the physis should have a follow-up of at least 2 years to assess for growth abnormalities.

PITFALLS:

- Physeal fractures should not be reduced after 7 days in order to prevent further damage to the physis.

- Try to avoid penetration of the physis by K-wires, and if needed preferable use smooth K-wires with the thinnest diameter (minimum 1 mm, maximum 1.6 mm).[46]
- Do not cut the K-wires too short to prevent subcutaneous migration.
- The K-wire should not cross each other in the fracture plane, this causes instability and gives a higher risk of secondary displacement (Fig. 7).

Continued

Panel 3: Pearls and Pitfalls—cont'd

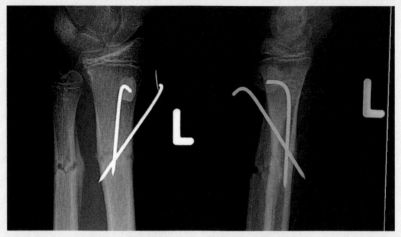

FIG. 7 Incorrect position of K-wires after operative treatment of a distal radius fracture (crossing K-wires in the fracture).

Editor's Tips & Tricks: Volar plating in children
Geert Alexander Buijze

In case of high degree of displacement such as the current physis-sparing metaphyseal antebrachial fracture, open reduction may be required (notably in older children) to remove incarcerated tissue and free periosteum to improve reduction. © Dr. Buijze 2020.

Although no superiority is shown in the literature—as pointed out by the authors of this chapter—for unstable fractures it can be advantageous to prebend the smallest available volar plate near-straight and fixate it with (nonlocking) screws well proximal to the physis. © Dr. Buijze 2020.

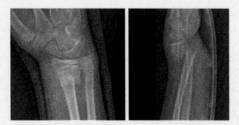

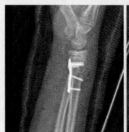 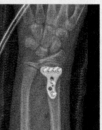

Continued

Editor's Tips & Tricks: Volar plating in children—cont'd

A splitted circular above-elbow cast may be necessary for the first 2 to 4 weeks postoperatively awaiting some early consolidation of the ulnar fracture, although in line with the author's findings a below-elbow cast may suffice. © Dr. Buijze 2020.

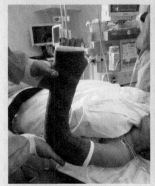
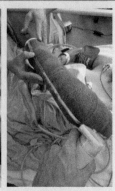

REFERENCES

1. Noonan KJ, Price CT. Forearm and distal radius fractures in children. *J Am Acad Orthop Surg*. 1998;6(3):146–156.
2. Landin LA. Epidemiology of children's fractures. *J Pediatr Orthop B*. 1997;6(2):79–83.
3. Larsen MC, Bohm KC, Rizkala AR, Ward CM. Outcomes of nonoperative treatment of Salter-Harris II distal radius fractures: a systematic review. *Hand (N Y)*. 2016;11 (1):29–35.
4. Houshian S, Holst AK, Larsen MS, Torfing T. Remodeling of Salter-Harris type II epiphyseal plate injury of the distal radius. *J Pediatr Orthop*. 2004;24(5):472–476.
5. Lee BS, Esterhai Jr. JL, Das M. Fracture of the distal radial epiphysis. Characteristics and surgical treatment of premature, post-traumatic epiphyseal closure. *Clin Orthop Relat Res*. 1984;185:90–96.
6. Gibbons CL, Woods DA, Pailthorpe C, Carr AJ, Worlock P. The management of isolated distal radius fractures in children. *J Pediatr Orthop*. 1994;14(2):207–210.
7. Do TT, Strub WM, Foad SL, Mehlman CT, Crawford AH. Reduction versus remodeling in pediatric distal forearm fractures: a preliminary cost analysis. *J Pediatr Orthop B*. 2003;12(2):109–115.
8. Dua K, Stein MK, O'Hara NN, et al. Variation among pediatric orthopaedic surgeons when diagnosing and treating pediatric and adolescent distal radius fractures. *J Pediatr Orthop*. 2019;39(6):306–313. https://doi.org/10.1097/BPO.0000000000000954.
9. Huetteman HE, Shauver MJ, Malay S, Chung TT, Chung KC. Variation in the treatment of distal radius fractures in the United States: 2010 to 2015. *Plast Reconstr Surg*. 2019;143(1):159–167.
10. Nietosvaara Y, Hasler C, Helenius I, Cundy P. Marked initial displacement predicts complications in physeal fractures of the distal radius: an analysis of fracture characteristics, primary treatment and complications in 109 patients. *Acta Orthop*. 2005;76(6):873–877.
11. Shah H, Chavali V, Daveshwar R. Adolescent volar barton fracture with open physis treated with volar plating using buttressing principle. *Malays Orthop J*. 2015;9(2):47–50.
12. Cha SM, Shin HD. Buttress plating for volar Barton fractures in children: Salter-Harris II distal radius fractures in sagittal plane. *J Pediatr Orthop B*. 2019;28(1):73–78.
13. Cannata G, De Maio F, Mancini F, Ippolito E. Physeal fractures of the distal radius and ulna: long-term prognosis. *J Orthop Trauma*. 2003;17(3):172–179 [discussion 179–180].
14. Luscombe KL, Chaudhry S, Dwyer JS, Shanmugam C, Maffulli N. Selective Kirschner wiring for displaced distal radial fractures in children. *Acta Orthop Traumatol Turc*. 2010;44(2):117–123.
15. Hove LM, Brudvik C. Displaced paediatric fractures of the distal radius. *Arch Orthop Trauma Surg*. 2008;128(1):55–60.
16. McQuinn AG, Jaarsma RL. Risk factors for redisplacement of pediatric distal forearm and distal radius fractures. *J Pediatr Orthop*. 2012;32(7):687–692.
17. Davis DR, Green DP. Forearm fractures in children: pitfalls and complications. *Clin Orthop Relat Res*. 1976;120: 172–183.
18. Handoll HH, Elliott J, Iheozor-Ejiofor Z, Hunter J, Karantana A. Interventions for treating wrist fractures in children. *Cochrane Database Syst Rev*. 2018;12:CD012470.
19. Pountos I, Clegg J, Siddiqui A. Diagnosis and treatment of greenstick and torus fractures of the distal radius in children: a prospective randomised single blind study. *J Child Orthop*. 2010;4(4):321–326.
20. Boutis K, Willan A, Babyn P, Goeree R, Howard A. Cast versus splint in children with minimally angulated fractures of the distal radius: a randomized controlled trial. *CMAJ*. 2010;182(14):1507–1512.
21. Zhu M, Lokino ES, Chan CS, Gan AJ, Ong LL, Lim KB. Cast immobilisation for the treatment of paediatric distal radius fracture: fibreglass versus polyolefin. *Singap Med J*. 2019;60 (4):183–187.

22. Silva M, Avoian T, Warnock RS, Sadlik G, Ebramzadeh E. It is not just comfort: waterproof casting increases physical functioning in children with minimally angulated distal radius fractures. *J Pediatr Orthop B*. 2017;26(5):417–423.

23. Ploegmakers JJ, Verheyen CC. Acceptance of angulation in the non-operative treatment of paediatric forearm fractures. *J Pediatr Orthop B*. 2006;15(6):428–432.

24. Karimi Mobarakeh M, Nemati A, Noktesanj R, Fallahi A, Safari S. Application of removable wrist splint in the management of distal forearm torus fractures. *Trauma Mon*. 2013;17(4):370–372.

25. Oakley EA, Ooi KS, Barnett PL. A randomized controlled trial of 2 methods of immobilizing torus fractures of the distal forearm. *Pediatr Emerg Care*. 2008;24(2):65–70.

26. Derksen RJ, Commandeur JP, Deij R, Breederveld RS. Swim cast versus traditional cast in pediatric distal radius fractures: a prospective randomized controlled trial. *J Child Orthop*. 2013;7(2):117–121.

27. West S, Andrews J, Bebbington A, Ennis O, Alderman P. Buckle fractures of the distal radius are safely treated in a soft bandage: a randomized prospective trial of bandage versus plaster cast. *J Pediatr Orthop*. 2005;25(3):322–325.

28. Davidson JS, Brown DJ, Barnes SN, Bruce CE. Simple treatment for torus fractures of the distal radius. *J Bone Joint Surg (Br)*. 2001;83(8):1173–1175.

29. Splint equal to cast for wrist buckle fracture in children. *J Fam Pract*. 2006;55(6):476.

30. Colaris JW, Biter LU, Allema JH, et al. Below-elbow cast for metaphyseal both-bone fractures of the distal forearm in children: a randomised multicentre study. *Injury*. 2012;43(7):1107–1111.

31. Schreck MJ, Hammert WC. Comparison of above- and below-elbow casting for pediatric distal metaphyseal forearm fractures. *J Hand Surg [Am]*. 2014;39(2):347–349.

32. Bohm ER, Bubbar V, Yong Hing K, Dzus A. Above and below-the-elbow plaster casts for distal forearm fractures in children. A randomized controlled trial. *J Bone Joint Surg Am*. 2006;88(1):1–8.

33. Paneru SR, Rijal R, Shrestha BP, et al. Randomized controlled trial comparing above- and below-elbow plaster casts for distal forearm fractures in children. *J Child Orthop*. 2010;4(3):233–237.

34. Webb GR, Galpin RD, Armstrong DG. Comparison of short and long arm plaster casts for displaced fractures in the distal third of the forearm in children. *J Bone Joint Surg Am*. 2006;88(1):9–17.

35. Sengab A, Krijnen P, Schipper IB. Risk factors for fracture redisplacement after reduction and cast immobilization of displaced distal radius fractures in children: a meta-analysis. *Eur J Trauma Emerg Surg*. 2020;46(4):789–800. https://doi.org/10.1007/s00068-019-01227-w.

36. Ploegmakers JJW, Groen W, Haverlag R, Bulstra SK. Predictors for losing reduction after reposition in conservatively treated both-bone forearm fractures in 38 children. *J Clin Orthop Trauma*. 2020;11(2):269–274.

37. Colaris JW, Allema JH, Biter LU, et al. Re-displacement of stable distal both-bone forearm fractures in children: a randomised controlled multicentre trial. *Injury*. 2013;44(4):498–503.

38. McLauchlan GJ, Cowan B, Annan IH, Robb JE. Management of completely displaced metaphyseal fractures of the distal radius in children. A prospective, randomised controlled trial. *J Bone Joint Surg (Br)*. 2002;84(3):413–417.

39. Sengab A, Krijnen P, Schipper IB. Displaced distal radius fractures in children, cast alone vs additional K-wire fixation: a meta-analysis. *Eur J Trauma Emerg Surg*. 2019;45(6):1003–1011.

40. Miller BS, Taylor B, Widmann RF, Bae DS, Snyder BD, Waters PM. Cast immobilization versus percutaneous pin fixation of displaced distal radius fractures in children: a prospective, randomized study. *J Pediatr Orthop*. 2005;25(4):490–494.

41. Ozcan M, Memisoglu S, Copuroglu C, Saridogan K. Percutaneous Kirschner Wire fixation in distal radius metaphyseal fractures in children: does it change the overall outcome? *Hippokratia*. 2010;14(4):265–270.

42. van Egmond PW, Schipper IB, van Luijt PA. Displaced distal forearm fractures in children with an indication for reduction under general anesthesia should be percutaneously fixated. *Eur J Orthop Surg Traumatol*. 2012;22(3):201–207.

43. Khandekar S, Tolessa E, Jones S. Displaced distal end radius fractures in children treated with Kirschner wires—a systematic review. *Acta Orthop Belg*. 2016;82(4):681–689.

44. van Egmond JC, Selles CA, Cleffken BI, Roukema GR, van der Vlies KH, Schep NWL. Plate fixation for unstable displaced distal radius fractures in children. *J Wrist Surg*. 2019;8(5):384–387.

45. Poublon AR, Walbeehm ET, Duraku LS, et al. The anatomical relationship of the superficial radial nerve and the lateral antebrachial cutaneous nerve: a possible factor in persistent neuropathic pain. *J Plast Reconstr Aesthet Surg*. 2015;68(2):237–242.

46. Kocher MS, Millis MB. *Pediatric Orthopaedic Surgery*. Philadelphia, PA: Elsevier/Saunders; 2011.

CHAPTER 26

Pediatric Forearm Fractures

A.E. VAN DER WINDT[a] • A.R. POUBLON[b] • J.H.J.M. BESSEMS[a] •
JOOST W. COLARIS[a]

[a]Orthopedics, Erasmus MC, Rotterdam, Netherlands, [b]Orthopedics, Elisabeth-TweeSteden Hospital, Tilburg, Netherlands

KEY POINTS

- Accept only minor fracture displacement in diaphyseal forearm fractures because the remodeling capacity is low and even mild malunion can result in impaired forearm rotation.
- Diaphyseal forearm fractures that are stable after reduction can be treated nonoperatively with an above-elbow cast followed by a below-elbow cast. Unstable fractures need additional fixation.
- Re-fractures occur frequently and give a higher change of impaired forearm rotation.

Panel 1: Case Scenario

A 10-year-old girl visits the emergency department after a fall from a trampoline on her outstretched right arm. Radiographs show a both-bone diaphyseal forearm fracture with angulation in the sagittal and coronal plane (Fig. 1).

After reduction in the emergency department, the maximum fracture angulation is still >10 degrees. This is accepted by the attending physician and she is treated with an above-elbow cast.

Six weeks later the cast is removed. The radiographs (Fig. 2) show a residual angulation and the girl has a limitation in pro- and supination. She is told this will improve as she ages. The girl is discharged from further care.

Three years later the girl attends your outpatient clinic with a persistent pro-supination impairment (Fig. 3). Is this going to improve with age?

A further 5 years later (Fig. 4), the patient is now 18 years old, and still has an impairment of pro-supination on the right side. Was the initial notion that the deformity and impairment will diminish with age correct?

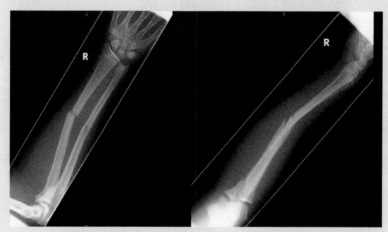

FIG. 1 Ten-year-old girl with a displaced both-bone diaphyseal forearm fracture.

Continued

Distal Radius Fractures. https://doi.org/10.1016/B978-0-323-75764-5.00031-7

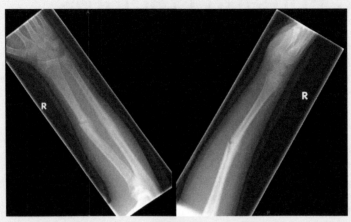

FIG. 2 Ten-year-old girl with residual deformity of a both-bone diaphyseal forearm fracture after reduction in the emergency room and treatment in an above-elbow cast.

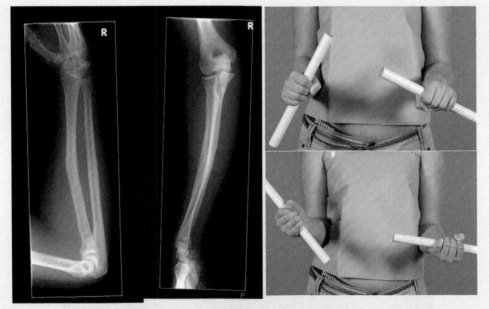

FIG. 3 Thirteen-year-old girl, who sustained a both-bone diaphyseal forearm fracture 3 years ago, with impaired forearm rotation and malunion after 3 years.

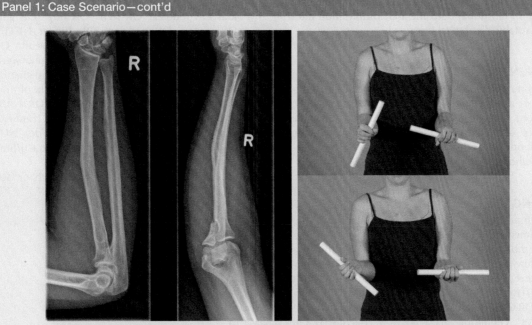

FIG. 4 Eighteen-year-old girl, who sustained a both-bone diaphyseal forearm fracture 8 years ago, with impaired forearm rotation and malunion after 8 years.

IMPORTANCE OF THE PROBLEM

Forearm fractures are the most common fractures among children between 0 and 14 years of age.[1] The most frequent mechanism of injury is a fall on the outstretched hand. Forearm rotation can be limited after a fracture and affects daily activities if pronation or supination is less than 50 degrees.[2] When treating pediatric forearm fractures, the basic principle is to accurately align, angularly and rotationally, both the radius and the ulna.

Both-bone forearm fractures can be anatomically divided in distal (metaphyseal), midshaft (diaphyseal), and proximal fractures. Distal fractures are the most common, while proximal fractures are rare. Furthermore, a differentiation is made between incomplete fractures typical for children (torus/buckle, greenstick, and bowing/plastic deformation) and complete fractures that occur in children as well as in adults. The treatment of both-bone forearm fractures depends on anatomical location, fracture displacement (minimally or severely displaced), and the expected growth remaining. Remodeling of an angulated fracture during the remaining growth is highest in young children with a fracture location close to the most active distal growth plate and an angulation in the sagittal plane.

MAIN QUESTION

What is the relative effect of closed reduction and cast immobilization versus closed reduction and internal fixation versus open reduction and internal fixation on functional outcome and complication rates in management of pediatric diaphyseal forearm fractures?

We divided the main question in the following three subquestions:

1. Is it safe to switch to a below-elbow cast after 3 weeks in the nonoperative treatment of minimally displaced diaphyseal fractures and displaced diaphyseal fractures that are stable after reduction?
2. What is the relative effect of closed reduction versus closed reduction and internal fixation (by intramedullary device) versus open reduction and internal fixation by plate on functional outcome and complication rates of unstable diaphyseal fractures?

3. Is single bone fixation as effective as both-bone fixation on functional outcome and complication rates of unstable diaphyseal fractures?

CURRENT OPINION

Both-bone diaphyseal forearm fractures which are minimally or nondisplaced can be treated nonoperatively. Displaced fractures need reduction and unstable fractures after reduction need additional fixation. Current opinion is divided with regard to the best fixation method.

FINDING THE EVIDENCE

- Cochrane search: Pediatric forearm fracture
- Pubmed (Medline):
  - Embase ('forearm fracture'/de OR 'radius fracture'/exp. OR 'ulna fracture'/exp. OR 'wrist fracture'/de OR 'distal radius fracture'/exp. OR (((forearm* OR fore-arm OR radius* OR ulna OR wrist* OR antebrach* OR both-bone* OR colles* OR monteggia*) NEAR/3 (fracture*)) OR ((salter-harris* OR epiphys*-plate* OR growth-plate* OR intra-articul* OR intraarticul*) AND (wrist* OR radius* OR ulna))):ab,ti,kw) AND ('fracture treatment'/exp. OR 'closed reduction (procedure)'/exp. OR 'open reduction (procedure)'/exp. OR 'bone resection'/de OR 'orthopedic surgery'/de OR (ORIF OR CRIF OR plaster* OR cast* OR k-wire* OR plate* OR nail* OR reduction* OR fixat* OR osteosynth* OR ilizarov* OR splint* OR ((therapy OR therapies OR treat* OR immobili*) NEAR/3 (fracture*)) OR ((orthoped*) NEAR/3 (surgic* OR surger* OR procedur*))):ab,ti,kw) AND ('Controlled clinical trial'/exp. OR 'Crossover procedure'/de OR 'Double-blind procedure'/de OR 'Single-blind procedure'/de OR 'review'/exp. OR 'meta-analysis'/de OR (meta-analys* OR meta-analys* OR review* OR random* OR factorial* OR crossover* OR (cross NEXT/1 over*) OR placebo* OR ((doubl* OR singl*) NEXT/1 blind*) OR assign* OR allocat* OR volunteer* OR trial OR groups):ab,ti,kw) AND (child/exp. OR adolescent/exp. OR adolescence/exp. OR pediatrics/exp. OR childhood/exp. OR 'child welfare'/de OR 'child development'/de OR 'child growth'/de OR 'child health'/de OR 'child health care'/exp. OR 'child care'/exp. OR 'childhood disease'/exp. OR 'pediatric ward'/de OR 'pediatric hospital'/de OR 'pediatric anesthesia'/de OR (adolescen* OR preadolescen* OR infan* OR child* OR kid OR kids OR toddler* OR teen* OR boy* OR girl* OR minors OR underag* OR (under NEXT/1 (age* OR aging OR ageing)) OR juvenil* OR youth* OR kindergar* OR puber* OR pubescen* OR prepubescen* OR prepubert* OR pediatric* OR paediatric* OR school* OR preschool* OR highschool* OR suckling* OR PICU OR NICU OR PICUs OR NICUs):ab,ti,kw) NOT ((animal/exp. OR animal*:de OR nonhuman/de) NOT ('human'/exp)) NOT ([Conference Abstract]/lim)
- Bibliography of eligible articles
- Articles that were not in the English, French, or German language were excluded.

QUALITY OF THE EVIDENCE

Level I:
Randomized controlled trials: 4
Level II:
Systematic review of observational studies: 2
Prospective studies: 2
Level III:
Retrospective comparative studies: 3

FINDINGS

In this chapter, we will discuss the evidence about the most effective treatment for both-bone diaphyseal forearm fractures. Fractures of the distal forearm are discussed in the previous chapter (pediatric distal radius fractures).

Nonoperative Treatment of Diaphyseal Both-Bone Forearm Fractures

Maximum acceptable angulations according to age for both-bone forearm fractures and plastic deformation were defined according to the graphs minus one standard deviation, shown in the metaanalysis by Ploegmakers et al.[3] (Graph 1A and B). In a prospective cohort study by Barvelink et al.,[4] fracture remodeling in relation to functional outcome is observed in nonreduced minimally displaced forearm fractures. After 1 year, the mean fracture angulation of 12 degrees measured at initial presentation was reduced to a mean residual angulation of 4 degrees. No significant differences for either grip strength or range of motion between the affected and the unaffected forearm were found. These results suggest that residual angulation of 4 degrees is of no functional concern. Nonoperative treatment without reduction could therefore be a good treatment option in minimally angulated forearm fractures.

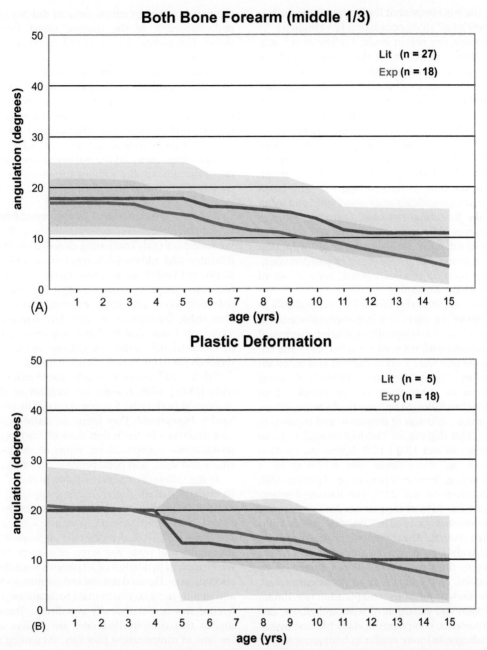

GRAPH 1 (A and B) Graphs showing age (years) plotted against angulation (degrees). The lines represent the limit of acceptance of deformity for both-bone diaphyseal fractures and plastic deformity for each age; pooled data from literature (Lit; *blue line*) and experts' opinion (Exp; *red line*) with one standard deviation.

However, the most important limitation of this study is the relatively small study population (26 children).

In a retrospective cohort study, Hadizie et al.[5] analyzed the long-term results of diaphyseal both-bone forearm fractures in children with a minimum of 4 years of growth remaining. In all patients, the fractures were reduced and treated in an above-elbow cast. The mean angular correction by growth for radius and ulna were 7.4 degrees (72% correction) and 6.7 degrees (75% correction), respectively, at skeletal maturity. The degree of angulation post reduction and at skeletal maturity did not influence the functional outcome at skeletal maturity. Age at the time of fracture was the only factor proven to have a significant association with, and influence on, the functional outcome. Seventeen patients were 10 years or older at time of the fracture and all of them developed some limitation in range of motion (supination/pronation). In the group of patients younger than 10 years at time of fracture, only 2 out of 27 developed any limitation.

Only one randomized controlled trial is available in literature about the effect of a below-elbow versus an above-elbow cast for minimally displaced diaphyseal forearm fractures without need for reduction.[6] The criteria for reduction were a priori defined and based on earlier studies.[3] The children were randomly allocated to 6 weeks of an above-elbow cast or 3 weeks of an above-elbow cast followed by 3 weeks of a below-elbow cast. The mean limitation of pronation and supination was 23.3 ± 22.0 degrees for children treated with an above-elbow cast and 18.0 ± 16.9 degrees for children treated with an above-elbow cast followed by a below-elbow cast. The overall percentage of patients with fracture displacement was 23%. The fracture displacement occurred in 91% of the patients during treatment with an above-elbow cast and in 73% of the patients during the first 3 weeks. Thus, even minimally displaced diaphyseal both-bone forearm fractures in children have a tendency to displace, and this is not prevented by immobilization of the elbow in an above-elbow cast. All other secondary outcomes (complication rate, limitation of flexion and extension of wrist and elbow, cast comfort, cosmetics, complaints in daily life and assessment of radiographs) were similar in both groups.

Only one randomized controlled trial was available in literature about the effect of a below-elbow versus an above-elbow cast for displaced diaphyseal both-bone forearm fractures that are stable after reduction. Colaris et al.[7] randomly allocated children to 6 weeks of an above-elbow cast or 3 weeks of an above-elbow cast followed by 3 weeks of a below-elbow cast. A fracture was defined as stable after reduction if full pronation and supination of the proximal forearm did not cause any re-displacement of the fracture under fluoroscopic vision. The authors found no differences in limitation of pronation or supination between groups after 6 months of follow-up and an overall re-displacement rate of 34%. All re-displacements occurred in the first 3 weeks of the treatment, and in 9 out of 43 children the fractures were reduced again. Interestingly, the slightly higher rate of re-displacement in fractures reduced at the emergency department (42% vs 30% in the operating room) led the authors to suspect that testing of fracture stability without anesthesia and fluoroscopy is less optimal.

Operative Treatment of Diaphyseal Forearm Fractures

We found no trials comparing closed reduction versus reduction and additional internal fixation of displaced diaphyseal both-bone forearm fractures. However, the consensus seems that fractures that are unstable after reduction need additional internal fixation because even stable fractures show secondary displacement in 34%.[7] We found one RCT and one systematic review of observational studies comparing different fixation methods for diaphyseal both-bone fractures.

Sahin et al.[8] compared elastic stable intramedullary nails (ESIN) with K-wires for fixation of displaced diaphyseal both-bone forearm fractures in 40 children aged 8–16 years old. They found no statistically significant difference in the union time of fractures, rate of postoperative complications, range of motion of the elbow and wrist, and postoperative symptoms.

In the systematic review by Baldwin et al.,[9] 12 level-III evidence observational studies comparing intramedullary (IM) nails with plate and screw fixation of displaced both-bone forearm fractures were analyzed. The literature fails to demonstrate a difference between IM nailing and plate and screw constructs. Outcomes were excellent in nearly 9 of 10 patients regardless of fixation strategy. Delayed unions and nonunions were rare and slightly more common in IM nails, although the difference was not statistically significant. These results suggest that complication rates are similar, although the type of complication may vary. IM nailing provides improved cosmetics but in general requires a second operation to remove hardware.

In addition, a prospective comparative study by Zhu et al.[10] compared the clinical outcomes of hybrid fixation using ESIN for the ulna and plate fixation for the radius (hybrid group) with dual plating fixation for both-bone forearm fractures in children between 10 and 16 years of age. Again, no differences were found in fracture union rates or functional outcome between groups. Complication rates were also similar between the groups. Incision length of ulna, duration of surgery, and hospital costs were significantly lower in the hybrid group ($P < .05$).

Zheng et al.[11] retrospectively compared three fixation techniques: dual ESIN, hybrid fixation, and dual plating in children aged 10–16 years. Surgeries and incisions were significantly shorter, and less intraoperative blood loss occurred, in the hybrid group compared with the double plate group ($P < .001$). The hybrid group was also characterized by less intraoperative fluoroscopy times and shorter duration of postoperative immobilization compared with the double ESIN group ($P < .001$). The union rate of the ulna at 3 months postoperatively was greater in the hybrid and double plate groups (86.7% and 90.9%, respectively) than in the dual ESIN group (64.6%, $P = .003$). The union rate of the radius was similar in all three groups ($P = .403$). All fractures of the radius had healed well at 6 months postoperatively. Two patients in the dual ESIN group showed nonunion of the ulna at 6 months postoperatively, and the mean time to union was longer in the dual ESIN group (10.3 weeks) than in the hybrid group (9.3 weeks) and the double plate group (9.1 weeks, $P = .020$). Again, no significant differences in functional outcome ($P = .822$) or complication rate ($P = .912$) were observed among the three groups.

Yong et al.[12] analyzed 1 RCT and 5 retrospective studies comparing single bone fixation with dual bone fixation in pediatric forearm fractures. There was substantial heterogeneity between the retrospective studies in terms of populations studied and interventions used. The authors of this systematic review suggest that single bone fixation might be a suitable treatment alternative for both-bone forearm fractures in children. Compared with the both-bone procedure, single bone fixation is less invasive, reduces both operative time, and fluoroscopy radiation exposure but the arm should be immobilized in cast postoperatively. However, pooled data from these studies suggest that patients managed with single bone fixation are at greater risk of re-displacement. The only RCT about this topic by Colaris et al.[13] showed that re-displacement of the fracture occurred in those fractures without an intramedullary nail in 4 out of 11 children. The authors of this RCT caution against the use of single-bone fixation in all both-bone forearm fractures.

This thought is supported by the more recent retrospective review of Crighton et al.[14] where their series show a propensity to increased angulation of fractures

fixed by single bone elastic intramedullary nail (7/13 in this group, compared to 0/23 in the dual bone fixation group).

RECOMMENDATION

In patients with a diaphyseal both-bone forearm fractures, evidence suggests:

Recommendation	Overall Quality
• Nonoperative treatment of minimally displaced diaphyseal forearm fractures gives good functional outcome, especially when a minimum of 4 years of growth remains.	⊕⊕○○ LOW
• It seems safe to convert to a below-elbow cast after 3 weeks of an above-elbow cast, in the nonoperative treatment of minimally displaced diaphyseal both-bone forearm fractures without need for reduction	⊕⊕○○ LOW
• Displaced diaphyseal both-bone forearm fractures that are stable after reduction can be treated nonoperatively. It is safe to convert to a below-elbow cast after 3 weeks. However, also minimally displaced and stable diaphyseal both-bone forearm fractures in children have a tendency to displace and frequent follow-up within the first 3 weeks is strongly recommended	⊕⊕⊕○ MODERATE
• Diaphyseal forearm fractures that are unstable after reduction need additional internal fixation. All fixation techniques (intramedullary nailing, plate and screw constructs, hybrid fixation) are safe and effective to use. There is a slight preference for intramedullary nailing because it is esthetically superior	⊕⊕⊕○ MODERATE
• It is recommended to use a double bone fixation technique to reduce the risk of re-displacement.	⊕⊕⊕○ MODERATE

CONCLUSION

Minimally displaced diaphyseal forearm fractures that do not need reduction according to maximum acceptable angulations (Graph 1A and B) can be treated nonoperatively, with 3 weeks of above-elbow casting followed by 3 weeks of below-elbow casting.

This nonoperative treatment of minimally displaced diaphyseal fractures gives overall good functional outcome. Age at the time of fracture is the most important factor to have a significant association with, and influence on, the functional outcome because of the ability to correct angular malunion during remaining growth.

Displaced diaphyseal both-bone forearm fractures should be tested for stability after reduction by passive pronation and supination of the forearm under fluoroscopy.[7] Displaced both-bone diaphyseal forearm fractures that are stable after reduction can be treated nonoperatively. It is safe to convert to a below-elbow cast after 3 weeks. However, even minimally displaced and stable diaphyseal both-bone forearm fractures in children have a tendency to displace (23%–34%), and this is not prevented by immobilization of the elbow in an above-elbow cast. Therefore, it is important to check for re-displacement during at least the first 3 weeks. Secondary displacement should be reduced and internally fixated.

Both-bone diaphyseal forearm fractures that are unstable during passive pronation and supination after reduction need additional internal fixation. Fixation of both bones reduces the risk for re-displacement compared to the single bone technique. All fixation techniques (intramedullary nailing, plate and screw constructs, hybrid fixation) seem safe and effective to use. The literature fails to show differences in union rate, functional outcome, or complication rate between the different fixation techniques.

Panel 2: Author's Preferred Technique

In the case described earlier, the girl sustained a displaced both-bone forearm fracture which was reduced in the emergency department. Preferably, reduction is performed in the operating theater with fluoroscopic control because repeated reductions are possible and because unstable fractures can be treated with internal fixation. This case demonstrates that only little remodeling of the malunion can be expected during the remaining growth because of the high distance to the most active distal growth plate. Thereby, even mild malunion of diaphyseal (both-bone) forearm fractures can result in impaired forearm rotation which will not improve during growth. If reduction in the operating theater reveals an unstable fracture, the authors prefer elastic stable intramedullary nailing for both the ulna and the radius. The intramedullary nail in the radius will be inserted retrograde, with the entry point just proximal to the physis at Lister's tubercle or 10–20 mm proximal to the physis on the radial styloid. In both locations care should be taken not to injure either the extensor pollicis longus (Fig. 5) or the superficial branch of the radial nerve. Careful blunt dissection is therefore advised.

The nails should be prebent to ensure three points of contact: the entry point, the fracture site, and the tip of the nail. The bowing of both nails should be in such a way that they have opposite concavities and that the elastic memory provides stabilization through interosseous membrane tightening. The tips of the nails should be buried underneath the skin. In general, there is no need for postoperative cast immobilization and the patient is allowed to exercise the wrist and elbow without loading the forearm. Remove the nails after 6–12 months.

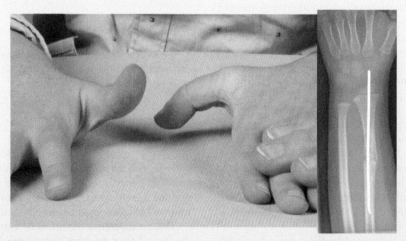

FIG. 5 Inability to extend the thumb caused by extensor pollicis longus rupture after treatment of a both-bone forearm fracture with ESIN.

PEARLS

- Preferably start with the most displaced bone first when performing the ESIN technique.
- The entry point for the ESIN should be guided under fluoroscopy as not to damage the physis.
- The skin incision is best placed slightly more distal to the entry point of the ESIN for the radius (and proximal for the ulna) as not to put pressure on the skin when the nail passes through the bone.

PITFALLS

- Pediatric diaphyseal forearm fractures will only minimally correct by growth and even mild malunion can result in impaired forearm rotation.[15]

- Risk factors for re-displacement in cast are: nondominant arm, complete fractures, translation of the ulna on the lateral radiographs, shortening of the bone, and the inability to obtain anatomic reduction.[16, 17] The casting indices do not correlate well as predictor of alignment loss.[17, 18]
- Re-fractures occur frequently and give an almost 12 times increased risk to end up with a limitation of pronation/supination of 20 degrees or more.[19]
- The use of a large diameter elastic nail can cause physeal arrest (Figs. 6 and 7).

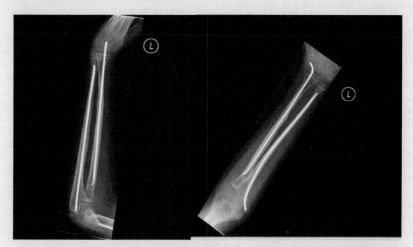

FIG. 6 Fixation of a both-bone diaphyseal forearm fractures with ESIN.

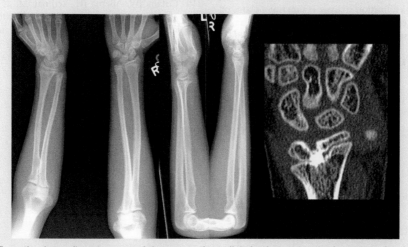

FIG. 7 The rather large diameter caused damage to the radial physis causing the formation of a physeal bar.

REFERENCES

1. Naranje SM, Erali RA, Warner Jr WC, Sawyer JR, Kelly DM. Epidemiology of pediatric fractures presenting to emergency departments in the United States. *J Pediatr Orthop.* 2016;36(4):e45–e48.
2. Morrey BF, Askew LJ, Chao EY. A biomechanical study of normal functional elbow motion. *J Bone Joint Surg Am.* 1981;63(6):872–877.
3. Ploegmakers JJ, Verheyen CC. Acceptance of angulation in the non-operative treatment of paediatric forearm fractures. *J Pediatr Orthop B.* 2006;15(6):428–432.
4. Barvelink B, Ploegmakers JJW, Harsevoort AGJ, et al. The evolution of hand function during remodelling in nonreduced angulated paediatric forearm fractures: a prospective cohort study. *J Pediatr Orthop B.* 2020;29(2): 172–178.
5. Hadizie D, Munajat I. Both-bone forearm fractures in children with minimum four years of growth remaining: can cast achieve a good outcome at skeletal maturity? *Malays Orthop J.* 2017;11(3):1–9.
6. Colaris JW, Reijman M, Allema JH, et al. Early conversion to below-elbow cast for non-reduced diaphyseal both-bone forearm fractures in children is safe: preliminary results of a multicentre randomised controlled trial. *Arch Orthop Trauma Surg.* 2013;133(10):1407–1414.
7. Colaris JW, Allema JH, Biter LU, et al. Conversion to below-elbow cast after 3 weeks is safe for diaphyseal both-bone forearm fractures in children. *Acta Orthop.* 2013;84 (5):489–494.
8. Sahin N, Akalin Y, Turker O, Ozkaya G. ESIN and K-wire fixation have similar results in pediatric both-bone diaphyseal forearm fractures. *Ulus Travma Acil Cerrahi Derg.* 2017;23(5):415–420.
9. Baldwin K, Morrison 3rd MJ, Tomlinson LA, Ramirez R, Flynn JM. Both bone forearm fractures in children and adolescents, which fixation strategy is superior—plates or nails? A systematic review and meta-analysis of observational studies. *J Orthop Trauma.* 2014;28(1): e8–e14.
10. Zhu S, Yang D, Gong C, Chen C, Chen L. A novel hybrid fixation versus dual plating for both-bone forearm fractures in older children: a prospective comparative study. *Int J Surg.* 2019;70:19–24.
11. Zheng W, Tao Z, Chen C, et al. Comparison of three surgical fixation methods for dual-bone forearm fractures in older children: a retrospective cohort study. *Int J Surg.* 2018;51:10–16.
12. Yong B, Yuan Z, Li J, et al. Single bone fixation versus both bone fixation for pediatric unstable forearm fractures: a systematic review and Metaanalysis. *Indian J Orthop.* 2018;52(5):529–535.
13. Colaris J, Reijman M, Allema JH, et al. Single-bone intramedullary fixation of unstable both-bone diaphyseal forearm fractures in children leads to increased re-displacement: a multicentre randomised controlled trial. *Arch Orthop Trauma Surg.* 2013;133 (8):1079–1087.
14. Crighton EA, Huntley JS. Single versus double intramedullary fixation of paediatric both bone forearm fractures: radiological outcomes. *Cureus.* 2018;10(4): e2544.
15. Colaris J, Reijman M, Allema JH, et al. Angular malalignment as cause of limitation of forearm rotation: an analysis of prospectively collected data of both-bone forearm fractures in children. *Injury.* 2014;45(6):955–959.
16. Colaris JW, Allema JH, Reijman M, et al. Risk factors for the displacement of fractures of both bones of the forearm in children. *Bone Joint J.* 2013;95-B(5):689–693.
17. Ploegmakers JJW, Groen W, Haverlag R, Bulstra SK. Predictors for losing reduction after reposition in conservatively treated both-bone forearm fractures in 38 children. *J Clin Orthop Trauma.* 2020;11(2):269–274.
18. Pretell Mazzini J, Rodriguez Martin J. Paediatric forearm and distal radius fractures: risk factors and re-displacement—role of casting indices. *Int Orthop.* 2010;34(3):407–412.
19. Colaris JW, Allema JH, Reijman M, et al. Which factors affect limitation of pronation/supination after forearm fractures in children? A prospective multicentre study. *Injury.* 2014;45(4):696–700.

CHAPTER 27

Distal Radius Fracture Fixation in the Elderly

GRACE XIONG[a] • CARL M. HARPER[b]

[a]Harvard Combined Orthopaedic Surgery Residency, Harvard Medical School, Boston, MA, United States, [b]Department of Orthopaedic Surgery, Harvard Medical School, Beth Israel Deaconess Medical Center, Boston, MA, United States

KEY POINTS

- Epidemiology: Fractures of the distal radius are the most common upper extremity fracture sustained in the elderly population. The incidence of these fractures is expected to increase in the future with increasing cost to the healthcare system.

- Nonsurgical Treatment: Conservative treatment has been shown to correlate with radiographic malunion, cosmetic deformity, and diminished grip strength. However, a number of studies have demonstrated that despite these issues, functional outcomes including DASH and PRWE are equivalent to operative treatment.

- Surgical Treatment: While operative treatment has been shown to result in superior radiographic outcomes and early improvement in grip strength, final functional outcomes were equivalent to conservative treatment. More recently, studies have shown not only improved radiographic outcomes but also functional improvement in the older population.

- Practice Patterns: While evidence remains unclear as to which patient would benefit from operative intervention, surveys demonstrate that a greater proportion of fractures are being treated operatively than would be expected based on outcomes data. The completion of a Hand Surgery fellowship strongly correlates with operative treatment.

- Contemporary Indications: More recent randomized controlled trials have demonstrated improved functional and radiographic outcomes following operative treatment as compared to conservative treatment in the more active older aged patient. It has been shown that in displaced, unstable fractures, both functional and radiographic outcomes are superior to nonoperative treatment with equivalent complication rates.

Panel 1: Case Scenario

A 72-year-old otherwise fit and active woman falls onto her outstretched right (dominant) arm while walking her dogs. She is seen in the ER where imaging is obtained demonstrating a right distal radius fracture (Fig. 1). She undergoes reduction and splinting and presents to clinic for repeat evaluation in 7 days. Her repeat imaging is shown (Fig. 2) with loss of height and worsening dorsal angulation. When discussing operative vs nonoperative treatment what are the expected outcomes for this patient?

Continued

Distal Radius Fractures. https://doi.org/10.1016/B978-0-323-75764-5.00004-4

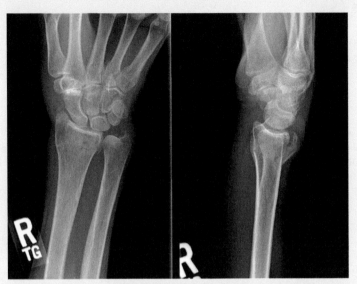

FIG. 1 Initial fracture demonstrating minimal displacement.

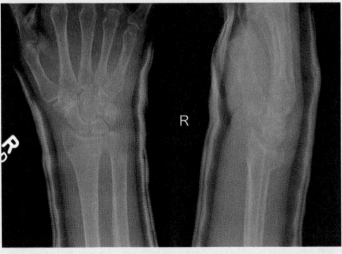

FIG. 2 Fracture at 1 week follow up demonstrating loss of radial length and dorsal angulation.

IMPORTANCE OF THE PROBLEM

Fractures of the distal radius are increasingly common, resulting in a cost of $170 million to Medicare alone.[1] They represent the most common fracture of the upper extremity and are the second most common fracture overall in women >60 years of age. With increasing life expectancy in most societies, the incidence of distal radius fractures (DRFs) has been steadily increasing over the past 40 years, particularly in the elderly population (defined as patients >65 years of age).[2] The lifetime risk of a Caucasian woman >60 sustaining a DRF is 15% (compared to 2% for men).[3] Thus, the injury burden imposed by fractures of the distal radius on society, particularly the elderly population, looms large. Radiographic parameters for operative vs nonoperative treatment have been well established for patients <65; however, consensus has yet to be reached regarding the optimal treatment for patients >65 years of age.[4] As clinical information continues to evolve, identifying evidence-based, cost-conscious practices will be essential for the sustainability of health systems worldwide.

MAIN QUESTION

What are the outcomes of operative vs nonoperative treatment of DRFs in the elderly population?

CURRENT OPINION

Historically, the majority of research has demonstrated that conservative treatment of DRFs resulted in equivalent clinical and functional outcomes with significantly fewer complications. Recently, several articles have supported operative intervention (with the use of anatomically shaped angular stable plate fixation) in these patients, challenging prior literature supporting conservative management.[5–7] In general, the incidence of operative treatment of DRFs in patients >65 years of age is increasing, particularly by surgeons with subspecialty train in hand surgery.[8] Proponents of conservative treatment cite equivalent functional outcome scores and a lower complication rate.[9] Proponents of operative fixation note increased grip strength and less cosmetic deformity (primarily with a volar locked plate), as well as earlier return to function.

FINDING THE EVIDENCE

The following Pubmed search algorithms were used to construct this chapter:

(((((((((("Radius fractures"[Mesh] OR distal radius fracture*[tiab]))) AND (("Geriatrics"[Mesh] OR elder* OR older*)))) AND ((*operative OR conservative OR *surgical)))))).

Articles were reviewed for relevance to the clinical question as well as study format and results. Articles were included if there was a full-text available in the English language.

QUALITY OF THE EVIDENCE

Thirty-three total studies were found which specifically addressed patient outcomes between operative and nonoperative management of DRFs in elderly patients. Owing to the comparative nature of the clinical question, no level IV studies were included. The level of evidence in relation to these studies were:

Level I:
- Randomized trials: 9

Level II:
- Prospective cohort studies: 3

Level III:
- Systematic Reviews/Metaanalyses of level I–III data: 5
- Retrospective cohort studies: 12

FINDINGS

Overview of Level I Evidence

There were no systematic reviews or metaanalyses which specifically focused on DRFs in the elderly and analyzed level I data. Nine randomized-controlled trials were included.

The RCTs included in the current review reflect overall trends of distal radius fixation. The two oldest studies compared external fixation with nonoperative treatment and found differences in radiographic but not functional outcomes. Moroni et al. (2004) randomized 40 elderly osteoporotic women with extraarticular DRFs and found that patients in the external fixation group had better preserved volar tilt and radial height at 6 weeks ($P = .008$) with no difference in SF-36 scores at 3 months.[10] Roumen et al. (1991), by contrast, randomized 101 Colles' fractures in patients greater than age 55 years and found similarly improved radiographic values based on the Lidstrom scale with no difference in functional outcomes, grip strength, nor any correlation between radiographic or functional parameters.[11]

Subsequent RCTs examined percutaneous pinning compared to nonoperative management with similar results compared with external fixation. Azzopardi et al. (2005) randomized 57 patients age 60 years or above with extraarticular DRFs to percutaneous pinning versus nonoperative management and found significant differences in radial height ($P=.03$), inclination ($P=.05$), and volar tilt ($P=.03$) at 1 year; however, no differences were reported in SF-36, pain, or activities of daily living scores.[12] Similarly, Wong et al. (2010) randomized 60 patients above age 65 years with extraarticular DRFs to pinning versus nonoperative management. They found higher rates of preserve radial height, inclination, and volar tilt in the percutaneous pinning group ($P<.05$), but no differences in quality of life or Mayo wrist scores.[13]

More recent RCTs have focused on volar locked plating in comparison with nonoperative management. Two studies found no significant advantage of surgical over nonoperative management. The earliest of these was Arora et al. (2011), who randomized 73 patients with AO type A or C DRFs to volar locked plating or nonoperative management.[14] Radiographic parameters were significantly improved in the operative group with improved volar tilt (3.0 vs −10.4 degrees, $P=.0001$), radial inclination (21.2 vs 15.9 degrees, $P<.0001$), ulnar variance (0.7 vs 3.2 mm, $P<.0001$), and articular stepoff (0.2 vs 0.6 mm, $P=.02$). Clinical outcomes at 1 year, however, showed no difference in DASH, PRWE scores, or range of motion, but did demonstrate improved grip strength in the operative group (22.2 vs 18.8 kg, $P=.02$). Of note, complications including tendon rupture or irritation because of screw or plate placement was significantly higher in the operative group ($P<.05$), while the nonoperative group had five cases of complex regional pain syndrome compared to two in the operative group. Bartl et al. (2014) found similar results in their study of 185 patients greater than 65 years of age with AO type C fractures. Radial inclination (20.3 vs 17.7 degrees, $P=.0005$), volar tilt (5.1 vs −3.7 degrees, $P<.001$) at 3 months were similarly improved in the operative group; however, SF-36, DASH, and ROM parameters were not significantly different between the two groups at 1 year.[15] Notably, 37 fractures randomized to nonsurgical treatment had subsequent loss of reduction requiring revision for a 41% conversion rate to surgical treatment, with C3 fractures having a 2.1 higher relative risk (95% CI 1.1 to 3.8) of conversion compared with C1 or C2 fractures.

By contrast, three more recent RCTs found advantages beyond radiographic improvement in volar locked plating compared with nonoperative treatment. Martinez-Mendez (2018) examined 90 patients above age 60 years with AO type C DRFs and found improved PRWE (17 vs 30, $P=.03$) and DASH (16 vs 28, $P=.04$) scores at 2 years, as well as improved supination (85 vs

72 degrees, $P=.01$) and pronation (84 vs 71 degrees, $P=.01$) in the operative group.[8] There was no difference in grip strength (64% casting vs 73% plating, $P=.15$). One patient in the nonoperative group developed CRPS. By contrast, two patients in the operative group required secondary operation, one for carpal tunnel syndrome and another for extensor pollicis longus tendon rupture. Saving et al. (2019) examined 140 patients above age 75 years with AO A or C DRFs types and similarly found better PRWE (7.5 vs 17.5, $P=.014$), DASH scores (8.3 vs 19.9, $P=.028$), and grip strength (96.8% vs 80.0%, $P=.001$) in the operative group which was accompanied by improved radiographic parameters.[9] They found no difference in complications between groups for either major (needing secondary operation, 14% operative, 11% nonoperative, $P=.6$) or minor complications (20% vs 11%, $P=.19$). Sirnio et al. (2019) found similar results in 80 patients over age 50 years with AO types A and C (excluding C3) fractures, with operatively treated patients exhibiting lower DASH scores compared with nonoperative treatment at 2 years (7.2 vs 14.4, $P=.0005$).[7] However, this difference may not be clinically significant. There was no significant difference in grip strength between the operative and nonoperative group (−1 kg, 95% −2 to 4). One case of Carpal tunnel syndrome required surgical release in the operative group, and three patients (two Carpal tunnel syndrome, one malunion) required secondary operation in the nonoperatively managed group.

Overview of Level II Evidence

There was one prospective cohort analysis that examined outcomes in elderly distal radius fractures in operative versus nonoperative management. The multicenter Wrist and Radius Injury Surgical Trial (WRIST) was a multicenter international study that was intended as a randomized controlled trial of surgical methods on DRFs in patients above age 60. Included fractures were unstable fractures which warranted surgical fixation, however, as part of the study, 117 of the 304 eligible participants opted for casting. Twelve-month follow-up demonstrated that the casting group had a relative risk of 1.88 (1.22–2.88) of developing any complication ($P<.01$);[16] however, this association was not significant when limited to moderate (requiring nonsurgical intervention) or severe (requiring surgical intervention) complications. The WRIST investigators also examined outcomes of the Michigan Hand Outcomes Questionnaire (MHQ) and found that opting for casting did not have a significant effect on 12-month outcomes,[17] nor did outcomes correlate with radiographic improvements (Table 1).[20]

TABLE 1
Randomized Controlled Trials Comparing Volar Locked Plating to Nonoperative Management.

Trial	Number of Subjects	DASH Scores (Operative Versus Nonoperative, P-value)	Grip Strength (Operative Versus Nonoperative, kg or %)	Complication Rate (Operative Versus Nonoperative)
Arora R. JBJS 2011	73	5.7 versus 8.0, $P = .34$	22.2 versus 18.8 kg, $P = .02$	13 versus 5, $P < .05$
Bartl C. Dtsch Arztebl Int. 2014	185	14.0 versus 19.0, $P = .102$	Not measured	84 versus 90, P-value not reported
Martinez-Mendez D. JHS Eur 2018	90	16 versus 28, $P = .04$	64% of unaffected side versus 73%, $P = .15$	2 versus 1, P-value not reported
Saving J. JBJS 2019	140	9.3 versus 19.9, $P = .028$	71.0% of unaffected side versus 53.9%, $P < .001$	11% versus 14%, $P = .606$ for major complications
Sirnio K. Acta Orthop. 2019	80	7.2 versus 14.4, $P = .0005$	27 versus 26 kg, $P = .2$	3 versus 5, P-value not reported

The differences shown by Aurora, Bartl and Sirnio while significant, may not be clinically relevant. The minimal clinically important DASH score has been shown to be ~10.[18] Minimal clinically important different for grip strength has been shown to be 6.5 kg.[19]

RECOMMENDATION

In elderly patients sustaining a fracture of the distal radius, evidence suggests:

Recommendation	Overall Quality
• Open reduction and internal fixation of DRFs in elderly patients have improved radiographic appearance at 1 year	⊕⊕⊕⊕ HIGH
• Open reduction and internal fixation can be associated with improved functional outcomes at 1 year compared with nonoperative treatment	⊕⊕○○ LOW
• Open reduction and internal fixation is associated with improved grip strength at 1 year compared with nonoperative treatment	⊕⊕○○ LOW
• Open reduction and internal fixation is associated with increased risk of secondary operation	⊕⊕○○ LOW

CONCLUSION

Fractures of the distal radius are increasingly common in the elderly population. Most historical studies agree that despite inferior radiographic outcomes, the functional outcomes of patients treated conservatively are equivalent to those patients treated operatively. Furthermore, the complication rate of operatively treated patients may be higher. More recent high-level studies have shown that operative treatment of elderly patients sustaining unstable, displaced, fractures of the distal radius may experience improved functional outcomes with equivalent complication rates. This finding is in keeping with current treatment trends, particularly among surgeons with subspecialty training in hand surgery. When possible, surgeons and patients should engage in shared decision making to ensure that realistic goals of treatment are discussed and appropriate expectations regarding outcomes are present.

Panel 2: Author's Preferred Technique

Prior to addressing treatment options we prefer to understand the patient's lifestyle and activity status. We then address the patients' goals and desired short- and long-term outcomes. These goals are contextualized with the radiographic findings. In the setting of a physiologically fit and active patient with an unstable DRF (meeting criteria for operative fixation in patients <65 years of age) who desires a faster return to function with the lowest degree of deformity, we recommend surgical fixation with a volar locked plate. Of note, we do not change our method of fixation (length of plate, number of locking screws, etc.) in the setting of a known diagnosis of osteoporosis. No difference has been shown in operative outcomes pertaining to load to failure, function, or radiologic outcomes in elderly patients with osteoporosis vs controls.[21, 22] In patients who lead relatively sedentary lifestyles and express an acceptance of clinical and radiographic deformity, we recommend short arm cast immobilization for 6 weeks with transition to a removable. Concurrent with cast immobilization we enact a rehabilitation protocol focusing on digital range of motion and edema control as well as shoulder and elbow range of motion to prevent stiffness.

Panel 3: Pearls and Pitfalls

PEARLS

- Developing a rapport and understanding of the goals of care with patients is essential. Educating patients and their families regarding the expected functional, radiographic and cosmetic outcomes of operative vs conservative treatment will help guide decision making.

- Extensive dorsal comminution, marked initial loss of radial length, associated ulnar neck fracture, dorsal angulation and known diagnosis of osteoporosis all predict subsequent loss of reduction with resultant malunion.

- Treatment with a low profile volar locked plate allows early mobilization with minimal soft tissue burden.

- Early finger mobilization and edema control is imperative in both methods of treatment. For patients treated operatively with stable fixation early wrist mobilization under the direction of occupational therapy is strongly advised.

PITFALLS

- Bone quality and the ability to achieve stable fixation is often compromised in the elderly population. Failure to address the compromised structural integrity of the operative construct through the liberal use of locking screws, application of longer plates, supra-periosteal dissection and bone graft/substitute can result in hardware failure (Fig. 3A and B).

- Positive ulnar variance following conservative treatment can result in discomfort through ulnocarpal impaction and limited forearm rotation. This may require a salvage procedure to address residual pain and disability (Fig. 4).

- Due to the propensity of the bone to "settle" in this population resulting in malreduction, tendon ruptures including the flexor pollicis longus and dorsal extensors may occur (Fig. 5). This may require subsequent tendon reconstruction and account for increased rates of re-operation.

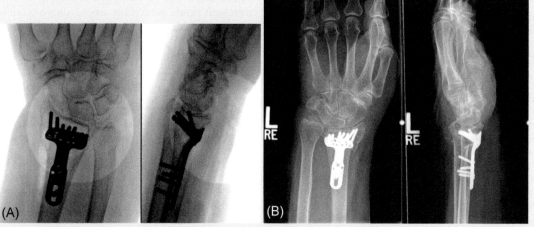

(A)

(B)

FIG. 3 (A) Intra operative imaging demonstrating restoration of radial length and volar tilt. (B) Six weeks follow up showing radial collapse.

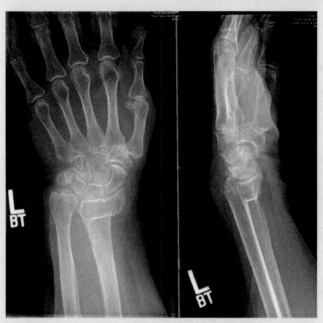

FIG. 4 Distal radius malunion showing significant ulnar positivity and ulnocarpal impaction.

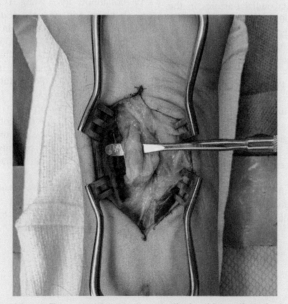

FIG. 5 Four months post operatively this patient lost ability to actively flex the thumb interphalangeal joint. Exploration demonstrated attritional rupture with intervening pseudotendon.

REFERENCES

1. Shauver MJ, Yin H, Banerjee M, Chung KC. Current and future national costs to medicare for the treatment of distal radius fracture in the elderly. *J Hand Surg [Am]*. 2011;36(8):1282–1287.
2. Nellans KW, Kowalski E, Chung KC. The epidemiology of distal radius fractures. *Hand Clin*. 2012;28(2):113–125.
3. Nguyen ND, Ahlborg HG, Center JR, Eisman JA, Nguyen TV. Residual lifetime risk of fractures in women and men. *J Bone Miner Res*. 2007;22(6):781–788.
4. Hammert WC, Kramer RC, Graham B, Keith MW. AAOS appropriate use criteria: treatment of distal radius fractures. *J Am Acad Orthop Surg*. 2013;21(8):506–509.
5. Sirnio K, Leppilahti J, Ohtonen P, Flinkkila T. Early palmar plate fixation of distal radius fractures may benefit patients aged 50 years or older: a randomized trial comparing 2 different treatment protocols. *Acta Orthop*. 2019;90(2):123–128.
6. Martinez-Mendez D, Lizaur-Utrilla A, de Juan-Herrero J. Intra-articular distal radius fractures in elderly patients: a randomized prospective study of casting versus volar plating. *J Hand Surg Eur Vol*. 2018;43(2):142–147.
7. Saving J, Severin Wahlgren S, Olsson K, et al. Nonoperative treatment compared with volar locking plate fixation for dorsally displaced distal radial fractures in the elderly: a randomized controlled trial. *J Bone Joint Surg Am*. 2019;101(11):961–969.
8. Chung KC, Shauver MJ, Birkmeyer JD. Trends in the United States in the treatment of distal radial fractures in the elderly. *J Bone Joint Surg Am*. 2009;91(8):1868–1873.
9. Salibian AA, Bruckman KC, Bekisz JM, Mirrer J, Thanik VD, Hacquebord JH. Management of unstable distal radius fractures: a survey of hand surgeons. *J Wrist Surg*. 2019;8(4):335–343.
10. Moroni A, Vannini F, Faldini C, Pegreffi F, Giannini S. Cast vs external fixation: a comparative study in elderly osteoporotic distal radial fracture patients. *Scand J Surg*. 2004;93(1):64–67.
11. Roumen RM, Hesp WL, Bruggink ED. Unstable Colles' fractures in elderly patients. A randomised trial of external fixation for redisplacement. *J Bone Joint Surg (Br)*. 1991;73(2):307–311.
12. Azzopardi T, Ehrendorfer S, Coulton T, Abela M. Unstable extra-articular fractures of the distal radius: a prospective, randomised study of immobilisation in a cast versus supplementary percutaneous pinning. *J Bone Joint Surg (Br)*. 2005;87(6):837–840.
13. Wong TC, Chiu Y, Tsang WL, Leung WY, Yam SK, Yeung SH. Casting versus percutaneous pinning for extra-articular fractures of the distal radius in an elderly Chinese population: a prospective randomised controlled trial. *J Hand Surg Eur Vol*. 2010;35(3):202–208.
14. Arora R, Lutz M, Deml C, Krappinger D, Haug L, Gabl M. A prospective randomized trial comparing nonoperative treatment with volar locking plate fixation for displaced and unstable distal radial fractures in patients sixty-five years of age and older. *J Bone Joint Surg Am*. 2011;93(23):2146–2153.
15. Bartl C, Stengel D, Bruckner T, Gebhard F. The treatment of displaced intra-articular distal radius fractures in elderly patients. *Dtsch Arztebl Int*. 2014;111(46):779–787.
16. Chung KC, Malay S, Shauver MJ, Kim HM. Assessment of distal radius fracture complications among adults 60 years or older: a secondary analysis of the WRIST randomized clinical trial. *JAMA Netw Open*. 2019;2(1):e187053.
17. Chung KC, Kim HM, Malay S, Shauver MJ. Predicting outcomes after distal radius fracture: a 24-center international clinical trial of older adults. *J Hand Surg [Am]*. 2019;44(9):762–771.
18. Sorensen AA, Howard D, Tan WH, Ketchersid J, Calfee RP. Minimal clinically important differences of 3 patient-rated outcomes instruments. *J Hand Surg [Am]*. 2013;38(4):641–649.
19. Bohannon RW, Wang YC, Noonan C. Relationships between grip strength, dexterity, and fine hand use are attenuated by age in children 3 to 13 years-of-age. *J Phys Ther Sci*. 2019;31(4):382–386.
20. Chung KC, Cho HE, Kim Y, Kim HM, Shauver MJ. Assessment of anatomic restoration of distal radius fractures among older adults: a secondary analysis of a randomized clinical trial. *JAMA Netw Open*. 2020;3(1):e1919433.
21. Lee JI, Park KC, Joo IH, Jeong HW, Park JW. The effect of osteoporosis on the outcomes after volar locking plate fixation in female patients older than 50 years with unstable distal radius fractures. *J Hand Surg [Am]*. 2018;43(8):731–737.
22. Mansuripur PK, Gil JA, Cassidy D, et al. Fixation strength in full and limited fixation of osteoporotic distal radius fractures. *Hand (N Y)*. 2018;13(4):461–465.

CHAPTER 28

Prevention of Distal Radius Fractures

LAURA SIMS[a] • YIYANG ZHANG[b] • RUBY GREWAL[b]
[a]University of Saskatchewan, Saskatoon Orthopedic and Sports Medicine Center, Saskatoon, SK, Canada, [b]Roth | McFarlane Hand and Upper Limb Center, St Joseph's Health Care, Western University, London, ON, Canada

KEY POINTS

- Distal radius fractures (DRFs) are common in patients' aged 50 and older, typically resulting from a low energy mechanism such as a fall from standing height.
- DRFs in this population offer an opportunity to identify patients with a high likelihood of osteoporosis or osteopenia and represent a potential to intervene and prevent future fragility fractures.
- Recognition of at risk adults using tools such as Fracture Risk Assessment Tool provides an opportunity to treat low bone density and implement fall prevention strategies, which may significantly decrease the incidence of subsequent fragility fractures in this population.
- Interventions for fall prevention are effective at decreasing falls on a population and individual level.

Panel 1: Case Scenario

A 61-year-old male fell while walking his dog, sustaining a left, displaced DRF (Fig. 1A). This was successfully treated with closed reduction (Fig. 1B), cast immobilization, and physiotherapy (Fig. 1C). Two years later, he slips on ice, fracturing his right distal radius (Fig. 2). What interventions could have been employed following his first fracture to decrease the risk of his second, contralateral fracture?

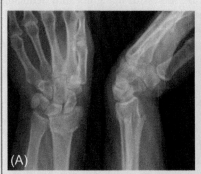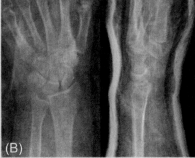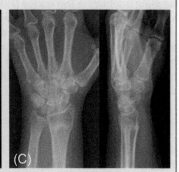

FIG. 1 Right distal radius fracture sustained following a ground level fall. Initial radiographs (A) showing a displaced fracture, which was managed nonsurgically (B and C).

Continued

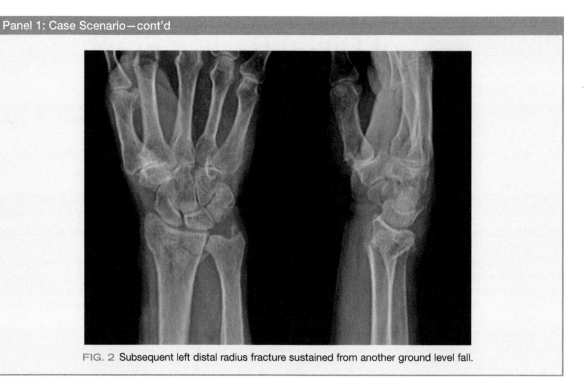

FIG. 2 Subsequent left distal radius fracture sustained from another ground level fall.

IMPORTANCE OF THE PROBLEM

Distal radius fractures (DRFs) are the second most common overall fracture type in elderly patients, typically occurring from low energy injuries such as a fall from standing height.[1, 2] A low energy DRF in patients 50 years and older is an indication of potential low bone density and suggests a significant risk for a future osteoporotic fracture.[2, 3] DRFs tend to occur earlier than other fragility fractures and typically in patients that are otherwise fairly healthy and mobile.[3] This makes a DRF an important sentinel event, offering an opportunity to optimize bone health and prevent future fractures. That is why patients over the age of 50 years, presenting with a DRF should be screened for osteoporosis and fall risk to prevent secondary fragility fractures such as hip fractures, which carry a higher morbidity and mortality rate as well as societal cost. Unfortunately, despite significant evidence suggesting the importance of this, screening for osteoporosis remains suboptimal and the rate of secondary fractures is significant.[4] Recent literature has suggested that secondary fracture prevention strategies are most often implemented when a bone mineral density (BMD) scan is ordered by the treating orthopedic surgeon or when a patient is directly referred to a fracture liaison service (FLS).[5, 6]

Although secondary prevention of future fractures is important, primary prevention of the initial DRF must not be overlooked. Fragility fractures result in significant patient morbidity and societal costs. Programs targeted at identifying at risk individuals and initiating screening for osteoporosis as well as falls education before a fracture occurs can be successful in significantly reducing DRF rates.[7] One useful method for identifying at-risk individuals is the Fracture Risk Assessment Tool (FRAX). The FRAX score predicts an individual's 10-year fragility fracture risk based on the following factors: age, sex, body mass index (weight to height ratio calculation), previous fracture, parental hip fracture, history of rheumatoid arthritis, glucocorticoid use, secondary conditions that contribute to bone loss, current smoking, osteoporosis, intake of more than three alcoholic drinks per day, and femoral neck bone mineral density.[8] As our population continues to age, low energy DRFs will continue to increase, placing strain on our healthcare resources. Preventative programs may help ease this burden, and more importantly reduce associated patient morbidity.

MAIN QUESTION

What strategies can be employed to prevent or decrease the risk of low energy DRFs from both a bone health and fall prevention perspective?

CURRENT OPINION

The majority of treating orthopedic surgeons view DRFs as an indication of low bone density and a risk factor for future fragility fractures. The responsibility of bone density investigation, ongoing treatment of osteoporosis, and referral to falls prevention programs is currently debated, with some suggesting this should be initiated by the treating orthopedic surgeon while others advocate for an alerting system or fracture liaison service. Furthermore, effective prevention of the initial DRF requires identification of at risk adults (from both a bone health and fall prevention perspective) and initiation of prevention strategies at the primary care level.

FINDING THE EVIDENCE

A Cochrane database search was carried out using the search terms "fall prevention" and "injury prevention."

Provided below is our Pubmed (Medline) search strategy employed to identify relevant literature used to construct this chapter:

For Osteoporosis:
- ("distal radius fracture" OR radial fracture [MeSH]) AND ("prevention") AND ("osteoporosis" OR "low bone density")

For Falls Prevention:
- ("fall prevention") AND ("radial fracture" [MeSH] OR "distal radius fracture" or colles fracture [MeSH] or "fragility fracture")

Bibliographies of eligible articles identified in our search were reviewed for additional relevant studies. Articles that were not in English were excluded.

QUALITY OF THE EVIDENCE

No randomized controlled trials or metaanalyses were found that specifically addressed our main question, however there were high quality systematic reviews and one randomized controlled trial that related to aspects of our main question. Four Cochrane reviews were identified that contained information addressing a component of our main question. We identified 22 studies with relevant information relating to DRF prevention through osteoporosis management and fall prevention education. The strength of this evidence is as follows:
- Level I:
  - Cochrane Reviews: 4
  - Systematic Reviews of RCTs: 4
  - Randomized Controlled Trial: 1
- Level II:
  - Cohort Studies: 4

- Level III:
  - Retrospective comparative studies: 9

FINDINGS

Evidence for Screening and Osteoporosis Management

There is substantial literature surrounding various aspects of DRFs and osteoporosis, with most of this focusing on screening and secondary prevention of fragility fractures (including distal radius fractures) following an initial fragility fracture. The majority of studies are level III evidence. There is a paucity of evidence which specifically examines routine screening of at-risk patients for osteoporosis as a means of preventing DRFs, with most primary prevention studies looking at overall fragility fracture reduction or reduction of hip fractures, which carry a higher mortality risk.

Pharmacologic Interventions

There are two Cochrane reviews and two level one studies examining the role of osteoporosis treatment in reducing fragility fracture risk. These studies examined both primary and secondary prevention of fractures, and while the studies included DRFs, they were not specific to DRFs and instead grouped "nonvertebral fractures" together. A 2010 Cochrane review by Wells et al. found that the use of Etidronate for 1 year did not reduce primary or secondary DRFs when compared to placebo treatment (which included patients on calcium and/or vitamin D) in patients with osteoporosis.[9] A subsequent 2016 Cochrane review examined the role of vitamin D and calcium supplementation in the prevention of future fractures, and found that when used in combination there was a significant reduction in nonvertebral fractures (10,380 participants, RR 0.86, 95% CI 0.78–0.96).[10] Furthermore, a systematic review by MacLean et al. compared fracture risk reduction among various pharmacologic treatments, finding significant evidence for alendronate, risedronate, and estrogen in the prevented nonvertebral fractures, suggesting that there may be differences between pharmacologic therapies.[11] Lastly, a 2014 systematic review by Crandal et al. found significant reductions in fragility fractures with the use of bisphosphonates, denosumab, and teriparatide compared to placebo (RRR 0.60–0.80 for nonvertebral fractures), but commented that comparative evidence between different treatment options is lacking.[12]

Osteoporosis as a Risk Factor for Distal Radius Fracture

Two studies highlighted osteoporosis as a clear risk factor for DRF (one level I and one level II). In a recent study by Uusi-Rasi et al., 197 women were followed prospectively for 20 years.[13] These women were divided into two groups based on whether they experienced a fall-related fracture over the study period. The authors found that those who had sustained a fracture had 4%–11% lower BMD than those who had not, suggesting that the presence of low BMD is a significant risk factor for fracture if a person falls.[13] Similarly, a case-control study by Kelsey et al. aimed to evaluate risk factors for DRFs.[3] These authors used a previous fragility fracture as a rough marker for osteoporosis, and found this to be a significant risk factor for a future DRF (OR = 1.48 [1.20–1.84] 95% CI).[3]

Secondary Prevention

Much of the literature surrounding osteoporosis and DRFs focuses on secondary prevention. A DRF is considered by many to represent a sentinel event indicating a person is at significant risk for further fragility fracture, distal radius, or otherwise. DRFs occur at a younger age, on average, compared to other fragility fractures making them an ideal catalyst for osteoporosis screening and treatment. There were three studies that highlight DRFs as a risk factor for secondary fracture (one level I and two level II). In a retrospective cohort study of 1288 participants, Cuddihy et al. showed that patients who

experience a DRF had a 55% incidence of another fracture at 10 years and 80% at 20 years.[14] This was significantly higher than expected fracture rates for all comers but was not specific to DRFs. Two retrospective reviews showed a high rate of subsequent fracture following and initial DRF. Benzvi et al. found that at an average of 25.2 months, 28% of patients had sustained a secondary fragility fracture, with only 21% of patients treated for osteoporosis at any time.[15] Similarly, Smith et al. found that in patients with a DRF and a subsequent femoral neck fracture, only 8% received investigation and treatment for osteoporosis following their DRF.[16]

Given the known risk of secondary fragility fracture following a DRF many studies have investigated the ideal protocol to ensure adequate screening and treatment of patients with these injuries. Five studies (Table 1) highlight poor screening and treatment of osteoporosis following DRFs (level II to IV evidence). These studies show that the rate of BMD scanning following a DRF ranges from 9% to 25% and the rate of medical treatment for osteoporosis ranges from 13% to 31%.[17–20] These numbers have been shown to be even lower in men.[21] In a systematic review of randomized controlled trials, Little et al. found that baseline rates of osteoporosis screening and treatment following fragility fractures was low (typically less than 20%) and

TABLE 1
Screening and Treatment of Osteoporosis Following a Fragility Fracture.

Study	Usual Screening for Osteoporosis (%)	Usual Treatment for Osteoporosis (%)	Intervention	Postintervention Screening for Osteoporosis (%)	Postintervention Treatment for Osteoporosis (%)
Ashe et al., 2004	23%	NR	Patient education Physician alerting system	92%	NR
Rozental et al., 2008	21%	28%	BMD scan ordered by treating orthopedic surgeon	93%	74%
Talbot et al., 2007	9%	31%	NR	NR	NR
Iba et al., 2018	NR	13%	Previously published literature indicating low treatment rates	25.3%	16%
Baba et al., 2015	9%	13%	NR	NR	NR

NR: not reported.

that while an intervention of any kind targeted at improving these rates did result in increased screening and treatment, overall rates remained suboptimal.[22] Baba et al. found that while overall screening rates were low, in cases where a BMD scan was ordered a significantly higher proportion of patients received treatment for osteoporosis (73.8% vs 8.2%).[18] This suggests that when adequate screening occurs, appropriate treatment ensues; therefore, targeting the best strategy for improved osteoporosis screening is paramount. Several studies have investigated the best means of ensuring appropriate screening. In a randomized controlled trial by Rozental et al. patients in whom the treating orthopedic surgeon ordered the BMD scan received significantly higher rates of screening (93% vs 30%), osteoporosis counseling (89% vs 35%), and osteoporosis treatment (74% vs 26%) compared to patients whose orthopedic surgeon sent a letter with screening guidelines to the primary care physician.[5] Aside from the treating orthopedic surgeon, a FLS has also been shown to be a reliable way to improve osteoporosis screening and treatment following DRFs, with an improvement in osteoporosis screening and treatment to 77.8% compared to 22.9% with usual care.[6]

Beyond simply improving screening and treatment of osteoporosis following DRFs, studies have demonstrated that this has translated to improved rates of secondary prevention. Two level III studies have demonstrated this. This first, by Astrand et al., showed a 42% lower risk of fracture in patients who were referred to a screening program following an initial fragility fracture.[23] Similarly, Huntjens et al. showed that implementation of a fracture liaison service translated to improved mortality and decreased subsequent non-vertebral fracture rates (HR 0.84 at 1 year 95% CI).[24] While these results are promising, improved primary prevention would result in the least morbidity for patients. There are few studies examining primary prevention specific to DRFs; however, a retrospective cohort study by Harness et al. utilized data available through Kaiser Permanente Southern California to investigate this.[7] They found that in at-risk patients treated with pharmacologic intervention, DRF risk was decreased by 48%.[7]

Evidence for Falls Prevention

Evidence for both population-based and individual-based interventions aimed at falls prevention has been shown to beneficially reduce fracture risk. This literature tends to focus on fragility fractures as a whole as opposed to individual fracture types such as DRFs.

Population-Based Interventions

A population-based intervention focuses on the countermeasures deployed with the community as a unit of analysis. This is in contrast to individual-based interventions where the unit of analysis is individuals. A Cochrane review in 2005 identified six population-based interventions carried out in communities in Australia, Taiwan, Denmark, Sweden, and Norway.[25] In Australia, the program was carried out in the New South Wales region. It was a 4 years intervention costing the government roughly $600,000 AUD.[26] It targeted knowledge, attitudes, behaviors, medication use, footwear, and home modifications through brochures, posters, and the media.[26] Denmark had a similar program in five municipalities which also included home visits, treatment of psychiatric conditions, and promotion of physical and mental well-being.[27] In Taiwan, a 2-year study was initiated in a rural town with the surrounding towns used as control.[28] In the first year, Tai chi was offered in public places 6 days of the week and the second year focused on posters and pamphlets promoting physical activity and environmental modifications.[28] The remaining three studies were based on the World Health Organization Safe Communities model of safety and injury prevention mostly involving the use of media to disseminate information, home visits, and promoting physical and mental health. It is difficult to determine the generalizability of each of these communities to other communities. In addition, there were no cluster randomized multiple community trials available to upgrade the level of evidence. However, given that there was consistency of reported reduction in fall-related injuries, the review concluded preliminarily that population-based interventions were effective.[25]

Individual-Based Interventions

Studies focusing on fracture risk through individual-based interventions have examined the role of exercise programs, pharmacotherapy, and multifactorial risk assessments including visual assessments and home safety assessments.

With respect to exercise, Sherrington et al. extended the Cochrane review in 2012 to examine the role of exercise in preventing falls in older people living in the community by including literature up to 2019.[29] This systematic review included only randomized controlled trials. They concluded that exercise reduce the rate of falls by 23% compared to controls.[29] Contrastingly, some authors have found that DRFs are actually increased in older adults who are more active as they tend to maintain quicker reaction times and are more likely to fall on an outstretched hand compared with less active patients.[3] These findings were mirrored in a study by Rikkonen et al. who found that higher levels of patient self-reported physical activity resulted in higher incidences of DRFs, but not other fragility fractures, compared to less active patients (HR 1.3 95% CI 1.14–1.69).[30] This highlights the need for education surrounding appropriate exercise programs and was examined in the subgroup analysis by Sherrington et al., where it was found that there was a larger effect of exercise when it was delivered by a healthcare professional (usually physiotherapist) rather than a nonhealthcare professional.[29] In addition, there was likely little or no difference in the effect of exercise (all types) on the rate of falls in trials where participants were aged 75 years or older compared with trials where participants were aged less than 75 years.[29] Moreover, "there was probably little or no difference in the effect of exercise on the rate of falls in trials where all participants were at an increased risk of falling compared with trials that did not use increased risk of falling as an entry criterion."[29]

Regarding pharmacologic interventions, Gillespie et al. concluded that vitamin D supplementation did not reduce the rate of falls, but may be effective in people with lower vitamin D levels before treatment.[31] A gradual withdrawal of psychotropic medication, however, was found to be beneficial in reducing falls.[31]

Lastly, multifactorial interventions can include risk assessment, vision assessment, and home safety assessment. This was shown in the Cochrane review in 2012 to reduce the rate of falls.[31] Home safety assessment and modification interventions alone can also reduce the rate of falls.[31]

RECOMMENDATION

In patients over 50 years of age with a low energy DRF, evidence suggests:

Recommendations	Overall Quality
• The presence of a low energy DRF is an indication of increased risk of future fragility fracture	⊕⊕⊕◯ MODERATE
• Screening for osteoporosis should be initiated by the treating orthopedic surgeon or through referral to a FLS	⊕⊕◯◯ LOW
• Screening and management of osteoporosis can significantly reduce secondary fracture risk	⊕⊕◯◯ LOW
• Primary prevention of low energy DRFs can be achieved through appropriate screening and treatment of low bone density in at risk individuals	⊕⊕⊕◯ MODERATE
• Population-based methods for fall prevention can be effective	⊕⊕⊕◯ MODERATE
• Exercise reduces the risk of falling	⊕⊕⊕◯ MODERATE

CONCLUSION

DRFs represent a population at-risk for future fractures, but also an opportunity for healthcare providers to intervene. The literature suggests that appropriate screening and treatment of osteoporotic patients and decreasing their fall risks can prevent future low energy DRFs. These same strategies can be used for primary prevention when at risk individuals are identified prior to any fracture.

Panel 2: Author's Preferred Technique

This case example highlights a missed opportunity for secondary fracture prevention. For patients with a low energy DRF, the authors recommend interventions aimed at reducing subsequent fracture risk in addition to appropriate management of the DRF. This requires a multimodal approach and will differ based on regional variation in available services. Based on the available evidence, the authors recommend referral to a FLS or ordering a BMD scan, communicating these results and providing up-to-date osteoporosis guidelines to the patients' primary care physician. Additional measures such as patient education on bone density, supplementation with calcium and vitamin D in combination, and referral to physiotherapy based exercise programs aimed at falls prevention are also suggested. These recommendations are outlined in Fig. 3. Had these strategies been implemented following the initial DRF in this case, the risk for a second fracture would have been significantly reduced.

Panel 2: Author's Preferred Technique—cont'd

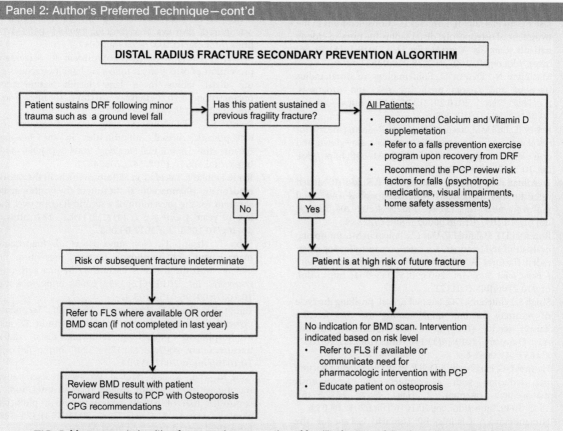

FIG. 3 Management algorithm for secondary prevention of fragility fractures following a distal radius fracture, based on best available evidence and guidelines set forth by osteoporosis Canada.[32] *DRF*, distal radius fracture; *PCP*, primary care physician; *FLS*, fracture liaison service; *BMD*, bone mineral density; *CGP*, clinical practice guideline.

Panel 3: Pearls and Pitfalls

PEARLS

- Patients experiencing a low energy DRF should be referred to a FLS when available.
- In centers without a FLS, we recommend that the treating physician order a BMD scan at the initial DRF visit. This should be followed by a discussion regarding low bone density with the patient and a copy of the BMD result forwarded to the primary care physician for ongoing management.
- Patients with low energy DRFs should be referred to local exercise programs once recovered, ideally those lead by a physiotherapist or healthcare professional.

PITFALLS

- Primary DRF prevention is superior to secondary prevention but is more challenging to achieve. Treating physicians should continue to advocate for programs that identify and treat at risk individuals before an initial fragility fracture is sustained.
- Males should not be overlooked as patients who are at risk for osteoporosis.
- Some patients may not have a primary care provider to follow them for bone density management. In these instances, Endocrinologists or Rheumatologists with an interest in osteoporosis may be able to fill this gap in care.

REFERENCES

1. Ostergaard PJ, Hall MJ, Rozental TD. Considerations in the treatment of osteoporotic distal radius fractures in elderly patients. *Curr Rev Musculoskelet Med*. 2019;12(1):50–56. https://doi.org/10.1007/s12178-019-09531-z.

2. MacIntyre NJ, Dewan N. Epidemiology of distal radius fractures and factors predicting risk and prognosis. *J Hand Ther*. 2016;29(2):136–145. https://doi.org/10.1016/j.jht.2016.03.003.

3. Kelsey JL, Prill MM, Keegan THM, et al. Reducing the risk for distal forearm fracture: preserve bone mass, slow down, and don't fall!. *Osteoporos Int*. 2005;16(6):681–690. https://doi.org/10.1007/s00198-004-1745-8.

4. Freedman BA, Potter BK, Nesti LJ, Cho T, Kuklo TR. Missed opportunities in patients with osteoporosis and distal radius fractures. *Clin Orthop*. 2007;454:202–206. https://doi.org/10.1097/01.blo.0000238866.15228.c4.

5. Rozental TD, Makhni EC, Day CS, Bouxsein ML. Improving evaluation and treatment for osteoporosis following distal radial fractures. A prospective randomized intervention. *J Bone Joint Surg Am*. 2008;90(5):953–961. https://doi.org/10.2106/JBJS.G.01121.

6. Singh S, Whitehurst DG, Funnell L, et al. Breaking the cycle of recurrent fracture: implementing the first fracture liaison service (FLS) in British Columbia, Canada. *Arch Osteoporos*. 2019;14(1):116. https://doi.org/10.1007/s11657-019-0662-6.

7. Harness NG, Funahashi T, Dell R, et al. Distal radius fracture risk reduction with a comprehensive osteoporosis management program. *J Hand Surg*. 2012;37(8):1543–1549. https://doi.org/10.1016/j.jhsa.2012.04.033.

8. Unnanuntana A, Gladnick BP, Donnelly E, Lane JM. The assessment of fracture risk. *J Bone Joint Surg Am*. 2010;92(3):743. https://doi.org/10.2106/JBJS.I.00919.

9. Wells GA, Cranney A, Peterson J, et al. Etidronate for the primary and secondary prevention of osteoporotic fractures in postmenopausal women. *Cochrane Database Syst Rev*. 2008;(1). CD003376 https://doi.org/10.1002/14651858.CD003376.pub3.

10. Avenell A, Mak JCS, O'Connell D. Vitamin D and vitamin D analogues for preventing fractures in post-menopausal women and older men. *Cochrane Database Syst Rev*. 2014;4:CD000227https://doi.org/10.1002/14651858.CD000227.pub4.

11. MacLean C, Newberry S, Maglione M, et al. Systematic review: comparative effectiveness of treatments to prevent fractures in men and women with low bone density or osteoporosis. *Ann Intern Med*. 2008;148(3):197–213. https://doi.org/10.7326/0003-4819-148-3-200802050-00198.

12. Crandall CJ, Newberry SJ, Diamant A, et al. Comparative effectiveness of pharmacologic treatments to prevent fractures: an updated systematic review. *Ann Intern Med*. 2014;161(10):711–723. https://doi.org/10.7326/M14-0317.

13. Uusi-Rasi K, Karinkanta S, Tokola K, Kannus P, Sievänen H. Bone mass and strength and fall-related fractures in older age. *J Osteoporos*. 2019; (2019). https://www.hindawi.com/journals/jos/2019/5134690/ Accessed 10 January 2020.

14. Cuddihy MT, Gabriel SE, Crowson CS, O'Fallon WM, Melton LJ. Forearm fractures as predictors of subsequent osteoporotic fractures. *Osteoporos Int*. 1999;9(6):469–475. https://doi.org/10.1007/s001980050172.

15. Benzvi L, Gershon A, Lavi I, Wollstein R. Secondary prevention of osteoporosis following fragility fractures of the distal radius in a large health maintenance organization. *Arch Osteoporos*. 2016;11:20. https://doi.org/10.1007/s11657-016-0275-2.

16. Smith MG, Dunkow P, Lang DM. Treatment of osteoporosis: missed opportunities in the hospital fracture clinic. *Ann R Coll Surg Engl*. 2004;86(5):344–346. https://doi.org/10.1308/147870804371.

17. Iba K, Dohke T, Takada J, et al. Improvement in the rate of inadequate pharmaceutical treatment by orthopaedic surgeons for the prevention of a second fracture over the last 10 years. *J Orthop Sci*. 2018;23(1):127–131. https://doi.org/10.1016/j.jos.2017.09.008.

18. Baba T, Hagino H, Nonomiya H, et al. Inadequate management for secondary fracture prevention in patients with distal radius fracture by trauma surgeons. *Osteoporos Int*. 2015;26(7):1959–1963. https://doi.org/10.1007/s00198-015-3103-4.

19. Talbot JC, Elener C, Praveen P, Shaw DL. Secondary prevention of osteoporosis: calcium, vitamin D and bisphosphonate prescribing following distal radial fracture. *Injury*. 2007;38(11):1236–1240. https://doi.org/10.1016/j.injury.2007.03.004.

20. Ashe M, Khan K, Guy P, et al. Wristwatch-distal radial fracture as a marker for osteoporosis investigation: a controlled trial of patient education and a physician alerting system. *J Hand Ther*. 2004;17(3):324–328. https://doi.org/10.1197/j.jht.2004.04.001.

21. Harper CM, Fitzpatrick SK, Zurakowski D, Rozental TD. Distal radial fractures in older men. A missed opportunity? *J Bone Joint Surg Am*. 2014;96(21):1820–1827. https://doi.org/10.2106/JBJS.M.01497.

22. Little EA, Eccles MP. A systematic review of the effectiveness of interventions to improve post-fracture investigation and management of patients at risk of osteoporosis. *Implement Sci*. 2010;5:80. https://doi.org/10.1186/1748-5908-5-80.

23. Åstrand J, Nilsson J, Thorngren K-G. Screening for osteoporosis reduced new fracture incidence by almost half. *Acta Orthop*. 2012;83(6):661–665. https://doi.org/10.3109/17453674.2012.747922.

24. Huntjens KMB, van Geel TACM, van den Bergh JPW, et al. Fracture liaison service: impact on subsequent nonvertebral fracture incidence and mortality. *J Bone Joint Surg Am*. 2014;96(4):e29. https://doi.org/10.2106/JBJS.L.00223.

25. McClure R, Turner C, Peel N, Spinks A, Eakin E, Hughes K. Population-based interventions for the prevention of fall-related injuries in older people. *Cochrane Database Syst Rev*. 2005;1:CD004441https://doi.org/10.1002/14651858.CD004441.pub2.

26. Kempton A, van Beurden E, Sladden T, Garner E, Beard J. Older people can stay on their feet: final results of a

community-based falls prevention programme. *Health Promot Int.* 2000;15(1):27–33. https://doi.org/10.1093/heapro/15.1.27.

27. Poulstrup A, Jeune B. Prevention of fall injuries requiring hospital treatment among community-dwelling elderly. *Eur J Pub Health.* 2000;10(1):45–50. https://doi.org/10.1093/eurpub/10.1.45.

28. Lin M-R, Hwang H-F, Wang Y-W, Chang S-H, Wolf SL. Community-based tai chi and its effect on injurious falls, balance, gait, and fear of falling in older people. *Phys Ther.* 2006;86(9):1189–1201. https://doi.org/10.2522/ptj.20040408.

29. Sherrington C, Fairhall N, Wallbank G, et al. Exercise for preventing falls in older people living in the community: an abridged Cochrane systematic review.

Br J Sports Med. 2019;https://doi.org/10.1136/bjsports-2019-101512.

30. Rikkonen T, Salovaara K, Sirola J, et al. Physical activity slows femoral bone loss but promotes wrist fractures in postmenopausal women: a 15-year follow-up of the OSTPRE study. *J Bone Miner Res.* 2010;25(11):2332–2340. https://doi.org/10.1002/jbmr.143.

31. Gillespie LD, Robertson MC, Gillespie WJ, et al. Interventions for preventing falls in older people living in the community. *Cochrane Database Syst Rev.* 2012;(9):CD007146 https://doi.org/10.1002/14651858.CD007146.pub3.

32. *Non-Hip Non-Spine Fractures | Osteoporosis Canada.* Fracture Liaison Service; 2020. (2020). *https://fls.osteoporosis.ca/appendix-i/non-hip-non-spine-fractures/* Accessed 11 January 2020.

CHAPTER 29

Diagnosing the Malunited Distal Radius

JESSE D. MEAIKE[a] • JOSHUA J. MEAIKE[b] • ALEXANDER Y. SHIN[b]
[a]Division of Plastic Surgery, Mayo Clinic, Rochester, MN, United States, [b]Department of Orthopaedic Surgery, Mayo Clinic, Rochester, MN, United States

---

KEY POINTS

- The diagnosis of a malunited distal radius fracture (DRF) must take into account both clinical symptoms and radiographic findings
- Standard radiographs of both the affected and contralateral wrist are usually sufficient to diagnose distal radius malunions, but CT scans can provide additional information for complex deformities

---

Panel 1: Case Scenario

A 72-year-old, right hand dominant, retired male presents to your office with chronic left wrist pain and decreased range of motion after conservative management of a distal radius fracture 10 years prior. Radiographs show a "malunited, impacted, intraarticular fracture of the left distal radius with dorsal tilt and decreased height and inclination of the distal radial articular surface (Fig. 1)." How would you proceed with your evaluation in order to identify a symptomatic malunion of his prior distal radius fracture?

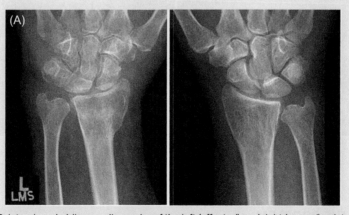

FIG. 1 (A–C) AP, lateral, and oblique radiographs of the left (affected) and right (normal) wrist demonstrating a malunited, impacted, intraarticular fracture of the left distal radius with dorsal tilt and decreased height and inclination of the distal radial articular surface. Scapholunate widening with DISI deformity. Moderate radioscaphoid narrowing and scattered moderate degenerative arthritis.

Continued

Distal Radius Fractures. https://doi.org/10.1016/B978-0-323-75764-5.00007-X

Panel 1: Case Scenario—cont'd

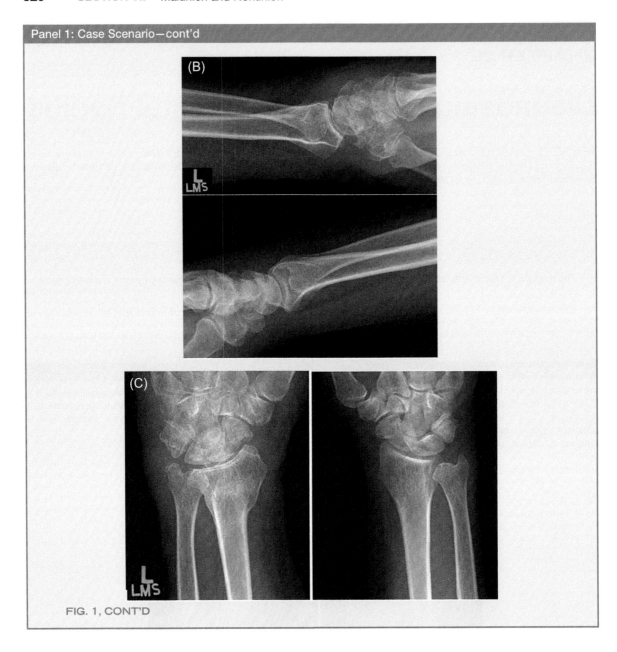

FIG. 1, CONT'D

IMPORTANCE OF THE PROBLEM

Distal radius fractures (DRFs) are among the most common fractures managed by trauma surgeons, accounting for approximately 17% of all fractures managed in an orthopedic trauma unit.[1] Malunion is fairly common following a DRF, with reported malunion rates of 23.6% and 10.6% after closed reduction with casting and surgical management, respectively.[2] Patients with symptomatic malunion after a DRF demonstrate persistent disability at 1 year, 2 years, and 12–14 years after fracture treatment.[3–5] Malunited DRFs alter the biomechanics of the distal radioulnar joint (DRUJ) as well as the radiocarpal, ulnocarpal, and midcarpal articulations, which may accelerate degenerative changes and produce pain as well as functional impairment.[6] Carefully planned corrective osteotomies can significantly improve the radiographic and functional outcomes in these patients,[7] and, therefore, it is paramount to recognize and appropriately diagnose this condition.

MAIN QUESTION

For all patients who have sustained DRFs, how is a symptomatic malalignment of the radius most accurately diagnosed, both clinically and radiologically?

CURRENT OPINION

The diagnosis of symptomatic distal radius malunion requires both clinical symptoms in addition to radiographic abnormalities. While plain radiographs are sufficient to diagnosis most distal radius malunions, computed tomography (CT) scans are extremely useful to diagnose rotational malunions as well as aid in surgical planning of the corrective osteotomies.

FINDING THE EVIDENCE

We provide below a list of search algorithms used to construct this chapter:

- Cochrane search: "distal radius"
- PUBMED (clinical queries: systematic reviews): "distal radius"
- PUBMED (Medline): "distal radius" AND "malunion"
- Bibliography review of the selected articles
- Articles that were not in the English were excluded.
- Articles involving anything other than human subjects were excluded.

QUALITY OF THE EVIDENCE

Overall, there were no randomized control trials or other Level I evidence that addressed the primary question. However, there were multiple articles of varying levels of evidence that are relevant to the main question. They are stratified into the following levels of evidence:

Level II: 4
Level III: 2
Level IV: 1
Level V: 8

FINDINGS

Evidence From Level II Studies

There were four studies that evaluated patient-reported outcomes in those with malunion of DRFs. Grewal and MacDermid[8] prospectively evaluated 216 patients with extraarticular DRFs with the goal of determining if individual radiographic parameters (dorsal angulation, radial inclination, and radial shortening) and the overall acceptability of alignment of the healed DRF influenced patient-reported pain and disability at 1 year, as measured by standardized patient-rated pain and disability scores [Patient-Rated Wrist Evaluation (PRWE) and Disabilities of Arm, Shoulder, and Hand (DASH)]. Alignment was deemed "unacceptable" if dorsal angulation was >10 degrees, if radial inclination was <15 degrees, or if there was ≥3 mm of ulnar positive variance. They found that in patients younger than 65 years of age, overall malalignment was associated with significantly higher pain and disability scores at 1 year. When examining radiographic parameters in isolation, radial inclination and radial shortening were associated with significantly higher PRWE scores and radial shortening was associated with a significantly higher DASH score (with dorsal angulation and radial inclination trending toward significance). In patients greater than 65 years of age, the presence of malalignment did not influence patient-reported outcomes.

Atroshi's group[3–5] in Sweden consecutively enrolled patients 18–65 years old who presented over a 15 months period with acute, extraarticular or intraarticular DRFs and were subsequently treated with casting, closed reduction and casting, or closed reduction and percutaneous fixation; those who underwent open reduction and internal fixation were excluded. These patients were prospectively enrolled and longitudinally followed with DASH scores and radiographs. Malunion was defined using the same criteria as describe above.[8] At 1 year,[3] 2 years,[4] and 12–14 years[5] follow-up, radiographic malunion was associated with higher arm-related disability. Specifically at 1 year, dorsal tilt and ulnar variance were found to significantly affect DASH score, while radial inclination had no significant effect. Patients with malunion involving dorsal tilt and/or ulnar variance were significantly more likely to have higher disability compared to patients with no malunion. Patients with malunion involving only dorsal tilt or only ulnar variance had lower DASH scores than patients with combined malunion. Again at 2 years follow-up, patients with malunion involving ulnar variance and dorsal tilt had worse disability than patients with no malunion. At the time of extended 12–14 years follow-up, increased dorsal angulation, increased ulnar variance, and decreased radial inclination were associated with higher DASH scores. The relationship between the DASH score and the radiographic variables of dorsal tilt, ulnar variance, and radial inclination were analyzed as continuous variables which demonstrated significant associations between a higher DASH score at time of follow-up and increased ulnar variance, increased dorsal angulation, and decreased radial inclination. The authors[4] advocate that patients with disability at 1 year after fracture and radiographic malunion with positive ulnar variance or substantial dorsal tilt should be considered for corrective osteotomy.

Evidence From Level III Studies

Miyake et al.[9] sought to estimate the accuracy of distal radius malunion assessment by comparing standard radiographic measurements (volar/dorsal tilt, radial inclination, and ulnar variance) with those from CT obtained 3-dimensional methods in 20 dorsally tilted malunions. They found that radiographic evaluation of dorsal tilt was reasonably accurate, but the radiographic evaluation of radial inclination and height were less accurate. With regards to radial inclination, the absolute difference between evaluations using the 3D method and plain radiographs was up to 21 degrees (average 5.7 degrees). When assessing ulnar variance, 8/20 cases had a discrepancy of ≥2 mm. The authors concluded that standard radiographic evaluation of volar/dorsal tilt was likely reliable for surgical planning, but measurements of radial inclination and shortening deformities may benefit from CT.

Prommersberger et al.[10] evaluated the rotational deformity of distal radius malunions. CT scans of both the normal and injured wrists were performed, and the radial torsion angle of both wrists was calculated. They found that 23/37 (62%), when compared to the uninjured wrist, demonstrated a rotational deformity. The supination deformity averaged 10 and 14 degrees in dorsally and volarly angulated malunions, respectively. The pronation deformity averaged 10 and 13 degrees in dorsally and volarly angulated malunions, respectively. The authors concluded that obtaining preoperative CT scans of both wrists may be helpful to identify a rotational malunion and to subsequently help plan the corrective osteotomy.

Evidence From Level IV Studies

Keizer et al.[7] performed a systematic review evaluating outcomes of 3D virtual planning of corrective osteotomies for distal radius malunions. The authors highlighted the anatomic variability among individuals and importance of imaging the contralateral forearm for a standard reference. The authors also discussed the utility of obtaining a CT scan to better understand the anatomy of complex deformities and to identify rotational deformities. They concluded that 3D-planned corrective osteotomy significantly improves both radiographic and functional outcomes in distal radius malunion reconstruction.

Evidence From Level V Studies

Multiple authors[6, 11–15] agree that the diagnosis of a distal radius malunion must take into account clinical symptoms, physical exam findings, and radiographic parameters. The standard radiograph to evaluate the distal radius should include anteroposterior (AP), lateral, and oblique views of the affected wrist, with contralateral wrist films for comparison. CT scans with 3D reconstructions may be helpful, especially to assess for rotational deformities. Radiographs do not always correlate with symptoms, and therefore the symptoms and resulting functional limitations should guide management rather than radiographic appearance alone.

Graham[16] proposed four radiographic criteria to assess the adequacy of healing of a DRF. Acceptable measurements were radial inclination ≥15 degrees, volar tilt <20 degrees, or dorsal tilt <15 degrees, radial shortening <5 mm at the DRUJ, and intraarticular incongruity <2 mm. Haase and Chung,[12] based upon their experience, expert opinion, and review of the literature, proposed the following criteria to radiographically define distal radius malunions: radial inclination <10 degrees, volar tilt >20 degrees, or dorsal tilt >20 degrees, radial height <10 mm, ulnar variance >2+, and intraarticular step or gap >2 mm. Slagel et al.[17] based upon their review of the literature and expert opinion, defined a malunited distal radius fracture as follows: dorsal tilt >20 degrees, displaced fractures with carpal malalignment (>15 degrees of dorsal angulation of lunate on lateral radiographs), incongruity of the DRUJ, and >5 mm of ulnar variance.

There are numerous biomechanical changes that may result from malunion of DRFs.[13–15] The resulting clinical sequelae are numerous and include pain (radiocarpal, midcarpal, or distal radioulnar), decreased range of motion (flexion/extension and pronation/supination), cosmetic deformity, and decreased grip strength.[6, 11–15, 17]

RECOMMENDATION

In patients with an intraarticular displaced distal radius fracture, evidence suggests:

Recommendation	Overall Quality
• The diagnosis of distal radius malunion requires consideration of both clinical symptoms and radiographic findings	⊕◯◯◯ VERY LOW
• Radiographic parameters suggesting distal radius malunion include deviations in volar tilt, radial inclination/radial height, ulnar variance, and articular congruity (Table 1)	⊕⊕⊕◯ MODERATE
• CT scans may be helpful to identify rotational malunions, understand complex deformities, and plan corrective osteotomy	⊕⊕◯◯ LOW

TABLE 1
Radiographic Evaluation of the Distal Radius—Normal Values and Proposed Malunion Criteria.[3–8, 12, 16, 17]

Parameter	Normal Value	Malunion
Dorsal angulation	11 degrees volar tilt	>10–20 degrees
Volar angulation	11 degrees volar tilt	>20 degrees
Radial inclination	21–25 degrees	<10–15 degrees
Radial height	10–13 mm	<10 mm vs >5 mm shortening
Ulnar variance	Neutral ± 1 mm	>2+ to 5+ mm
Intraarticular step-off	Congruous	>2 mm

CONCLUSION

The diagnosis of a symptomatic distal radius malunion begins with a thorough physical exam. Exam findings of a distal radius malunion can include signs or symptoms of radiocarpal, intercarpal, and distal radioulnar joint arthritis and instability as well as decreased range of motion and grip strength. AP, lateral, and oblique radiographs of the affected wrist should be compared to radiographs of the contralateral wrist and to normative values, noting changes in volar tilt, radial inclination/height, and ulnar variance. CT scans can be obtained for a more detailed evaluation and for surgical planning.

Panel 2: Author's Preferred Technique

In the case of chronic wrist pain and immobility after a previously treated DRF, the work-up for malunion proceeds with a detailed history and physical examination followed by radiographic evaluation. The authors assess for pain about the wrist, decreased range of motion, cosmetic deformity, and decreased grip strength. The authors preferred initial radiographic evaluation includes AP, lateral, and oblique views of both the injured and normal wrists, assessing for changes in volar/dorsal tilt, radial inclination/height, and ulnar variance. The authors will obtain CT scans to further evaluate complex deformities or to assist with operative planning (Figs. 2 and 3). In the senior author's practice, 3D reconstructions are obtained if the deformity cannot be fully appreciated on the CT scan or if there is concern for rotational deformity.

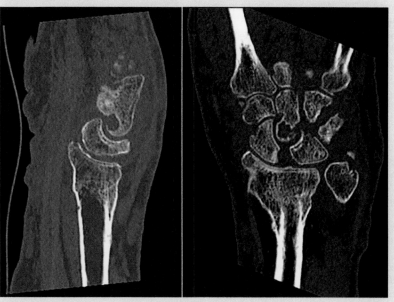

FIG. 2 CT scan of the left upper extremity with saggital *(left)* and coronal *(right)* views of a distal radius malunion demonstrating excess dorsal tilt and scapholunate widening with DISI deformity.

Continued

Panel 2: Author's Preferred Technique—cont'd

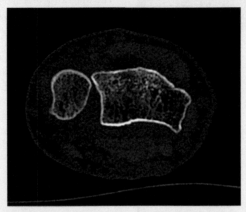

FIG. 3 CT scan of the left upper extemity with axial view of the distal radioulnar joint (DRUJ).

In the case of this patient, the decision was made to proceed with an opening wedge osteotomy of the distal radius with volar plate fixation and allograft bone grafting to address the radial shortening and dorsal angulation.

Panel 3: Pearls and Pitfalls

PEARLS:

- Carefully listen to the patient's complaints regarding loss of motion (flexion, extension, forearm rotation) after they are "healed" from a DRF. When applicable, compare motion to the uninjured side.
- Appropriate radiographs of the wrist can identify a majority of malunions of the distal radius.
- Do not forget about the DRUJ.

PITFALLS:

- Failure to identify malunion early can result in irreversible arthritic changes at multiple joint of the wrist or lead to adaptive carpal instability.
- Consider the patients physiologic age, not chronologic age, when considering treatment for malunions.

REFERENCES

1. Court-Brown CM, Caesar B. Epidemiology of adult fractures: a review. *Injury.* 2006;37(8):691–697.
2. Fernandez DL. Surgical management of malunited distal radius fractures. In: Cooney WP, ed. *The Wrist: Diagnosis and Operative Treatment.* 2nd ed. Philadelphia, PA: LWW; 2010:347.
3. Brogren E, Hofer M, Petranek M, Wagner P, Dahlin LB, Atroshi I. Relationship between distal radius fracture malunion and arm-related disability: a prospective population-based cohort study with 1-year follow-up. *BMC Musculoskelet Disord.* 2011;12:9.
4. Brogren E, Wagner P, Petranek M, Atroshi I. Distal radius malunion increases risk of persistent disability 2 years after fracture: a prospective cohort study. *Clin Orthop Relat Res.* 2013;471(5):1691–1697.
5. Ali M, Brogren E, Wagner P, Atroshi I. Association between distal radial fracture malunion and patient-reported activity limitations: a long-term follow-up. *J Bone Joint Surg Am.* 2018;100(8):633–639.
6. Bushnell BD, Bynum DK. Malunion of the distal radius. *J Am Acad Orthop Surg.* 2007;15(1):27–40.
7. de Muinck Keizer RJO, Lechner KM, Mulders MAM, Schep NWL, Eygendaal D, Goslings JC. Three-dimensional virtual planning of corrective osteotomies of distal radius malunions: a systematic review and meta-analysis. *Strategies Trauma Limb Reconstr.* 2017;12(2):77–89.
8. Grewal R, MacDermid JC. The risk of adverse outcomes in extra-articular distal radius fractures is increased with malalignment in patients of all ages but mitigated in older patients. *J Hand Surg [Am].* 2007;32(7):962–970.

9. Miyake J, Murase T, Yamanaka Y, Moritomo H, Sugamoto K, Yoshikawa H. Comparison of three dimensional and radiographic measurements in the analysis of distal radius malunion. *J Hand Surg Eur Vol.* 2013;38(2):133–143.

10. Prommersberger KJ, Froehner SC, Schmitt RR, Lanz UB. Rotational deformity in malunited fractures of the distal radius. *J Hand Surg [Am].* 2004;29(1):110–115.

11. Mathews AL, Chung KC. Management of complications of distal radius fractures. *Hand Clin.* 2015;31(2):205–215.

12. Haase SC, Chung KC. Management of malunions of the distal radius. *Hand Clin.* 2012;28(2):207–216.

13. Prommersberger KJ, Pillukat T, Mühldorfer M, van Schoonhoven J. Malunion of the distal radius. *Arch Orthop Trauma Surg.* 2012;132(5):693–702.

14. Patton MW. Distal radius malunion. *J Am Soc Surg Hand.* 2004;4(4):266–274.

15. Evans BT, Jupiter JB. Best approaches in distal radius fracture Malunions. *Curr Rev Musculoskelet Med.* 2019;12(2):198–203.

16. Graham TJ. Surgical correction of malunited fractures of the distal radius. *J Am Acad Orthop Surg.* 1997;5(5):270–281.

17. Slagel BE, Luenam S, Pichora DR. Management of post-traumatic malunion of fractures of the distal radius. *Orthop Clin North Am.* 2007;38(2):203–216 [vi].

CHAPTER 30

Treatment of the Extraarticular Malunited Distal Radius

NICK JOHNSON • JOSEPH DIAS
University Hospitals of Leicester, Leicester, United Kingdom

KEY POINTS

- The relationship between malunion and functional outcome following distal radius fracture (DRF) is not well understood.
- Some patients tolerate malunion well, whereas others have poor functional outcome.
- Evidence evaluating operative and nonoperative treatment of extraarticular malunion is largely of low quality.
- Distal radius osteotomy is likely to improve symptoms in carefully selected patients with a symptomatic malunion following DRF.
- Complication rate and need for re-operation is considerable.
- Careful consideration and adequate patient counseling should be carried out before deciding optimum treatment for a patient with extraarticular DRF malunion.

Panel 1: Case Scenario

A 67-year-old, fit and well woman slipped and fell onto her outstretched dominant right hand. Initial radiographs showed a distal radius fracture (DRF) with neutral angulation and slight shortening (Fig. 1). This was treated in a plaster cast for 6 weeks with no further radiographs taken. After cast removal, the wrist was stiff, painful with an obvious dorsal deformity. After several months of hand therapy, the patient still described ongoing symptoms of pain, reduced grip strength, and was concerned about the appearance of the wrist. What would be the optimal management for this patient?

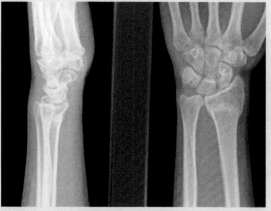

FIG. 1 Radiographs demonstrating an extraarticular distal radius fracture malunion with shortening and neutral angulation.

Distal Radius Fractures. https://doi.org/10.1016/B978-0-323-75764-5.00002-0

IMPORTANCE OF THE PROBLEM

DRFs are a very common injury and a huge burden on healthcare resources worldwide.[1, 2] Despite the frequency in which these injuries are encountered, there is still many unanswered questions regarding which fractures require intervention, optimum treatment methods, and long-term outcome. The evidence regarding fracture displacement and functional outcome after DRF is varied. Some studies have previously suggested only a small amount of displacement may lead to poor outcomes, whereas others have reported that significant displacement leads to minimal long-term functional problems.[3–6] Increasing evidence has suggested that in older patients malunion is well tolerated.[7, 8]

Up to 24% of patients develop malunion following a conservatively treated DRF and 10% of those treated surgically.[9] Unsatisfactory position in 58% of patients who underwent closed reduction of a displaced fracture has been reported, with 68% of those which were initially reduced satisfactorily subsequently displacing.[10] Despite this, most patients make a satisfactory recovery with only a small number of patients suffering significant symptoms because of malunion. Which patients are most affected by malunion is not well understood. The commonest and most effective surgical intervention for a symptomatic malunion following a DRF is a distal radius osteotomy although the evidence base is limited.[11].

MAIN QUESTION

Key Question: What is the most effective treatment (operative vs nonoperative) for extraarticular malunion in terms of short-term outcomes and long-term consequences?

CURRENT OPINION

Many patients may tolerate extraarticular malunion well following DRF, especially the elderly and those with less functional demand. If symptomatic malunion occurs following DRF, then intervention such as distal radius osteotomy should be considered taking into account the patient's functional status and general health.

FINDING THE EVIDENCE

We searched Cochrane Database of systematic reviews, MEDLINE and EMBASE.

Example of MEDLINE search terms:

(((distal ADJ3 (radius OR radial)) OR (wrist OR colles OR smith*)) ADJ3 fracture*).ti,ab
exp "RADIUS FRACTURES"/

exp "WRIST INJURIES"/
    EXTRA-ARTICULAR FRACTURES
    FRACTURES, MALUNITED
    (malunited fracture*).ti,ab
    (abnormal union fracture*).ti,ab

"CONSERVATIVE TREATMENT"/
"FRACTURE HEALING"/
TREATMENT OUTCOME/
"SURGICAL PROCEDURES, OPERATIVE"/

QUALITY OF THE EVIDENCE

Level I: 1 (comparison of planning techniques not operative and conservative management)
Level IV: 40

FINDINGS

No studies compare operative treatment with nonoperative treatment for extraarticular malunion following DRF. Forty-one studies were identified which report outcome following operative treatment for extraarticular malunion. One RCT reported outcome following osteotomy for extraarticular DRF but the aim of the study was to compare 3D computer-assisted planning with conventional two-dimensional (2D) planning for corrective osteotomy.

Thirty-nine of the studies reported on distal radius osteotomy with two describing ulnar shortening osteotomy. Thirty-seven studies were retrospective case series with three prospective series.

Most studies described new techniques such as the type of osteotomy, fixation method, use of different bone grafts, measurement or planning methods and supplemental procedures such as arthroscopy.

The decision about which DRF require surgical intervention is difficult. A huge amount of evidence on the subject has been produced but most of it is poor quality with conflicting findings. Significant variation in treatment currently exists.[12, 13] Recently, an international Delphi study has provided guidance about radiographic thresholds of intervention for different age groups (Table 1).[14] Guidance has also been produced by several national specialist groups.[15, 16] Despite this, malunion is not uncommon; however, the effect of this on a patient's functional outcome appears variable.

Distal radius osteotomy is a well described and popular treatment for patients with a symptomatic malunion following DRF.[11, 17] The evidence identified is of low quality and heterogenous with a wide variety of techniques studied. There is no strong evidence regarding the optimum timing for surgery or surgical technique.

TABLE 1
Delphi Study
Radiographic Threshold at Which Surgeon's Would Intervene.

| | | Parameter | | |
Age	Ulnar variance (mm)	Dorsal tilt (degrees)	Radial inclination (degrees)	Radial height (mm)
38	3	10	10	5
agreement	84%	79%	90%	85%
58	3	10	10	5
agreement	74%	87%	82%	90%
75	4 / >5	20	10	5
agreement	50% / 42%	87%	91%	88%

Agreement denotes the percentage of the expert panel who would intervene at this measurement.

Pillukat et al. prospectively reviewed 48 patients who underwent corrective osteotomy for malunion following DRF. Seventeen patients were aged 65 years and over and 31 were aged less than 65.[18] Range of motion, grip strength, pain, and radiographic parameters improved in both groups, although the younger age group had greater improvement. They concluded that osteotomy was beneficial for all age groups but older patients may not gain as much benefit. In a separate nonrandomized study, Pillukat et al. prospectively studied 34 consecutive patients with extraarticular DRF malunion and compared outcome for those who underwent early correction (less than 14 weeks following injury) and later correction.[19] At 2 year follow-up, Mayo scores improved significantly in both groups. The only difference between the groups was less requirement for bone grafting in those corrected early. Jupiter and Ring felt earlier reconstruction was technically simpler and resulted in a reduced period of disability when comparing 10 patients who underwent osteotomy at a mean time of 8 weeks following injury with 10 who underwent surgery at 40 weeks following injury.[20]

El-Karef et al. prospectively assessed the outcomes of 26 symptomatic patients with malunited DRF. A staged reconstructive approach was used and outcome measured using the Fernandez score. Satisfactory functional scores were achieved by 20 of the 26 patients after distal radial osteotomy alone, and 24 of the 26 after

subsequent ulnar shortening osteotomies and arthroscopy after 54 months. In their RCT comparing patient-reported outcome measures (PROMs) after corrective osteotomy for malunited DRF with and without 3-dimensional planning and use of patient-specific surgical guides, Buijze et al. found a trend toward a minimal clinically important difference in PROMs in favor of 3D-assisted group, although it did not attain significance because of (post-hoc) insufficient power.[21] Radiographic analysis showed minimal significant differences in the mean residual volar angulation and radial inclination, in favor of 3D planning and guidance. However, both groups gained significant improvement in DASH and PRWE scores.

Mulders et al. retrospectively reviewed 48 patients who underwent corrective osteotomy at a median of 27 months.[11] VAS pain scores decreased significantly from 6.5 preoperatively to 1.0 postoperative and grip strength recovered to 85% of the uninjured side. Postoperatively, they found a median PRWE score of 18.5 (IQR 6.5–37.0) and a DASH score of 10.0 (IQR 5.8–23.3), which is equal to the estimated score of the general population. Preoperative scores were not available. Eighteen patients (38%) had a complication for which additional treatment was required.

Disseldorp et al. retrospectively reviewed 132 corrective osteotomies of DRF malunions at mean follow-up of 92 months (range 13–252 months).[17] All but two osteotomies healed within 4 months and no nonunions occurred. Radiographic parameters improved significantly after surgery. They did not collect PROM data. Wound or soft tissue complications occurred in 21 (15.9%) patients. Seventy-three (55.3%) patients subsequently underwent metalwork removal because of complications, functional impairment, or pain.

There is minimal evidence regarding outcome after nonoperative treatment of extraarticular DRF malunion. Concern exists regarding the development of arthritis or problems related to carpal malalignment and altered wrist kinematics. Forward et al. assessed patients 38 years following nonoperative management of a DRF.[5] Sixty-six patients were examined who had sustained an extraarticular DRF. Patient evaluation measure score was 5% less than the uninjured side, with range of movement 98% and grip strength 96% of the uninjured side.

There is evidence that older patients tolerate malunion well with satisfactory functional outcome despite imperfect position.[7,8,22] Anzurat et al. prospectively graded DRF in patients aged over 50 as acceptable or unacceptable reduction according to radiographic parameters. At 6 months follow-up, there was no difference in SF12 and DASH scores between the groups. Several metaanalyses have reported no improvement in functional outcome when comparing surgical intervention and closed reduction in older patients despite superior radiological outcome with surgery.[23,24]

RECOMMENDATIONS

In patients with an intraarticular displaced distal radius fracture, evidence suggests:

Recommendations	Overall Quality
• Distal radius osteotomy is likely to improve symptoms in *carefully selected patients* with a symptomatic malunion following DRF	⊕⊕⊕⊕ HIGH
• Patient factors including preinjury functional status must be considered	⊕⊕◯◯ LOW
• Complication rate and need for further surgery is high. Most secondary surgery is for implant removal	⊕⊕⊕◯ MODERATE
• Older patients tolerate malunion well and may be less likely to require and benefit from osteotomy	⊕⊕⊕◯ MODERATE
• Optimal timing of surgery and surgical technique is not established	⊕◯◯◯ VERY LOW

CONCLUSION

There is a vast amount of evidence investigating outcome after DRF and DRF osteotomy but the majority is low quality. Multiple studies that suggest osteotomy will improve outcome after DRF malunion. There are few high quality studies using PROMs but the evidence from lower quality studies generally suggests a benefit from osteotomy. Many variables are not well understood such as surgical approach, adjunct procedures, use and type of bone graft, and timing of surgery. Complication rate and need for re-operation is considerable. There is evidence that older patients tolerate malunion well. Therefore, careful consideration and adequate patient counseling should be carried out before deciding optimum treatment for a patient with DRF malunion.

Panel 2: Author's Preferred Technique (Related to Case Scenario)

In this case of a DRF in an independent, active patient who is symptomatic following extraarticular malunion, surgical management was chosen. The patient had undergone extensive conservative therapy with minimal benefit. Symptoms were consistent with ulnar sided impaction and radiographs revealed carpal malalignment secondary to loss of volar tilt. After discussion with the patient regarding risks and benefits of the treatment options it was decided to carry out distal radius osteotomy to lengthen the radius and restore volar tilt to improve carpal alignment. Preoperative planning involved plain radiographs and a CT scan of the injured side only. Measurements were made from these images to estimate the amount of correction required but

these are used as a planning guide only and definitive decisions were made intraoperatively based on image intensifier findings. A volar opening wedge osteotomy was performed (Fig. 2). In this case, correcting the tilt improved length without a large amount of distraction therefore bone grafting was not required as there was adequate bony contact at the osteotomy site. If bone grafting is required our preference is to pack the defect with synthetic bone graft after plate application. This method is simple and quick and avoids donor site problems. The patient reported a significant improvement in symptoms, the osteotomy healed uneventfully and radiographic parameters were satisfactory.

Panel 2: Author's Preferred Technique (Related to Case Scenario)—cont'd

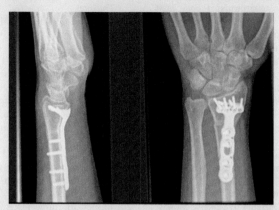

FIG. 2 Radiographs following volar opening wedge osteotomy with improvement in length and angulation.

Panel 3: Pearls and Pitfalls

PEARLS

- Careful counseling of patients is essential prior to carrying out any osteotomy. Many patients will be older people and need to understand the possible complications, lengthy rehabilitation, and potential need for further surgery.
- When performing a volar osteotomy for a dorsally angulated or neutral short malunion fix, the plate to the radius distally before carrying out any bone cuts. Place several screws distally then remove all but one. Loosen the remaining screw and move the plate away from the distal radius to allow the osteotomy cut to be made. Following this, the screws can be replaced and tightened. Otherwise fixing the plate to the mobile, loose distal radius fragment after osteotomy can be difficult.
- The most common technique to correct a volar angulated malunions is a volar opening wedge osteotomy. Another option is a sliding osteotomy which involves an oblique osteotomy to recreate the fracture. The distal fragment is slid dorsally and stabilized.
- A laminar spreader placed in the osteotomy site and gradually opened can provide a significant amount of distraction and help lengthen shortened fractures.

Placing the lamina spreader on the radial side of the osteotomy site will also help increase radial inclination.

PITFALLS

- Metalwork should be placed carefully to try and avoid the need for further surgery. In some cases, particularly with significant malunion, it may be difficult to place metalwork in an ideal position. Patients should be warned prior to surgery that they may require metalwork removal.
- Lengthening the radius significantly (>8 mm) is difficult and can lead to problems such as postoperative pain and nerve injury. If a large lengthening is required consider an alternative technique or combine with an ulnar shortening procedure.
- In older patients with osteoporotic bone, the malunion will often involve shortening. Lengthening of fragile bone is difficult and may need to be combined with an ulnar shortening procedure.
- Careful assessment of distal radioulnar joint (DRUJ) congruence is required. Failure to address this may lead to ongoing pain and future arthritis.

REFERENCES

1. Stirling ER, Johnson NA, Dias JJ. Epidemiology of distal radius fractures in a geographically defined adult population. *J Hand Surg Eur Vol.* 2018;43(9):974–982.
2. O'Neill TW, Cooper C, Finn JD, et al. Incidence of distal forearm fracture in British men and women. *Osteoporos Int.* 2001;12(7):555–558.
3. Catalano LW, Cole RJ, Gelberman RH, Evanoff BA, Gilula LA, Borrelli J. Displaced intra-articular fractures of the distal aspect of the radius. Long-term results in young adults after open reduction and internal fixation. *J Bone Joint Surg Am.* 1997;79(9):1290–1302.
4. Chung KC, Kotsis SV, Kim HM. Predictors of functional outcomes after surgical treatment of distal radius fractures. *J Hand Surg [Am].* 2007;32(1):76–83.

5. Forward DP, Davis TR, Sithole JS. Do young patients with malunited fractures of the distal radius inevitably develop symptomatic post-traumatic osteoarthritis? *J Bone Joint Surg.* 2008;90(5):629–637.

6. Kopylov P, Johnell O, Redlund-Johnell I, Bengner U. Fractures of the distal end of the radius in young adults: a 30-year follow-up. *J Hand Surg (Br).* 1993;18(1):45–49.

7. Synn AJ, Makhni EC, Makhni MC, Rozental TD, Day CS. Distal radius fractures in older patients: is anatomic reduction necessary? *Clin Orthop Relat Res.* 2009;467 (6):1612–1620.

8. Anzarut A, Johnson JA, Rowe BH, Lambert RG, Blitz S, Majumdar SR. Radiologic and patient-reported functional outcomes in an elderly cohort with conservatively treated distal radius fractures. *J Hand Surg [Am].* 2004;29(6):1121–1127.

9. McGrory B, Amadio P. Malunion of the distal radius. In: *The Wrist: Diagnosis and Operative Treatment.* Mosby; 1998:365–384.

10. Arora R, Lutz M, Deml C, Krappinger D, Haug L, Gabl M. A prospective randomized trial comparing nonoperative treatment with volar locking plate fixation for displaced and unstable distal radial fractures in patients sixty-five years of age and older. *JBJS.* 2011;93(23):2146–2153.

11. Mulders MA, d'Ailly P, Cleffken B, Schep N. Corrective osteotomy is an effective method of treating distal radius malunions with good long-term functional results. *Injury.* 2017;48(3):731–737.

12. Johnson NA, Stirling E, Dias JJ. Variation in surgical fixation rate for distal radial fracture in England. *J Hand Surg Eur Vol.* 2019;16. https://doi.org/10.1177/1753193419849765 [Epub 2019/05/18].

13. Walenkamp MMJ, Mulders MAM, Goslings JC, Westert GP, Schep NWL. Analysis of variation in the surgical treatment of patients with distal radial fractures in the Netherlands. *J Hand Surg Eur Vol.* 2017;42(1):39–44.

14. Johnson N, Leighton P, Pailthorpe C, Dias J, Distal Radius Fracture Delphi Study Group. Defining displacement thresholds for surgical intervention for distal radius fractures–a Delphi study. *PLoS ONE.* 2019;14(1):e0210462.

15. Salling N, Andreasen TS, Foldager-Jensen AD, et al. *National Clinical Guideline on the Treatment of Distal Radial Fractures.*

16. Lichtman DM, Bindra RR, Boyer MI, et al. Treatment of distal radius fractures. *J Am Acad Orthop Surg.* 2010;18 (3):180–189.

17. Disseldorp DJ, Poeze M, Hannemann PF, Brink PR. Is bone grafting necessary in the treatment of malunited distal radius fractures? *J Wrist Surg.* 2015;4(3):207–213.

18. Pillukat T, Prommersberger K. Is corrective osteotomy for malunited distal radius fractures also indicated for elderly patients? *Handchir Mikrochir Plast Chir.* 2007;39 (1):42–48.

19. Pillukat T, Schädel-Höpfner M, Windolf J, Prommersberger K. The malunited distal radius fracture-early or late correction? *Handchir Mikrochir Plast Chir.* 2013;45(1):6–12.

20. Jupiter JB, Ring D. A comparison of early and late reconstruction of malunited fractures of the distal end of the radius. *JBJS.* 1996;78(5):739–748.

21. Buijze GA, Leong NL, Stockmans F, et al. Three-dimensional compared with two-dimensional preoperative planning of corrective osteotomy for extra-articular distal radial malunion: a multicenter randomized controlled trial. *J Bone Joint Surg.* 2018;18100 (14):1191–1202.

22. Diaz-Garcia RJ, Oda T, Shauver MJ, Chung KC. A systematic review of outcomes and complications of treating unstable distal radius fractures in the elderly. *J Hand Surg.* 2011;36 (5):824–835.

23. Navarro CM, Brolund A, Ekholm C, et al. Treatment of radius or ulna fractures in the elderly: a systematic review covering effectiveness, safety, economic aspects and current practice. *PLoS ONE.* 2019;14(3):e0214362.

24. Chen Y, Chen X, Li Z, Yan H, Zhou F, Gao W. Safety and efficacy of operative versus nonsurgical management of distal radius fractures in elderly patients: a systematic review and meta-analysis. *J Hand Surg [Am].* 2016;41 (3):404–413.

CHAPTER 31

Treatment of the Intraarticular Malunited Distal Radius

NICK JOHNSON • JOSEPH DIAS
University Hospitals of Leicester, Leicester, United Kingdom

KEY POINTS

- Intraarticular malunion following distal radius fracture (DRF) leads to radiographic arthritis, but the effect on functional outcome is not well understood.
- Evidence evaluating operative and nonoperative treatment of intraarticular malunion is of low quality.
- Some small, retrospective case series suggest osteotomy will improve outcome after intraarticular DRF malunion.
- Surgery is challenging with high complication rate and need for re-operation.
- There is insufficient evidence to establish whether osteotomy for intraarticular malunion prevents the development of arthritis.

Panel 1: Case Scenario

A 42-year-old, fit and well man was involved in a high-speed road traffic accident. He required an extended ICU admission and surgery for intraabdominal injuries. Following a good recovery from these injuries and discharge to a general surgical ward, he described pain in his dominant left wrist. Radiographs were obtained 3 weeks after his initial injury and these demonstrated a distal radius fracture with dorsal angulation and a depressed and rotated lunate fossa fragment with a 2 mm intraarticular step (Fig. 1). What would be the optimal management for this patient?

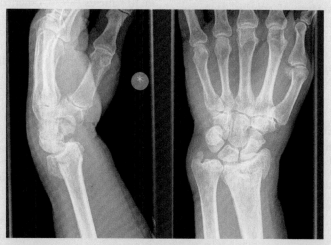

FIG. 1 Radiographs demonstrating an intra and extra articular distal radius fracture malunion with loss of dorsal angulation and a depressed, rotated lunate fossa fragment.

Distal Radius Fractures. https://doi.org/10.1016/B978-0-323-75764-5.00037-8

IMPORTANCE OF THE PROBLEM

Persistent articular incongruity of the distal radius after fracture healing is known to lead to early degenerative changes of the radiocarpal joint. Cadaveric experiments have shown that an articular step affects the biomechanics of the joint with a step of 1 mm causing a significant increase in contact stresses.[1, 2] Despite the evidence that articular incongruity leads to radiologically proven arthritis, the correlation with symptoms and poor outcome is debatable. Studies by Trumble et al. and Chung et al. showed that residual articular displacement was associated with a poorer outcome.[3, 4] Others have shown minimal long term functional impairment.[5]

Intraarticular malunion can be measured as a step and/or gap. Step is thought to be the most important parameter to affect functional outcome and many surgeons would recommend intervention for a step of 2 mm or more in younger patients.[6] Correcting intraarticular malunion is challenging and involves the risk of rare but disastrous complications such as nonunion or avascular necrosis. Complexity of surgery is compounded by associated extra-articular malunion.

MAIN QUESTION

What is the most effective treatment (operative vs nonoperative) for intraarticular malunion in terms of short-term outcomes and long-term consequences?

CURRENT OPINION

Patients with an intraarticular step following DRF develop radiographic evidence of arthritis. However, this may not lead to significant functional impairment. Surgery to correct intraarticular displacement is complex with a risk of significant complications. It may be considered for younger patients with a significant intraarticular step taking into account the patient's functional status and general health.

FINDING THE EVIDENCE

We searched the Cochrane Database of systematic reviews, MEDLINE and EMBASE.

The following MEDLINE search terms were used: (((distal ADJ3 (radius OR radial)) OR (wrist OR colles OR smith*)) ADJ3 fracture*).ti,ab
exp "RADIUS FRACTURES"/

exp "WRIST INJURIES"/
   INTRA-ARTICULAR   FRACTURES,   ARTICULAR
FRACTURES, MALUNITED, (malunited fracture*).ti,ab
(abnormal union fracture*).ti,ab

"CONSERVATIVE TREATMENT"/
"FRACTURE HEALING"/
TREATMENT OUTCOME/
"SURGICAL PROCEDURES, OPERATIVE"/

QUALITY OF THE EVIDENCE

Level IV: 14

FINDINGS

No studies compared operative treatment with nonoperative treatment for intraarticular malunion following DRF. Fourteen studies were identified which report outcome following operative treatment for intraarticular malunion. All studies were retrospective case series and the largest case series involved 23 patients.

Ring et al. evaluated 23 patients at an average of 38 months after corrective osteotomy for an intraarticular malunion following DRF.[7] Average articular incongruity was reduced from 4 to 0.4 mm. The rate of excellent or good results was 83% according to the rating systems of Fernandez and of Gartland and Werley. No patient had evidence of nonunion or avascular necrosis.

Buijze et al. assessed 18 patients at an average of 78 months after corrective osteotomy for a combined intra- and extra-articular malunion of the distal radius.[8] All patients healed uneventfully, and final articular incongruity was reduced to 2 mm or less. Rate of excellent or good results was 72% according to the Mayo Modified Wrist Score. Hardware removal was required in 10 patients (56%), other complications occurred in 5 patients (28%), of which transient de Quervain tenosynovitis was the most common (3 patients, 17%).

Luo et al. evaluated seven consecutive patients with a mean age of 38 years who underwent corrective osteotomy for intraarticular malunion after DRF.[9] Mean time from injury to corrective surgery was 10 weeks. At mean follow-up of 44 months, significant improvements in pain scores, QuickDASH, and grip strength were seen. One patient had evidence of degenerative change at final follow up but was asymptomatic. No significant complications were reported. The authors recommended that early corrective osteotomies should be considered in young patients with intraarticular distal radius malunions.

Arthroscopic assistance has been reported to help guide osteotomy and reduction by allowing direct visualization of the joint surface. In a study of 11 patients with intraarticular malunion following DRF, del Pinal et al. carried out an osteotomy from inside the joint outward under arthroscopic guidance.[10] At follow-up ranging from 12 to 48 months, there were 4 excellent and 7 good results according to the Gartland and Werley score.

Correction of intraarticular malunions is desirable to prevent the development of radiocarpal degenerative evolution. Knirk and Jupiter showed a step of 2 mm or more led to a 100% incidence of radiological arthritis in 40 young adults at mean follow-up of 6.7 years.[11]

Catalano et al. found 76% of patients with residual intraarticular displacement 7 years after internal fixation of DRF had evidence of arthritis which had progressed when reassessed after 15 years by radiographs and computerized tomography (CT) scans.[12, 13]

A total of 93% of the patients in Knirk and Jupiter's study were symptomatic. However, 61% reported a good or excellent outcome, and only one patient who had bilateral fractures had to stop work due to their injury.[11] The only functional limitation seen in the 15-year review of Catalano's original study, was an insignificant reduction in wrist flexion.[13]

Forward et al. retrospectively reviewed 40 young adults with intraarticular distal radius fractures at a mean of 38 years and found DASH (Disabilities of Arm, Shoulder, and Hand) scores were not different to population norms and functional impairment was less than 10% when assessed by the Patient Evaluation Measure.[5] Kopylov et al. evaluated patients who had sustained a DRF 30 years, previously. Radiographic osteoarthritis was related to articular incongruity, but complaints were limited; 87% of patients reported no difference between their injured and uninjured sides.[14]

RECOMMENDATIONS

In patients with an intraarticular displaced distal radius fracture, evidence suggests:

Recommendation	Overall Quality
• There is weak evidence that distal radius osteotomy may improve symptoms in carefully selected patients.	⊕⊕○○ LOW
• There is insufficient evidence to establish whether osteotomy for intraarticular malunion prevents the development of arthritis.	⊕⊕○○ LOW
• Surgery is complex with significant potential complications and the need for further surgery is high.	⊕⊕○○ LOW
• Optimal timing of surgery and surgical technique is not established.	⊕○○○ VERY LOW
• Intraarticular malunion invariably leads to arthritis but the effect on functional outcome may be minimal.	⊕⊕○○ LOW

CONCLUSION

There is minimal evidence investigating outcome after interventions for intraarticular malunion following DRF. Some small, retrospective case series suggest osteotomy will improve outcome after intraarticular DRF malunion. Surgery is challenging with a high complication rate and common need for re-operation, notably hardware removal. Long-term evidence demonstrates that intraarticular malunion does lead to arthritis. Some studies have reported that this leads to poor functional outcome whereas other long-term studies have suggested functional impairment is minimal even in younger patients.

Panel 2: Author's Preferred Technique (Related to Case Scenario)

In this case of a distal radius fracture in a fit patient with extra and intraarticular malunion surgical management was chosen. The patient was extensively counseled prior to surgery about the risks and benefits of surgery and the lack of understanding about long-term outcome with conservative or surgical management. Due to concerns about long-term outcome and early arthritis he decided to undergo surgical intervention. A CT scan was obtained to aid surgical planning. The procedure was performed through a volar approach. Two osteotomy cuts were made using osteotomes to enable the lunate fossa fragment to be elevated and the dorsal angulation to be corrected. The fragment was relocated using gentle levering with an osteotome under image intensifier guidance to reduce the articular step. It was held temporarily with two K-wires then fixed rigidly with a volar locking plate in the desired position. The defect proximal to the elevated fragment was packed with synthetic bone graft (Fig. 2). The patient made a good recovery with no early complications and the osteotomy united. The metalwork was placed in a satisfactory position, but the patient has been advised to seek early medical attention if he develops signs or symptoms of hardware problems such as tendon irritation.

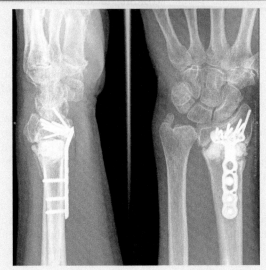

FIG. 2 Radiographs following osteotomy demonstrating elevation of the lunate fossa fragment and correction of dorsal angulation.

Panel 3: Pearls and Pitfalls

PEARLS

- Careful counseling of patients is essential prior to carrying out an intraarticular osteotomy. Patients must be aware that the long-term functional outcome is not well understood. There is a risk of serious complications and a potential need for further surgery.
- Intraarticular step is believed to lead to more long-term problems than gap.
- Further imaging such as a CT or MRI scan is extremely useful to fully understand the three-dimensional anatomy of the malunion and aid surgical planning.
- Volar, dorsal, or combined approaches may be used. This may depend on the unique anatomy of the malunion and individual surgeon preference.
- After performing the osteotomy gentle levering with an osteotome or other small, flat instrument can help reduce the fragment. Manoeuvre such as traction and extension or flexion can also assist reduction. When reduced the fragment can be held with temporary K-wires. Once satisfactory position has been confirmed with an image intensifier or arthroscopy, definitive fixation can be carried out.

PITFALLS

- Surgery for intraarticular surgery is complex and relatively uncommon. This type of surgery should be carried out by experienced surgeons in specialist units.
- Arthroscopic procedures require considerable surgical skills and experience. An experienced assistant is extremely valuable and can help reduce operating time.
- Metalwork should be placed carefully to try and avoid the need for further surgery but in some cases it is unavoidable that metalwork is placed in a prominent, distal position to enable fixation of a reduced fragment. Patients should be warned prior to surgery that they may require metalwork removal and advised of signs and symptoms to look out for which may suggest metalwork problems.
- Whilst focusing on intraarticular malunion, it is also likely that a combined extra-articular malunion will be present following distal radius fracture. This must be identified and may also require correcting to prevent ongoing symptoms.
- Additional simultaneous procedures may be necessary. Most frequently for the distal ulna and distal radioulnar joint. These areas must be carefully assessed and treatment options considered prior to commencing an intraarticular osteotomy.

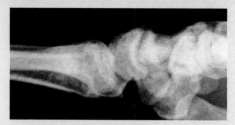

Fig. 1A. Correcting a combined intra- and extra-articular such as this patient, is slightly more complex and has to be "broken down" in their respective components.

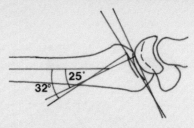

Fig. 1B. A schematic drawing is helpful to show the extra-articular component, a dorsal angulation of 32 degrees of the scaphoid fossa and 25 degrees of the lunate fossa, 6 months postinjury.

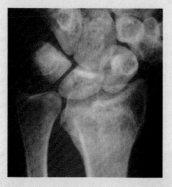

Fig. 1C. The posteroanterior radiograph shows a 7 mm ulnar-positive variance and a 6 mm step-off and gap.

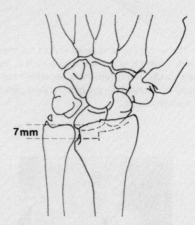

Fig. 1D. Again a corresponding schematic drawing is made.

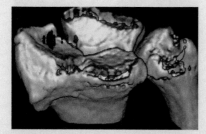

Fig. 1E. It consists of three malunited fracture components, a dorso-ulnar part, a volar-ulnar part, and a radial styloid part.

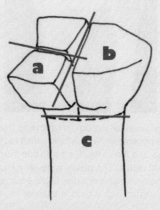

Fig. 2A. Schematic drawing from the dorsal view of the three osteotomy lines that follow the fracture pattern.

Continued

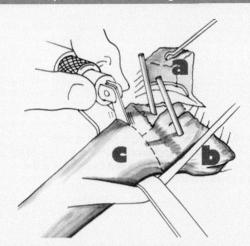

Fig. 2B. The volar-ulnar and radial styloid fragments were pinned with 1.5 mm K-wires, and a skin hook is used to open the capsule. The osteotomies separated the dorso-ulnar component (a), the radial styloid part (b), and the metaphysis (c).

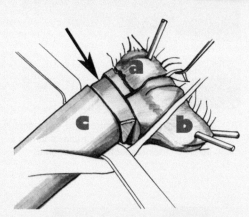

Fig. 3. To provide fracture fragment mobilization, the fragments were dorsally pinned with stout K-wires for mobilization with a joystick-type control. Once the optimal anatomical position was achieved, the parts were temporarily fixed with smooth Kirschner wires, and a cortico-cancellous bone graft from the iliac crest was introduced at the metaphyseal osteotomy *(arrow)*.

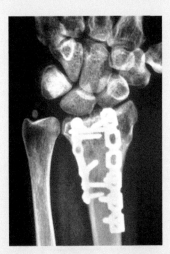

Fig. 4. Posteroanterior radiograph showing that the articular components were then fixed with a radially inserted 2.0 mm screw and the metaphysis with one 1.5 mm and one 2.0 mm dorsal plates. The plates were removed because of dorsal tenosynovitis and index finger extensor tendons rupture and treated with a tendon transfer.

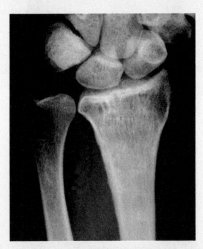

Fig. 5. At 11-year follow-up, the patient had excellent function, full range of motion, and no signs of osteoarthritis in the wrist.

REFERENCES

1. Baratz ME, Des Jardins JD, Anderson DD, Imbriglia JE. Displaced intra-articular fractures of the distal radius: the effect of fracture displacement on contract stresses in a cadaver model. *J Hand Surg [Am]*. 1996;21(2):183–188.
2. Wagner WF, Tencer AF, Kiser P, Trumble TE. Effects of intra-articular distal radius depression on wrist joint contact characteristics. *J Hand Surg [Am]*. 1996;21(4):554–560.
3. Trumble TE, Schmitt SR, Vedder NB. Factors affecting functional outcome of displaced intra-articular distal radius fractures. *J Hand Surg [Am]*. 1994;19(2):325–340.
4. Chung KC, Kotsis SV, Kim HM. Predictors of functional outcomes after surgical treatment of distal radius fractures. *J Hand Surg [Am]*. 2007;32(1):76–83.
5. Forward DP, Davis TR, Sithole JS. Do young patients with malunited fractures of the distal radius inevitably develop symptomatic post-traumatic osteoarthritis? *J Bone Joint Surg Br Vol*. 2008;90(5):629–637.
6. Johnson N, Leighton P, Distal Radius Fracture Delphi Study Group, Pailthorpe C, Dias J. Defining displacement thresholds for surgical intervention for distal radius fractures—Delphi study. *PLoS One*. 2019;14(1), e0210462 [Epub 2019/01/09].
7. Ring D, Prommersberger K-J, Del Pino JG, Capomassi M, Slullitel M, Jupiter JB. Corrective osteotomy for intra-articular malunion of the distal part of the radius. *JBJS*. 2005;87(7):1503–1509.
8. Buijze GA, Prommersberger K-J, del Pino JG, Fernandez DL, Jupiter JB. Corrective osteotomy for combined intra- and extra-articular distal radius malunion. *J Hand Surg [Am]*. 2012;37(10):2041–2049.
9. Luo TD, Nunez Jr FA, Newman EA, Nunez Sr FA. Early correction of distal radius partial articular malunion leads to good long-term functional recovery at mean follow-up of 4 years. *Hand*. 2020;15(2):276–280.
10. del Piñal F, Cagigal L, García-Bernal FJ, Studer A, Regalado J, Thams C. Arthroscopically guided osteotomy for management of intra-articular distal radius malunions. *J Hand Surg [Am]*. 2010;35(3):392–397.
11. Knirk JL, Jupiter JB. Intra-articular fractures of the distal end of the radius in young adults. *J Bone Joint Surg Am*. 1986;68(5):647–659.
12. Catalano LW, Cole RJ, Gelberman RH, Evanoff BA, Gilula LA, Borrelli J. Displaced intra-articular fractures of the distal aspect of the radius. Long-term results in young adults after open reduction and internal fixation. *J Bone Joint Surg Am*. 1997;79(9):1290–1302.
13. Goldfarb CA, Rudzki JR, Catalano LW, Hughes M, Borrelli J. Fifteen-year outcome of displaced intra-articular fractures of the distal radius. *J Hand Surg [Am]*. 2006;31(4): 633–639.
14. Kopylov P, Johnell O, Redlund-Johnell I, Bengner U. Fractures of the distal end of the radius in young adults: a 30-year follow-up. *J Hand Surg Br Eur Vol*. 1993;18(1):45–49.

CHAPTER 32

Three-Dimensional Planning and Surgical Guidance of Malunion Correction

MAARTJE MICHIELSEN[a,b] • MATTHIAS VANHEES[a,b] • FREDERIK VERSTREKEN[a,b]
[a]Orthopedic Department, AZ Monica Hospital, Antwerp, Belgium, [b]Orthopedic Department,
Antwerp University Hospital, Edegem, Belgium

KEY POINTS

- Malunion is the most common complication following a distal radius fracture.
- Restoration of anatomy is a key factor in obtaining good functional outcome, but this can be technically challenging.
- Next to radiographs and CT-scans, three-dimensional (3D) visualization and printed bone models can further improve understanding of the malunion pattern.
- The use of three-dimensional (3D) computer planning and the production of patient-specific instruments allow accurate and reproducible correction, especially in complex malunion patterns.
- The additional cost is one of the major disadvantages of the 3D technique.
- Further clinical investigations are necessary to better define the added value, the indications, and cost-effectiveness of 3D technology in the treatment of malunions.

Panel 1: Case Scenario

A 48-year old woman sustained a severely displaced intra- and extra-articular fracture of the left distal radius. She was initially treated at another facility with closed reduction, additional external fixation, and K-wires.

She presented 8 months later, with an intra- and extra-articular malunion, causing persistent wrist pain (VAS 8/10) and severe functional impairment (Quick-DASH 62).

Physical examination revealed residual pain at the radio-carpal and distal radioulnar joint, restricted wrist movement, and decreased grip strength. The Modified Mayo Wrist score was poor (MMWS 10).

Can 3D technology provide a more accurate reduction and better outcome of her complex distal radius malunion (Fig. 1)?

Continued

Distal Radius Fractures. https://doi.org/10.1016/B978-0-323-75764-5.00035-4

Panel 1: Case Scenario—cont'd

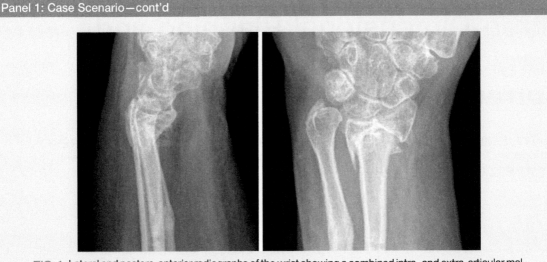

FIG. 1 Lateral and postero-anterior radiographs of the wrist showing a combined intra- and extra-articular malunion of the distal radius.

IMPORTANCE OF THE PROBLEM

Malunion of the distal radius is a common complication, with a reported incidence of up to 23% of nonsurgically treated distal radius fractures.[1–4] It often causes persistent wrist pain and functional impairment. Additionally, secondary carpal malalignment and intraarticular deformities can lead to early degenerative changes.[5–9]

When surgical treatment is deemed necessary, a corrective osteotomy is the procedure of choice, and clinical studies have shown a significant correlation between the precise reconstruction of normal anatomy and the clinical outcome.[10–15]

Planning and performing a corrective osteotomy can be a technically challenging procedure. Conventional two-dimensional radiographs are limited in the visualization of complex intraarticular or rotational deformities of the malunited wrist.[16, 17] And studies have shown that even following careful planning, restoration of bony alignment was only obtained in 40% of patients.[14] A complication rate of up to 42% has been reported following corrective osteotomy, with tendon injuries and delayed or nonunion being the most commonly reported problems.[3, 18]

Three-dimensional technology might address some of these problems, and improve outcome following corrective surgery (Box 1).

MAIN QUESTION

What is the added value of three-dimensional (3D) planning and surgical guidance compared to more conventional techniques in the correction of distal radius malunions?

Current Opinion

Most surgeons are confident that preoperative planning with two-dimensional (2D) imaging for corrective osteotomy of distal radius malunions leads to acceptable results and complication rates in the majority of cases. They argue that 3D technology complicates the procedure without proven added value or cost effectiveness.

Finding the Evidence

- Cochrane library: Distal radius malunion
- Pubmed (Medline): ((Colles' fracture* [tiab] OR distal radius fracture* [tiab]) AND (Three-dimensional [tiab] OR 3D [tiab] OR 3-D [tiab] OR computer assisted [tiab] OR computer simulated [tiab] OR computer aided [tiab] OR virtual planning) AND (Malunited fracture* [tiab] OR malunion [tiab] OR osteotomy [tiab] OR corrective osteotomy [tiab]))
- Randomized controlled trials (RCTs), systematic reviews, case series, and case reports published between January 1, 2000, and January 20, 2020 were considered

---

BOX 1
The 3 Steps of 3D Technology.

Step 1 DICOM (Digital Imaging and Communications in Medicine) data are collected through computed tomography (CT) scans of the malunited and the contralateral forearm. This can be done simultaneously with the patient in the prone position, shoulders in full extension and both arms overhead, to decrease radiation exposure. To allow precise 3D reconstruction of bony anatomy, a specific scanning protocol needs to be followed with scanning parameters set at a tube current of 10–30 mA and voltage of 90–120 kV, a slice thickness of <0.625 mm and a field of view of 200 mm × 200 mm or smaller.

Step 2 Virtual 3D models (STL files) are created, using dedicated medical image processing software. Precise assessment of the deformity in all planes is now possible

and corrective surgery can be planned in detail, based on the healthy contralateral side.[19]

Step 3 3D technology will allow this virtual plan to be translated to the operation room, and multiple methods have been developed to do this: virtual and three-dimensional printed bone models,[20] optical tracking devices,[21, 22] synthetic or bony prefabricated wedges that fit into the osteotomy gap,[23–25] and the use of patient-specific surgical cutting and drilling guides.[20, 26–33] The last one appears to be the most promising technique.[4] The drilling and cutting guides are designed based on the surgical plan, and 3D printed in medical-grade material that can be sterilized.

- Review of references of eligible studies
- Articles that were not in English, French, German or Dutch were excluded

Quality of the Evidence

Level I:
Randomized controlled trial: 1
Level IV:
Clinical application review: 1
Systematic review of case series and metaanalysis: 1
Case series: 17
Level V:
Case reports: 6

FINDINGS

Evidence From Level I Studies

Buijze et al. included 40 patients in a randomized controlled trial to compare conventional 2D planning with 3D computer-assisted planned corrective osteotomies for extra-articular distal radius malunion. They found a significantly improved radiographic outcome (radial tilt and volar angulation) ($P < .05$), and a trend toward better PROMs (DASH and PRWE) in favor of the 3D planning group, which did not attain significance because of (post hoc) insufficient power of the study. However, there were no significant differences in pain, satisfaction, range of motion, and grip strength.[34]

Evidence From Level IV Studies

In a systematic review including 15 studies and 68 patients treated with 3D virtual planning for both extra- and intraarticular malunions, de Muinck Keizer et al.[17] found a statistically significant improvement

($P < .05$) of the radiographic parameters in 96% of the patients, in whom anatomy was restored to within 5 degrees (angulation) or 2 mm (ulnar variance) of their normal values. This is clearly better than the 40% achieved with meticulous two-dimensional preoperative planning, using the same criteria for restoration of anatomy.[14] Furthermore, a significant ($P < .05$) improvement of wrist range of motion and grip strength was noted, with an overall complication rate of 16%, compared to a reported complication rate of up to 42% with conventional techniques..[17, 18] Three more recent case series on three-dimensional corrective osteotomies of the distal radius showed comparable results, reinforcing the growing evidence in support of three-dimensional technology.[35–37]

The use of three-dimensional technology and patient-specific guides allows precise reconstruction of intraarticular step-offs,[31, 36, 38] and seems to be of most benefit for complex deformities of the distal radius.[17, 30, 32]

Besides this growing evidence for better clinical and radiographic results, three-dimensional technology allows for a reproducible and safe correction of distal radius malunion and reduces operation time, blood loss volume, and radiation exposure during surgery.[6, 39] The reported complication rates following 3D-assisted osteotomies of the distal radius compare favorably to those following conventional techniques.[3, 17, 18, 20]

The disadvantages of 3D technology are the need for specialized computer software, radiation exposure during CT-scanning, the time and effort for preoperative planning and the additional cost of the custom-made surgical guides and implants.[17, 27] These existing costs currently prevent everyday clinical use.[40] To address some of these issues, Caiti et al. have proposed a software solution to streamline the design of patient-specific instruments to make 3D technology more accessible.[40]

Evidence From Level V studies

Other authors have suggested that in-hospital planning and 3D printing of guides can decrease the cost of 3D technology.[41, 42]

RECOMMENDATION

In patients with symptomatic malunion of the distal radius, evidence suggests the following:

Recommendation	Overall Quality
• A corrective osteotomy is the treatment of choice and significantly improves functional and radiographic outcomes.	⊕⊕⊕⊕ HIGH
• The use of 3D technology allows better correction of radiographic parameters: angulation and rotation.	⊕⊕⊕⊕ HIGH
• There is no significant difference in clinical outcome when 3D technology is used, but a trend toward better PROMs exists.	⊕⊕⊕○ MODERATE
• Complex deformities of the distal radius, in particular, will benefit from three-dimensional planning and guidance.	⊕○○○ VERY LOW

- Intraarticular congruency can be reliably restored using 3D technology. ⊕⊕○○ LOW
- The use of 3D technology allows for a lower complication rate compared to conventional techniques. ⊕⊕○○ LOW
- The use of 3D technology increases the cost of treatment and has not been shown to be cost-efficient. ⊕⊕⊕○ MODERATE

CONCLUSION

Although the added value and cost-effectiveness of three-dimensional technology need to be confirmed, three-dimensional planning and surgical guidance facilitate restoration of normal anatomy. It allows accurate, reproducible, and safe correction of the malunited radius. Especially complex deformities: multidirectional malalignment and intraarticular deformations of the distal radius will benefit from the use of three-dimensional techniques. Further clinical investigations are necessary to find the correct indications to use this technology and determine its cost-efficiency. New technical developments, including lower-dose scanning technology, software improvements, artificial intelligence, and in-hospital printing may lower the associated costs and improve cost efficiency.

Panel 2: Authors' Preferred Treatment

We have a low threshold to use 3D evaluation of deformity when a patient presents with symptomatic malunion of the distal radius. It allows precise assessment of deformity in all planes and intraarticular incongruency. If surgical correction is deemed necessary, the decision to further use 3D technology can be based on the deformity that is present. In our experience, preoperative planning and the use of patient-specific instruments facilitate the precise restoration of anatomy, especially in complex cases. Besides that, we have found that it lowers operating time and fluoroscopy use.

In the aforementioned patient, a three-dimensional corrective osteotomy was performed given the complexity of the malunion. Following precise planning or extra- and intraarticular correction, surgical guides were designed, 3D printed and used during the procedure. This allowed for precise restoration of anatomy and articular congruency. The osteotomy healed uneventfully and at 1 year postoperatively, she had significant improvement of wrist pain (VAS 1/10) and function, with a Quick-DASH of 23 and a Modified Mayo Wrist score of 70 (Figs. 2–6).

Panel 2: Authors' Preferred Treatment—cont'd

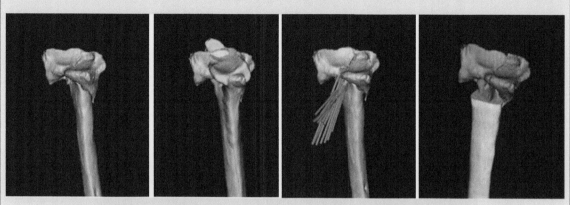

FIG. 2 Three-dimensional images of a mirrored version of the contralateral healthy side are superimposed on the malunited radius and both an intra- and extra-articular correction is planned.

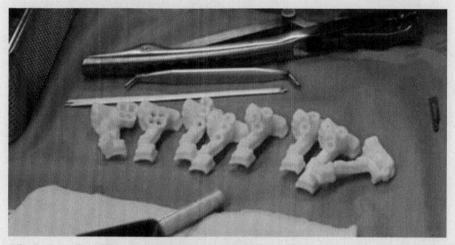

FIG. 3 Patient-specific drilling and cutting guides are printed in a medical-grade material (polyamide) that can be sterilized for use in the operating room.

Continued

Panel 2: Authors' Preferred Treatment—cont'd

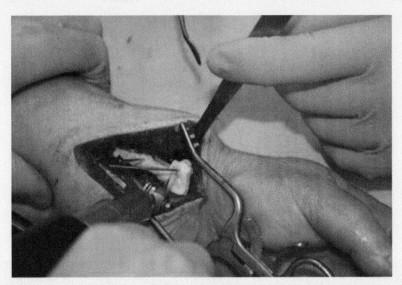

FIG. 4 The patient-specific cutting guide is precisely positioned on the distal radius using a standard distal Henry approach.

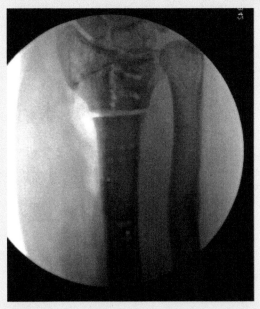

FIG. 5 Fluoroscopy images following intra- and extraarticular osteotomy and predrilling of the screw holes for later plate and screw fixation.

Panel 2: Authors' Preferred Treatment—cont'd

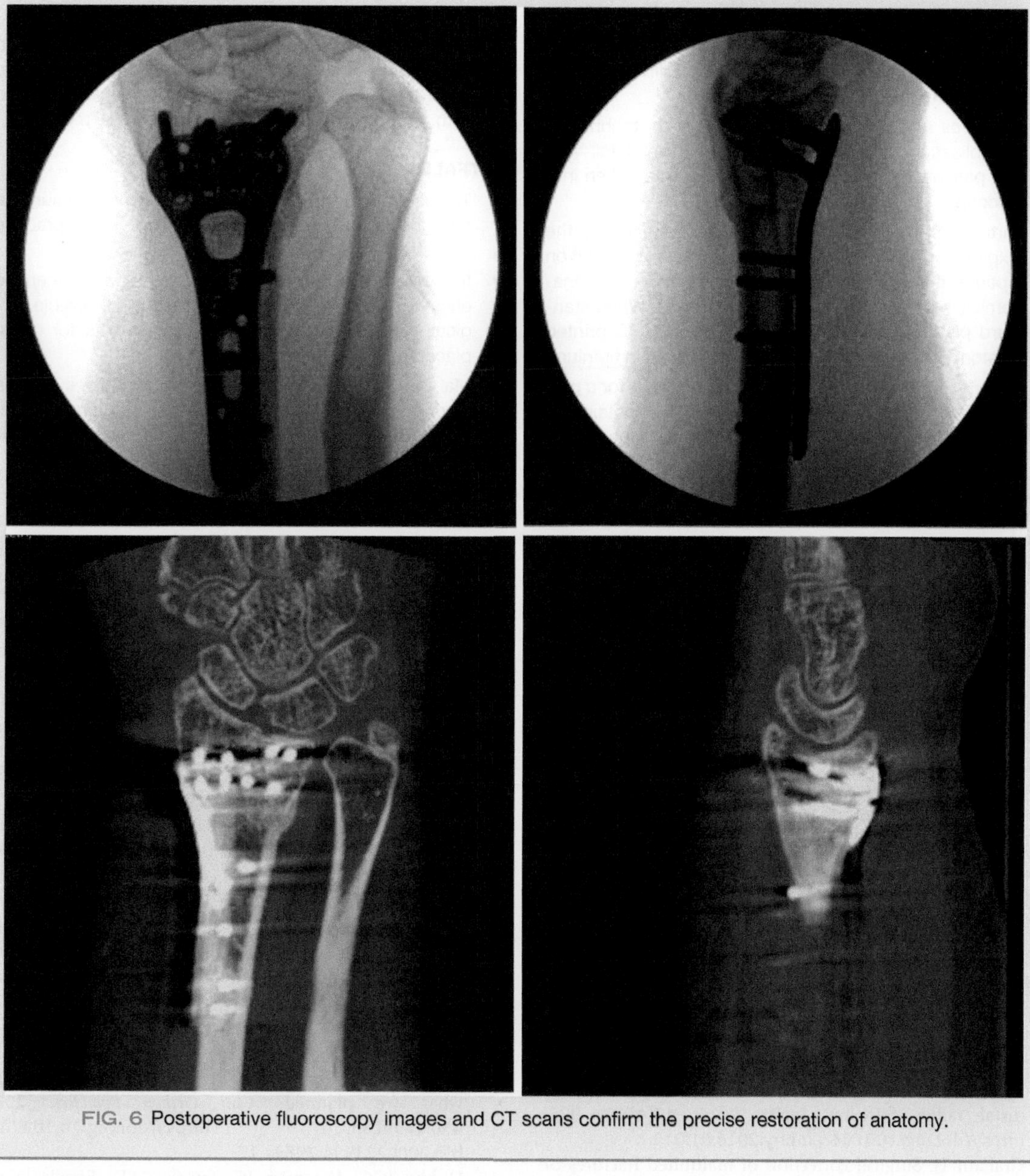

FIG. 6 Postoperative fluoroscopy images and CT scans confirm the precise restoration of anatomy.

Panel 3: Pearls and Pitfalls

PEARLS

- In symptomatic patients with a complex multidirectional or intraarticular malunion of the distal radius, the use of 3D technology may be beneficial to facilitate surgical correction when indicated.

- The pros and cons of the procedure with its inherent complication rate should be discussed in detail with the patient. The additional cost needs to be taken into account.

- Virtual 3D planning of corrective surgery allows the exploration of different osteotomy planes and fixation options. If needed, plates can be prebent on printed anatomical models for optimal fit on the bone. When standard plates don't allow adequate fixation, 3D printed custom plates can be designed and printed in titanium.

- Clear exposure of bony landmarks is essential for a precise fit of the surgical guides, in order to obtain the planned result. The availability of 3D printed anatomical models of the distal radius helps to check the correct placement of the surgical guides.

- If needed, fluoroscopy can confirm the correct position of the guide. The guide itself will not show clearly, but the K-wires used to fix it will. Their position can be compared with K-wires placed in a printed anatomical model.

PITFALLS

- The use of 3D technology can facilitate complex surgical procedures but does not replace good clinical practice and standard surgical techniques.

- In the planning process, close collaboration between the engineer and treating surgeon is essential. Possible surgical approaches and soft tissue restraints for guide placement need to be taken into account.

- Mal-positioning of the patient-specific guides causes incorrect placement of drill holes and cutting planes, possibly leading to an incomplete restoration of anatomy and a compromised clinical outcome.

REFERENCES

1. Slagel BE, Luenam S, Pichora DR. Management of post-traumatic malunion of fractures of the distal radius. *Hand Clin.* 2010; https://doi.org/10.1016/j.hcl.2009.08.013.

2. Lodha S, Wyscocki R, Cohen M. Malunions of the distal radius. In: *Hand Surgery Update V.* Chicago, IL, USA: American Society for Surgery of Hand; 2011:125–138.

3. Mulders MAM, d'Ailly PN, Cleffken BI, Schep NWL. Corrective osteotomy is an effective method of treating distal radius malunions with good long-term functional results. *Injury.* 2017; 48(3):731–737. https://doi.org/10.1016/j.injury.2017.01.045.

4. Caiti G, Dobbe JGG, Strackee SD, Strijkers GJ, Streekstra GJ. Computer-assisted techniques in corrective distal radius osteotomy procedures. *IEEE Rev Biomed Eng.* 2019; https://doi.org/10.1109/RBME.2019.2928424.

5. Cooney WP, Dobyns JH, Linscheid RL. Complications of Colles. *J Bone Joint Surg.* 1980; 62(4):613–619. Retrieved from:(1980). https://insights.ovid.com/pubmed?pmid=6155380.

6. Bizzotto N, Tami I, Tami A, et al. 3D printed models of distal radius fractures. *Injury.* 2016; 47(4):976–978. https://doi.org/10.1016/j.injury.2016.01.013.

7. Graham TJ. Surgical correction of malunited fractures of the distal radius. *J Am Acad Orthop Surg.* 1997; 5 (5):270–281. https://doi.org/10.5435/00124635-199709000-00005.

8. Park MJ, Cooney WP, Hahn ME, Looi KP, An KN. The effects of dorsally angulated distal radius fractures on carpal kinematics. *J Hand Surg.* 2002; 27(2):223–232. https://doi.org/10.1053/jhsu.2002.32083.

9. Bushnell BD, Bynum DK. Malunion of the distal radius. *J Am Acad Orthop Surg.* 2007; https://doi.org/10.5435/00124635-200701000-00004.

10. Fernandez DL. Correction of post-traumatic wrist deformity in adults by osteotomy, bone-grafting, and internal fixation. *J Bone Joint Surg Am Vol.* 1982; 64A (8):1164–1178.

11. Villar RN, Marsh D, Rushton N, Greatorex Ra. Three years after Colles' fracture. A prospective review. *J Bone Joint Surg Br Vol.* 1987; 69(4):635–638. https://doi.org/10.1016/0268-0033(88)90160-X.

12. McQueen M, Caspers J. Colles fracture: does the anatomical result affect the final function? *J Bone Joint Surg (Br).* 1988; 70:649–651. https://doi.org/10.1016/S0140-6736(61)91292-2.

13. Prommersberger KJ, Van Schoonhoven J, Lanz UB. Outcome after corrective osteotomy for malunited fractures of the distal end of the radius. *J Hand Surg.* 2002; 27B(1):55–60. https://doi.org/10.1054/jhsb.2001.0693.

14. Von Campe A, Nagy L, Arbab D, Dumont CE. Corrective osteotomies in malunions of the distal radius: do we get what we planned? *Clin Orthop Relat Res.* 2006; 450:179–185. https://doi.org/10.1097/01.blo.0000223994.79894.17.

15. Dobbe JGG, Vroemen JC, Strackee SD, Streekstra GJ. Corrective distal radius osteotomy: including bilateral differences in 3-D planning. *Med Biol Eng Comput.* 2013; 51(7):791–797. https://doi.org/10.1007/s11517-013-1049-2.

16. Cirpar M, Gudemez E, Cetik O, Turker M, Eksioglu F. Rotational deformity affects radiographic measurements

in distal radius malunion. *Eur J Orthop Surg Traumatol.* 2011; 21(1):13–20. https://doi.org/10.1007/s00590-010-0653-1.

17. de Muinck Keizer RJO, Lechner KM, Mulders MAM, Schep NWL, Eygendaal D, Goslings JC. Three-dimensional virtual planning of corrective osteotomies of distal radius malunions: a systematic review and meta-analysis. *Strateg Trauma Limb Reconstr.* 2017; https://doi.org/10.1007/s11751-017-0284-8.

18. Haghverdian JC, Hsu JWY, Harness NG. Complications of corrective osteotomies for extra-articular distal radius malunion. *J Hand Surg.* 2019; 44(11):987.e1–987.e9. https://doi.org/10.1016/j.jhsa.2018.12.013.

19. Gray RJ, Thom M, Riddle M, Suh N, Burkhart T, Lalone E. Image-based comparison between the bilateral symmetry of the distal radii through established measures. *J Hand Surg.* 2019; 44(11):966–972. https://doi.org/10.1016/j.jhsa.2019.05.021.

20. Walenkamp MMJ, de Muinck Keizer RJO, Dobbe JGG, et al. Computer-assisted 3D planned corrective osteotomies in eight malunited radius fractures. *Strateg Trauma Limb Reconstr.* 2015; 10(2):109–116. https://doi.org/10.1007/s11751-015-0234-2.

21. Athwal GS, Ellis RE, Small CF, Pichora DR. Computer-assisted distal radius osteotomy. *J Hand Surg.* 2003; 28 (6):951–958. https://doi.org/10.1016/S0363-5023(03)00375-7.

22. Croitoru H, Ellis RE, Small CF, Pichora DR. Fixation-based surgery: a new technique for distal radius osteotomy. *Lect Notes Comput Sci.* 2000; 1935:1126–1135.

23. Rieger M, Gabl M, Gruber H, Jaschke WR, Mallouhi A. CT virtual reality in the preoperative workup of malunited distal radius fractures: preliminary results. *Eur Radiol.* 2005; 15(4):792–797. https://doi.org/10.1007/s00330-004-2353-x.

24. Honigmann P, Thieringer F, Steiger R, Haefeli M, Schumacher R, Henning J. A simple 3-dimensional printed aid for a corrective palmar opening wedge osteotomy of the distal radius. *J Hand Surg.* 2016; https://doi.org/10.1016/j.jhsa.2015.12.022.

25. Shintani K, Kazuki K, Yoneda M, et al. Computer-assisted three-dimensional corrective osteotomy for malunited fractures of the distal radius using prefabricated bone graft substitute. *J Hand Surg Asian Pac Vol.* 2018; 23 (4):479–486. https://doi.org/10.1142/S2424835518500467.

26. Murase T, Oka K, Moritomo H, Goto A, Yoshikawa H, Sugamoto K. Three-dimensional corrective osteotomy of malunited fractures of the upper extremity with use of a computer simulation system. *J Bone Joint Surg.* 2008; 90 (11):2375–2389. https://doi.org/10.2106/JBJS.G.01299.

27. Miyake J, Murase T, Moritomo H, Sugamoto K, Yoshikawa H. Distal radius osteotomy with volar locking plates based on computer simulation. *Clin Orthop Relat Res.* 2011; 469(6):1766–1773. https://doi.org/10.1007/s11999-010-1748-z.

28. Kunz M, Ma B, Rudan JF, Ellis RE, Pichora DR. Image-guided distal radius osteotomy using patient-specific instrument guides. *J Hand Surg.* 2013; https://doi.org/10.1016/j.jhsa.2013.05.018.

29. Dobbe JGG, Vroemen JC, Strackee SD, Streekstra GJ. Patient-specific distal radius locking plate for fixation and accurate 3D positioning in corrective osteotomy. *Strateg Trauma Limb Reconstr.* 2014; 9(3):179–183. https://doi.org/10.1007/s11751-014-0203-1.

30. Oka K, Moritomo H, Goto A, Sugamoto K, Yoshikawa H, Murase T. Corrective osteotomy for malunited intra-articular fracture of the distal radius using a custom-made surgical guide based on three-dimensional computer simulation: case report. *J Hand Surg.* 2008; 33 (6):835–840. https://doi.org/10.1016/j.jhsa.2008.02.008.

31. Schweizer A, Fürnstahl P, Nagy L. Three-dimensional correction of distal radius intra-articular malunions using patient-specific drill guides. *J Hand Surg.* 2013; 38 (12):2339–2347. https://doi.org/10.1016/j.jhsa.2013.09.023.

32. Stockmans F, Dezillie M, Vanhaecke J. Accuracy of 3D virtual planning of corrective osteotomies of the distal radius. *J Wrist Surg.* 2013; 2(212):306–314. https://doi.org/10.1055/s-0033-1359307.

33. Zimmermann R, Gabl M, Arora R, Rieger M. Computer-assisted planning and corrective osteotomy in distal radius malunion. *Handchir Mikrochir Plast Chir.* 2003; 35 (5):333–337. https://doi.org/10.1055/s-2003-43115.

34. Buijze GA, Leong NL, Stockmans F, et al. Three-dimensional compared with two-dimensional preoperative planning of corrective osteotomy for extra-articular distal radial malunion. *J Bone Joint Surg.* 2018; 100(14):1191–1202. https://doi.org/10.2106/JBJS.17.00544.

35. Michielsen M, Van Haver A, Bertrand V, Vanhees M, Verstreken F. Corrective osteotomy of distal radius malunions using three-dimensional computer simulation and patient-specific guides to achieve anatomic reduction. *Eur J Orthop Surg Traumatol.* 2018; 28 (8):1531–1535. https://doi.org/10.1007/s00590-018-2265-0.

36. Pillukat T, Osorio M, Prommersberger KJ. Correction of intraarticular malunion of the distal radius based on a computer-assisted virtual planning. *Handchir Mikrochir Plast Chir.* 2018; 50(5):310–318. https://doi.org/10.1055/a-0751-2959.

37. Abe S, Oka K, Miyamura S, et al. Three-dimensional in vivo analysis of malunited distal radius fractures with restricted forearm rotation. *J Orthop Res.* 2019; 37(9):1881–1891. https://doi.org/10.1002/jor.24332.

38. Oka K, Shigi A, Tanaka H, Moritomo H, Arimitsu S, Murase T. Intra-articular corrective osteotomy for intra-articular malunion of distal radius fracture using three-dimensional surgical computer simulation and patient-matched instrument. *J Orthop Sci.* 2019; https://doi.org/10.1016/j.jos.2019.11.005.

39. Chen C, Cai L, Zhang C, Wang J, Guo X, Zhou Y. Treatment of die-punch fractures with 3D printing technology. *J Investig Surg*. 2017; 1–8. https://doi.org/10.1080/08941939.2017.1339150.

40. Caiti G, Dobbe JGG, Loenen ACY, et al. Implementation of a semiautomatic method to design patient-specific instruments for corrective osteotomy of the radius. *Int J Comput Assist Radiol Surg*. 2019; 14(5):829–840. https://doi.org/10.1007/s11548-018-1896-2.

41. Inge S, Brouwers L, Van Der Heijden F, Bemelman M. 3D printing for corrective osteotomy of malunited distal radius fractures: a low-cost workflow. *BMJ Case Rep*. 2018; 2018https://doi.org/10.1136/bcr-2017-223996.

42. Temmesfeld MJ, Hauksson IT, Mørch T. Intra-articular osteotomy of the distal radius with the use of inexpensive in-house 3D printed surgical guides and arthroscopy: a case report. *JBJS Case Connect*. 2020; 10(1):e0424. https://doi.org/10.2106/JBJS.CC.18.00424.

FURTHER READING

Schweizer A, Fürnstahl P, Harders M, Székely G, Nagy L. Complex radius shaft malunion: osteotomy with computer-assisted planning. *Hand*. 2010; 5(2):171–178. https://doi.org/10.1007/s11552-009-9233-4.

Michielsen M, Van Haver AV, Vanhees M, van Riet R, Verstreken F. Use of three-dimensional technology for complications of upper limb fracture treatment. *EFORT Open Rev*. 2019; 4(6):302–312. https://doi.org/10.1302/2058-5241.4.180074.

Oka K, Murase T, Moritomo H, Goto A, Sugamoto K, Yoshikawa H. Corrective osteotomy using customized hydroxyapatite implants prepared by preoperative computer simulation. *Int J Med Robot Comput Assist Surg*. 2010; 6(2):186–193. https://doi.org/10.1002/rcs.305.

Miyake J, Murase T, Yamanaka Y, Moritomo H, Sugamoto K, Yoshikawa H. Three-dimensional deformity analysis of malunited distal radius fractures and their influence on wrist and forearm motion. *J Hand Surg Eur Vol*. 2012; 37(6):506–512. https://doi.org/10.1177/1753193412443644.

CHAPTER 33

Nonunion of Distal Radius Fractures

JOSHUA J. MEAIKE[a] • JESSE D. MEAIKE[b] • ALEXANDER Y. SHIN[a]
[a]Department of Orthopedic Surgery, Mayo Clinic, Rochester, MN, United States, [b]Division of Plastic Surgery, Mayo Clinic, Rochester, MN, United States

KEY POINTS

- While the cause of nonunion is often multifactorial, both injury (open fracture, severe comminution, soft tissue interposition) and patient (diabetes, smoking, obesity, substance abuse, malnutrition, peripheral vascular disease, social situation) factors play a role.
- Treatment is based on the history of previous surgical attempts, the status of the radiocarpal joint, and the status of the distal radioulnar joint.
- Commonly utilized methods include orthogonal plating, nonvascularized bone grafting, vascularized bone grafting, modified Sauve-Kapandji procedure, and radiocarpal arthrodesis.

Panel 1: Case Scenario

A 67 year-old, right-handed female with a history of poorly controlled type II diabetes and cerebral palsy with associated spasticity presented to an outside hospital following a ground level fall with a closed distal radius fracture (Fig. 1A and B). Closed reduction and casting was attempted, however she was referred to our clinic approximately 3 months status post injury with concern for nonunion with associated loss of reduction, shortening, radial deviation, and volar subluxation (Fig. 1C and D). What is the most effective approach for management of this clinical scenario?

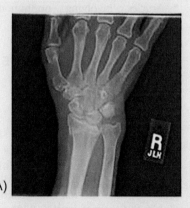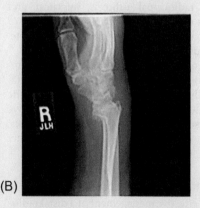

(A)   (B)

FIG. 1 Injury AP (A) and lateral (B) radiographs of a patient following a distal radius fracture.

Continued

Distal Radius Fractures. https://doi.org/10.1016/B978-0-323-75764-5.00011-1

Panel 1: Case Scenario—cont'd

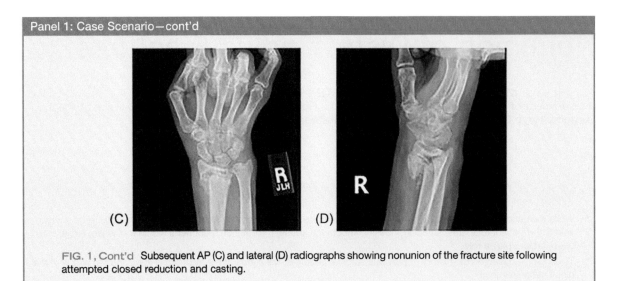

(C)   (D)

FIG. 1, Cont'd   Subsequent AP (C) and lateral (D) radiographs showing nonunion of the fracture site following attempted closed reduction and casting.

IMPORTANCE OF THE PROBLEM

Distal radius fractures are a commonly encountered injury in orthopedic surgery, representing the most common upper extremity fracture encountered in the emergency department and accounting for approximately 20% of all fractures occurring in adults.[1] Common complications include median nerve neuropathy, extensor pollicis longus tendon rupture, flexor pollicis longus tendon rupture, radiocarpal arthrosis, infection, and malunion. A less commonly observed complication of distal radius fractures is nonunion of the fracture site, estimated to occur in 0.03%–1.6% of cases (Fig. 2).[2–4]

Though rare, nonunions can be a devastating complication, resulting in severe pain and functional limitation. Additionally, even those that are able to be successfully treated often require multiple operative interventions, resulting in increased health care costs, time away from work, and risk of infection or other complications.

MAIN QUESTION

What is the most effective management of a distal radius fracture nonunion?

CURRENT OPINION

Nonunion of a distal radius fracture is historically a topic of debate. Some argue for definitive treatment in the form of arthrodesis while others attempt fixation in order to preserve function.

FINDING THE EVIDENCE

- Cochrane search: "distal rad*" AND "nonunion"
- Pubmed (Medline): "distal rad*" AND "nonunion."
- Bibliography review of eligible articles.
- Articles that were not in English were excluded.
- Articles involving nonhuman subjects were excluded.

QUALITY OF THE EVIDENCE

Level IV:
Case series: 7
Case report: 8

FINDINGS

Fifteen studies were identified for inclusion in this review. Seven of 15 selected studies were case series (Table 1), and the remaining eight were case reports (Table 2). Segalman et al. (1998) evaluated 10 females and 1 male with nonunion after distal radius fracture and found that all had significant associated co-morbidities, most notably diabetes, peripheral vascular disease (PVD), psychiatric disease, alcoholism, and/or morbid obesity.[5] They ultimately recommended

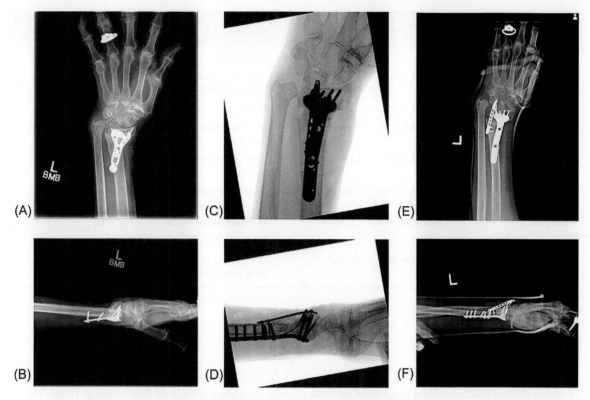

FIG. 2 A commonly encountered clinical scenario in which a patient presents with a malunion (A,B), requiring a revision ORIF with osteotomy for deformity correction (C,D), that subsequently goes on to nonunion (E,F).

TABLE 1
Case Series.

Study	N[a]	Complications	Average Age (Years)	Union Rate[b]
Segalman 1998	6 (arthrodesis cohort)	NR[c]	58.7	6/6
	3 (ORIF cohort)	NR[c]	41.7	3/3
Smith 1999	5	NR[c]	44	3/5
Fernandez 2001	10	4	46	10/10
Eglseder 2002	10	4	47.75	8/10
Prommersberger 2002	10 (small fragment cohort)	5	53	10/10
	13 (large fragment cohort)	4	56	12/13
Mithani 2014	8	1	68	8/8
Henry 2017	6	1	52	6/6

[a]N = number of subjects.
[b]Union rate = number of patients that went on to union/number of patients in cohort.
[c]NR = not reported.

TABLE 2
Case Reports.

Study	Patient	Initial Injury	Treatment	Time to Union
Kwa 1997	10-Year-old female	Closed	Open reduction, ICBG[a] autograft, SAC[b]	4 months
Song 2003	10-Year-old male	Closed	ORIF[c]	4 months
Crow 2005	51-Year-old female	Open	ORIF with vascularized autograft	7.5 months
Henry 2007	53-Year-old male	Open	ORIF with vascularized autograft	5 weeks
Villamor 2008	53-Year-old female	Closed	Modified Sauve-Kapandji	Union achieved, time frame not reported
Karuppiah 2010	41-Year-old female	Open	Modified Sauve-Kapandji	7 months
Shinohara 2017	59-Year-old male	Closed	ORIF with ICBG	3 months
Pedrazzini 2018	15-Year-old male	Closed	ORIF with proximal radius bone autograft	2 months

[a]ICBG (iliac crest bone graft).
[b]SAC (short arm cast).
[c]ORIF (open reduction, internal fixation).

that wrist arthrodesis be performed in those with <5 mm of subchondral bone distal to the nonunion site in order to decrease complication and failure rates. From 1990 to 1997, Smith et al. (1999) identified 5 patients with an average age of 44 years and nonunion of a distal radius fracture.[6] All were treated with open reduction, internal fixation (ORIF), and iliac crest bone autograft. Two achieved union with the index procedure, and one required a second ORIF before achieving union. Two patients ultimately were treated with wrist arthrodesis after an average of 3 additional procedures. All five patients were noted to be active smokers. In a study of 10 patients with nonunion, Fernandez et al. (2001) noted that patients typically presented with gross malalignment, pain, and severely limited function.[7] Forty percent of their cohort was found to have arthrosis of the distal radioulnar joint (DRUJ) requiring either a Bowers hemiresection with interposition or a Darrach procedure. Of note, cases in which a Darrach procedure was utilized also had extreme angular deformity and shortening at the nonunion site. A 100% union rate was achieved by 3 months and 7/10 functional outcomes were rated as excellent or good after undergoing ORIF with either a volar or dorsal approach.

Eglseder et al. (2002) evaluated 758 distal radius fractures over a 5-year span, identifying 12 (1.6%) that went on to nonunion.[3] They found that 7/12 were

initially open fractures, stating that an open injury was associated with a 10-fold increase (6.4% versus 0.6%) of nonunion. Data were available on 10/12 patients, who were treated with ORIF plus iliac crest bone autograft, resulting in an 80% union rate. In the largest identified case series, Prommersberger et al. (2002), studied 23 patients, 10 with <5 mm of subchondral bone distal to the nonunion site (small fragment cohort) and 13 with >5 mm (large fragment cohort).[8] All underwent ORIF with distraction and autograft use with plating systems, aside from 1 patient who was treated with Kirschner wires for fixation. Again, treatment of the DRUJ was performed in several patients. The entire small fragment cohort achieved union and 12/13 in the large fragment cohort achieved union. There were no clinical differences between the cohorts with an average follow-up of >20 months. Mithani et al. (2014) studied the use of dorsal bridge plating in the setting of distal radius nonunion. Union was achieved in 8/8 cases resulting in a 76 degrees arc of flexion/extension, >150 degrees arc of pronation/supination, and significantly improved DASH scores.[9] One patient went on to arthrodesis in the setting of persistent pain. The authors concluded that the optimal use of dorsal bridge plating is in the setting of severe shortening with a distal fragment inadequate for reliable fixation. In a consecutive case series of 6 patients, Henry et al.

(2017) reviewed the efficacy of a custom-designed medial femoral condyle (MFC) bone flap.[10] Again, multiple comorbidities were present including tobacco use, alcoholism, and osteomyelitis, as was a history of multiple prior surgeries (average 3.7). At a mean of 6.8 months postsurgery, all patients achieved radiographic union. DASH scores improved from a preoperative mean of 63 to a postoperative mean of 18.

Eight case reports were identified, with publication dates ranging from 1997 to 2018. The average age of the involved patients was 36.5 years, ranging from 10 to 59 years. All patients underwent open, operative intervention, though with a variety of techniques. One patient was treated with irrigation and debridement, iliac crest bone autograft, and immobilization without hardware placement.[11] Two patients were treated with ORIF and a plating system for fixation, with one patient also receiving nonvascularized bone autograft.[12, 13] Pedrazzini et al. (2018) used cancellous autograft from the proximal radius and achieved fixation with one cannulated screw and one Kirschner wire.[14] Vascularized bone autograft was utilized in 2 cases, with the medial femoral condyle being the donor site in one case and the second metacarpal in the second.[15, 16] Both Villamor et al. (2008) and Kapruppiah et al. (2010) performed modified Sauve-Kapandji procedures, in which the distal segment of the ulna was used to span the nonunion site of the radius.[17, 18] Union was achieved in all 8 cases. Time to union was documented in 7 cases, with union occurring at an average of 5.1 months postsurgery (range 1.25–7.5 months).

The importance of achieving bony healing at the union site lies in the significant limitations of upper extremity function when one loses motion about the wrist joint.[7, 19] Improving construct stability increases the chances of a successful outcome, and this can be achieved with fixed angle constructs and/or by applying multiple plates in orthogonal planes.[7, 20] Careful handling of soft tissues and avoiding extensive periosteal stripping can play an important role in healing as well, especially given the fact that this is often a highly traumatized area that has already undergone previous surgical intervention.[21] As mentioned previously, focus must not solely be at the site of nonunion, as DRUJ involvement is often present. If DRUJ stability is of concern, often times re-establishing normal length of the radius will correct instability.[7, 22, 23] Alignment and length

may be challenging to restore, as these injuries have often had months to form scar tissue and contractures, therefore lengthening or release of the brachioradialis, flexor carpi radialis, joint capsule, or other soft tissues may be necessary.[5, 7, 24–26]

RECOMMENDATION

In patients with nonunion of a distal radius fracture, the data suggests that:

Recommendation	Overall Quality
• Open reduction and internal fixation with the use of bone autograft provides a high likelihood of achieving union.	⊕⊕◯◯ LOW
• In more complex cases, including significant bone loss and/or resistant nonunion, one should consider more advanced procedures such as the modified Sauve-Kapandji procedure or vascularized bone grafting.	⊕◯◯◯ VERY LOW
• Careful evaluation of the DRUJ must be performed with consideration of targeted operative intervention in the setting of stiffness or arthrosis via Bowers hemiresection with interposition, Darrach procedure, or arthrolysis.	⊕◯◯◯ VERY LOW
• No one method of fixation is universally agreed upon as the gold standard. With the vast array of surgical approaches and modalities of fixation that currently exist, it is advised that careful consideration is applied to surgical planning in order to ensure that adequate bony fixation is achieved to result in a stable construct that promotes healing.	⊕⊕◯◯ LOW

CONCLUSION

Nonunion of a distal radius fracture is an event that rarely occurs, though is of significant concern as it often requires multiple operations and causes significant pain and functional limitations. Though no high-level evidence currently exists in the literature, nonunion should initially be managed with ORIF with utilization of bone autograft and a fixation device that provides reliable stability. For resistant or more complex cases, one should consider more extensive measures, such as a vascularized bone graft.

Panel 2: Author's Preferred Technique

In the case of a minimally operated on (0–2 previous operations) distal radius fracture nonunion, such as case 1 discussed previously, the senior author prefers the use of nonvascularized bone autograft and a construct with increased stability (Fig. 3). This can be achieved by the use of multiple plates or fixed angle devices.

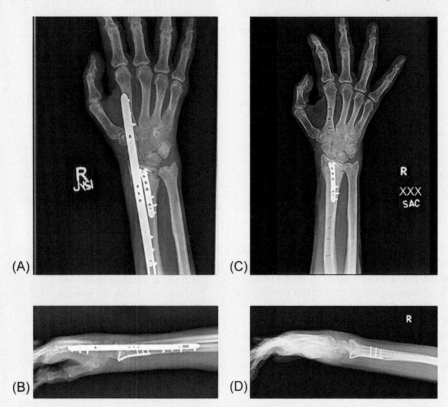

(A)   (C)

(B)   (D)

FIG. 3 Treatment AP (A) and lateral (B) radiographs following volar hook plate and dorsal bridge plate placement. Final AP (C) and lateral (D) radiographs demonstrating successful union and dorsal bridge plate removal.

Panel 3: Pearls and Pitfalls

PEARLS

- In cases of spasticity, such as case 1 above, consider the use of botox injections to decrease tension forces on the nonunion site and construct. Similarly, soft tissue releases can be performed in cases of deformity with contracture formation.

- When able, time should be taken to optimize patient comorbidities via a multidisciplinary approach, as these are often times modifiable and have a significant impact on healing.

- The use of a vascularized bone graft provides its own supply of substantial healing potential and has been shown to be extremely valuable in resistant or complex cases of distal radius nonunion.

- In the setting of multiple failed reconstructions, one should consider endocrine evaluation. If endocrine evaluation does not reveal any abnormalities, carefully evaluate social situation for iatrogenic, self-induced, abuse-induced, or abuse-related causes.

Panel 3: Pearls and Pitfalls—cont'd

PITFALLS

- The flexor and extensor muscles/tendons lie in close relationship to the radial cortex. One must be aware of any prominences, especially when using grafts or multiple fixation devices, as irritation or even rupture of these structures has been reported.

- Vascularized bone grafts are a technically demanding procedure, and one must ensure that the anastomoses occurs at a site of good vessel health, which can be challenging given the nearly universal history of significant trauma and multiple previous surgeries in these cases.

Additionally, one must take care in selecting where to place the vessels as kinking or compression can jeopardize blood flow and supply.

- Frequently cited causes of nonunion or failed healing of a nonunion include inadequate postoperative immobilization (quality and/or duration), poor construct stability, excessive distraction, soft tissue interposition, and iatrogenic disruption of surrounding soft tissues and blood supply. Care and particular attention to detail must be employed throughout preoperative planning, surgical execution, and postoperative follow-up.

REFERENCES

1. Chung KC, Spilson SV. The frequency and epidemiology of hand and forearm fractures in the United States. *J Hand Surg [Am]*. 2001;26(5):908–915.
2. Bacorn RW, Kurtzke JF. Colles' fracture; a study of two thousand cases from the New York State Workmen's Compensation Board. *J Bone Joint Surg Am Vol*. 1953;35-A(3):643–658.
3. Eglseder Jr WA, Elliott MJ. Nonunions of the distal radius. *Am J Orthop (Belle Mead NJ)*. 2002;31(5):259–262.
4. Jones RW. Fractures and Other bone and joint injuries. *Am J Phys Med Rehabil*. 1942;21(1):54.
5. Segalman KA, Clark GL. Un-united fractures of the distal radius: a report of 12 cases. *J Hand Surg [Am]*. 1998;23(5):914–919.
6. Smith VA, Wright TW. Nonunion of the distal radius. *J Hand Surg (Br)*. 1999;24(5):601–603.
7. Fernandez DL, Ring D, Jupiter JB. Surgical management of delayed union and nonunion of distal radius fractures. *J Hand Surg [Am]*. 2001;26(2):201–209.
8. Prommersberger KJ, Fernandez DL, Ring D, Jupiter JB, Lanz UB. Open reduction and internal fixation of un-united fractures of the distal radius: does the size of the distal fragment affect the result? *Chir Main*. 2002;21(2):113–123.
9. Mithani SK, Srinivasan RC, Kamal R, Richard MJ, Leversedge FJ, Ruch DS. Salvage of distal radius nonunion with a dorsal spanning distraction plate. *J Hand Surg [Am]*. 2014;39(5):981–984.
10. Henry M. Vascularized medial femoral condyle bone graft for resistant nonunion of the distal radius. *J Hand Surg Asian Pac Vol*. 2017;22(1):23–28.
11. Kwa S, Tonkin MA. Nonunion of a distal radial fracture in a healthy child. *J Hand Surg (Br)*. 1997;22(2):175–177.
12. Shinohara T, Hirata H. Distal radius nonunion after volar locking plate fixation of a distal radius fracture: a case report. *Nagoya J Med Sci*. 2017;79(4):551–557.
13. Song KS, Kim HK. Nonunion as a complication of an open reduction of a distal radial fracture in a healthy child: a case report. *J Orthop Trauma*. 2003;17(3):231–233.
14. Pedrazzini A, Bastia P, Bertoni N, et al. Distal radius nonunion after epiphyseal plate fracture in a 15 years old young rider. *Acta Biomed*. 2018;90(1-s):169–174.
15. Crow SA, Chen L, Lee JH, Rosenwasser MP. Vascularized bone grafting from the base of the second metacarpal for persistent distal radius nonunion: a case report. *J Orthop Trauma*. 2005;19(7):483–486.
16. Henry M. Genicular corticoperiosteal flap salvage of resistant atrophic non-union of the distal radius metaphysis. *Hand Surg*. 2007;12(3):211–215.
17. Karuppiah SV, Johnstone AJ. Sauve-Kapandji as a salvage procedure to treat a nonunion of the distal radius. *J Trauma*. 2010;68(5):E123–E125.
18. Villamor A, Rios-Luna A, Villanueva-Martinez M, Fahandezh-Saddi H. Nonunion of distal radius fracture and distal radioulnar joint injury: a modified Sauve-Kapandji procedure with a cubitus proradius transposition as autograft. *Arch Orthop Trauma Surg*. 2008;128(12):1407–1411.
19. Adams BD, Grosland NM, Murphy DM, McCullough M. Impact of impaired wrist motion on hand and upper-extremity performance(1). *J Hand Surg [Am]*. 2003;28(6):898–903.
20. Perren SM. Evolution of the internal fixation of long bone fractures. The scientific basis of biological internal fixation: choosing a new balance between stability and biology. *J Bone Joint Surg (Br)*. 2002;84(8):1093–1110.
21. Fernandez FF, Eberhardt O, Langendorfer M, Wirth T. Nonunion of forearm shaft fractures in children after intramedullary nailing. *J Pediatr Orthop B*. 2009;18(6):289–295.
22. Prommersberger KJ, VANS J, Lanz UB. A radiovolar approach to dorsal malunions of the distal radius. *Tech Hand Up Extrem Surg*. 2000;4(4):236–243.

23. Shea K, Fernandez DL, Jupiter JB, Martin Jr C. Corrective osteotomy for malunited, volarly displaced fractures of the distal end of the radius. *J Bone Joint Surg [Am]*. 1997;79(12):1816–1826.

24. McKee MD, Waddell JP, Yoo D, Richards RR. Nonunion of distal radial fractures associated with distal ulnar shaft fractures: a report of four cases. *J Orthop Trauma*. 1997;11 (1):49–53.

25. Ring D. Nonunion of the distal radius. *Hand Clin*. 2005;21 (3):443–447.

26. Saleh M, Ribbans WJ, Meffert RH. Bundle nailing in nonunion of the distal radius: case report. *Handchir Mikrochir Plast Chir*. 1992;24(5):273–275.

CHAPTER 34

Tendon Ruptures After Distal Radius Fracture

JIN BO TANG

Department of Hand Surgery, Affiliated Hospital of Nantong University, Nantong, Jiangsu, China

KEY POINTS

- The incidence of tendon ruptures after distal radius fracture is rare, currently 1%–3%, and generally occur within the first year after surgery. The extensor pollicis longus (EPL) or flexor pollicis longus (FPL) are most often involved tendons, and rupture of flexor or extensor tendons to the fingers were also reported.
- The key to prevent flexor tendon rupture is to properly position the plate, and Soong classification offers practical guide to ideal plate position.
- The key to prevent extensor tendon rupture is to avoid too long screws that dorsally protrude. The dorsal tangential/horizon/skyline or carpal shoot-through view offers a reliable verification intraoperatively, and/or a CT scan, postoperatively.
- Once clinical diagnosis is established, surgical exploration should proceed and hardware should be removed before proceeding to tendon reconstruction.
- Tendon transfer or grafting are two common option of surgical treatment and prognosis of these surgeries are believed to be reliable in achieving a satisfactory result.

Panel 1: Case Scenario

A 63 year-old, right hand dominant male presents with a spontaneous inability to flex his thumb after several months of pain along the course of the FPL. His medical history include a volar plate osteosynthesis of a distal radius fracture 2 years earlier after a skiing trauma (Fig. 1). Clinical examination confirms an FPL tendon rupture and ultrasound identifies a rupture at the CMC-1 joint with a retracted proximal tendon stump that cannot be localized. What is the most effective approach for management of his rupture and how could it have been prevented?

Continued

Panel 1: Case Scenario—cont'd

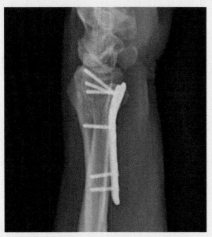 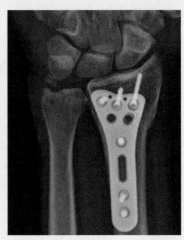

FIG. 1 Preoperative radiographs show a standard volar locking plate slightly proud to the volar rim, classified as Soong grade 1. (Courtesy of Leo Chiche.)

IMPORTANCE OF THE PROBLEM

Tendon rupture after distal radius fractures were found with or without surgical treatment. The timing of the tendon rupture varies from days or months after fracture or many years after surgical treatment. The most common incidence is associated with open reduction and internal fixation when the plate is not placed in a correct position and most commonly involved tendons are extensor tendons. DeGeorge et al.[1] reported among 647 cases of distal radius fractures (636 patients) with open treatment of extra-articular and intraarticular distal radius fractures with internal fixation between May 2000 and May 2015, there is 2 extensor pollicis longus (EPL) ruptures and 1 flexor pollicis longus (FPL) tendon rupture. The mean time to tendon rupture was 481 days with a range from 21 to 1599 days. This is a rather uncommon complications compared with other complications such as loose or painful hardware (48 cases) and tendinopathy (flexor tendon irritation in 16 cases, extensor tendon irritation in 11 cases). In a survey of distal radius fractures treated with volar plating in a prefecture in Japan, Naito et al.[2] reported 10 FPL ruptures (0.35%), 8 EPL ruptures (0.29%), 1 rupture of the flexor digitorum profundus (FDP) tendon to index finger (0.04%) and 1 rupture of the extensor digitorum communis (EDC) (0.04%) out of a total

of 2787 cases. Thorninger et al.[3] followed 576 patients with distal radius fractures treated with volar plating and found 5 flexor tendon ruptures and 12 extensor tendon ruptures. The incidence of tendon rupture was 2.9%.[3]

In a systematic review of the 56 studies (6278 patients) before 2017, Azzi et al.[4] reported overall tendon-related adverse events were recorded in 420 patients (6.8%). The incidence of tendon ruptures (EPL, FPL, FDP plus flexor digitorum superficialis, or EDC) was 1.5% with volar plates and 1.7% with dorsal plates. The incidence of tenosynovitis was 4.5% with volar plates and 7.5% with dorsal plates. Other reported detailed the ruptures of the flexor carpi radialis tendon or all finger flexors, or patients with late ruptures or the ruptures in nonoperative patients.[5–15]

The incidence of tendon rupture was reported in 1%–3% of the cases with volar or dorsal plating according to the recent large patient cohorts,[1–3, 16, 17] which appears not differ from the data in earlier publications (1%–2%).[4] Though tendon rupture was seen in distal radius fracture without open reduction and surgical plating, our chapter will focus on questions and evidence of tendon rupture relating to surgical treatment.

MAIN QUESTION

How are tendon ruptures after distal radius fracture most effectively prevented, diagnosed, and treated?

CURRENT OPINION

Tendon rupture secondary to conservatively treated distal radius fractures are excessively rare and may go unnoticed if a high index of suspicion is not maintained. The vast majority of tendon ruptures following distal radius fractures are related to hardware malposition, have an insidious onset postoperatively after surgery and are preventable.

FINDING THE EVIDENCE

- Cochrane search: Distal Radius Fracture
- Pubmed (Medline): ("Radius Fractures" [Mesh] OR distal radius fracture*[tiab]) AND (tendon rupture*)
- Bibliography of eligible articles that were not in the English language were excluded.

QUALITY OF THE EVIDENCE

Level II:
Prospective study: 1
Level III:
Systematic review and metaanalysis: 1
Retrospective comparative studies: 3
Level IV:
Case series: 13

FINDINGS

Prevention

The EPL tendon is at risk for spontaneous rupture even in the absence of identifiable predisposing risk factor.[18] It has been suggested that rather than pure mechanical irritation, vascular, and metabolic factors may also play a substantial role in the etiology of this exceedingly rare diagnosis. Spontaneous EPL rupture with conservative treatment of a usually nondisplaced fracture as a result of retinaculum remaining intact—with increased pressure in EPL compartment leading to ischemia—often will occur within 4–8 weeks post injury. Signs and symptoms include initial discomfort with thumb use and soon tenderness over EPL compartment. The patient is best informed from outset that there is low risk but if discomfort persists to return as may need to have compartment opened.

With regard to (post-)operative prevention, Soong et al. proposed a grading system to classify the palmar prominence of the plate relative to the watershed line.[19] Soong classification is based on standard lateral plain radiographs: (a) Grade 0: The plate is dorsal to the volar critical line and proximal to the volar rim. (b) Grade 1: The plate is palmar to the volar critical line, but proximal to the volar rim. (c) Grade 2: The plate extends beyond the level of the volar rim.

Recent reports[20–23] of the Soong classification with incidence of plate removal and tendon ruptures were summarized in Table 1. The cohort with the largest number of patients (113 patients) showed a statistically significant correlation between FPL rupture as well as flexor tenosynovitis and the plate position according to the Soong classification.[23] Soong grading is a valuable tool to classify the position of palmar plates relative to the watershed line and to detect patients at risk of tendon injuries (Figs. 1 and 2). Elective removal of implants after union should be considered in patients with a higher Soong grade (1 and 2) (Box 1).[23]

With regard of prevention of tendon rupture of the FPL tendon, following two measures should be taken: (1) carefully determine the position of volar plates and avoid project the plate beyond the volar rim (watershed line) as well as keep the plate dorsal to the volar cortical line (Figs. 3 and 4); (2) if the plate was found to project palmar to the volar cortical line (Soong grade

TABLE 1

Soong Grades of Palmar Plates Removed After Distal Radial Fracture.

Authors	years	Patients With Implant Removal	Grade 0	Grade 1	Grade 2	Tendon Ruptured
Snoddy et al.	2015	33	14 (42%)	10 (30%)	9 (27%)	1
Lutsky et al.	2015	37	4 (11%)	28 (76%)	2 (5%)	0
Selles et al.	2018	54	10 (19%)	20 (37%)	24 (44%)	0
Goren et al.	2020	113	28 (25%)	48 (42%)	37 (33%)	16

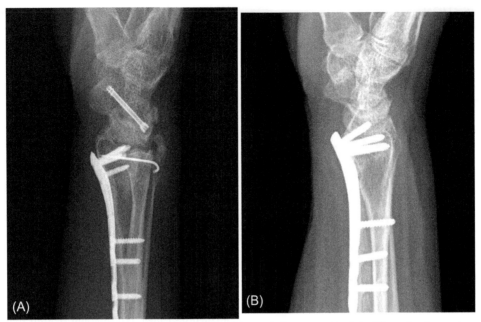

FIG. 2 Two positions of the volar locking plates which may induce a greater risk of flexor tendon rupture: (A) Soong grade 1; (B) Soong grade 2. Both may irritate the flexor tendons, especially in the patients with Soong grade 2 (shown in B) the tendons have a greater chance to glide over the distal rim of the plate.

BOX 1
Prevention and Clinical Diagnosis of Tendon Rupture.

1. Proper position of a plate is a measure to decrease the risk of tendon rupture. Avoid placing the distal rim of a standard volar plate palmar and distal to the watershed line. (Figs. 3 and 4).

2. Do not project the screws over the dorsal cortical surface of the distal radius in the standard lateral view. An additional dorsal tangential/horizon/skyline or carpal shoot-through is more accurate and reliable to identify protruding screws (Fig. 5).

3. Soft tissue coverage over the plate is recommended.

4. If intraoperative reduction of the fracture requires the plate to locate in a position of Soong grade 2 or 3, early removal of the plate after fracture healing should be

considered. If tendon irritation presents, removal is highly suggested.

5. Loss of active thumb interphalangeal flexion (or extension) indicates rupture of the FPL (or EPL) tendon, and loss of finger flexion at the distal interphalangeal joint indicates injuries to the finger flexor tendons. Weakness in finger extension suggest the possible rupture of finger extensor tendons.

6. The median reported interval to rupture after surgery is 9 months with exceptional cases being reported up to 10 years. Most patients have prodromal symptoms of crepitus, pain with finger motion, clicking or a rubbing sensation prior to rupture.

---

1) or distal to the volar rim (Soong Grade 2), removal of the plate after fracture healing is recommended. (3) protection of the plate with coverage of soft tissues such as repair of the pronator quadrates. Newer designed volar rim plates which are curved to cover the distal rim are intended to wrap over the projected volar rim of the distal radius. The design may reduce contact of the plates with the tendons (such as the FPL tendon), thereby theoretically reduce the chance of tendon irritation and risk of tendon rupture.[24]

Extensor tendon ruptures can spontaneously occur due to a laceration, diminished posttraumatic vascularity or a bone spur in case of conservative treatment and are exceedingly rare. The vast majority of extensor

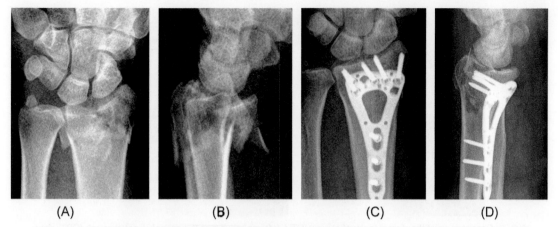

FIG. 3 It is ideal to place the volar plate proximal cortical line and dorsal to the volar rim of the distal radius and to project screws at different angles to fix the fracture fragments (A–D).

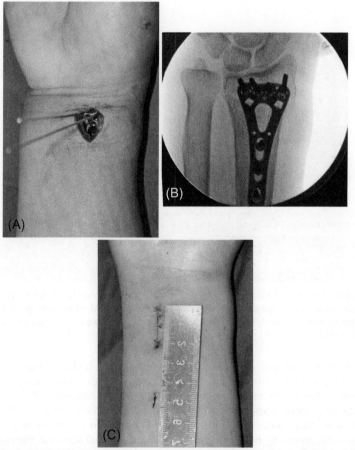

FIG. 4 If a mini-incision is used (shown in A), it is essential to check plate position with a C-arm fluoroscope (B), because the plate position is not easily visible through the mini-incision. (C) Mini-incisions are too small to allow direct visualization of the plate location in relating to distal radial rim.

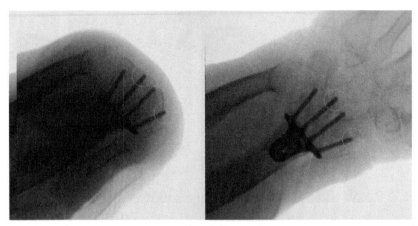

FIG. 5 Comparison of the dorsal tangential view (DTV, *left image*) versus the carpal shoot-through (CST, *right image*). Note the two protruding screws *(encircled in blue)*. Caution in interpretation of the over projection of the lunate and scaphoid distal to the dorsal radial rim is needed. (Courtesy of Geert Alexander Buijze.)

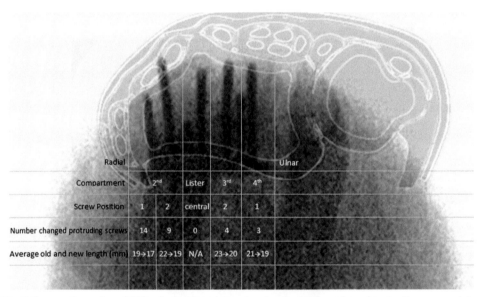

	Radial			Ulnar	
Compartment	2nd	Lister	3rd	4th	
Screw Position	1	2	central	2	1
Number changed protruding screws	14	9	0	4	3
Average old and new length (mm)	19→17	22→19	N/A	23→20	21→19

FIG. 6 Prospective series of 100 volar locking plates showing the total number of protruding screws intraoperatively changed for shorter lengths. (With permission from Bergsma M, et al. Volar plating in distal radius fractures: a prospective clinical study on efficacy of dorsal tangential views to avoid screw penetration. *Injury*. 2018;49(10):1810–1815.)

tendon ruptures are related to dorsally protruding screws as lateral views tends to underestimate the true protrusion of the dorsal cortex in the radial grooves adjacent to Lister's tubercle. Hence, a specific fluoroscopic view to diagnose screw tip prominence is recommended. A recent systematic review by Bergsma et al. showed that of all additional fluoroscopic views, the dorsal tangential/horizon/skyline view (DTV) was most studied and proved to be practical and time

efficient, with higher efficacy, accuracy, and reliability compared with conventional views.[25] A prospective study in 100 patients, obtaining additional DTV was found to be efficacious as it led to change in intraoperative strategy in one-third of patients.[26] Screws in the two most radial screws in the plate were at the highest risk of being revised (Fig. 6). In diagnostic work-up, CT and ultrasound are also considered accurate modalities.

Diagnosis

Diagnosis of relevant tendon rupture is not different from those in traumatic tendon rupture. Inability of active flexion of the interphalangeal joint of the thumb indicate the rupture of the FPL tendon. In the patients with distal radius fracture receiving volar plating fixation, and no other trauma history in the hand, FPL tendon rupture caused by the plate should be highly suspected. Tenderness at the distal forearm along the course of the FPL can lead to clinical diagnosis of the FPL tendon. Plain radiographs of the distal forearm should be taken to rule out any other bone related pathologies as well as assess the Soong classification of the plate.

Surgical Treatment

Once the clinical diagnosis is established, surgical exploration is indicated. Depending on the tendons ruptured, a volar or dorsal incision is made. A longitudinal incision is preferred, centered with the distal rim of the plate. The incision usually needs to be extended proximally, as the proximal tendon end retract. The distal stump of the tendon can be found rather easily with the change of thumb or finger position. A tendon graft is recommended, as a graft can ease the tension and avoid placing the junction site close to the rim of the distal radius (Fig. 7). The plate has to be removed in most cases and the author strongly suggest plate removal before tendon grafting, so the tension of the graft can be properly set. The ideal length of the graft is about 15 cm, usually taken from palmaris longus tendon. For the EPL tendon rupture, transfer of the extensor indicis proprius (EIP) is a valid option (Fig. 7), and in fact it is a better option than a graft to the EPL. Separate incisions in the dorsal wrist, proximal to the thumb metacarpophalangel (MP) joint, and index finger MP joints should be used for EIP tendon transfer. An FPL tendon repair is usually repaired using a palmaris longus graft (Fig. 8), although harvesting an EIP tendon as a donor of a free graft is also a valid option. The tension of the EIP transfer or graft should be set with the thumb MP and interphalangeal joint in full extension and basal joint dorsally extended and moderately abducted. A Pulvertaft weave suture is used for all tendon junctions secured with 4-0 monofilament nylon or Ethibond sutures (Fig. 7).

Rupture of the flexor digitorum profundi or extensor digitorum communis tendons are even rarer. If suspected, tendon grafting is indicated using a palmaris longus tendon. A flexor digitorum superficialis tendon rupture does not need to repair.

Postoperatively, the thumb or fingers need to be protected with a splint holding the tendon in tension-reducing position. There is no need to perform any motion in the first 1 or 2 weeks. However, passive joint motion with limited partial range active motion of the thumb (or finger) MP and interphalangeal joints can be started from the middle or end of week 2. The splint can be discarded at the end of week 5, and gentle full-range active hand motion can start, and the patient can return to normal use of the hand around week 8–10.

EVIDENCE TO SUPPORT SPECIFIC TREATMENT (BOX 2)

Because tendon rupture is a rare complication, there are no case series of sufficient sample size to support any one specific surgical method against the others. There is no report about benefits of any specific surgical details which may improve the outcomes.

OUTCOMES AND PROGNOSIS

In general, the outcomes of the tendon transfer or grafting in the forearm are good and reliable. There are not sufficient number of samples to determine any factors affecting the prognosis. However, as the tendon transfer or grafting is not different from those without a distal radius fracture, and in the cases with tendon rupture, the fracture is already healed, there are no reasons to expect that tendon grafting or transfer likely has a notably different prognosis than those commonly seen.

White et al.[27] reported 6 tendon ruptures in 1359 patients (0.4%) with the distal radius fractures treated nonoperatively for the fracture and 8 tendon ruptures in 999 patients (0.8%) treated with volar plate fixation. At the time of final follow-up, these patients had minimal pain and excellent motion and grip strength. Mean Disabilities of the Shoulder, Arm, and Hand scores were 6 for patients treated nonoperatively for the fracture and 4 for those treated with volar plating. White et al.[27] were unable to verify volar plate or dorsal screw prominence as independent risk factors for tendon rupture after distal radius fractures. However, it is still recommended to continue follow-up and plate removal for symptomatic patients who have volar plate prominence or dorsal screw prominence. In the event of tendon rupture, clinical outcomes after tendon repair or tendon transfer are predictably good.

Rubensson et al.[28] reported 17 consecutive ruptures in 14 patients with distal radius fractures with plates. The incidence was 1.4%. Analysis of radiographs demonstrated sub-optimal placement of plate or screws in all cases. Three patients declined tendon surgery. Eleven patients were treated with a free tendon graft. Only two

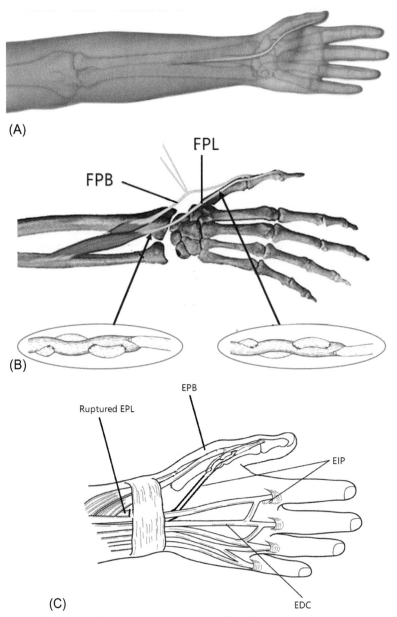

(A)

(B)

(C)

FIG. 7 Drawings illustrating (A) anatomical course of the FPL, (B) a tendon graft for the ruptured FPL tendon, and (C) EIP tendon transfer to repair the EPL tendon. Proper tension is a surgical key for either transferred or grafted tendon.

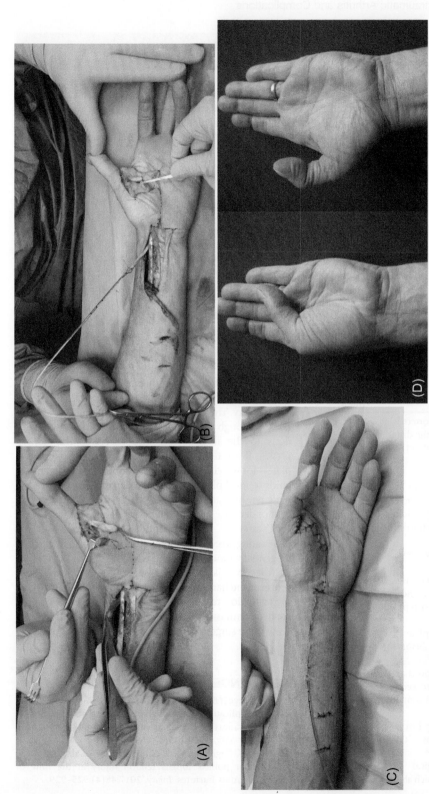

FIG. 8 Case scenario continued (A) hardware removal, intraoperative localization, A1-pulley sectioning and tenolysis of the proximal and distal FPL tendon stumps, held by the forceps and clamp, respectively. (B) Tunneling of a palmaris longus graft through the carpal tunnel guided by a silicone rod. (C) After both-sided Pulvertaft tendon weaves, tendon gliding, and tenodesis effects are verified to obtain optimal tension and functional motion. Proper tension on the tendon with the wrist in neutral position results in palmar abduction of the thumb volar of the index finger metacarpal and the interphalangeal joint of the thumb in 30 degrees of flexion. (D) At 4 months, a good active functional outcome and strength recovery is achieved with a Kapandji score of 8, which is consistent with the average result of this procedure. (Courtesy of Leo Chiche.)

BOX 2
Keys in Surgical Treatments.

1. Tendon transfer or tendon grafting is recommended for any ruptured single tendon such as EPL, FPL, or other tendons.
2. A Pulvertaft weave tendon junction is recommended, with these junctions away from the region of the distal radius.
3. Implants (such as plates) should be removed at the time of surgery if having not been removed previously.

4. Proper tension should be maintained through the transferred or grafted tendons as the tendons tend to be loose as the muscle tone recovers.
5. Gentle active motion can be initiated 2 weeks after tendon transfer or grafting and splint can be discarded 5 weeks after surgery.

---

patients showed excellent results regarding mobility in the thumb and/or fingers. They recommend that early removal of the plate when the placement is suboptimal or when local volar tenderness appears would prevent the ruptures.

RECOMMENDATIONS

In patients with an intraarticular displaced distal radius fracture, evidence suggests:

Recommendation	Overall Quality
• Positioning the volar plate in a correct position not projecting distal to the distal radial rim or cortical rim is important in preventing the tendon-related complications including rupture or irritation.[29, 30] Repair of the pronator quadratus is also recommended to protect the tendons. Removal of the ill-positioned plates or screws are also recommended after fracture healing.	⊕⊕◯◯ LOW
• In preventing dorsally protruding screws at risk for extensor tendon rupture, the intraoperative dorsal tangential view is practical and time efficient, with higher efficacy, accuracy, and reliability compared with conventional views.	⊕⊕◯◯ LOW
• Soong classification of the volar plate positioning provide clue for risk factors for flexor tendon rupture.	⊕⊕◯◯ LOW
• Recognize the rupture of the tendons as early as possible clinically and proceed to surgical exploration and repair as soon as possible after clinical diagnosis	⊕◯◯◯ VERY LOW
• EPL and FPL are most commonly involved, though flexor or extensor tendons of the fingers may very rarely rupture.	⊕⊕⊕◯ MODERATE
• Plate removal at the time of surgical exploration is recommended, which should	⊕◯◯◯ VERY LOW

be performed before tendon grafting or transfer.

• Tendon transfer or grafting are common surgical options. ⊕⊕◯◯ LOW

• Postoperative mobilization starting from the end of week 2 is recommended, with splinting for a total of 5 weeks. ⊕◯◯◯ VERY LOW

CONCLUSIONS

The incidence of tendon ruptures after distal radius fracture is rare, currently less than 1%, but can occur up to 10 years after surgery. The EPL or FPL are most often involved tendons, although rupture of other flexor and extensor tendons to the fingers were also reported. The key to prevent flexor tendon rupture is to properly position the plate—for which the Soong classification offers a practical guide to ideal plate position and determining the need of plate removal after fracture healing. This can help to prevent or decrease the risk of tendon rupture. The key to prevent extensor tendon rupture is to avoid dorsally penetrating screws or other hardware—for which a dorsal tangential view can be utilized intraoperatively. Once clinical diagnosis is established, surgical exploration should proceed, and hardware should be removed before proceeding to tendon reconstruction. Tendon transfer or grafting are two common option of surgical treatment and prognosis of these surgeries are believed to be reliably good.

REFERENCES

1. DeGeorge Jr BR, Brogan DM, Becker HA, Shin AY. Incidence of complications following volar locking plate fixation of distal radius fractures: an analysis of 647 cases. *Plast Reconstr Surg.* 2020;145(4):969–976.
2. Naito K, Sugiyama Y, Dilokhuttakarn T, et al. A survey of extensor pollicis longus tendon injury at the time of distal radius fractures. *Injury.* 2017;48(4):925–929.

3. Thorninger R, Madsen ML, Wæver D, Borris LC, Rölfing JHD. Complications of volar locking plating of distal radius fractures in 576 patients with 3.2 years follow-up. *Injury.* 2017;48(6):1104–1109.

4. Azzi AJ, Aldekhayel S, Boehm KS, Zadeh T. Tendon rupture and tenosynovitis following internal fixation of distal radius fractures: a systematic review. *Plast Reconstr Surg.* 2017;139(3):717e–724e.

5. Monda MK, Ellis A, Karmani S. Late rupture of flexor pollicis longus tendon 10 years after volar buttress plate fixation of a distal radius fracture: a case report. *Acta Orthop Belg.* 2010;76(4):549–551.

6. de Boer SW, van Kooten EO, Ritt MJ. Extensor pollicis longus tendon rupture with concomitant rupture of the extensor digitorum communis II tendon after distal radius fracture. *J Hand Surg Eur Vol.* 2010;35(8):679–681.

7. Valbuena SE, Cogswell LK, Baraziol R, Valenti P. Rupture of flexor tendon following volar plate of distal radius fracture. Report of five cases. *Chir Main.* 2010;29(2):109–113.

8. Caruso G, Vitali A, del Prete F. Multiple ruptures of the extensor tendons after volar fixation for distal radius fracture: a case report. *Injury.* 2015;46(Suppl. 7):S23–S27.

9. Proubasta IR, Lamas CG, Natera L, Arriaga N. Delayed rupture of all finger flexor tendons (excluding thumb) following nonoperative treatment of Colles' fracture: a case report and literature review. *J Orthop.* 2014;12 (Suppl. 1):S65–S68.

10. Rivlin M, Fernández DL, Nagy L, Graña GL, Jupiter J. Extensor pollicis longus ruptures following distal radius osteotomy through a volar approach. *J Hand Surg [Am].* 2016;41(3):395–398.

11. Chen PJ, Liu AL. Concurrent flexor carpi radialis tendon rupture and closed distal radius fracture. *BMJ Case Rep.* 2014;2014 pii: bcr2014204196.

12. Song D, Evans R, Arneja JS. Delayed extensor pollicis longus tendon rupture following nondisplaced distalradius fracture in a child. *Hand.* 2013;8(2):242–244.

13. Kitay A, Swanstrom M, Schreiber JJ, et al. Volar plate position and flexor tendon rupture following distal radius fracture fixation. *J Hand Surg [Am].* 2013;38 (6):1091–1096.

14. Roth KM, Blazar PE, Earp BE, Han R, Leung A. Incidence of extensor pollicis longus tendon rupture after nondisplaced distal radius fractures. *J Hand Surg [Am].* 2012;37(5):942–947.

15. Al-Najjim M, Fenton C, Scott T. Closed rupture of abductor pollicis longus and extensor pollicis brevis associated with fracture of the distal radius. *J Hand Surg Eur Vol.* 2012;37 (2):176–177.

16. Alter TH, Ilyas AM. Complications associated with volar locking plate fixation of distal radial fractures. *JBJS Rev.* 2018;6(10):e7.

17. Sato K, Murakami K, Mimata Y, Doita M. Incidence of tendon rupture following volar plate fixation of distal radius fractures: a survey of 2787 cases. *J Orthop.* 2018;15 (1):236–238.

18. Hu C-H, Fufa D, Hsu C-C, Lin Y-T, Lin C-H. Revisiting spontaneous rupture of the extensor pollicis longus tendon: eight cases without identifiable predisposing factor. *Hand (N Y).* 2015;10(4):726–731.

19. Soong M, Earp BE, Bishop G, Leung A, Blazar P. Volar locking plate implant prominence and flexor tendon rupture. *J Bone Joint Surg Am.* 2011;93(4):328–335.

20. Lutsky KF, Beredjiklian PK, Hioe S, Bilello J, Kim N, Matzon JL. Incidence of hardware removal following volar plate fixation of distal radius fracture. *J Hand Surg [Am].* 2015;40(12):2410–2415.

21. Selles CA, Reerds STH, Roukema G, van der Vlies KH, Cleffken BI, Schep NWL. Relationship between plate removal and Soong grading following surgery for fractured distal radius. *J Hand Surg Eur Vol.* 2018;43 (2):137–141.

22. Snoddy MC, An TJ, Hooe BS, Kay HF, Lee DH, Pappas ND. Incidence and reasons for hardware removal following operative fixation of distal radius fractures. *J Hand Surg [Am].* 2015;40(3):505–507.

23. Gören Y, Sauerbier M, Arsalan-Werner A. Impact of Soong grading on flexor tendon ruptures following palmar plating for distal radial fractures. *J Hand Surg Eur Vol.* 2020;45(4):348–353.

24. Stepan JG, Marshall DC, Wessel LE, et al. The effect of plate design on the flexor pollicis longus tendon after volar locked plating of distal radial fractures. *J Bone Joint Surg Am.* 2019;101(17):1586–1592.

25. Bergsma M, Denk K, Doornberg JN, et al. Volar plating: imaging modalities for the detection of screw penetration. *J Wrist Surg.* 2019;8(6):520–530.

26. Bergsma M, Doornberg JN, Duit R, et al. Volar plating in distal radius fractures: a prospective clinical study on efficacy of dorsal tangential views to avoid screw penetration. *Injury.* 2018;49(10):1810–1815.

27. White BD, Nydick JA, Karsky D, Williams BD, Hess AV, Stone JD. Incidence and clinical outcomes of tendon rupture following distal radius fracture. *J Hand Surg [Am].* 2012;37(10):2035–2040.

28. Rubensson CC, Ydreborg K, Boren L, Karlander LE. Flexor tendon repair after rupture caused by volar plate fixation of the distal radius. *J Plast Surg Hand Surg.* 2015;49 (2):112–115.

29. Selvan DR, Machin DG, Perry D, Simpson C, Thorpe P, Brown DJ. The role of fracture reduction and plate position in the aetiology of flexor pollicis longus tendon rupture after volar plate fixation of distal radius fractures. *Hand.* 2015;10(3):497–502.

30. Agnew SP, Ljungquist KL, Huang JI. Danger zones for flexor tendons in volar plating of distal radius fractures. *J Hand Surg [Am].* 2015;40(6):1102–1105.

CHAPTER 35

Chronic DRUJ Instability After Distal Radius Fractures

VICENTE CARRATALÁ BAIXAULI[a] • FRANCISCO J. LUCAS GARCÍA[a] •
IGNACIO MIRANDA GÓMEZ[b] • FERNANDO CORELLA MONTOYA[c,d]
[a]Hand and Upper Limb Surgery Unit, Quirónsalud Valencia Hospital, Valencia, Spain, [b]Orthopedic
Surgery and Traumatology Department, Arnau de Vilanova Hospital, Valencia, Spain, [c]Hand Surgery
Unit, Infanta Leonor Hospital, Madrid, Spain, [d]Hand Surgery Unit, Quirónsalud Madrid Hospital, Madrid,
Spain

KEY POINTS

- The triangular fibrocartilage complex (TFCC) and its proximal component, the radioulnar ligaments, constitute the primary intrinsic stabilizer of the distal radioulnar joint (DRUJ).
- TFCC injuries are frequently associated (in up to 78% of cases) with distal radius fractures, although the vast majority heals without long-term sequalae.
- Chronic lesions of the proximal component of the TFCC can cause pain and DRUJ instability.
- The volar and dorsal radioulnar ligaments have an important stabilizing effect in forearm rotation, with an isometric point of insertion in the fovea.
- Symptomatic nonrepairable or chronic TFCC tears can be treated by ligament reconstruction if the articular cartilage is in good condition.
- Wrist arthroscopy is the most reliable method for diagnosis and decision making in this type of injury, and also enables treatment by ligament reconstruction.

Panel 1: Case Scenario

A 35-year-old male patient with a history of left distal radius fracture 7 years previously, which was treated using external fixation (Figs. 1 and 2).

As fracture sequelae, he presented chronic scapholunate instability and DRUJ instability.

The scapholunate instability was successfully treated by arthroscopic ligamentoplasty but an attempt to repair the TFCC failed. Nonrepairable TFCC tissue and the absence of arthritis at the DRUJ level and ulnar side of the wrist were previously confirmed. What is the most effective treatment to restore DRUJ instability, and what is the role for arthroscopic assistance?

Continued

Panel 1: Case Scenario—cont'd

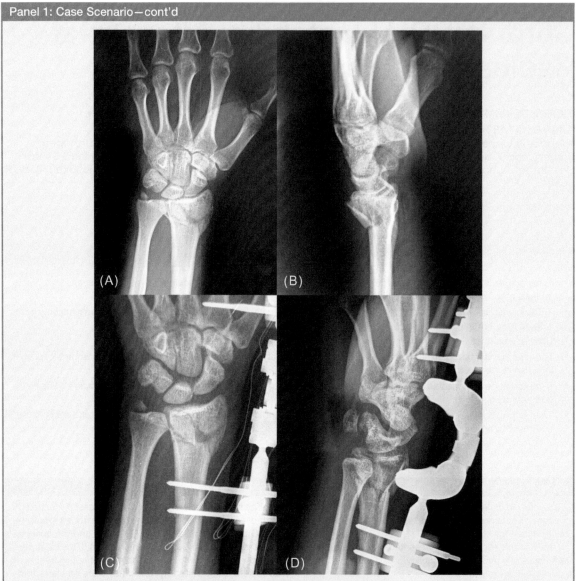

FIG. 1 Clinical case. (A) and (B) Distal radius fracture in 35 years old man. (C) and (D) Treatment of the fracture using external fixation. Postop radiographs.

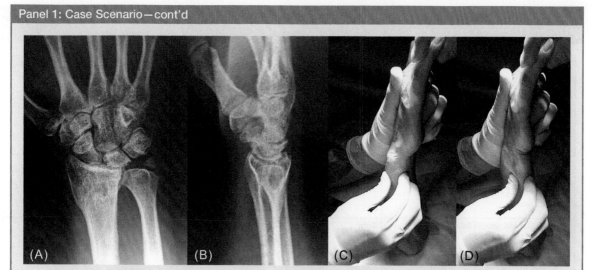

Panel 1: Case Scenario—cont'd

FIG. 2   (A) and (B) Radiographs 1 year after the fracture. The patient reported ulnar sided wrist pain with DRUJ instability and also symptomatic scapholunate (SL) instability. The SL instability was treated performing an arthroscopic ligamentoplasty (C) and (D) Clinical examination, DRUJ ballottement test before surgery.

IMPORTANCE OF THE PROBLEM

Peripheral tears of the triangular fibrocartilage complex (TFCC) can cause pain and distal radioulnar joint (DRUJ) instability. There are several techniques for the repair or reconstruction of these lesions, which vary depending on the location, healing capacity, and tissue viability.

TFCC injuries are frequently associated (in up to 78% of cases) with distal radius fractures.[1] The volar and dorsal radioulnar ligaments form the proximal component of the TFCC.[2] Lesions of this component can cause pain and DRUJ instability, with functional and mobility limitations.

In chronic nonrepairable TFCC tears with clinical DRUJ instability in which the articular cartilage is in good condition, ligament reconstruction with tendon graft is the treatment of choice, either by open or arthroscopy-assisted surgery. It is also the preferred treatment in cases of previous failed repair surgeries in patients with clinical DRUJ instability.

Atzei and Luchetti published a new classification of Palmer class 1-B injuries, in which they differentiated these types of nonrepairable tears of the proximal component with DRUJ instability, designating them as class 4[3] (Table 1).

Numerous procedures have been described to restore the stability of the DRUJ through nonanatomic reconstructions, and include extra-articular ulnocarpal plasty, direct radioulnar fixation plasty to the joint[4–6] and dynamic muscle transfers using the pronator quadratus muscle.[7] The role of the distal oblique bundle in DRUJ stability has also been studied recently, but is present in only 40% of cases.[8] These techniques are less effective compared to anatomic reconstruction of the DRUJ ligaments using a tendon graft.

The growth and refinement of arthroscopy has led to a considerable qualitative leap in the diagnosis and treatment of wrist injuries, and many classic surgical techniques have been converted to arthroscopic procedures, including those aimed at restoring stability in the DRUJ. The main advantages of arthroscopy over open procedures are better intraarticular visualization and reduced morbidity.

In order to correctly indicate TFCC reconstruction with tendon graft, it is important to be able to diagnose a nonrepairable injury to the proximal component of the TFCC, ensure that the articular surfaces are in good condition, and confirm the correct functioning of the interosseous membrane (to rule out Essex-Lopresti injury). Wrist arthroscopy is the gold standard for

TABLE 1
Atzei and Luchetti Classification.

	Class 1: Repairable distal tear	Class 2: Repairable complete tear	Class 3: Repairable proximal tear	Class 4: Non repairable tear	Class 5: Arthritic DRUJ
Clinical DRUJ instability	None/slight	Mild/severe	Mild/ severe	Severe	Mild/ severe
Status distal component TFCC (RC arthroscopy)	Torn	Torn	Intact	Torn	Variable
Status TFCC proximal component (Hook test, DRUJ arthroscopy)	Intact	Torn	Torn	Torn	
Healing potential of TFCC tissue	Good	Good	Good	Poor	
Status of DRUJ cartilage	Good	Good	Good	Good	Poor
TREATMENT	**Repair** Suture (lig to capsule)	**Repair** Foveal refixation	**Repair** Foveal refixation	**Reconstruction tendon graft**	**Salvage** Arthroplasty or joint replacementg

Comprehensive classification of TFCC peripheral tears and associated ulnar styloid fracture. Class 4, nonrepairable TFCC tears. Suggested treatment: tendon graft ligamentoplasty.

accurate diagnosis and guidance, and very often for the application of the appropriate treatment in a given case.[9–12]

MAIN QUESTION

"What is the most effective ligament reconstruction for management of chronic DRUJ instability associated with a (healed) distal radius fracture?"

CURRENT OPINION

Anatomic DRUJ ligament reconstruction using a tendon graft is an effective method for restoring DRUJ stability. The ideal candidate is a patient with clinically significant chronic DRUJ instability, nonrepairable TFCC and healthy articular cartilage. Evidence will need to establish whether there is an advantageous role for arthroscopic and minimally invasive techniques to potentially reduce soft tissue morbidity including periarticular scarring and fibrosis.

FINDING THE EVIDENCE

A systematic review was carried out in accordance with Preferred Reporting Items for Systematic Reviews and Meta-Analyses (PRISMA) guidelines.[13] On March 2, 2020, a search was conducted on the PubMed and Cochrane databases with the terms "DRUJ instability" or "chronic distal radioulnar joint instability" (Fig. 3). Abstracts and subsequently full-text articles were analyzed by two senior orthopedic surgery and traumatology specialists. Relevant articles from the bibliography of the selected articles were included. Articles that were not available in English or Spanish were excluded.

Quality of the Evidence

Level IV:
Clinical case series: 14

Findings

Fourteen level IV studies with case series (of 5–95 patients) of chronic DRUJ instability treated using some

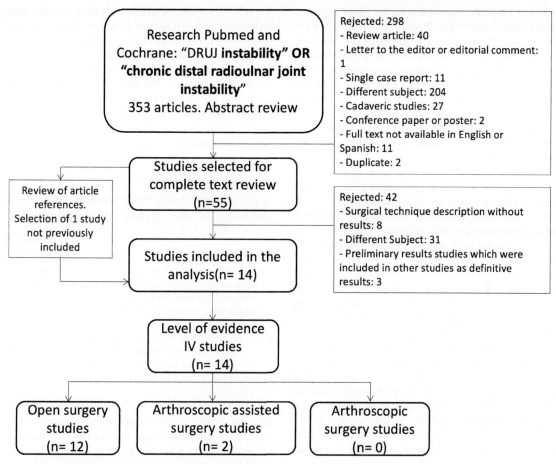

FIG. 3 Systematic review. The search was conducted on the PubMed and Cochrane databases with the terms "DRUJ instability" or "chronic distal radioulnar joint instability."

type of graft to restore stability were identified (Table 1). The older studies employed different types of open reconstruction techniques,[14–17] while more recent ones included case series of patients treated with open reconstruction procedures and others using arthroscopy-assisted reconstruction.[18,19,20,21]

In 1983, Mansat et al. described an anatomic ligamentoplasty using a *palmaris longus* tendon graft reconstructing the distal volar and dorsal radioulnar ligaments.[14] In 1994, Scheker[15] presented a series of 15 patients treated by open distal radioulnar ligamentoplasty with a *palmaris longus* tendon graft, reconstructing only the dorsal distal radioulnar ligament; pain was eliminated in 80% of the patients, with an increase in grip strength and no loss of mobility compared to before the surgery. In 2000, Adams[22] modified the more anatomic open reconstruction technique by Mansat, in

which he reconstructed the distal volar and dorsal radioulnar ligaments using a *palmaris longus* graft, publishing his results in 2002.[16] His modification of the original technique[16,22] became the gold standard for treatment. In addition to the initial study, four more series have been published using this method,[17–19,23] most of which modify it in some way. The five series of results using the Adams modification (9, 14, 16, 74 and 95 patients) showed good outcomes in 86%–100% of patients, with recovery of wrist stability (78%–100%), disappearance of pain or mild pain only (76%–89%) and improved grip strength in the functional evaluations.[16–19,23] Meyer et al.[24] presented a further modification of the Adams technique in which they created a second tunnel in the ulna, allowing the graft to be tied over a bone bridge, giving more resistant fixation and possibly allowing shorter and less strict immobilization;

the authors describe results similar to those reported with the Adams technique. Three other techniques have been published using pronator quadratus interposition (volar stabilization),[25] the dorsal capsule and extensor retinaculum (dorsal stabilization)[26] and *palmaris longus* tendon graft but located more proximal to the diaphysis (extra-articular ligament reconstruction).[27] Although the authors reported good results, and the procedures have the advantage of being technically simpler, the reconstruction is less anatomic and they are less frequently used.

Three patient series have also been published in which wrist arthroscopy was performed to confirm the diagnosis prior to open reconstruction surgery. Pürisa et al.[27] performed diagnostic arthroscopy and then extra-articular ligament reconstruction. Shih et al.[28] performed a diagnostic arthroscopy and, once the diagnosis was confirmed, open reconstruction 1 week later, with tunnels similar to those used in the Adams technique but with *extensor carpi ulnaris* tendon graft. The results reported were worse, with the drawback of performing the surgery in two stages. Henry[29] carried out wrist arthroscopy to confirm the diagnosis and, in the same procedure, performed the reconstruction using a *palmaris longus* graft. He made two tunnels in the radius in an attempt to replicate the insertion of the distal radioulnar ligaments in the sigmoid notch, suturing the graft over the bone bridge of the radius; outcomes were good, with joint stability in all patients in the series, improved grip strength, and no loss of motion with respect to the preoperative scores in the functional tests.

A further step has been taken more recently, and two series have been published with arthroscopy-assisted open surgery reconstruction techniques. These allow more accurate localization of the exit point of the ulnar tunnel in the fovea, as well as smaller (and therefore more cosmetic) incisions and less injury to soft tissues. Mak et al.[20] (part of this series previously published by

Tse et al.[30]) performed a procedure similar to the Adams technique, adding a second tunnel in the ulna to fix the graft over a bone bridge. Luchetti and Atzei[21] presented their case series, where they created the same tunnels as in the Adams technique, fixing the graft on the ulna with a bio-tenodesis screw. The authors reported results comparable to the Adams open technique in terms of stability, grip strength, and functional scores, showing an improvement in postoperative mobility, as well as a cosmetic advantage (Table 2).

RECOMMENDATION

In patients with chronic DRUJ instability associated to a (healed) distal radius fractures, evidence suggest:

Recommendation	Overall Quality
Anatomic distal radioulnar ligament reconstruction based on tendon grafting is a valid and reproducible technique providing satisfactory outcomes in absence of osteoarthritis.	⊕⊕○○ LOW
Potential advantages of arthroscopy over open procedures are better intraarticular visualization and lower morbidity at the expense of advanced technical training.	⊕○○○ VERY LOW

CONCLUSION

For the treatment of chronic nondegenerative DRUJ instability, anatomic distal radioulnar ligament reconstruction based on tendon grafting is a valid and reproducible technique with good reported functional outcomes and reduction of pain in several series. No superiority has been shown for any particular technique or modification as comparative studies are lacking. With popularization of wrist arthroscopy, there seems a trend toward arthroscopic-assisted techniques with potential advantages for surrounding soft tissues, though this not (yet) evidence based.

TABLE 2
Case Series of TFCC Reconstruction.

Authors	Year	N	Kind of Surgery	Graft	Tunnels and Fixation	Stability (% Patients)	Grip Strength (% of Contralateral)	ROM (°)	Pain	Functional Scores	Complications. Satisfaction
Scheker et al.	1994	15	OS	PL or plantaris or EDC	3 in R; 3 in C. Fix. 2 sutures over bone bridge (R, U).		80	F 61; E 62; RD 24; UD 31; P 82; S 80	86% none, 14% minor discomfort		1 Postblock brachial plexus neuritis 1 Mild reflex sympathetic dystrophy 1 Recurrence of instability
Adams and Berger	2000	14	OS	PL	PA in R; Ob in U. Fix. around U neck.	86	85	P72; S70	64% none, 36% mild pain		2 Recurrence of instability 2 Paraesthesia (healed)
Teoh and Yam	2005	9	OS	PL	PA in R; Ob in U. Fix. around U neck.	78	86	P–S (in % of contralateral): 92%	66% mild pain	MMWS 87	1 Paraesthesia (healed) 1 Stiffness
Shih and Lee	2005	37	DA+OS (1 week after)	ECU	PA in R; Ob in U.		65–90		None patients pain in daily activity	MMWS: 29.7% excellent 59.5% good 10.8% fair	3 Superficial wound infections
Seo et al.	2009	16	OS	PL	PA in R; Ob in U. Fix. around U neck.	75		F 70.9; E 72.8; RD 13.4; UD 30.3; P 76.3; S 82.5	PRWE (pain): 9.1/ 50	MMWS 92.8 DASH 10.5 PRWE 11.2	3 Laxity 1 Subluxation
Pürisa et al.	2011	5	DA+OS	PL	PA in R diaphysis. Fix. around U diaphysis	100		F 42; E 45; P 49; S 47	VAS 1.88	DASH 6.81	
Henry	2012	25	DA+OS	PL	2 in sigmoid notch in R. Ob in U. Suture over bone bridge (R).	100	79	F 61; E 62; P 71; S 74		DASH 7	
Lee et al.	2016	21	OS	PQ	3–4 in U. Suture over bone bridges.	100	91	F 72; E 69; P 77; S 82		DASH 12.5 PRWE 14.7	None

Continued

TABLE 2
Case Series of TFCC Reconstruction.—cont'd

Authors	Year	N	Kind of Surgery	Graft	Tunnels and Fixation	Stability (% Patients)	Grip Strength (% of Contralateral)	ROM (°)	Pain	Functional Scores	Complications. Satisfaction
Luchetti and Atzei	2017	11	AAS	PL	PA in R; Ob in U. Interference screw in U.	91	96	F 60; E 67; P 80; S 81	VAS (rest) 2 VAS (stress) 4	MWS 82 DASH 25 PRWE 33	1 Fracture ulnar styloid (healed) 3 Ulnar paraesthesia (healed) 1 Graft rupture 1 Instability recurrence
El-Haj et al.	2017	17	OS	ER+DC	Fix. Anchor suture in R.	100		P-S "full"	VAS 2.21	DASH 13.39	None
Meyer et al.	2017	48	OS	PL or FCU or LTE	PA in R; 2 Ob in U. Fix. Suture over bone bridge (U).	91	80.3	F 67.1; E 70.1; RD 19.6; UD 32.9; P 67.9; S 66.1	VAS 1.3		2 Subluxation persisted 2 Recurrent instability
Mak and Ho	2017	28	AAS	PL	PA in R, Ob in U+PA in U. Suture over bone bridge (U).		71.6	In % of contralateral: P+S: 91.1% E+F: 83.7% RD+UD: 83.5%	VAS 3	MWS 79	35.7%: 4 graft rupture 3 nerve injuries (healed) 3 discomfort over scar 1 breakage KW
Kootstra et al.	2018	22[a]	OS	PL or toe extensor or plantaris	PA in R; Ob in U. Fix. around U neck.	100	89.7	F 67; E 71.8; UD 30.9; RD 17.7; P 73; S 71.4		DASH 13.1 PRWE 20.3	4% Recurrent instability
Gillis et al.	2019	95	OS	PL or plantaris or TS or gracilis or semitendinosus	PA in R; Ob in U. Fix. around U neck or fix. anchors or Fix. interference screw	90.8	77.4	F 52.1; E 58.6; RD 19.8; UD 28.6; P 71.3;S 62.7	27.5% none, 48.4% mild pain	MMWS 68.9	31.6%: neuroapraxia, neuroma, recurrent instability, generative disease Satisfaction: VAS 8.1. 86.3%

AAS, arthroscopy assisted surgery; DA, diagnostic arthroscopy; DASH, disabilities of the arm, shoulder, hand score; DC, dorsal capsule; E, extension; ECU, extensor carpi ulnaris; EDC, extensor digitorum communis; ER, extensor retinaculum; F, flexion; FCU, flexor carpi ulnaris; Fix., fixation of the graft; KW, Kirschner-wire; LTE, long toe extensor; MMWS, modified mayo wrist score; MWS, mayo wrist score; Ob, oblique; OS, open surgery; P, pronation; PA, posteroanterior; PL, palmaris longus; PQ, pronator quadratus; PRWE, patient-rated wrist and hand evaluation score; R, radius; RD, radial deviation; ROM, range of movement; S, supination; TS, triceps surae; U, ulna; UD, ulnar deviation; Vas, visual analogue scale.

[a]74 Patients operated, of whom 22 patients responded to the invitation for clinical follow up (outcomes related to this 22 patients).

All-arthroscopic TFCC reconstruction with tendon graft:

If wrist arthroscopy material and implants are available and the surgeon is technically trained, the authors recommend an arthroscopy-assisted technique[20,21] or, ideally, an all-arthroscopic technique with fixation of the grafts with implants in their anatomic insertions.[31]

The procedure presented by the authors[31] is, to our knowledge, the first technique for performing fully arthroscopic TFCC ligament reconstruction. As we have seen in the historical progression of the series presented herein, increasing attempts have been made to perform more anatomic reconstruction, with more stable fixation. The introduction of arthroscopic techniques has led to smaller (and therefore more esthetic) incisions, a more anatomic location of the tunnel position and less soft tissue insult, leading to improved mobility without worsening outcomes in terms of pain, stability, grip strength, or functional scores.

The authors analyzed the results of nine patients who underwent arthroscopic ligamentoplasty with a minimum follow-up of 12 months (12–52 months). The following outcomes were observed: good or excellent results in the Mayo Wrist Score in eight cases (88.8%), with DRUJ stability in all cases; improvement in pain (previous visual analogue scale [VAS] 5.88[4–8] vs. VAS at 12 months 1.77 (0–4)); full range of motion or improvement from previous score in eight patients (88.8%); and QuickDash score at 12 months of 11.18 (6.75–18) compared to a presurgery score of 44.70 (36.25–54).

The main advantages of arthroscopy over open procedures are better intraarticular visualization and lower morbidity, particularly when operating in the ulnar compartment of the wrist. An arthroscopy-assisted technique for the reconstruction of nonrepairable peripheral TFCC tears is intended not only to minimize the surgical trauma in order to reduce postoperative pain and to facilitate rehabilitation, but also to allow greater precision and thus improve both the quality of the reconstruction and the functional outcome.

PORTALS EMPLOYED AND TENDON GRAFT

There are essentially three portals used to perform the TFCC reconstruction technique: radiocarpal portals 3–4 and 6R, and a Volar Distal Radioulnar Portal that gives direct access to the DRUJ similar to the direct foveal portal, but slightly volar and distal, having volar access at the level of the 6R portal. This portal is located ulnar to the *flexor carpi ulnaris* tendon.[32,33] A proximal ulnar mini-incision is also made to create the ulnar tunnel (Fig. 4).

The *palmaris longus* tendon of the homolateral forearm is used as a tendon graft. A *flexor carpi radialis* (FCR) hemitendon, approximately 2–3 mm thick and 10 cm long, may also be obtained.

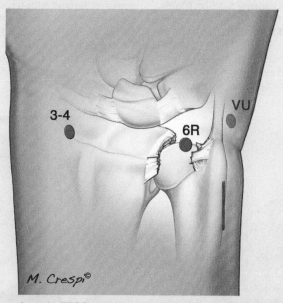

FIG. 4 Portals used to perform the TFCC reconstruction technique: 3–4 and 6R portal, and a Volar Distal Radioulnar Portal that gives direct access to the DRUJ. A proximal ulnar mini-incision is also made to create the ulnar tunnel.

Continued

Panel 2: Author's Preferred Technique—cont'd

CREATING THE ULNAR TUNNEL

With the scope in the 3–4 portal, the position of the ulnar fovea is visualized. The TFCC tissue remnants must first be debrided. A C-shaped guide is introduced through the 6R portal. The tip of the guide is placed in the position of the fovea; the extra-articular portion marks the position of the ulnar incision required to create the bone tunnel. Care must be taken to protect the dorsal sensory branch of the ulnar nerve. The guide wire is inserted from outside to inside under arthroscopic control (Fig. 5), drilling over the guide wire to create a 4-mm tunnel.

CREATING THE RADIAL TUNNELS IN THE VOLAR AND DORSAL INSERTION

The scope in the 3–4 portal provides a good view for inserting the guide wires for subsequent drilling of the tunnels in the volar and dorsal insertions of the radioulnar ligaments.

The guide wires should be placed at the volar and dorsal edges of the radius, in a convergent direction and slightly angled (about 30–45 degrees) toward the radial metaphysis (Fig. 6). The correct position of the wires should be confirmed before creating the bone tunnels. It is also important to check that enough bone wall is retained in the tunnels after drilling, in order to avoid breaking the wall when inserting the graft and implants.

The radial tunnels are created using a 3-mm cannulated drill bit, drilling to a depth of approximately 1–1.5 cm (Fig. 6).

PASSING THE TENDON GRAFT TO THE ULNAR TUNNEL

With the scope in the 3–4 portal, a Micro SutureLasso (Arthrex®, Naples, FL) is inserted straight through the ulnar tunnel (Fig. 7), leaving the nitinol loop open over the DRUJ.

A grasper or arthroscopic clamp is advanced from the 6R portal to the volar portal through the nitinol loop. The grasper is retrieved, grasping one end of the tendon graft and passing it through the loop, leaving one end in the volar ulnar portal, the other in the 6R portal, and the graft introduced in the nitinol loop (Fig. 7).

Pulling the nitinol loop from the ulnar tunnel, a tendon loop is pulled out through the ulnar tunnel, leaving a dorsal end in the 6R portal and a volar end in the volar distal radioulnar portal (Fig. 8).

FIXING THE TENDON GRAFT IN THE RADIAL TUNNELS

With a view from the 3–4 portal, keeping the nitinol loop with the tendon loop in the ulnar tunnel, the two ends of the tendon graft (in which a Krackow-type stitch has previously been made) are introduced in the corresponding volar and dorsal radial tunnels using a Suture Passer needle (Arthrex®, Naples, FL).

Maintaining the tension of the sutures exiting at the radial edge of the wrist, the graft is fixed using 3-mm interference screws (Fig. 9). The dorsal radial interference screw is inserted from the 6R portal and the volar screw from the volar distal radioulnar portal.

FIXING THE TENDON GRAFT IN THE ULNAR TUNNEL

With a direct view from the 3–4 or 6R portal, maintaining the tension of the graft in the ulnar tunnel, the graft is fixed using a 4-mm interference screw (Arthrex®, Naples, FL), thuscompleting the reconstruction of the proximal portion of the TFCC (Fig. 10).

The tension to be applied to the graft is previously tested, enabling correct pronosupination without excessive compression on the DRUJ.

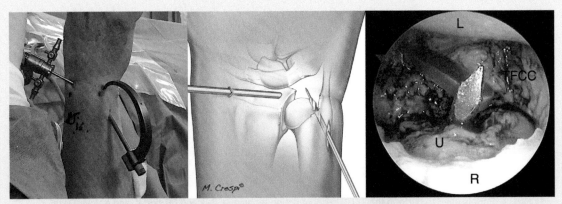

FIG. 5 With the scope in the 3–4 portal, a C-shaped guide is introduced through the 6R portal. The guide wire is inserted from outside to inside under arthroscopic control drilling over the guide wire to create a 4-mm tunnel. L (Lunate), R (Radius), TFCC (Triangular Fibrocartilage Complex), U (Ulnar head).

Panel 2: Author's Preferred Technique—cont'd

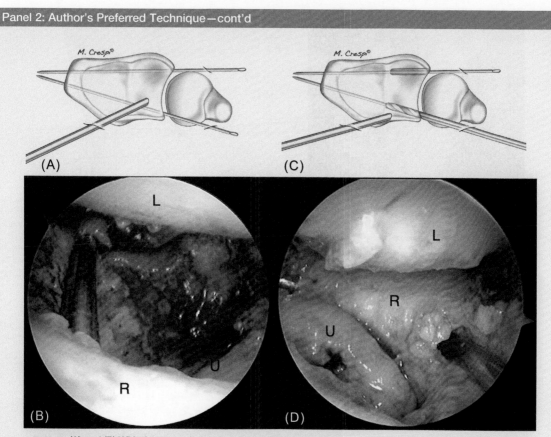

FIG. 6 (A) and (B) With the scope in the 3–4 portal, the guide wires are inserted at the volar and dorsal edges of the radius, in a convergent direction and slightly angled (about 30–45 degrees) toward the radial metaphysis. (C) Subsequent drilling of the tunnels is performed in the volar and dorsal insertions of the radioulnar ligaments. (D) Checking from the volar distal radioulnar portal that enough bone wall is retained in the tunnels after drilling. L (Lunate), R (Radius), U (Ulnar head).

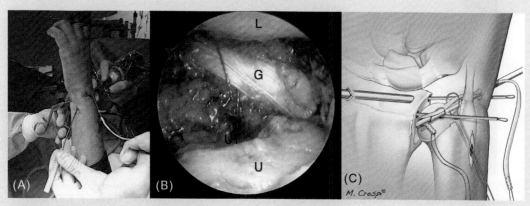

FIG. 7 Passing the tendon graft to the ulnar tunnel. (A) A grasper is advanced from the 6R portal to the volar portal through the nitinol loop previously introduced in the ulnar tunnel. (B) and (C) The grasper is retrieved, grasping one end of the tendon graft and passing it through the loop, leaving one end in the volar distal radioulnar portal, the other in the 6R portal. G (Tendon Graft), L (Lunate), U (Ulnar head), UT (Ulnar tunnel).

Continued

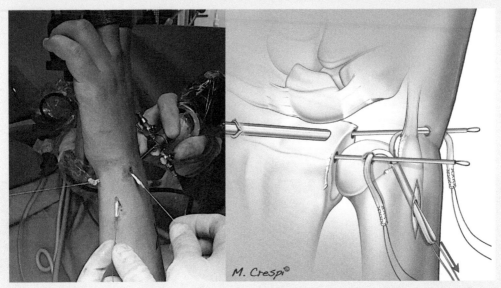

FIG. 8 Pulling the nitinol loop, a tendon loop is pulled out through the ulnar tunnel. Tendon graft disposition after the passage through the ulnar tunnel. The volar and dorsal ends of the graft remain in the volar distal radioulnar portal and in 6R portal.

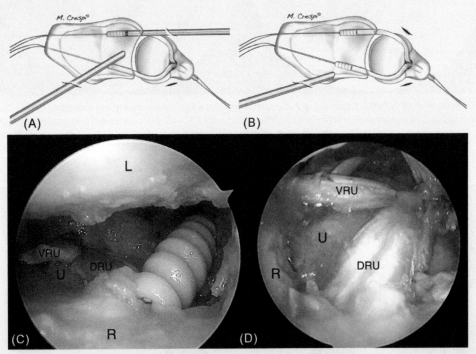

FIG. 9 (A) and (B) With a view from the 3–4 portal, the two ends of the tendon graft are introduced in the corresponding volar and dorsal radial tunnels using a Suture Passer needle (Arthrex®, Naples, FL). (C) Maintaining the tension of the sutures exiting at the radial edge of the wrist, the graft is fixed from the 6R and volar distal radioulnar portals using 3-mm interference screws. (D) View from 3 to 4 portal, both ends of the graft have been fixed in the radial tunnels. DRU (Dorsal Radioulnar Ligament), L (Lunate), R (Radius), U (Ulnar head), VRU (Volar Radioulnar Ligament).

Panel 2: Author's Preferred Technique—cont'd

POSTOPERATIVE CARE

After the portals and incisions have been closed, a long-arm splint is applied with the forearm in neutral pronosupination.

The splint should be worn for 2 weeks, after which it is replaced with a forearm splint, leaving the elbow free, for another week.

After removing the forearm splint, a removable orthosis is fitted, and the patient starts the specific rehabilitation protocol.[30]

This was the technique used in the clinical case presented, with a favorable outcome just 2 months after surgery (Fig. 11).

COMPLICATIONS

The main complications that may appear are as follows:

- Nerve injuries: the dorsal cutaneous branch of the ulnar nerve is the nervous structure at greatest risk. By avoiding anteroposterior tunnels at the level of the sigmoid cavity of the radius, the risk of injury to the ulnar neurovascular bundle is avoided.

- Bone injuries: there is a risk of ulnar styloid or distal ulnar fracture after the bone tunnel is made and after the introduction of a plasty or an interferential screw that is too thick. It is important to ensure the existence of a bone-bridge of at least 1.5 cm from the ulnar styloid to the entrance of the bone tunnel.

- Chondral injuries: chondral injuries may appear when creating the convergent bone tunnels at the level of the sigmoid cavity of the radius if they are too distal.

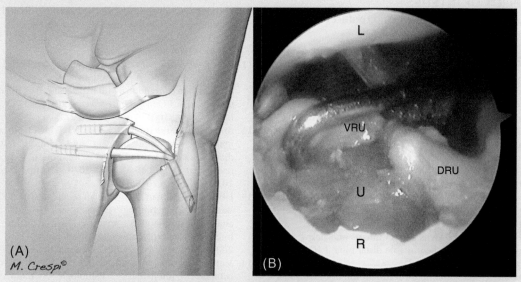

FIG. 10 (A) Finishing the reconstruction of the proximal portion of the TFCC after ulnar tunnel fixation using 4-mm interference screw. (B) Completed TFCC ligamentoplasty, view from 3 to 4 portal. DRU (Dorsal Radioulnar Ligament), L (Lunate), R (Radius), U (Ulnar head), VRU (Volar Radioulnar Ligament).

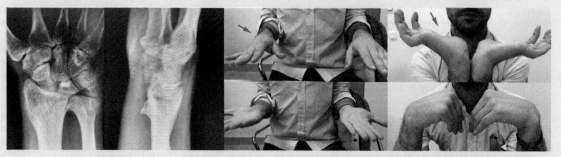

FIG. 11 Clinical case. X-Ray and clinical results 3 months after the arthroscopic TFCC ligamentoplasty. *Red arrow marks* the injured wrist.

Panel 3: Pearls and Pitfalls

PEARLS

- The volar and dorsal radioulnar ligaments have an important stabilizing effect in forearm rotation, with an isometric point of insertion in the fovea.
- Arthroscopy enables a more precise diagnosis and better therapeutic decision making.
- Anatomic reconstruction of the radioulnar ligaments achieves good clinical outcomes.
- Minimally invasive surgery and arthroscopy reduce soft tissue insult and can help improve outcomes.

PITFALLS

- In chronic TFCC injuries, with friable tissue and DRUJ instability, direct repair has a high degree of clinical failure.
- The presence of advanced DRUJ arthritis contraindicates ligament reconstruction and should be ruled out before surgery is performed.
- Precision in the position of bone tunnels is critical to the success of the technique and to avoid intraoperative fractures.
- Prolonged immobilization after surgery increases joint stiffness and makes functional recovery difficult.

CONFLICT OF INTEREST

The authors declare that there is no conflict of interest.

REFERENCES

1. Lindau T, Arner M, Hagberg L. Intraarticular lesions in distal fractures of the radius in young adults. A descriptive arthroscopic study in 50 patients. *J Hand Surg (Br)*. 1997;22:638–643. https://doi.org/10.1016/s0266-7681(97)80364-6.
2. Nakamura T, Makita A. The proximal ligamentous component of the triangular fibrocartilage complex. *J Hand Surg (Br)*. 2000;25:479–486. https://doi.org/10.1054/jhsb.1999.0329.
3. Atzei A, Luchetti R. Foveal TFCC tear classification and treatment. *Hand Clin*. 2011;27:263–272. https://doi.org/10.1016/j.hcl.2011.05.014.
4. Breen T, Jupiter J. Extensor carpi ulnaris and flexor carpi ulnaris tenodesis of the unstable distal ulna. *J Hand Surg [Am]*. 1989;14:612–617.
5. Eliason EL. An operation for recurrent inferior radioulnar dislocation. *Ann Surg*. 1932;96:27–35.
6. Hui F, Linscheid R. Ulnotriquetral augmentation tenodesis: a reconstructive procedure for dorsal subluxation of the distal radioulnar joint. *J Hand Surg [Am]*. 1982;7:230–236.
7. Johnson R, Shrewsbury M. The pronator quadratus in motions and in stabilization of the radius and ulna at the distal radioulnar joint. *J Hand Surg [Am]*. 1976;1:205–209.
8. Marès O. Distal radioulnar joint instability. *Hand Surg Rehabil*. 2017;36:305–313. https://doi.org/10.1016/j.hansur.2017.08.001.
9. Park J, Ahn K, Chang A, Kwon Y, Choi I, Park J. Changes in the morphology of the triangular fibrocartilage complex (TFCC) on magnetic resonance arthrography related to disruption of ulnar foveal attachment. *Skelet Radiol*. 2020;49:249–256. https://doi.org/10.1007/s00256-019-03278-x.
10. Mutimer J, Green J, Field J. Comparison of MRI and wrist arthroscopy for assessment of wrist cartilage. *J Hand Surg Eur Vol*. 2008;33:380–382. https://doi.org/10.1177/1753193408090395.
11. Boer B, Vestering M, van Raak S, van Kooten E, Huis In 't Veld R, Vochteloo A. MR arthrography is slightly more accurate than conventional MRI in detecting TFCC lesions of the wrist. *Eur J Orthop Surg Traumatol*. 2018;28:1549–1553. https://doi.org/10.1007/s00590-018-2215-x.
12. Andersson J, Andernord D, Karlsson J, Fridén J. Efficacy of magnetic resonance imaging and clinical tests in diagnostics of wrist ligament injuries: a systematic review. *Art Ther*. 2015;31:2014–2020. e2. https://doi.org/10.1016/j.arthro.2015.04.090.
13. Liberati A, Altman DG, Tetzlaff J, et al. The PRISMA statement for reporting systematic reviews and meta-analyses of studies that evaluate health care interventions: explanation and elaboration. *PLoS Med*. 2009;6. https://doi.org/10.1371/journal.pmed.1000100.
14. Mansat M, Mansat C, Martinez C. L'articulation radio-cubitale inférieure. Pathologie traumatique. In: Razemon JP, Fisk GR, eds. *Le poignet. Monographies du Groupe d'Etude de la Main*. Paris: Expansions Scientifiques Francaise; 1983:187–195.
15. Scheker L, Belliappa P, Acosta R, German D. Reconstruction of the dorsal ligament of the triangular fibrocartilage complex. *J Hand Surg (Br)*. 1994;19:310–318. https://doi.org/10.1016/0266-7681(94)90079-5.
16. Adams BD, City I, Berger RA. An anatomic reconstruction of the distal radioulnar ligaments for posttraumatic distal radioulnar joint instability. *J Hand Surg [Am]*. 2002;243–251. https://doi.org/10.1053/jhsu.2002.31731.
17. Teoh LC, Yam AKT. Anatomic reconstruction of the distal radioulnar ligaments: long-term results. *J Hand Surg (Br)*. 2005;30:185–193. https://doi.org/10.1016/j.jhsb.2004.10.017.
18. Gillis JA, Soreide ÃE, Khouri ÃJS, Berger RA, Moran SL. Outcomes of the Adams–Berger ligament reconstruction

for the distal radioulnar joint instability in 95 consecutive cases. *J Wrist Surg.* 2019;1:268–275.

19. Kootstra TJM, Van DMH, Schuurman A. Functional effects of the Adams procedure: a retrospective intervention study. *J Wrist Surg.* 2018;7:331–335. https://doi.org/10.1055/s-0038-1660812.

20. Mak MC, Ho P. Arthroscopic-assisted triangular fibrocartilage complex reconstruction. *Hand Clin.* 2017;33:625–637. https://doi.org/10.1016/j.hcl.2017.07.014.

21. Luchetti R, Atzei A. Arthroscopic assisted tendon reconstruction for triangular fibrocartilage complex irreparable tears. *J Hand Surg Eur Vol.* 2017;42:346–351. https://doi.org/10.1177/1753193417690669.

22. Adams D. Anatomic reconstruction of radioulnar ligaments for DRUJ instability. *Tech Hand Up Extrem Surg.* 2000;4:154–160.

23. Seo KN, Park MJ, Kang HJ. Anatomic reconstruction of the distal radioulnar ligament for posttraumatic distal radioulnar joint instability. *Clin Orthop Surg.* 2009;138–145. https://doi.org/10.4055/cios.2009.1.3.138.

24. Meyer D, Schweizer A, Nagy L. Anatomic reconstruction of distal radioulnar ligaments with tendon graft for treating distal Radioulnar joint instability: surgical technique and outcome. *Tech Hand Up Extrem Surg.* 2017;21:107–113. https://doi.org/10.1097/BTH.0000000000000163.

25. Lee SK, Lee JW, Choy WS. Volar stabilization of the distal radioulnar joint for chronic instability using the pronator quadratus. *Ann Plast Surg.* 2016;76:1–5. https://doi.org/10.1097/SAP.0000000000000354.

26. El-Haj M, Baughman C, Thirkannad S. A technique for treating dorsal instability of the distal radioulnar joint. *Tech Hand Up Extrem Surg.* 2017;21:67–70. https://doi.org/10.1097/BTH.0000000000000157.

27. Pürisa H, Sezer İ, Kabakaş F, Tunçer S, Ertürer E, Yazar M. Ligament reconstruction using the Fulkerson-Watson method to treat chronic isolated distal radioulnar joint instability: short-term results. *Acta Orthop Traumatol Turc.* 2011;45:386–390. https://doi.org/10.3944/AOTT.2011.2380.

28. Shih J, Lee H. Functional results post-triangular fibrocartilage complex reconstruction with extensor carpi ulnaris with or without ulnar shortening in chronic distal radioulnar joint instability. *Hand Surg.* 2005;10:169–176. https://doi.org/10.1142/S0218810405002759.

29. Henry M. Anatomic reconstruction of the radioulnar ligament. *Hand.* 2012;7:413–419. https://doi.org/10.1007/s11552-012-9456-7.

30. Tse W, Lau S, Yee W, Cheng H, Chow C. Arthroscopic reconstruction of triangular fibrocartilage complex (TFCC) with tendon graft for chronic DRUJ instability. *Injury.* 2013;44:386–390. https://doi.org/10.1016/j.injury.2013.01.009.

31. Carratalá Baixauli V, Lucas García FJ, Martínez Andrade C, Carratalá Baixauli R, Guisasola Lerma E, Corella Montoya F. All-arthroscopic triangular fibrocartilage complex ligamentoplasty for chronic DRUJ instability. *Tech Hand Up Extrem Surg.* 2019;23:44–51. https://doi.org/10.1097/BTH.0000000000000222.

32. Carratalá Baixauli V, Lucas García F, González Jofré C, Carratalá Baixauli R, Sánchez Alepuz E. Técnica de reinserción foveal artroscópica sin nudos del fibrocartílago triangular con visión directa de la articulación radiocubital distal. *Rev Iberoam Cir Mano.* 2016;44:39–46. https://doi.org/10.1016/j.ricma.2016.02.002.

33. Lucas FJ, Carratalá V, Miranda I, Martínez C. The Volar Distal Radioulnar Portal in wrist arthroscopy: an anatomical study. *J Wrist Surg.* 2020. https://doi.org/10.1055/s-0040-1720964.

CHAPTER 36

Posttraumatic DRUJ Arthritis

SIMON FARNEBO[a,b] • SANDRA LINDQVIST[c] • PETER AXELSSON[c]
[a]Department of Hand Surgery and Plastic Surgery, and Burns, Linköping University, Linköping, Sweden,
[b]Department of Biomedical and Clinical Sciences, Linköping, Linköping University, Linköping, Sweden,
[c]Department of Hand Surgery, Institute of Clinical Sciences, Sahlgrenska Academy, University
of Gothenburg, Gothenburg, Sweden

KEY POINTS

- Salvage procedures of distal radioulnar joint (DRUJ) arthritis after distal radius fractures (DRFs) can be divided in resection arthroplasties and implant arthroplasties.
- Corrective osteotomy, ulnar shortening, ligament—reinsertion or reconstruction should be considered before reconstruction of the joint.
- Specific indications for the different reconstructive procedures after DRFs have not been established, and the scientific evidence for any treatment is weak.
- Decision on what operative treatment to choose for DRUJ osteoarthritis is primarily based on factors related to; patient demands, especially on loading of the forearm, DRUJ morphology, and stability provided by constraining soft tissues.

Panel 1: Case Scenario

A 64-year-old female with osteoporosis presents at your clinic. She has retired since a few years after knee arthroplasties, but is still living an active lifestyle, including a wish to continue playing golf.

A year earlier she was treated at a nearby hospital with external fixation and pinning for a distal radius fracture (DRF) (Fig. 1). Upon initial consultation, she complains of ulnar-sided wrist pain while lifting or moving her arm.

Her grip strength is reduced by 50%, compared to the uninjured side, but range of motion is less affected, with a pronosupination of 130 degrees (Table 1).

She experiences pain on palpation and compression of the DRUJ as well as on resisted forearm rotation. There is a minor instability on the shear test of the DRUJ in fully pronated position. Radiographs reveal ulnocarpal impaction, because of radial shortening, and a 10 degree dorsal tilt compared to the uninjured wrist (Fig. 1C and D).

What treatment will you suggest to this patient?

Continued

Distal Radius Fractures. https://doi.org/10.1016/B978-0-323-75764-5.00001-9

Panel 1: Case Scenario—cont'd

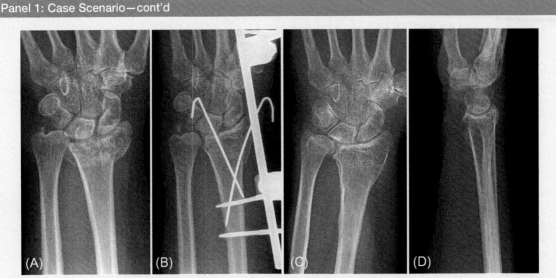

FIG. 1 (A) Initial fracture, (B) primary treatment, (C and D) presentation at 1 year.

TABLE 1
Recordings of PROMs and physical measures before and after surgery

	VAS S	VAS R	VAS A	DASH	PRWE	ROM S°	ROM P°	Grip (kg)	Lift N (kg)	Lift S (kg)	Lift P (kg)	Torque S (Nm)	Torque P (Nm)
Preop.		55	75	25	71	60	70	20	5.6	6.2	5.8	3.9	3.9
Latest	96	17	40	24	31	70	80	30	10.1	10	8.7	3.9	3
Contral.						70	85	40	10.6	12.5	8.9	4.2	3.9

Preop., preoperative recordings. *Latest*, latest follow-up measurements. *Contral.*, recordings from the unaffected side. *VAS*, visual analogue scale; *VAS S*, satisfaction; *VAS R*, VAS pain at rest; *VAS A*, VAS pain during activity; *ROM S*, range of motion-supination; *VAS P*, pronation; *Grip*, grip strength; *Lift N*, lifting strength in neutral forearm position; *Lift S*, lifting strength in fully supinated position; *LIFT P*, lifting strength in pronated position. *Torque S*, torque in supinated direction. *Torque P*, torque in pronating direction.

IMPORTANCE OF THE PROBLEM

Involvement of the sigmoid notch of the distal radio ulnar joint (DRUJ) is known to be as high as 80% in intraarticular distal radius fractures (DRF).[1,2] How many of these injuries that actually progresses to symptomatic OA and disability is not known, however data from Cooney et al. in the 70s show a prevalence of DRUJ osteoarthritis in Colles' fractures of 5%.[3] Diagnostic modalities and treatment techniques has changed considerably since then, and the frequency of DRUJ involvement in DRF may also be underestimated, as it has been shown that displacement of the sigmoid notch of intraarticular fractures is often missed with plain radiographs.[4] Nevertheless, it seems like involvement of the

sigmoid notch with DRF does not necessarily lead to development of OA, and a poor result. Vitale et al. hypothesize that the DRUJ may be a more tolerant joint for articular injury and malalignment than the radiocarpal joint.[5]

Not only involvement of the sigmoid notch, but also direct injury to the joint surfaces, will cause joint degeneration. It is likely that associated ligament injuries, or a combination of ligamentous injuries and fracture later on will lead to OA. Therefore, depending on how the OA developed different treatment modalities need to be considered when the joint is reconstructed.

Patients that are affected by DRUJ arthritis may suffer from substantial physical morbidity with; disabling ulnar-sided wrist pain, decreased ability to load the wrist in all static positions, as well as during forearm rotation. Conservative treatment with pronosupination locking splints may offer some relief, but is a poor option as restriction of forearm movements is not well tolerated. Selective denervation of the DRUJ is rarely performed and current literature is sparse for this treatment. Other surgical treatments for disabling DRUJ arthritis range from simple low-cost resection arthroplasties to complex and expensive implant arthroplasties. The paucity of data—not only on the prevalence of symptomatic DRUJ OA following DRF—is even more striking when it comes to comparing treatment modalities.

MAIN QUESTION

What is the optimal surgical treatment for a patient with a painful osteoarthritic DRUJ after a DRF?

CURRENT OPINION

To sort out what treatment option is best for the individual patient, some critical factors need to be addressed. Most importantly, the patient's functional demands and expectations, specifically regarding the ability to bear load, needs to be assessed. This is often, but not necessarily, related to the patient's age. Previous multiple surgeries will usually affect the outcome in a negative way, why they need to be taken into consideration. DRUJ characteristics, the localization of the OA, any remaining malalignment, and signs of ligamentous injuries are other key elements that need to be identified.

If a bony deformity remains, it should usually be treated first. Not only does a corrected malalignment reduce symptoms and potentially prevent further deterioration of the DRUJ, but also enable a better starting point for later salvage procedures if needed. Corrective osteotomy of the radius is usually first considered, but an ulnar shortening might be sufficient in certain cases, such as when there is a positive ulnar variance and a suitable type of joint geometry.

Second to addressing malunion is determining if there is a concomitant ligamentous injury that can be fixed, or needs to be accounted for when the treatment strategy is decided upon. In general, surgery to repair or reconstruct ligaments can be done simultaneously to a corrective osteotomy, but many times it is better left to a later point when the outcome of the osteotomy can be evaluated.

If the primary procedures to correct for malunion or joint instability fail, or in case of a remaining severe DRUJ arthritis, salvage procedures are to be considered.

For many decades, the only surgical intervention that could be offered for an arthritic DRUJ was some kind of resection arthroplasty. Functionally, the main drawback of resection arthroplasties is the loss of solid support to the loaded hand and wrist which will affect the ability to grip and lift. As the ulnar head is removed also the separation of the distal radius and ulna is lost, sometimes causing painful dynamic impingement of the bones. Only solid DRUJ prostheses have the possibility to solve this problem, as the distal ulnar buttress is restored. This treatment option became available in the late 90s, primarily as salvage procedures for failed resection arthroplasties. Biomechanical studies which show superior properties compared to resection arthroplasties[6,7] and with favorable clinical results, that seems to last, has made the joint replacements gain approval with increased popularity. In most institutions though, resection arthroplasty, with or without soft tissue stabilization of the ulnar stump remains as standard treatment of care for the osteoarthritic DRUJ.

SURGICAL TREATMENT OPTIONS

Denervation

When doing our literature search, we have not found any reports on outcomes of selective denervation of the DRUJ, although the anatomical prerequisites are described.[8]

DRUJ Resection Arthroplasties

Darrach's Procedure

The easiest way to remove an arthritic DRUJ surface is through simple complete ulnar head resection, popularized as the Darrach procedure. There is a great disparity in the published long-term results after Darrach's procedure, and the majority of the literature is on patients with rheumatoid arthritis. Most studies recognize the risk for mechanical impingement, and a loss of grip strength up to 50%,[9–11] and several studies have shown that only about 50% of posttraumatic patients are satisfied with the results of the procedure,[12,13] especially in slightly younger age groups (Fig. 2).

Some recent reports[10,14] show reasonably good pain relief in the long term, but data on outcome after treatment secondary to DRF is scarce.

A magnitude of technical modifications of the procedure has been described, including, whether or not the styloid should be spared, if there should be an extraperiosteal

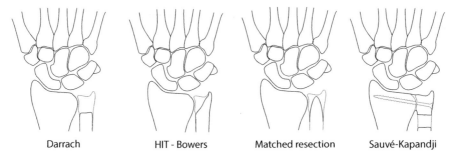

| Darrach | HIT - Bowers | Matched resection | Sauvé-Kapandji |

FIG. 2 Schematic sketches of the different resection arthroplasties.

or intraperiosteal resection or whether or not the distal ulna should be stabilized or not.

Partial Ulnar Head Resection/Hemiresection Interposition Technique (Bowers Procedure or HIT)

The technique is designed to preserve ulnocarpal ligamentous structures, and thereby theoretically provide a more stable distal ulnar end. Although there is some evidence supporting this assumption, based primarily on in vitro studies (see below—"Complications to Resection Arthroplasties" section), clinical follow-up show marginally better stabilizing effects of the ulnar head compared to unsupported S-K and Darrach´s procedures.[11] The main benefit compared to Darrach's procedure is the increase in grip strength, and ability to return to work.[11]

There is no consensus on what capsular interposition flap should be used for optimal results. A modified approach to the initial procedure has been advocated by Bain et al.,[15] where a more robust, single ulnar compound capsular flap is used. The ECU is mobilized within its sheath to a more dorsal position, possibly acting as a dynamic stabilizer to the distal ulna.

Matched Resection

The main difference from the HIT-procedure lies in the reshaping of the distal ulna over a 5 cm length, with no need for interposition of tissue in the articular space.

The distal ulna is shaped to match the distal curvature of the radius, with the aim to decrease the risk for impingement. Also, the ligamentous insertions of the distal ulna are relieved to produce a broad noncontact area to radius throughput full pronation and supination.

There is very little, or no, literature supporting this procedure for posttraumatic osteoarthritis after DRF, however it is likely that the results would be similar to the Darrach's procedure.[16]

Sauvé-Kampandji Procedure

This procedure combines DRUJ arthrodesis with a segmental resection of the distal ulna, resulting in a pseudarthrosis which allows forearm rotation.

The procedure is designed to remove the arthritic surfaces while maintaining ulnar support for the carpus as well as, for instance, the extensor carpi ulnaris tendon sheath. Thereby, the S-K procedure reduces the risk of carpal translation and permits the function of soft tissue constraints to work in a more native way. This maintains a more normal translation of forces from the hand to the forearm and is likely the reason for the consistent increase in grip strength that is seen in several studies,[11,17–19] and the high rate of return to work.[11]

Complications to Resection Arthroplasties

The main complication after partial- or complete resection of the distal ulna is associated with loss of the buttress function of the ulnar head. Typically, this leads to unpredictable results, because of stump instability and ensuing pathological motion in the medio-lateral and dorso-palmar planes. Most commonly this instability causes radio-ulnar convergence and impingement of the radial metaphysis to the fixed ulnar shaft. In vitro studies comparing radio-ulnar convergence between Darrach procedures and HIT procedures consistently show smaller amounts of displacement in the HIT group compared to the Darrach group.[6] Similarly, Minami et al.[11] showed a high ratio of instability of the ulnar stump in Darrach and S-K group, but not to the same extent after HIT procedure, or after ECU tendon stabilization of the S-K patients.

In reality, the increased convergence seen radiologically, typically presents as a "click," or mild pain at the ulnar stump, which only requires additional surgery in a smaller number of patients.

Various stabilization procedures have been promoted to overcome the problems with radio-ulnar convergence. Slips from the extensor carpi ulnaris tendon,[11] the flexor carpi ulnaris tendon,[20] or both[21] have been used to stabilize the shaft of the ulna.

Other common complications after resection arthroplasty include hardware problems and symptoms of the dorsal sensory branch of the ulnar nerve. Hardware problems that require removal in the S-K group is as common as 6%–16%.[17,18,22]

DRUJ Implant Arthroplasties
Partial Ulnar Head Prosthesis
There are currently two partial ulnar head prostheses (Partial-UHPs) in the market. In this concept, only the articular portion of the ulnar head is substituted while part of the TFCC and other soft tissue restraints are left intact. This is an attractive solution which may lower the risk for postoperative instability-related complications compared to a total UHP. Unfortunately, there are only a few reports about these implants[23,24] which cannot be ground for comparison. Therefore, it is, at the moment, not possible to make valid distinctions on when this type of implant should be preferred over the total UHPs (Fig. 3).

Total Ulnar Head Prosthesis
There are several designs of total ulnar head prostheses (Total-UHPs). All are modular designs, based on a solid metal ulnar stem. The first and most well documented implant is commonly used with a ceramic head while others use metal heads. Some metal heads include the opportunity to reattach the TFCC but if this of clinical importance is debated and not proven. As total ulnar head implants prevent firm attachment of ligaments, they are heavily dependent on the stability provided by the remaining soft tissue envelope. The shape of the sigmoid notch and the contact area on the ulnar side of the radius is also important.[25] Rigorous preoperative assessment, preferably using a CT scan, is therefore usually of great value. Any remaining malalignment of the distal radius after a previous DRF should also be recognized as this may force the UHP out of position.

Outcome after total UHP is generally good, with significant improvement in pain as seen in several studies.[25–28] Additionally, low complication rates are seen,[25,26,28–30] with survival rates up to 83% at 6 years[31] and 90% at 15 years follow-up.[30]

Although complications related to instability are a major concern regarding total UHPs,[28,29,32] it is not directly correlated to failure or impairment.[25,27] In a recent systematic review, Calcagni and Giesen also reported a high frequency of radiographic instability, while at the same time concluding that clinically relevant instability seems to be rare.[33]

Symptomatic instability of the distal ulna can usually be avoided by careful patient selection and soft tissue handling. Minor preoperative DRUJ instability can be managed by appropriate sizing of the ulnar head and additionally sometimes by contouring of the sigmoid notch and the adjacent area during the procedure. Gross instability, or persistent instability after multiple procedures, are however considered relative contraindications to UHP.

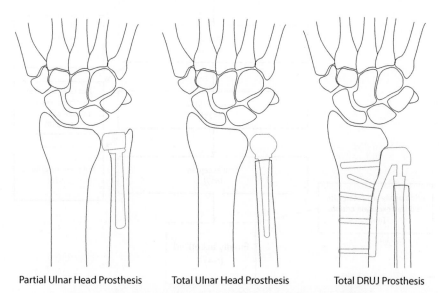

Partial Ulnar Head Prosthesis   Total Ulnar Head Prosthesis   Total DRUJ Prosthesis

FIG. 3 Schematic sketches of the different implant arthroplasties.

Total Distal Radioulnar Joint Prosthesis

The total DRUJ implant is of a linked design with components that are fixed both to the ulna and the radius. It replaces not only the joint, but also the TFCC and other stabilizing soft tissues. Controversy exists if it should be classified as a constrained prosthesis, or possibly semi-constrained because of its large degree of freedom of motion.

The total DRUJ prosthesis available today appears to be the most commonly used of all implants and it is the most well documented on the market. The general impression is that this implant provides satisfactory results even in the most complicated cases[31,34–36] but high complication rates have been reported.[33,35,37] As many of the complications occur early, and appear to be avoidable, it is likely that these complications are related to the fact that this type of arthroplasty is technically demanding.

Gross instability, for any reason, in addition to DRUJ arthritis is the main indication for the total DRUJ implant. It is especially useful after previous multiple failed procedures and after failed implant arthroplasties. Malunions in the distal—radius or ulna, osteoporosis, as well as possible future need for a total wrist replacement, are relative contraindications.

FINDING THE EVIDENCE

Search Strategy

The search was made in Cochrane, Medline, and Embase (Fig. 4) electronic databases. We based the search on following terms; Distal radioulnar joint, DRUJ, implant, arthroplasty, denervation, resection, replacement, prosthesis, and salvage.

Exclusion criteria were articles with cohorts less than 10 cases, follow-up less than 1 year, reviews, biomechanical, and cadaveric studies. Articles including inflammatory arthritis and congenital disorders were also excluded, if the results for posttraumatic DRUJ osteoarthritis were not separated. Only articles written after year 2000 and published in English, German, or French were considered.

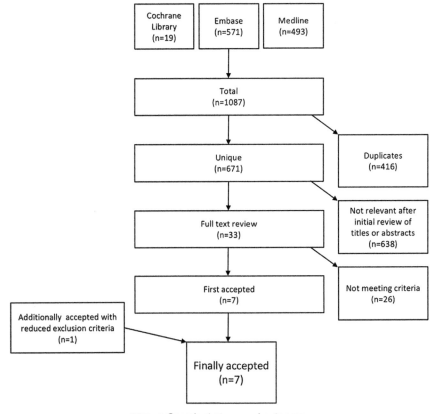

FIG. 4 Search strategy and outcome.

The search generated 671 hits after removing duplicates. An independent, blinded review of titles and abstracts were then conducted by the three authors using the Rayyan online software (Qatar Computing Research Institute, Qatar). This rendered 33 articles of interest. After further review, excluding language other than English, only 7 articles remained. Later, during the review process we found additional relevant articles of which two were finally accepted as primary sources of information. These articles were Schoonhoven et al.[28] written in German with power analysis and Minami et al.[11] with a comparative study between different resection arthroplasties.

There were extremely few studies specifically referring to salvage after a previous DRF. Therefore, we also included a few articles primarily related to DRUJ salvage following unspecified trauma.

QUALITY OF EVIDENCE

Level III: Retrospective comparative studies: 3 (Outcome research)

Level IV: Case series: 6

FINDINGS

There were no prospective comparative clinical studies that fulfilled our inclusion criteria.

We found no clinical studies comparing resection arthroplasties with implant arthroplasties and no comparative studies between different prostheses. Most of the studies were retrospective reviews without preoperative recordings, and for some the follow-up was done online, or by phone.

The most common reason for exclusion of articles was a lack of details regarding the underlying reason for the DRUJ osteoarthritis. Most of the papers included a mixed cohort of patients, and did not discriminate for etiology, for example, between rheumatoid and posttraumatic patients. Also, in some articles, if the indication for surgery was described, the outcome was not detailed accordingly. Other limitations, although not for exclusion, were lack of stratification for factors, like age, sex, working status, number of previous surgeries, preoperative instability, etc. The lack of standard for outcome assessment added further to the difficulties in comparing results for different procedures. Patient-reported outcome measures (PROMs) were occasionally used, with DASH and PRWE being most frequent. Some articles also used Mayo wrist score, however the latter is not validated

Our results are outlined in Table 2, and recommendations based on the literature and our experience is outlined below as well as in Fig. 5.

RECOMMENDATIONS

In patients with an intraarticular displaced distal radius fracture, evidence suggests:

Recommendation	Overall Quality
• Several studies show that prior procedure, and number of previous procedures tends to affect outcome negatively.[10,25,27,30] Therefore, we question a stepwise operative approach to DRUJ arthritis. A treatment philosophy that always starts with a resection arthroplasty that later can be saved with an implant arthroplasty, if needed, is therefore not used.	⊕⊕⊕○ MODERATE
• There are no clinical studies that compare a resection arthroplasty with an implant arthroplasty, but biomechanical studies have shown that implant arthroplasties are superior in restoring DRUJ kinematics, compared to ablative procedures.[6,7,38]	NOT APPLICABLE
• Bowers procedure, or matched resection, are likely better reconstructive options (lower VAS for pain, better grip strength)[11,17] than Darrach's procedure, provided that the DRUJ is stable preoperatively and that there is zero, or negative ulnar variance.	⊕⊕○○ LOW
• Darrach's procedure should be limited to older patients with low-demand on grip strength and is rarely indicated after DRFs. When used, the ulnar head excision should be kept to a minimum.	⊕⊕⊕○ MODERATE
• The optimal treatment option for a younger patient with higher demands for loading is difficult to foresee. The risk of failure for resection arthroplasties is high. As S-K enables better grip strength it is likely to be the best choice for this group.[11] In the case that the DRUJ is stable and the joint looks suitable, a partial- or total UHP could be considered as a primary solution.	⊕⊕○○ LOW
• If implants are not available, or if the joint is substantially unstable, a S-K procedure is a better choice, especially in cases with positive ulnar variance. In case of failure,	⊕⊕○○ LOW

salvage is more demanding, requiring a total DRUJ implant or possibly the Fernandez salvage technique.

- The choice of joint replacement is mainly dependent on the constraining soft tissue conditions and to some extent on the sigmoid notch morphology. Careful preoperative evaluation of the quality of soft tissue constraints is thus of utmost importance especially in cases of posttraumatic DRUJ arthritis were there may be a concomitant ligament injury. ⊕⊕⊕○ MODERATE

- When full stability cannot be achieved during total-UHP arthroplasty the implant can be left in place combined with a stricter rehabilitation protocol. The rationale for this approach is the fact that instability is not always symptomatic. If instability persists over time, and causes impairment there are three options; (i) simply remove the implant and hope that the Darrach will ⊕⊕○○ LOW

lead to acceptable symptoms, (ii) try to stabilize it with a tendon sling, that is, the Brachioradialis as described by Gupta et al.,[39] (iii) revise to a total DRUJ prosthesis.

- Total DRUJ implant can be used as a last resort option for the more complicated cases—where DRUJ arthritis is combined with gross instability—or as a primary solution in multioperated patients. ⊕○○○ VERY LOW

- Last-resort options such as one-bone forearm, radioulnar fusion, wide resection, and achilles tendon allograft interposition have poorly documented outcomes but they could be considered in extreme situations. ⊕○○○ VERY LOW

- For younger patients, new techniques using perichondrium allografts, interposition of biodegradable spacers, and reconstruction with meniscal cartilage have shown good results in small case series.[40–42] ⊕○○○ VERY LOW

TABLE 2

Summary of included papers in the review related to resection arthroplasties and implant arthroplasty.

Publication	Study design level of evidence	Number of cases	Technique	Follow up	Mean age	Pain	Grip strength	Pronation/supination	Outcome	COMPLICATIONS Reoperations	Other
Verhiel et al. (2019)[22]	Retrospective comparative study (III)	PT 85 S-K 28 (18 to F-U) D 57 (34 to F-U)	S-K or Darrach	8.4Y survey	S-K 48Y D 53Y	VAS (scale 0–10) S-K 2.5 D 2.5			PROMIS UE: S-K 39 D 39	Reop: S-K 39% D 16% S-K 14% screw S-K* 11% heterotopic ossification	Instability of stump: S-K 7% D 14%
George et al. (2004)[17]	Retrospective comparative study (III)	48 DRF S-K: 18 (12 to F-U survey, 9 in clinic) D: 30 (21 to F-U survey, 13 in clinic)	S-K or Darrach	S-K: clinic 2Y S-K: survey 4Y D: clinic 6Y D: survey 4Y	S-K 34Y D 39Y	MMWS: (pain) S-K 20 (Mild) D 19 (Moderate)	S-K postop 103% of CL D postop 82% of CL	Pron: S-K 74° D 80° Sup: S-K 82° D 77°	MMWS: S-K 78 (Fair) D 72 (Fair) DASH: S-K 23 D 23	Reop: S-K 17% D 0%	S-K 8 D 9
Carter and Stuart (2000)[18]	Retrospective case series (IV)	41 DRF (37 to F-U)	S-K	2.7Y	55Y	None 32% Mild 41% Moderate 16% Severe 11%	Postop: 62% of CL	Pron: 82° Sup: 89°	MMWS: 10 Excellent 12 Good 6 Fair 9 Poor	No reported reop.	25 with symptoms
Zimmermann et al. (2003)[19]	Retrospective case series (IV)	105 PT (81 DRF)	Modified S-K	8Y	58Y	VAS (scale 0–100) 16	Preop: 38% of CL Postop: 55% of CL	Pron: 55%–78% of CL Sup: 50%–85% of CL	DASH 28 (43 cases)	Reop: 6% screw 2% heterotopic ossification 74% ulnar convergence	
Mansat et al. (2010)[44]	Retrospective case series (IV)	20 DRF	Modified Darrach	11Y	45Y	VAS (scale 0–4) Preop: 2.2 Postop: 0.5	Postop: 81% of CL	Pron: 66°–84° Sup: 37°–80°	Satisfaction rate 95% at 11Y (6.75–18.6)	No reported reop.	1 CRPS
Grawe et al. (2012)[14]	Retrospective case series (IV)	(98 PT) 27 to F-U, 15 in clinic	Darrach	13Y	53Y	VAS (scale 0–4) Rest 0.1 Loading 0.6		Pron: 101% of CL Sup: 91% of CL	QDASH: 17 PRWE: 14	Reop: 22%	

Continued

TABLE 2
Summary of included papers in the review related to resection arthroplasties and implant arthroplasty—cont'd

Publication	Study design level of evidence	Number of cases	Technique	Follow up	Mean age	Pain	Grip strength	Pronation/ supination	Outcome	COMPLICATIONS Reoperations	Other
Minami et al. (2005)[11]	Retrospective comparative study (III)	61 (23 PT): D:20 (15 PT) S-K:25 (5 PT) HIT:16 (3 PT)	S-K or Darrach or HIT	10Y	60Y	None: D 40% S-K 60% HIT 37,5% Slight: D 20% S-K 20% HIT 50% Moderate: D 25% S-K 20% HIT 12,5% Severe: D 15% S-K 0% HIT 0%	S-K preop 58% of CL postop 70% of CL* D preop 57% of CL postop 43% of CL HIT preop 45% of CL postop 80% of CL*	Pron: S-K 64–80°* D 50–70°* HIT 65–83°* Sup: S-K 69–86°* D 52–71°* HIT 64–86°*		No reported reop.	
van Schoonhoven et al. (2003)[45]	Retrospective case series (IV)	PT 51 (36 to F-U)	HIT	2.8Y	53Y	VAS (scale 1–10) Preop: 7.8 Postop: 3.9*	Preop: 40% of CL Postop: 64% of CL*	Pron: 74–76° ns Sup: 54–69°*	DASH: 35	Reop: 39%	Radioulnar impingement 21
Sabo et al. (2014)[30]	Retrospective case series (IV)	79 (PT 32) F-U 47 (in clinic 21)	Ulnar head arthroplasty (54 Herbert, 6 First choice, 21 unknown)	7Y	50Y		Postop: 67% of CL	Pron: 80° Sup: 53°	PRWE 56 in PT PEM 42 in PT WWS 74 in PT EQ5D 9 in PT	Reop: 41% 9% implant revision 32% other non-implant Implant survival: 5Y and 15Y both 90%	

PT, posttraumatic; PROMIS UE, Patient-Reported Outcomes Measurement Information System Upper Extremity; F–U, follow up; MMWS, Modified Mayo Wrist Score; VAS, visual analog scale; DRF, distal radius fracture; DASH, disability of the arm, shoulder and hand; QDASH, quick DASH; PRWE, Patient-Rated Wrist Evaluation (scale 0–100); PEM, patient evaluation measure (scale 11–77); WWS, Wrightington wrist score (0–130); EQ5D, queries patient mobility, self-care, pain, activities, anxiety/depression (scale 5–15); HIT, hemiresection-interposition arthroplasty; ns, not statistically significant change.
*Statistically significant difference P < .05.

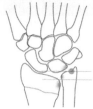

1. Age - loading/demand?
2. Malunion?
3. Previous surgery?
4. Stable DRUJ - intact TFCC?
5. Ulnar variance?

		Age *and/or* loading/demand		
		Young age *and/or* High demand	Middle age *and/or* Middle demand	Old age *and/or* Low demand
OA (early)	Conservative	Splints, NSAID, Cortison	Splints, NSAID, Cortison	Splints, NSAID, Cortison
OA - stable	Resection arthroplasty	S-K	Bowers	Bowers or Darrach
	Implant arthroplasty	Partial UHP	Partial- or total UHP	Partial- or total UHP
OA-unstable	Resection arthroplasty	S-K	S-K	Bowers or Darrach
	Implant arthroplasty	x	Total DRUJ arthroplasty	Total DRUJ arthroplasty

FIG. 5 Schematic algorithm to outline choice of procedure that may be proposed as salvage in radio-ulnar osteoarthritis after distal radius fractures. Recommendations are primarily based on experts' opinion, rather than scientific evidence after our literature search. Procedures, depending on age and demand, as well as morphological features. X—indicates that implant arthroplasty in young patients that will use the arm for heavy loading is highly controversial, and is not recommended.

Panel 2: Author's Preferred Treatment

The radiographs (Fig. 1C and D) demonstrated a positive ulnar variance with ulnocarpal impaction. To further visualize geometry and joint congruity a CT scan was made which revealed widespread OA in the volar part of the DRUJ, and a sigmoid notch which had a Tolat C-shape morphology[43] (Fig. 6)

This type of sigmoid notch, which provides some osseous stability, and thus is suitable for arthroplasty. Flat face or ski slope morphology are less suitable for ulnar head replacement arthroplasty. In such cases, the sigmoid notch may need to be deepened and contoured with a burr at surgery. The sigmoid notch also displayed a reversed angulation in the coronal plane, with OA in the proximal portion (Fig. 7A) and a depression of about 3/4 of the lunate fossa of the radius (Fig. 7B)

Combined, these findings indicated that; (i) the remaining radial malalignment did not obstruct any procedure, and that a corrective osteotomy would seemingly make little difference, (ii) that the morphology of the sigmoid notch would make an ulnar shortening less likely to be successful while contouring might make it able to retain a partial- or total UHP, (iii) that the stability of the soft tissues would probably allow a total UHP.

Other factors that were considered was that the patient's osteoporosis constituted a risk in regards to a total DRUJ implant which would also obstruct a future total wrist arthroplasty which could be warranted by the radiocarpal injury.

A Bowers procedure was also discussed, although with a positive ulnar variance and the patient's functional demands, this would be a risk for ulnocarpal impaction and dynamic radio-ulnar and ulnocarpal impingement.

The patient was operated on with an ulnar head arthroplasty (Fig. 8).

Outcomes are summarized in Table 1. Note how lifting-strength in all positions return to levels near to what is seen in the contralateral arm, indicating that the arthritic pain from the joint was no longer present and that its stability was adequate.

Continued

Panel 2: Author's Preferred Treatment—cont'd

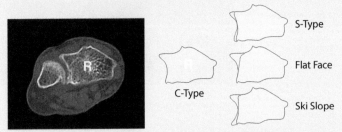

FIG. 6 Preop CT, and sagittal plane schematic drawings of the radius (*R*), with emphasis of the sigmoid notch, combined with different morphology *(red dotted lines)* according to Tolat et al.[43]

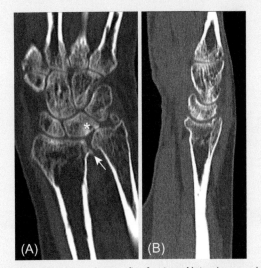

FIG. 7 CT images 1 year after fracture. Note ulnocarpal impaction (*) and a sigmoid notch, in the coronal plane, less suitable for ulnar shortening, due to reversed angulation and arthritic changes in the proximal portion of the sigmoid notch *(arrow)*.

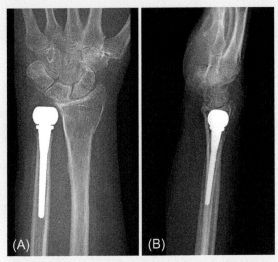

FIG. 8 Postoperative X-rays after total UHP placement.

Panel 3: Pearls and Pitfalls Resection Arthroplasty

PEARLS

- Resections arthroplasties, S-K and Darrach procedures, should always be supplemented with a tenodesis or other stabilizing soft tissue procedure.
- Always, keep ulnar resections limited to keep as much as possible of the ulnar shaft.

PITFALLS

- The superficial branch of the ulnar nerve is at great risk of injury during salvage procedures for the DRUJ.
- Resection arthroplasties should primarily be used in older patients, or patients with low demand for loading.

PEARLS AND PITFALLS IMPLANT ARTHROPLASTY
Pearls

- Meticulous soft tissue evaluation is needed for implant arthroplasties except for the total DRUJ procedure.

- Contouring of the sigmoid notch could increase the osseous constraint of a total UHP.
- For the total DRUJ implant, exact alignment of the radial component is of paramount importance. Meticulous screw length measurement is another crucial step, they should barely grip the radial cortex. Preoperative templating provides considerable help.

Pitfalls

- Remaining malalignment after the DRF may lead to failure of implant arthroplasties.
- Gross instability—or persistent instability after multiple procedures—are considered relative contraindications to UHP
- Osteoporosis is a relative contraindication for the total DRUJ procedure because of risk of periprosthetic fracture

---

CONCLUSION

Reconstruction of the DRUJ remains one of the most challenging in hand surgery, especially after severe wrist injuries, such as after DRFs. Not only is the biomechanics of this loaded joint complex, injuries to the cartilage are commonly accompanied by ligamentous injuries, and malalignment of the bone structures. As the evidence for superior performance of any salvage procedure is weak, it is reasonable to adopt a strategy where the least invasive, and least expensive procedures are considered first. Recent advances in arthroplasty procedures and customized rehabilitation protocols however hold great promise for this group of patients.

REFERENCES

1. Tanabe K, Nakajima T, Sogo E, Denno K, Horiki M, Nakagawa R. Intra-articular fractures of the distal radius evaluated by computed tomography. *J Hand Surg Am.* 2011; 36(11):1798–1803.
2. Nakanishi Y, Omokawa S, Shimizu T, Nakano K, Kira T, Tanaka Y. Intra-articular distal radius fractures involving the distal radioulnar joint (DRUJ): three dimensional computed tomography-based classification. *J Orthop Sci.* 2013; 18(5):788–792.
3. Cooney 3rd WP, Dobyns JH, Linscheid RL. Complications of Colles' fractures. *J Bone Joint Surg Am.* 1980; 62(4): 613–619.
4. Heo YM, Roh JY, Kim SB, et al. Evaluation of the sigmoid notch involvement in the intra-articular distal radius fractures: the efficacy of computed tomography compared with plain X-ray. *Clin Orthop Surg.* 2012; 4(1):83–90.
5. Vitale MA, Brogan DM, Shin AY, Berger RA. Intra-articular fractures of the sigmoid notch of the distal radius: analysis of progression to distal radial ulnar joint arthritis and impact on upper extremity function in surgically treated fractures. *J Wrist Surg.* 2016; 5(1):52–58.
6. Sauerbier M, Hahn ME, Fujita M, et al. Dynamic radioulnar convergence after Darrach operation, soft tissue stabilizing operations of the distal ulna and ulnar head prosthesis implantation—an experimental biomechanical study. *Unfallchirurg.* 2002; 105(8):688–698.
7. Gordon KD, Dunning CE, Johnson JA, King GJ. Kinematics of ulnar head arthroplasty. *J Hand Surg Br.* 2003; 28(6):551–558.
8. Hohenberger GM, Maier MJ, Dolcet C, Weiglein AH, Schwarz A, Matzi V. Sensory nerve supply of the distal radio-ulnar joint with regard to wrist denervation. *J Hand Surg Eur Vol.* 2017; 42(6):586–591.
9. Geissler WB, Fernandez DL, Lamey DM. Distal radioulnar joint injuries associated with fractures of the distal radius. *Clin Orthop Relat Res.* 1996; 327:135–146.
10. Jochen-Frederick H, Pouyan Y, Khosrow BA, et al. Long-term functional outcome and patient satisfaction after ulnar head resection. *J Plast Reconstr Aesthet Surg.* 2016; 69(10):1417–1423.
11. Minami A, Iwasaki N, Ishikawa J, Suenaga N, Yasuda K, Kato H. Treatments of osteoarthritis of the distal radioulnar joint: long-term results of three procedures. *Hand Surg.* 2005; 10(2–3):243–248.
12. af Ekenstam F, Engkvist O, Wadin K. Results from resection of the distal end of the ulna after fractures of the lower end of the radius. *Scand J Plast Reconstr Surg.* 1982; 16(2):177–181.

13. Field J, Majkowski RJ, Leslie IJ. Poor results of Darrach's procedure after wrist injuries. *J Bone Joint Surg Br*. 1993; 75(1):53–57.

14. Grawe B, Heincelman C, Stern P. Functional results of the Darrach procedure: a long-term outcome study. *J Hand Surg Am*. 2012; 37(12):2475–2480 e2471–2472.

15. Bain GI, Pugh DM, MacDermid JC, Roth JH. Matched hemiresection interposition arthroplasty of the distal radioulnar joint. *J Hand Surg Am*. 1995; 20(6):944–950.

16. Watson HK, Manzo RL. Modified arthroplasty of the distal radio-ulnar joint. *J Hand Surg Br*. 2002; 27(4):322–325.

17. George MS, Kiefhaber TR, Stern PJ. The Sauve-Kapandji procedure and the Darrach procedure for distal radio-ulnar joint dysfunction after Colles' fracture. *J Hand Surg Br*. 2004; 29(6):608–613.

18. Carter PB, Stuart PR. The Sauve-Kapandji procedure for post-traumatic disorders of the distal radio-ulnar joint. *J Bone Joint Surg Br*. 2000; 82(7):1013–1018.

19. Zimmermann R, Gschwentner M, Arora R, Harpf C, Gabl M, Pechlaner S. Treatment of distal radioulnar joint disorders with a modified Sauve-Kapandji procedure: long-term outcome with special attention to the DASH questionnaire. *Arch Orthop Trauma Surg*. 2003; 123(6):293–298.

20. Syed AA, Lam WL, Agarwal M, Boome R. Stabilization of the ulna stump after Darrach's procedure at the wrist. *Int Orthop*. 2003; 27(4):235–239.

21. Breen TF, Jupiter JB. Extensor carpi ulnaris and flexor carpi ulnaris tenodesis of the unstable distal ulna. *J Hand Surg Am*. 1989; 14(4):612–617.

22. Verhiel S, Ozkan S, Chen NC, Jupiter JB. Long-term outcomes after extensor carpi ulnaris subsheath reconstruction with extensor retinaculum. *Tech Hand Up Extrem Surg*. 2020; 24(1):2–6.

23. Garcia-Elias M. Eclypse: partial ulnar head replacement for the isolated distal radio-ulnar joint arthrosis. *Tech Hand Up Extrem Surg*. 2007; 11(1):121–128.

24. Adams BD, Gaffey JL. Non-constrained implant arthroplasty for the distal radioulnar joint. *J Hand Surg Eur Vol*. 2017; 42(4):415–421.

25. Kakar S, Swann RP, Perry KI, Wood-Wentz CM, Shin AY, Moran SL. Functional and radiographic outcomes following distal ulna implant arthroplasty. *J Hand Surg Am*. 2012; 37(7):1364–1371.

26. Sauerbier M, Arsalan-Werner A, Enderle E, Vetter M, Vonier D. Ulnar head replacement and related biomechanics. *J Wrist Surg*. 2013; 2(1):27–32.

27. Axelsson P, Sollerman C, Karrholm J. Ulnar head replacement: 21 cases; mean follow-up, 7.5 years. *J Hand Surg Am*. 2015; 40(9):1731–1738.

28. van Schoonhoven J, Muhldorfer-Fodor M, Fernandez DL, Herbert TJ. Salvage of failed resection arthroplasties of the distal radioulnar joint using an ulnar head prosthesis: long-term results. *J Hand Surg Am*. 2012; 37(7):1372–1380.

29. Warwick D, Shyamalan G, Balabanidou E. Indications and early to mid-term results of ulnar head replacement. *Ann R Coll Surg Engl*. 2013; 95(6):427–432.

30. Sabo MT, Talwalkar S, Hayton M, Watts A, Trail IA, Stanley JK. Intermediate outcomes of ulnar head arthroplasty. *J Hand Surg Am*. 2014; 39(12):2405–2411 e2401.

31. Kakar S, Fox T, Wagner E, Berger R. Linked distal radioulnar joint arthroplasty: an analysis of the APTIS prosthesis. *J Hand Surg Eur Vol*. 2014; 39(7):739–744.

32. Herbert TJ, van Schoonhoven J. Ulnar head replacement. *Tech Hand Up Extrem Surg*. 2007; 11(1):98–108.

33. Calcagni M, Giesen T. Distal radioulnar joint arthroplasty with implants: a systematic review. *EFORT Open Rev*. 2016; 1(5):191–196.

34. Reissner L, Bottger K, Klein HJ, Calcagni M, Giesen T. Midterm results of semiconstrained distal radioulnar joint arthroplasty and analysis of complications. *J Wrist Surg*. 2016; 5(4):290–296.

35. Rampazzo A, Gharb BB, Brock G, Scheker LR. Functional outcomes of the Aptis-Scheker distal radioulnar joint replacement in patients under 40 years old. *J Hand Surg Am*. 2015; 40(7):1397–1403 e1393.

36. Moulton LS, Giddins GEB. Distal radio-ulnar implant arthroplasty: a systematic review. *J Hand Surg Eur Vol*. 2017; 42(8):827–838.

37. Bellevue KD, Thayer MK, Pouliot M, Huang JI, Hanel DP. Complications of semiconstrained distal radioulnar joint arthroplasty. *J Hand Surg Am*. 2018; 43(6):566 e561–566, e569.

38. Douglas KC, Parks BG, Tsai MA, Meals CG, Means Jr. KR. The biomechanical stability of salvage procedures for distal radioulnar joint arthritis. *J Hand Surg Am*. 2014; 39 (7):1274–1279.

39. Burke CS, Zoeller KA, Waddell SW, Nyland JA, Voor MJ, Gupta A. Assessment of distal radioulnar joint stability after reconstruction with the brachioradialis wrap. *Hand (N Y)*. 2018; 13(4):455–460.

40. Vedung T, Vinnars B. Resurfacing the distal radioulnar joint with rib perichondrium—a novel method. *J Wrist Surg*. 2014; 3(3):206–210.

41. Nilsson K, Farnebo S. Artelon spacer for post-traumatic distal radioulnar joint post-traumatic osteoarthritis: 10 years follow-up in five patients. *J Hand Surg Eur Vol*. 2020; :1753193420924261.

42. Clark NJ, Munaretto N, Elhassan BT, Kakar S. Ulnar head replacement and sigmoid notch resurfacing arthroplasty with minimum 12-month follow-up. *J Hand Surg Eur Vol*. 2019; 44(9):957–962.

43. Tolat AR, Stanley JK, Trail IA. A cadaveric study of the anatomy and stability of the distal radioulnar joint in the coronal and transverse planes. *J Hand Surg Br*. 1996; 21(5):587–594.

44. Mansat P, Ayel JE, Bonnevialle N, Rongières M, Mansat M, Bonnevialle N, Rongières M, Mansat M, Bonnevialle P. Long-term outcome of distal ulna resection—stabilisation procedures in post-traumatic radio-ulnar joint disorders. *Orthop Traumatol Surg Res*. 2010; 96:216–221.

45. van Schoonhoven J, Kall S, Schober F, Pommersberger KJ, Lanz U. Die hemiresektions-interpositionsarthroplastik als Rettungsoperation bei arthrose des distalen radioulnargelenkes. *Handchir Mikrochir Plast Chir*. 2003; 35:175–180.

CHAPTER 37

Posttraumatic Radiocarpal Arthritis

MICHEL E.H. BOECKSTYNS[a,b] • PER FREDRIKSON[c] • PETER AXELSSON[c]

[a]Department of Orthopedic Surgery, Section of Hand Surgery, Herlev-Gentofte Hospital, Hellerup, Denmark, [b]Capio Private Hospital, Hellerup, Denmark, [c]Department of Hand Surgery, Institute of Clinical Sciences, Sahlgrenska Academy, University of Gothenburg, Gothenburg, Sweden

KEY POINTS

- Before embarking for salvage procedures, conservative treatment and corrective osteotomy should have been considered.
- If these measures are inapplicable or fail, partial or extensive wrist denervation should be considered.
- Partial or total wrist (TW)[1] arthrodesis or arthroplasty are the next options to be considered, arthroplasties being more suited for the low-demand/elderly patients.
- If the midcarpal joint is intact, a radioscapholunate (RSL) arthrodesis is another option. In low-demand patients, hemi-arthroplasty might be an alternative.
- In patients who request a final procedure, or in the case of panarthritis, TW arthrodesis (or as an alternative in the elderly/low-demand patient: TW arthroplasty) is preferred.

Panel 1: Case Scenario

A 26-year-old construction worker sustained an intraarticular distal radial fracture (DRF) in his dominant right hand side. The fracture was conservatively treated and healed with a step-off in the radial joint surface. Some pain remained but this was tolerable and he returned to his previous employment.

Thirteen years later, he complained of increasing wrist pain and episodes of numbness in his radial sided fingers. After carpal tunnel decompression and resection of the terminal posterior interosseous nerve, the symptoms radiating to the fingers disappeared. However, his wrist pain persisted despite a change of profession, use of splints, analgesics, and intraarticular steroid injections. Radiographs revealed moderate osteoarthritis in the radiocarpal joint including the lunate fossa (Fig. 1). How would you counsel him?

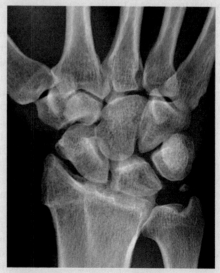

FIG. 1 Radiocarpal osteoarthritis 13 years after a distal radial fracture. Preserved midcarpal joint.

IMPORTANCE OF THE PROBLEM

Wrist degeneration after intraarticular DRFs is caused either by a direct blow to the cartilage, or joint surface disruption with step-offs and gaps. Joint degeneration can also develop as a result of extra-articular malunited fractures with altered angulations. Concurrent ligament injuries, if present, contribute to carpal incongruence and altered pressure areas.

In younger, nonosteoporotic patients, the prevalence of OA following DRFs has been reported as high as 32%–50%[2-4] and frequently causes impairment.[5] Ultimately the condition may end in a partial or TW arthrodesis and sometimes in inability for the patient to return to his or her habitual occupation.[6-9] In elderly, low-demand patients posttraumatic wrist arthritis is better tolerated.[10]

MAIN QUESTION

Which procedures can we offer to a patient with a painful osteoarthritic wrist after a DRF and which outcomes can we expect?

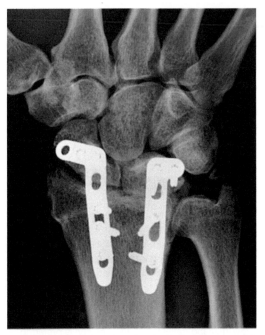

FIG. 2 Radioscapholunate arthrodesis. In this case, plates and screws were used for fixation and no distal scaphoidectomy was performed.

CURRENT OPINION

Conservative treatment is the first action to be taken in order to relieve the symptoms of painful posttraumatic OA. This includes nonsteroid antiinflammatory drugs, analgesics, cortisone injections, and splinting. There is time to carefully choose the right surgical option since spontaneous improvement of symptoms may occur as time goes by and the wrist stiffens. Some ligament injuries can also stabilize by time and, furthermore, proprioceptive training may reduce symptoms. However, even though splints and orthoses usually work well, they cannot always be used during work and are seldom a long-term solution. If severe symptoms persist, surgical treatment is indicated.

Wrist denervation could be the first surgical move before embarking for salvage procedures. RSL arthrodesis is an option if the midcarpal joint is preserved (Fig. 2). TW arthrodesis is indicated in young patients who want a final solution, or as a salvage procedure in case of RSL failure (Fig. 3). Prosthetic TW replacement is an alternative to TW arthrodesis especially in elderly, low-demand patients (Fig. 4). In recent years, hemi-arthroplasty[11-17] and interpositional pyrocarbon arthroplasty[18] have been proposed as alternatives.

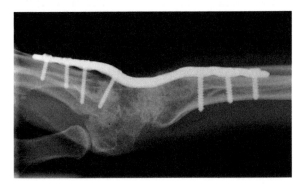

FIG. 3 Total wrist arthrodesis

Other salvage procedures for the wrist, including four corner arthrodesis and proximal row carpectomy, are less common options after DRF since a prerequisite for these procedures is an intact lunate facet of the radius. However, these procedures might be advised if the lunate facet is intact, or has been properly restored, while a concurrent scapholunate injury has caused a carpal collapse and subsequent OA.

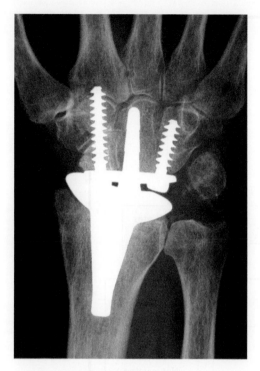

FIG. 4 Total wrist arthroplasty.

Prosthetic replacement of the wrist may offer reduction of pain, preserved range of motion, and improved function but the long-term durability in different subgroups of patients is not well established. Although by many considered a panacea, TW arthrodesis is not a guarantee for freedom of pain and return to work.[6–9]

FINDING THE EVIDENCE

Search Strategy

Articles were selected through searches made in Cochrane, Embase, and Medline databases (Fig. 5). The searches were based on the following terms: wrist, radiocarpal joint, osteoarthritis, arthroplasty, hemiarthroplasty, replacement, implant, denervation, styloidectomy, carpectomy, fusion, arthrodesis, salvage. Only articles written in English, German, or French were considered. Anatomical and cadaver studies were excluded as well as articles published before the year of 2000 in order to avoid obsolete methods and implants. Cohorts with less than 10 cases and (review) articles without original data were excluded. Series that also

included rheumatoid arthritis or Kienböck's disease were also excluded if the DRFs could not be assessed separately. A total of 2831 articles were identified (Cochrane $n = 120$, Embase $n = 1370$, and Medline $n = 1858$). After deleting duplicates ($n = 973$), 1858 articles were accepted for further review by using Rayyan® online software. The articles were reviewed independently and blindly by three reviewers. Two hundred and nine abstracts rendered interest by at least one of the three reviewers. After joined discussion, 37 abstracts were accepted for full-text review. A considerable amount of articles were excluded because of mixed patient cohorts, without specification of the data for DRFs. Finally, only four articles were found to meet inclusion and exclusion criteria.[19–22] One more article dealt specifically with wrist arthritis after DRF.[23] It was a review article without original data but made reference to a previous publication with relevant data. We decided to include that publication instead.[24] By further reducing the restrictions and accepting articles that included posttraumatic OA in general and not solely on the basis of DRF, eight additional articles were selected.[14,25–31]

QUALITY OF EVIDENCE

All selected articles had methodical flaws, including low number of patients and low quality of evidence (Tables 1–4). Generally, preoperative patient-reported outcome measures (PROMs) were missing. Reported postoperative PROMs were not easily comparable between studies.

FINDINGS

The principal findings are summarized in Tables 1–4. Clinically relevant pain reduction seems to be obtainable after denervation in about two thirds of patients with posttraumatic wrist degeneration. Extensive denervation yields better results than partial denervation but the mean disability of the arm, shoulder, and hand (DASH) questionnaire scores after partial denervation still indicate moderate disability.[22,30] It is to be noted that the partial denervation in the series of Radu et al. was not merely a resection of the terminal posterior and anterior interosseous nerves but also included branches of the superficial radial nerve to the wrist joint, branches of the radial antebrachial cutaneous nerve, divisions of the palmar branch of the median nerve, divisions of the dorsal branch of the ulnar nerve,

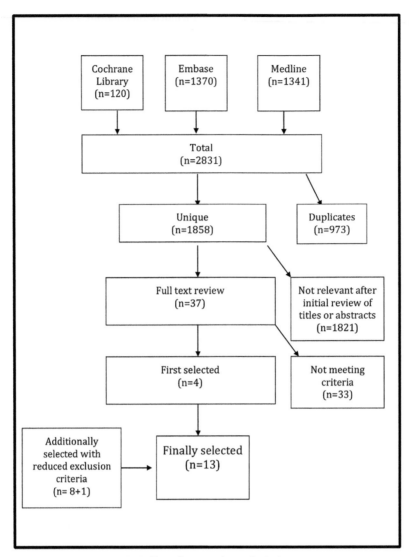

FIG. 5 Flow diagram of search strategy.

and branches of the posterior antebrachial cutaneous nerve. The extensive denervation furthermore included the perforant branches of the ulnar nerve. Seventy-six percent of the patients with extensive (complete) denervation reported pain relief in contrast to 57% of the partially denervated.[30]

RSL arthrodesis has the advantage over TW arthrodesis of preserving some wrist motion. Mean range of motion is better if the distal scaphoid is resected.[20,21,29] Some series indicate that mid-carpal (MC) OA develops more frequently if no distal scaphoidectomy is performed,[20,24] while one series, not resecting the distal scaphoid, did not find MC OA at all[32] and two series found that distal scaphoidectomy did not influence the development of OA.[27,29] It seems that resecting the distal scaphoid also reduces the risk of nonunion.[27,29] Sixty-seven to eighty percent obtained clinical relevant pain reduction.[20,24,27] Residual pain on activity was reported as 2–4.5 on a visual analogue scale (VAS).[21,29,32] The scores of the DASH questionnaire or its short version (QuickDASH) at follow-up indicated slight disability[21,32] or moderate disability[27,29] but with considerable ranges up to severe disability in some cases.

TABLE 1
Summary of Findings Related to Denervation Procedures.

Publication	Study Design	Number of Cases	Technique	Follow-Up	Pain	PROM
Schweizer et al. (2006)[14]	Retrospective	71 (11 DRF, no RA)	Extensive (complete)	9.6 (1–23) years	35 None or little 20 Moderate 15 Considerable or severe	DASH-score 33 for DRF
Radu et al. (2010)[22]	Retrospective	70 (43 to f.u., 30 hereof PT)	29 Extensive, 14 partial	51 (18–97) months	63%–64% PT had pain reduction. Better in extensive denervation	DASH-score 38–46 for PT

DASH, disabilities of arm, shoulder and hand questionnaire; *DRF*, distal radial fracture; *f.u.*, follow-up; *PT*, posttraumatic; *RA*, rheumatoid arthritis.

TW arthrodesis was reported to yield good functional outcomes with slight disability in most patients but up to 80% still had some pain, 18% having severe pain.[25]

Patients with TW arthroplasty mostly had functional ranges of motion, although some wrists were very rigid.[26,28] (Quick)DASH-scores indicated slight to moderate disability. Pain scores on VAS were generally low but some patients indicated severe pain.[26] Implant survival was more than 90% at 7–8 years.

Most papers reporting on hemi-arthroplasty did not qualify to our selection because they included diagnoses not related to DRF or acute DRFs. This was also the case of pyrocarbon interpositional arthroplasty. Only one paper reported on reconstruction after posttraumatic wrist arthritis in general.[14] This particular series had a substantial failure incidence despite promising early results.

RECOMMENDATIONS

In patients with posttraumatic RSL arthritis, evidence suggests:

Recommendations	Overall Quality
• To consider joint denervation before embarking for more radical, extensive surgeries. It is not clear whether terminal anterior and posterior interosseous nerve resection alone should be preferred to more extensive denervation.	⊕⊕○○ LOW
• To resect the distal scaphoid when performing RSL arthrodesis, in order to	⊕⊕⊕○ MODERATE

achieve greater range of motion and reduce the risk for nonunion.

• To avoid TW arthroplasty in younger, physically active patients because of increased risk for early loosening.	⊕⊕⊕○ MODERATE
• To inform the patient that ROM may not be markedly changed after TW arthroplasty, that the longevity is limited and that later conversion to TW arthrodesis may be needed.	⊕⊕⊕○ MODERATE
• Primary hemi-arthroplasty may be recommended for the elderly low-demand patients with severely comminuted DRF. This could shorten the rehabilitation period and prevent repeated surgeries. However, documentation for its use in reconstruction surgery for posttraumatic OA is very limited and so far not favorable.	⊕⊕○○ LOW
• TW arthrodesis is a final solution but contrary to common opinion it does not guarantee freedom of pain.	⊕⊕⊕○ MODERATE
• RSL arthrodesis requires an intact midcarpal joint. Preoperative evaluation by CT scanning or arthroscopy may reveal osteoarthritic changes not readily visible on standard radiographs (Fig. 7) but patients should be aware that the final decision sometimes has to be made intraoperatively.	⊕⊕⊕○ MODERATE
• To consider the condition of the contralateral wrist and of other joints in the upper extremities as it may influence the choice of procedure. For instance, bilateral TW fusion is not well tolerated in case of multiple joint disease.	⊕○○○ VERY LOW

TABLE 2
Summary of Findings Related to Radioscapholunate Arthrodesis.

Publication	Study Design	Number of Cases	Technique	Follow-Up	Union	Wrist Motion Degrees Mean (Range)	Pain	OA at FU	Outcome
Beyermann and Prommersberger (2000)[24]	Retro	18 DRF	No DS. K-wire fixation	19 (6–66) months	1 Required reoperation	F: 23 (5–40)[a] E: 24 (10–40)[a] R: 9 (0–20) U: 16 (10–25)	VAS score in activity: 3.6 (0–9) VAS score at rest: 0.6 (0–20)	No MC-joint OA	DASH score 26 (3–55)
Degeorge et al. (2019)[19]	Retro	85 PT, 75 at FU	Locking T-plate/ screws/ staplers/K-wires 25 with DS, 50 without DS	9 (1–21) years	24% nonunion (less after DS)	45% had functional mobility[b]	33% had no or slight pain	MC OA in 44% (independent of DS)	QDASH score 31–40 Good in 80% with DS, 40% without DF[b]
Garcia-Elias et al. (2005)[12]	Retro (comparing with literature)	16 (13 DRF)	K-wires. All with DS in own series, no DS in selected literature	34 (12–70) months	All united	F: 36 (16–52) E: 36 (25–50) R: 16 (10–28) U: 29 (5–32) (F better than in literature)	13/16 no or slight pain. 3 occasional pain (better than in literature)	No MC OA after DRF. (1/3 in literature had MC OA)	NA

Study	Type	Patients	Fixation	Follow-up	Nonunions	Range of motion	VAS	MC OA	DASH
Muhldorfer-Fodor et al. (2012)[21]	Retro	61, 35 for f.u. (hereof 32 DRF)	K-wires 20 DS, 15 no DS	23–28 (10–47) months	3 nonunions (all without DS)	F with DS: 25 (25–50) F without DS: 20 (0–45) E with DS: 28 (0–50) E without DS: 28 (0–40) R with DS: 12 (0–25) R without DS: 7 (0–15) U with DS: 17 (5–35) U without DS: 16 (0–30)	VAS score with DS: 4.5 (0–8.5) VAS score without DS: 3.6 (0–8)	6 MC OA with DS 6 MC OA without DS 14 of the initial 61 patients had a TW arthrodesis	DASH score with DS: 43 (12–83) DASH score without DS: 44 (9–81)
Nagy and Büchler (1997)[16]	Retro	15 DRF	Plates and screws, no DS	8 (7–12) years	4 nonunions (2 converted to TW arthrodesis, 1 re-RSL)	F: 18 (6–356) E: 32 (20–55) R: 3 (−25 to 10) U: 25 (5–45)	11 no pain 1 occasional pain 3 considerable pain	3 progressive OA 5 nonprogressive OA	NA
Quadlbauer et al. (2017)[13]	Retro	11 DRF	Locking frame plate. DS in all	63 (30–97) months	No nonunions	F: 63 (30–97)[c] E: 42 (20–60)[c] R: 10 (0–20) U: 25 (20–30)	VAS score 2 (0–5)	No MC OA	DASH score 24 (4–68)

DS, distal scaphoidectomy; *MC*, midcarpal; *OA*, osteoarthritis; *TW*, total wrist; *VAS*, visual analogue scale; *DASH*, disability of the arm, shoulder and hand questionnaire; *QDASH*, QuickDASH = short version of the DASH; *F*, wrist flexion; *E*, wrist extension; *R*, wrist radial deviation; *U*, wrist ulnar deviation; *f.u.*, follow-up; *Retro*, retrospective study.

[a]Clinical relevant decrease as compared to preoperatively. (F + E: 21 degrees).

[b]According to modified Cooney classification.

[c]Improved F + E.

TABLE 3
Summary of Findings Related to Total Wrist Arthrodesis.

Publication	Study Design	Number of Cases	Technique	Follow-Up Mean/Median (Range)	Union	Pain	Outcome
Adey et al. (2005)[17]	Retro	22 PT (13 DRF)	Plate and screws (sparing CMC3-joint)	6 (1.5–15) years	All united	14 with pain, hereof 4 severe	DASH score 25 (4–43)
Steckel et al. (2006)[23]	Retro	22 PT (17 DRF)	Plate and screws	11 (11–19) years (incl 22 RA cases)	3 require re-arthrodesis	15 no pain 7 occasional pain	8 very good[a] 11 good 3 satisfactory 0 bad

PT, posttraumatic; *DRF*, distal radial fracture; *CMC3*, third carpometacarpal; *RA*, rheumatoid arthritis; *DASH*, disability of the arm, shoulder and hand questionnaire; *Retro*, retrospective study.
[a]According to Lohmann/Buck-Gramcko classification.

TABLE 4
Summary of Findings After Total Wrist Arthroplasty.

Publication	Study Design	Number of Cases	Technique	Follow-Up	Mobility Mean (Range)	Pain	Outcome	Implant Survival
Boeckstyns et al. (2013)[18]	Prospective	35 PT (hereof 11 DRF)	Remotion	39 (24–96) months	F: 33 (0–80)[a] E: 34 (0–80)[a] R: 9 (0–25)[a] U: 22 (0–46)[a]	VAS score 2.3 (0–8.2)	QDASH score: 33 (0–77)	92% at 8 years
Froschauer et al. (2019)[20]	Retrospective	21 PT (also 39 RA)	Remotion	7 (3–12) years (incl. RA-cases)	F: 40 (SD 9)[b] E: 35 (SD10)[b] R: 10 (SD 5)[b] U: 30 (SD 10)[b]	VAS score 2 (IQR 1.7)	DASH score: 31 (IQR 1.7)	97% at 7 years

PT, posttraumatic; *DRF*, distal radial fracture; *RA*, rheumatoid arthritis; *DASH*, disability of the arm, shoulder and hand questionnaire; *QDASH*, short version of the DASH; *IQR*, interquartile range; *F*, wrist flexion; *E*, wrist extension; *R*, wrist radial deviation; *U*, wrist ulnar deviation; *Remotion*, Stryker, Kalamazoo, MI, USA.
[a]No clinical relevant change in mobility compared to preoperatively.
[b]Mobility statistically significantly improved compared to preoperatively.

CONCLUSION

Specific documentation of salvage procedures for wrist arthritis after DRF is remarkably scarce and the methodology of the studies identified by our search is generally poor. It seems reasonable to attempt wrist denervation before more invasive surgical procedures. Relevant pain relief is obtained in two thirds of cases. If denervation fails but the midcarpal joint is in good condition, the next step could be to perform an RSL arthrodesis, which reduces wrist pain effectively in most cases but carries a risk of up to 25% of nonunion, especially if the distal scaphoid is not resected. Nonunion may eventually require TW arthrodesis. TW arthrodesis is always a possible solution if other procedures fail but freedom of pain is not guaranteed. TW arthroplasty is an alternative in elderly and low-demand patients or in patients with multiple joint involvement in the upper extremities. However, the durability of TW arthroplasty is not well-documented in different subgroups as for age or physical load.

Panel 2: Author's Preferred Treatment

We propose the treatment algorithm shown in Fig. 6. Following our algorithm for the patient presented in the case scenario, we performed an RSL arthrodesis with plate fixation and bone grafting from the iliac crest, without distal scaphoidectomy (Fig. 2). Union between the radius and the scaphoid was delayed but was achieved about one year after surgery (Fig. 7). Due to continuous pain and tenderness on the radial aspect of the wrist, the hardware was removed 2.5 years after the arthrodesis (Fig. 8) and pain improved to some extent.

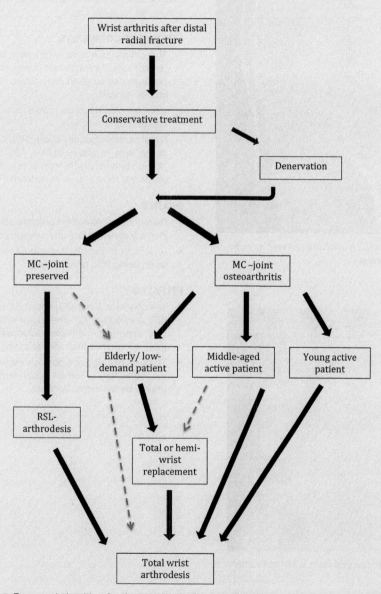

FIG. 6 Proposed algorithm for the treatment of wrist osteoarthritis after distal radial fractures.

Continued

Panel 2: Author's Preferred Treatment—cont'd

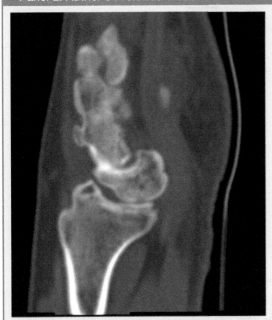

FIG. 7 CT-scan showing midcarpal as well as radio-carpal joint degeneration.

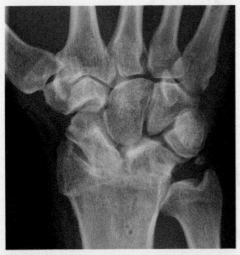

FIG. 8 Healed radioscapholunate arthrodesis after hardware removal.

The patient was again referred for disabling pain centrally located in the carpal region. Pain was aggravated upon deviating the hand and there is tenderness over the midcarpal joint. Grip strength was 52 kg, wrist extension 30 degrees and wrist flexion 15 degrees. An MRI scan showed degeneration in the midcarpal joint. The patient was then scheduled for a TW fusion.

HINDSIGHT COMMENTS

- The course of events might have been different if an (arthroscopic) intraarticular corrective osteotomy had been performed at an early stage, before osteoarthritis had developed.
- Complete denervation could have been attempted before RSL arthrodesis.
- Distal scaphoidectomy during RSL arthrodesis, or even at the time of plate removal, had been preferable to obtain a better range of motion, to reduce the risk of non-union and maybe even of midcarpal osteoarthritis.

PEARLS

- Denervation, preferably complete, should be considered in many cases before any salvage procedure.
- Resection of the distal scaphoid should be performed when doing RSL arthrodesis.

PITFALLS

- The condition of the MC joint is crucial when considering RSL arthrodesis. CT-imaging or arthroscopy may provide important, additional information and is usually more informative than MRI scanning.
- The patient's age and physical requirements as well as the condition of other upper-extremity joints must always be taken into account.

REFERENCES

1. Moher D, Cook DJ, Eastwood S, Olkin I, Rennie D, Stroup DF. Improving the quality of reports of meta-analyses of randomised controlled trials: the QUOROM statement. Quality of reporting of meta-analyses. *Lancet.* 1999;354(9193):1896–1900.
2. Forward DP, Davis TR, Sithole JS. Do young patients with malunited fractures of the distal radius inevitably develop symptomatic post-traumatic osteoarthritis? *J Bone Joint Surg Br.* 2008;90(5):629–637.
3. Lameijer CM, Ten Duis HJ, Dusseldorp IV, Dijkstra PU, van der Sluis CK. Prevalence of posttraumatic arthritis and the association with outcome measures following distal radius fractures in non-osteoporotic patients: a systematic review. *Arch Orthop Trauma Surg.* 2017;137(11):1499–1513.
4. Lameijer CM, Ten Duis HJ, Vroling D, Hartlief MT, El Moumni M, van der Sluis CK. Prevalence of posttraumatic arthritis following distal radius fractures in non-osteoporotic patients and the association with radiological measurements, clinician and patient-reported outcomes. *Arch Orthop Trauma Surg.* 2018;138(12):1699–1712.
5. Knirk JL, Jupiter JB. Intra-articular fractures of the distal end of the radius in young adults. *J Bone Joint Surg Am.* 1986;68(5):647–659.
6. De Smet L, Truyen J. Arthrodesis of the wrist for osteoarthritis: outcome with a minimum follow-up of 4 years. *J Hand Surg Am.* 2003;28(6):575–577.
7. Reigstad O, Holm-Glad T, Korslund J, Grimsgaard C, Thorkildsen R, Rokkum M. High re-operation and complication rates 11 years after arthrodesis of the wrist for non-inflammatory arthritis. *Bone Joint J Am.* 2019;101-B(7):852–859.
8. Sauerbier M, Kluge S, Bickert B, Germann G. Subjective and objective outcomes after total wrist arthrodesis in patients with radiocarpal arthrosis or Kienbock's disease. *Chir Main.* 2000;19(4):223–231.
9. Weiss AC, Wiedeman Jr. G, Quenzer D, Hanington KR, Hastings 2nd H, Strickland JW. Upper extremity function after wrist arthrodesis. *J Hand Surg Am.* 1995;20(5):813–817.
10. Nelson GN, Stepan JG, Osei DA, Calfee RP. The impact of patient activity level on wrist disability after distal radius malunion in older adults. *J Orthop Trauma.* 2015;29(4):195–200.
11. Adams BD. Surgical management of the arthritic wrist. *Instr Course Lect.* 2004;53:41–45.
12. Adams BD. Wrist arthroplasty: partial and total. *Hand Clin.* 2013;29(1):79–89.
13. Herzberg G, Burnier M, Marc A, Izem Y. Primary wrist hemiarthroplasty for irreparable distal radius fracture in the independent elderly. *J Wrist Surg.* 2015;4(3):156–163.
14. Huish Jr. EG, Lum Z, Bamberger HB, Trzeciak MA. Failure of Wrist Hemiarthroplasty. *Hand.* 2017;12(4):369–375.
15. Ichihara S, Diaz JJ, Peterson B, Facca S, Bodin F, Liverneaux P. Distal radius isoelastic resurfacing prosthesis: a preliminary report. *J Wrist Surg.* 2015;4(3):150–155.
16. Roux JL. Replacement and resurfacing prosthesis of the distal radius: a new therapeutic concept. *Chir Main.* 2009;28(1):10–17.

17. Vergnenegre G, Hardy J, Mabit C, Charissoux JL, Marcheix PS. Hemiarthroplasty for complex distal radius fractures in elderly patients. *J Wrist Surg.* 2015;4(3):169–173.
18. Bellemère P, Maes-Clavier C, Loubersac T, Gaisne E, Kerjean Y, Collon S. Pyrocarbon interposition wrist arthroplasty in the treatment of failed wrist procedures. *J Wrist Surg.* 2012;1(1):31–38.
19. Beyermann K, Prommersberger KJ. Simultaneous management of multi-fragment distal radius fractures with palmar and dorsal approach. *Handchir Mikrochir Plast Chir.* 2000;32(6):404–410.
20. Garcia-Elias M, Lluch A, Ferreres A, Papini-Zorli I, Rahimtoola ZO. Treatment of radiocarpal degenerative osteoarthritis by radioscapholunate arthrodesis and distal scaphoidectomy. *J Hand Surg Am.* 2005;30(1):8–15.
21. Quadlbauer S, Leixnering M, Jurkowitsch J, Hausner T, Pezzei C. Volar radioscapholunate arthrodesis and distal scaphoidectomy after malunited distal radius fractures. *J Hand Surg Am.* 2017;42(9):754 e751–754.e758.
22. Schweizer A, von Kanel O, Kammer E, Meuli-Simmen C. Long-term follow-up evaluation of denervation of the wrist. *J Hand Surg Am.* 2006;31(4):559–564.
23. Nagy L. Salvage of post-traumatic arthritis following distal radius fracture. *Hand Clin.* 2005;21(3):489–498.
24. Nagy L, Buchler U. Long-term results of radioscapholunate fusion following fractures of the distal radius. *J Hand Surg Am.* 1997;22(6):705–710.
25. Adey L, Ring D, Jupiter JB. Health status after total wrist arthrodesis for posttraumatic arthritis. *J Hand Surg Am.* 2005;30(4):932–936.
26. Boeckstyns ME, Herzberg G, Sorensen AI, et al. Can total wrist arthroplasty be an option in the treatment of the severely destroyed posttraumatic wrist? *J Wrist Surg.* 2013;2(4):324–329.
27. Degeorge B, Montoya-Faivre D, Dap F, Dautel G, Coulet B, Chammas M. Radioscapholunate fusion for radiocarpal osteoarthritis: prognostic factors of clinical and radiographic outcomes. *J Wrist Surg.* 2019;8(6):456–462.
28. Froschauer SM, Zaussinger M, Hager D, Behawy M, Kwasny O, Duscher D. Re-motion total wrist arthroplasty: 39 non-rheumatoid cases with a mean follow-up of 7 years. *J Hand Surg Eur.* 2019;44(9):946–950.
29. Muhldorfer-Fodor M, Ha HP, Hohendorff B, Low S, Prommersberger KJ, van Schoonhoven J. Results after radioscapholunate arthrodesis with or without resection of the distal scaphoid pole. *J Hand Surg Am.* 2012;37(11):2233–2239.
30. Radu CA, Schachner M, Trankle M, Germann G, Sauerbier M. Functional results after wrist denervation. *Handchir Mikrochir Plast Chir.* 2010;42(5):279–286.
31. Steckel H, Stankovic O, Klinger HM, Baums MH, Schmid A, Schultz W. Current status of wrist arthrodesis. *Z Orthop Grenzgeb.* 2006;144(2):212–217.
32. Beyermann K, Prommersberger KJ, Lanz U. Radioscapholunate fusion following comminuted fractures of the distal radius. *Eur J Trauma.* 2000;26:169–175.

CHAPTER 38

Wrist Contracture After Distal Radius Fractures

MARCO GUIDI[a] • MAURIZIO CALCAGNI[a] • RICCARDO LUCHETTI[b]
[a]Department of Plastic Surgery and Hand Surgery, University Hospital Zurich, Zurich, Switzerland,
[b]Rimini Hand and Upper Limb Surgery and Rehabilitation Center, Rimini, Italy

KEY POINTS

- The origin of a posttraumatic wrist joint stiffness can be either extra-articular, intraarticular, or both.
- Surgical arthrolysis is a viable option that can be performed via open or arthroscopic surgery.
- A poor articular surface may be responsible for failure or recurrence of painful stiffness after arthrolysis
- Arthroscopy of the DRUJ can be challenging.

Panel 1: Case Scenario

- **Case 1:** A 24-year-old male manual worker presented with a painful stiffness of left wrist. He had an extra-articular distal radius fracture (DRF) treated with reduction and above elbow to hand cast with the wrist flexed and pronated. One month later the cast was removed. Rehabilitation was done for 3 months without satisfactory results (Fig. 1A–F): wrist ROM (FE=15 degrees/PS=0 degrees) and pain 8 according with VAS scale 0–10.

- **Case 2:** A 33-year-old male presented with right wrist stiffness after ORIF (volar plate) for an intraarticular DRF. Rehabilitation was done for 4 months but wrist stiffness persisted (Fig. 2A–F).

  How can you come to an evidenced-based decision in the management of these two similar cases?

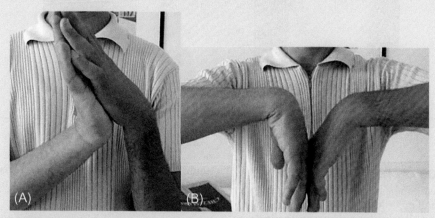

FIG. 1 33-Year-old male presents with painful stiffness in the left wrist after a distal radius fracture treated in a cast. Preoperative clinical function of wrist extension (A), flexion (B), supination (C) and pronation (D) and preoperative radiographic imaging of the wrist (E, F).

Continued

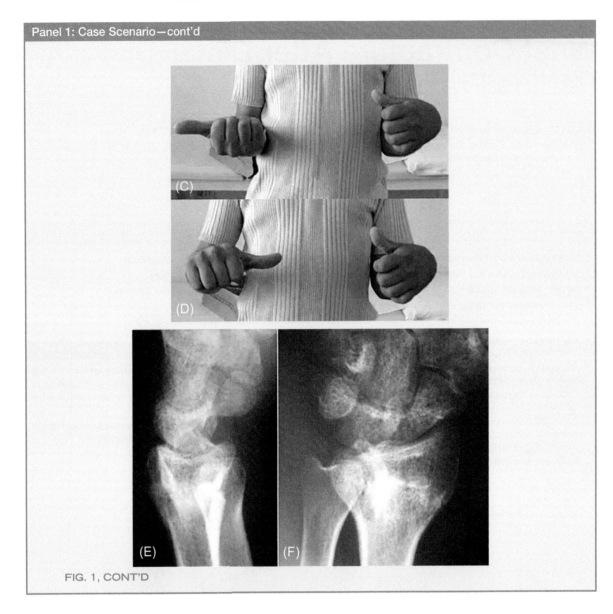

FIG. 1, CONT'D

IMPORTANCE OF THE PROBLEM

Wrist contracture can be a disabling complication after trauma or surgical procedures.[1-4] Intraarticular and capsular injuries as well as prolonged immobilization may cause arthrofibrosis.[3, 4] This could lead to a limited range of motion (ROM), pain, and long-lasting disability.[3, 4] Usually a good rehabilitation program of the wrist is the first treatment. In case the rehabilitation regime fails to increase wrist ROM, wrist manipulation under general anesthesia or peripheral regional blocks may be attempted with a potential risk of ligament or bone avulsions.

MAIN QUESTION

What is the best surgical method for wrist stiffness after distal radius fractures (DRFs) treated by cast or volar plate fixation?

Is the same question valid for stiffness of the DRUJ?

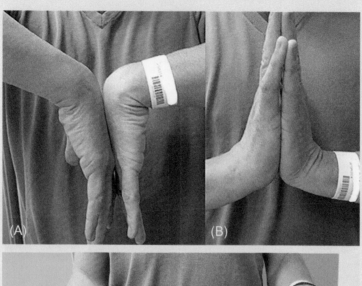

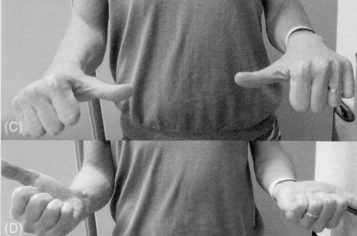

FIG. 2 36-Year-old male with painful stiffness to the right wrist after a distal radius intraarticular fracture treated with palmar plate fixation (A–F) in association with ulnar fracture and ulnar styloid fracture. Clinical function of the wrist flexion (A), extension (B), pronation (C) and supination (D) and preoperative radiographic imaging showing the position of the palmar plate to the distal radius with healing of all fractures (E, F)

Continued

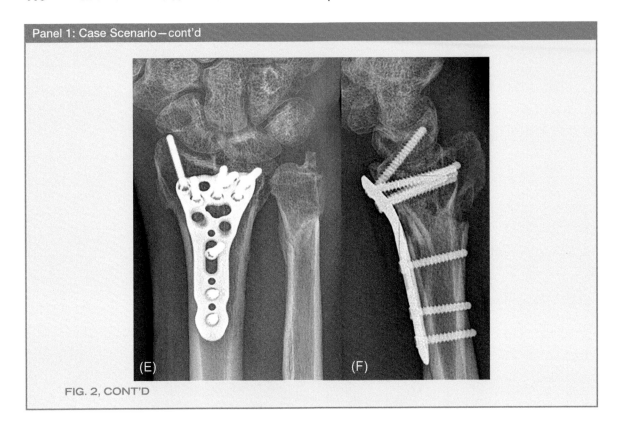

(E)   (F)

FIG. 2, CONT'D

Current Options

Surgical arthrolysis is a viable option that can be performed via open surgery or arthroscopy. Arthrolysis of the radio-carpal (RC) joint can be useful in flexion-extension stiffness, while distal radio ulnar joint (DRUJ) arthrolysis is indicated in cases with limited pronation-supination. The aim of this chapter is to compare the results of open and arthroscopic arthrolysis of the radio-carpal (RC) joint and DRUJ in posttraumatic stiffness of the wrist.

Finding the Evidence

A comprehensive search strategy was created in collaboration with an independent research librarian and was designed to capture all relevant articles relating to wrist arthrolysis. The search strategy was applied to the Pubmed-MEDLINE databases from database inception until 15th January 2020 with the following keywords: "open wrist arthrolysis," "arthroscopic wrist arthrolysis," "posttraumatic wrist stiffness," "arthroscopic wrist capsular release," "DRUJ arthrolysis."

Quality of the Evidence

We followed the graded ranking proposed by Sackett[5] concerning the studies obtained through the literature search. Five levels of degrees were considered from Level I to Level V (Table 1). Each accepted study was evaluated according with the Schünemann[6] and also graded based on the quality of evidence on the Grade Working Group system (Tables 2 and 3).[7]

No randomized controlled trials, systematic reviews, or metaanalysis were found which specifically answered to the initial questions. Overall the studies on wrist arthrolysis were selected for the outcomes of a single technique: open or arthroscopic surgery. Only eight studies of some importance related to the surgical technique of wrist arthrolysis were found. All but one of these studies had an evidence of Level IV (GRADE 3B). The final study was Level V (GRADE 4).

TABLE 1
Level of Evidence.

Level of Evidence	
I	Large randomized controlled trials
II	Small randomized controlled trials
III	Cohort and case-control studies
IV	Case series
V	Expert opinion

TABLE 2
Assigning Grades of Evidence by GRADE Working Group.

Level of Evidence	
1A	Systematic review of randomized controlled trials
1B	Individual randomized controlled trial
2A	Systematic review of cohort studies
2B	Individual cohort study
3A	Systematic review of case-control studies
3B	Individual case-control study
4	Case series
5	Expert opinion without explicit critical appraisal or based on physiology or bench research

TABLE 3
Overall Quality by GRADE Working Group.

Quality	
High	Further research is very unlikely to change our confidence in the estimate of effect
Moderate	Further research is likely to have an important impact on our confidence in the estimate of effect and may change the estimate
Low	Further research is very likely to have an important impact on our confidence in the estimate of effect and is likely to change the estimate
Very low	Any estimate of effect is very uncertain

FINDINGS

Evidence From Level IV–V Studies

In eight included studies, three reported results on open technique (two articles on open DRUJ arthrolysis and one article on open volar wrist (RC) capsulotomy) (Table 4). Five articles studied the results of the arthroscopic arthrolysis (four on RC joint, and one on DRUJ arthrolysis) (Table 5).

Radio-Carpal Joint

Open Volar Arthrolysis. Open arthrolysis is done with a resection of the radio-carpal (RC) volar capsule[8] (Level IV/GRADE 3B). It can be combined with a volar distal radioulnar joint (DRUJ) capsule release if there is lack of supination.[8] Carpal stability is maintained after release, likely secondary to the presence of other extrinsic ligaments that stabilize the carpus to the distal radius and ulna (the remnant of the short radio-lunate (SRL), ulno-lunate, ulno-triquetral, and dorsal radiocarpal ligaments). In one study,[8] 11 patients with an average age of 45 years (21–62 years) were treated with a mean follow-up of 4.5 years. ROM improved in all aspects (Table 4).

Arthroscopic Arthrolysis. Arthroscopic release of the volar capsule may include the radio-scapho-lunate (RSL) ligament, the long radio-lunate (LRL) ligament, and the radio-scapho-capitate (RSC) ligament. The ulno-triquetral and ulno-lunate ligament were left intact[9] (Level V/GRADE 4). The most important finding in this technique was that sectioning of numerous ligaments did not result in ulnar or palmar translation.[10] With the addition of ulnar carpal (UC) sectioning palmar translation of the carpus occurred. The addition of sectioning of the dorsal ulnar (DUL) and palmar ulnar (PUL) ligaments led to ulnar translation as well. Although the numbers were small, the study described the safety of this technique to neighboring structures, along with improved wrist ROM flexion-extension, grip strength, and pain at 6 months after surgery. They also demonstrated that the median nerve and the radial artery are at a safe distance from the site of ligament resection (from 5 to 6 mm).

Another interesting arthroscopic study found three different types of radiocarpal septa[11] (Level IV/GRADE 3B): Type A, a single fibro-membranous structure completely divides the radiocarpal joint between the lunate and the scaphoid fossae (9 cases); Type B, membranous structures with a fenestration that partially divides the radiocarpal joint between the lunate and the scaphoid fossae (1 case); Type C, multiple bands

TABLE 4
Studies With Open Arthrolysis.

No.	Author	Year	Journal	Technique	No. of Cases	Age (yr)	Sex	Dominant hand	Follow up	Previous Surgeries	Measurements	Results		
1	af Ekenstam[14]	1988	Scandinavian Journal of Plastic and Reconstructive Surgery	Capsulotomy DRUJ	18	44 (17–67)	15 Women and 3 men	10 Dominant, 8 nondominant	1–6 years	15 Patients in 5 of whom the radius previously had been osteotomized. In the other 3 cases the TFCC was injured. In one case the ligament Injury was combined with an epiphysiolysis of the ulnae and in another it was combined with a complex transscaphoid perilunar dislocation.	Forearm rotation, pronation, supination. Grip strength, pain		Preop	Postop
												Forearm rotation	92 (40–125)	138 (70–175)
												Supination	45 (0–80)	66 (20–90)
												Pronation	46 (15–90)	71 (50–90)
												Grip strength	50%	70% (injured/uninjured hand)
												Pain: improved in 15, unchanged in 2, worse in 1.		
2	Kleinman and Graham[15]	1998	The Journal of Hand Surgery	Capsulotomy DRUJ–"Silhouette" resection	9	40 (25–48)	5 Women and 4 men	6 Dominant, 3 non dominant	Not reported	Eight of the 9 patients sustained displaced fractures of the distal radius and underwent open reduction and internal fixation. In 6 of these 8 patients, the original radius fracture extended into the sigmoid fossa of the distal radius.	Pain, extension, flexion, pronation, supination	Wrist extension and flexion improved approximately 20 degrees. Likewise, radial and ulnar deviation increased 5 and 9 degrees, respectively. Grip strength improved from an average of 36% of the contralateral side to 55%. Postoperative VAS was 3. The surgery was rated successful by all patients.		
3	Kamal and Ruch[8]	2017	J Hand Surg Am	Open Volar Capsular Release	11	45 (21–62)	6 Women and 5 men	Not reported	4.5 years	Volar plating for a distal radius fracture.	DASH, wrist flexion, extension, pronation, supination, VAS, ulnocarpal translocation		Preop	Postop
												Flexion	35.9±9.2	62.7±18.8
												Extension	24.8±15.5	58.6±13.4
												Pronation	61.5±12.6	75.9±9.2
												Supination	49.3±16.8	72.3±13.1
												DASH	45.9±15.5	9.6±12.9
												VAS	2.6±1.0	2.2±1.2

TABLE 5
Studies With Arthroscopic Arthrolysis.

No.	Author	Year	Journal	Technique	No. of Cases	Age (yr)	Sex	Dominant Hand	Follow Up	Previous Surgeries	Measurements	Results
1	Verhellen and Bain[9]	2000	Arthroscopy	Arthroscopic wrist arthrolysis	2	29 (23–35)	1 Woman and 1 man	Not reported	6 months	Case 1: excision of a large right lunate intraosseous ganglion and bone grafting from the ipsilateral distal radius metaphysis. Case 2: intraarticular distal radial fracture that was treated by closed reduction and percutaneous K-wire fixation.	Flexion-extension, pronation-supination, Grip strength, VAS.	Case 1: Flexion improved from 20 to 45 degrees. Extension improved from 10 to 50 degrees. Grip strength improved from 15 kg preoperatively to 42 kg postoperatively. Pain score measured on a visual analogue scale changed from 0 to 1 on a scale of 10. Case 2: Flexion improved from 15 to 50 degrees. Extension improved from 10 to 50 degrees. Grip strength improved from 12 kg preoperatively to 21 kg postoperatively. Visual analogue pain score decreased from 3 preoperatively to 1 postoperatively.
2	Hattori et al.[11]	2006	Arthroscopy	Arthroscopic wrist arthrolysis	11	40 (16–65)	2 Women and 9 men	Not reported	13 months (4–24)	Patients had previous surgeries for 8 fractures of the distal radius (6 intraarticular and 2 extra-articular), 1 Galeazzi fracture, 1 perilunate dislocation, and 1 carpal bone contusion. Internal fixation was carried out in 2 of 8 fractures of the distal radius, external fixation in 2.	Forearm rotation, pronation-supination, flexion, extension. Grip strength.	<table><tr><td></td><td>Preop</td><td>Postop</td></tr><tr><td>Forearm rotation</td><td>92 (40–125)</td><td>138 (70–175)</td></tr><tr><td>Supination</td><td>45 (0–80)</td><td>66 (20–90)</td></tr><tr><td>Pronation</td><td>46 (15–90)</td><td>71 (50–90)</td></tr><tr><td>Extension</td><td>47 (5–65)</td><td>56 (30–77)</td></tr><tr><td>Flexion</td><td>29 (5–53)</td><td>42 (15–62)</td></tr><tr><td>Grip strength</td><td>50%</td><td>70%</td></tr></table>
3	Luchetti et al.[12]	2007	Arthroscopy	Arthroscopic wrist arthrolysis	22 Patients	Mean age of 37 yr	6 Women and 16 men	22 Dominant	28 months (9–144)	All of the cases had incurred wrist rigidity as a result of prolonged Immobilization after wrist fracture.	Pain, flexion-extension, radial-ulnar deviation, pronation-supination. Grip strength, Mayo wrist score, DASH.	Flexion-extension Preop 83.6 (SD 28.8) Post op 98.68 (SD 10.5) Radio-ulnar Preop 42.82 (SD10.88) Post op 47.18 (SD 10.93). Prono-Supination Preop 143.95 (SD 34.44) Post op 159.09 (SD 18.23) Grip (kg) Preop 22.36 (10.36) Post op 28.36 (SD9 .65) Pain Preop 7.73 (SD 1.86) Post op 2.09 (SD 2.64) The mean modified Mayo wrist score improved from 28 preoperatively to 79 postoperatively, and the mean score on the DASH questionnaire was 21 points.

Continued

TABLE 5
Studies With Arthroscopic Arthrolysis—cont'd

No.	Author	Year	Journal	Technique	No. of Cases	Age (yr)	Sex	Dominant Hand	Follow Up	Previous Surgeries	Measurements	Results
4	Bain et al.[13]	2008	Techniques In Hand & Upper Extremity Surgery	Arthroscopic dorsal capsular release	12	Not reported	Not reported	Not reported	Not reported	Not reported	ROM, grip strength	A 75% improvement in range of motion and grip strength was reported by 9 of the 12 patients.
5	del Pinal et al.[16]	2018	J Hand Surg Am	Arthroscopic arthrolysis of the DRUJ	6	15–71 years	4 Women and 2 men	4 Dominant, 2 non dominant	3.3 years (1–6.4)	Five of them had sustained a distal radius fracture: 3 had been treated with a volar plate (1 of them for an extra-articular malunion), 1 with an external fixator and K-wires, and 1 had been treated in a cast.	Pain, flexion-extension, radial-ulnar, pronation-supination. Grip strength Mayo wrist score	Full effortless passive pronosupination was achieved in all patients. The mean supination was 76 degrees at the latest follow-up (50–90 degrees). Improvement in supination was 80 degrees (50–100 degrees). Pronation also improved by a mean of 17 degrees. The total arc of improvement in pronosupination was 97 degrees (70–120 degrees). There were no cases of DRUJ instability, ulnar wrist pain, or other complications

of fibrous tissue are formed between radiocarpal articulations. They did a simple section of the radiocarpal septum obtaining a significant increase of ROM. No complications were observed. We also found increased in ROM after arthroscopic arthrolysis without any complications[12] (Level IV/GRADE 3B).

Dorsal arthroscopic capsular release is another interesting option with a 75% improvement in ROM and grip strength[13] (Level V/GRADE 4). The structures most at risk when performing this procedure are the extensor tendons and structures surrounding the arthroscopy portals. It has been advised to use a nylon tape passed through the 3–4 portal to the level of the tendon-capsule interface, then along this plane and out again via the 6R portal.[13] With traction on this tape, you can pull the tendons away from the capsule increasing the safe zone for the capsular release.

Distal Radio-Ulnar Joint

Open Arthrolysis. In wrist stiffness after DRFs it has been known for many years that if there is deficit of pronation, a dorsal capsulotomy should be used, while in restricted supination you should use a volar approach[14] (Level IV/GRADE 3B). In cases of combined restricted pronation and supination, you can combine volar and dorsal approach.[14] In this historic paper, no complications were found and ROM improved as well as grip strength.[14]

A so-called "silhouette" capsulectomy of the volar capsule of the DRUJ is an interesting option for the loss of supination and of the dorsal DRUJ capsule for the loss of pronation[15] (Level IV/GRADE 3B). The technique is to excise the DRUJ capsule from its insertions into the radius, TFCC and ulna with improved ROM, grip strength and without complications.[15]

Arthroscopic Arthrolysis. We have described a method to perform an arthroscopic release of DRUJ contractures by using DRUJ portals[12] (Level IV/GRADE 3B). We introduced a dissector into the proximal portal and released the adhesions between the ulnar head and the sigmoid fossa with a significant increase in pronosupination.[12]

In extreme losses of 90 degrees supination there is a specialized technique using a curved periosteal elevator inserted through the 6R portal into the volar-radial corner of the TFCC and advanced proximally gliding on the anterior ulnar head surface[16] (Level IV/GRADE 3B). The volar capsule and the ulnar head are thereby released. The arthroscopic arthrolysis can be combined with a manipulation by the surgeon. Postoperatively full supination was maintained in an orthosis for 2–3 days and a significant improvement can be expected without DRUJ instability or other complications[16] (Level IV/GRADE 3B).

RECOMMENDATION

All studies were Level IV and Level V, therefore achieving only low GRADE of evidence (3B-4). No studies compared open and arthroscopic arthrolysis of the RC joint or DRUJ, hence the evidence for these procedures is weak. However, all of them demonstrated that wrist arthrolysis works well, giving an improvement of motion of the RC joint and DRUJ, without causing instability.

Panel 2: Author's Preferred Technique

In cases of RC wrist stiffness due to a DRF treated with cast (Case scenario 1) the authors prefer the arthroscopic arthrolysis after a proper rehabilitation period.

This procedure is called an "in-out progressive technique." The first step of this technique is the resection of the fibrotic bands (Fig. 3) and the adherences between the dorsal capsule and the lunate and scaphoid (Fig. 4). After the first step, the wrist motility is checked and if the motion is sufficiently improved the second step is not necessary.

The second step is to consider resection of the volar capsular contracture (Fig. 5).

The patient presented in Case scenario 1 obtained an important but incomplete improvement of wrist ROM (FE = 50 degrees / PS = 120 degrees) and pain 1 (according with VAS scale 0–10) at 3 years of follow-up (Fig. 6A–D).

In case of RC wrist stiffness due to previous distal radius volar plate fixation (Case scenario 2) the authors prefer open surgery which we call an "out-in progressive technique":

The first step is to remove the plate. The second step is to resect the volar RC ligaments (Fig. 7) with scalpel and internal fibrotic band resection and dorsal capsular adherences detachment with a curved periosteal elevator.

Even during this technique the wrist motility is checked after each step. It means that if the wrist motion is totally or sufficiently improved after the first step the procedure is stopped.

Continued

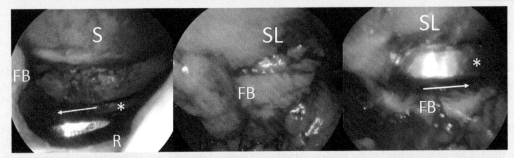

FIG. 3 Resection of the fibrotic band with a hook blade (A–C) introduced into the RC joint through the 3–4 portal under arthroscopic control in 6R portal. [(FB=fibrotic band, R=radius, S=scaphoid, L=lunate, SL=scapho-lunate ligament, *=hook blade, *white arrows* that show the direction of the hook blade at the entrance into the RC joint (A) and at the fibrotic band resection (C).

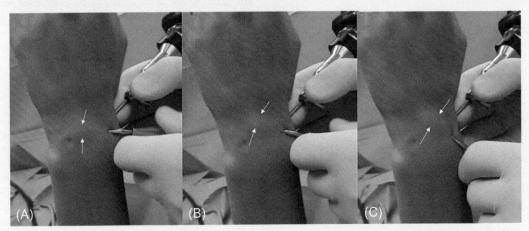

FIG. 4 Arthroscopic detachment of the adherences between the dorsal capsule and the carpal bones (A–C). Note the position of the tip of the periosteal elevator *(white arrows)* under the skin of the dorsal wrist and the direction by which it is moved: from ulnar to radial in a round and curved fashion. Arthroscope in 1–2 portal and periosteal elevator in 3–4 portal.

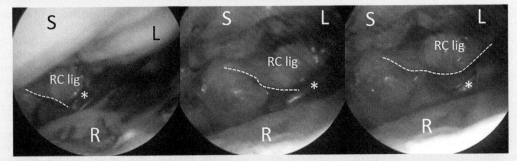

FIG. 5 Arthroscopic images showing the resection of the radio carpal volar ligament. The hook blade, introduced into the RC joint through the 6R portal, reaches the most radial part of the volar RC ligament and inserted into the RC ligament with a progressive retraction produce the resection of this ligament. [R=radius, S=scaphoid, L=lunate, RC lig=radio-carpal ligament, *=hook blade, dotted white line corresponds to the margin of the most lateral side of the RC ligament.

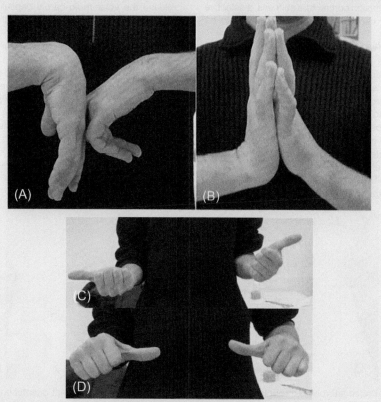

FIG. 6 Clinical result of open arthrolysis of the radio-carpal joint and the DRUJ. Wrist motion recovered almost completely at 3 months of follow-up (A–D).

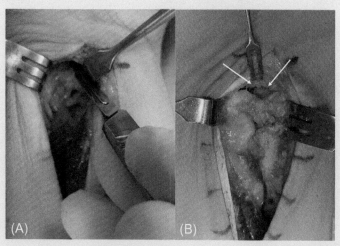

FIG. 7 Intraoperative images showing (A) the technique of resection of the RC ligaments after plate removed; (B) RC joint becomes evident through the RC ligaments resected.

Continued

In cases with extension contracture stiffness, a selective arthroscopic dorsal capsule resection (Fig. 4) should be sufficient.

In cases with DRUJ stiffness, the volar and/or dorsal capsule resection is performed by open surgery through dedicated anterior and/or posterior approaches. Isolated pronation stiffness is treated with a dorsal approach to the DRUJ (Fig. 8): the dorsal capsule is released improving the pronation. Through the dorsal approach it is possible to release the volar capsule, too.

If the stiffness involves only supination, a selective volar approach is suggested. If the supination stiffness isassociated with wrist extension stiffness (flexion-pronation contracture), the volar DRUJ capsule contracture could be resected (Fig. 9) through the same approach adopted to release the volar radio-carpal capsule (and remove, for example, a DR palmar plate) (Fig. 7), without using a second more ulnar approach.

The patient presented in Case scenario 2 obtained an improvement of wrist ROM and pain 0 (according with VAS scale 0–10) at 1 year of follow-up (Fig. 10A–D).

Arthroscopic DRUJ arthrolysis is frequently adopted in association with RC arthrolysis. Improvement of the prono-supination may be obtained through the release of the volar and dorsal adherence using the periosteal elevator under arthroscopic control (Fig. 11).

Isolated arthroscopic DRUJ arthrolysis is rare and more difficult than the open approach but allows achieving similar results.

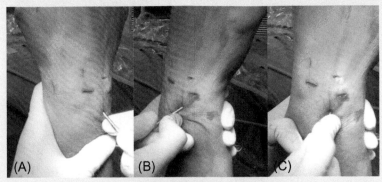

FIG. 8 DRUJ open arthrolysis through the dorsal approach (A–C). Note the different orientations of the periosteal elevator into the DRUJ and around the ulnar head.

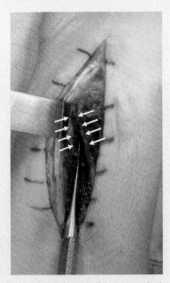

FIG. 9 Intraoperative image which shows that it is possible to reach the DRUJ through the volar approach used to remove the palmar plate from the distal radius. The resection of the DRUJ volar capsule *(white arrows)* has been done and with the periosteal elevator introduced deeply into the joint the surgeon tries to detach the dorsal adherences with resection of the dorsal capsule improving both the supination and the pronation.

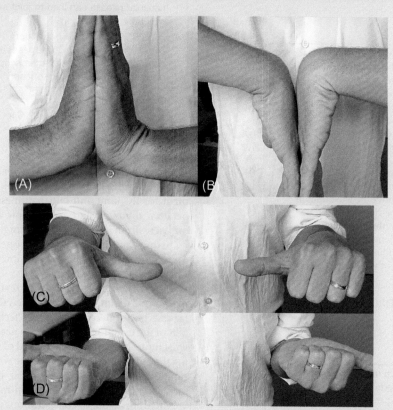

FIG. 10 Clinical result of the patient presented in case scenario 2 after open RC joint and DRUJ arthrolysis.

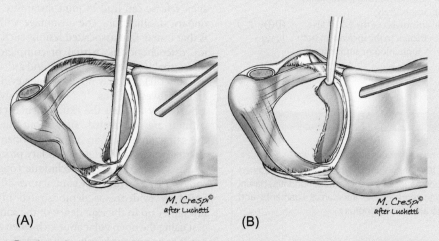

FIG. 11 Drawings showing the technique of the arthroscopic dorsal and volar capsule adherences of the DRUJ.

In patients with RC wrist joint stiffness after DRF, evidence suggests:

Recommendation	Overall Quality
• Open arthrolysis with volar approach for RC joint rigidity can be useful to obtain an improvement in wrist extension and pain.	⊕⊕◯◯ LOW
• Open arthrolysis with dorsal approach should be used for wrist stiffness in which flexion has to be improved.	⊕⊕◯◯ LOW
• Arthroscopic arthrolysis is also valid for both flexion and extension stiffness of the RC joint.	⊕⊕◯◯ LOW
• Arthroscopic arthrolysis allows resection to start with the internal fibrotic bands. This resection can improve the wrist motion without adding the capsular resection.	⊕⊕◯◯ LOW
• Volar and dorsal arthroscopic capsular resection can be done in isolation or in association to the fibrotic bands to complete the improvement of wrist extension or flexion, or both.	⊕⊕◯◯ LOW

In patients with DRUJ stiffness after DRF, evidence suggests:

Recommendation	Overall Quality
• The volar approach used for RC joint volar capsular open resection, allows resection of the volar DRUJ capsule providing a good improvement of supination.	⊕⊕◯◯ LOW
• Selective volar or dorsal open approach to the DRUJ allows release of the volar or the dorsal DRUJ capsule improving supination or pronation, respectively.	⊕⊕◯◯ LOW
• Arthroscopic arthrolysis of the DRUJ also proved to be efficient in the increase of both pronation and supination or supination in isolation.	⊕⊕◯◯ LOW

Panel 3

PEARLS

OPEN: lower costs, shorter surgical time, safe.

ARTHROSCOPY: arthroscopy may find associated lesions such as loose bodies, osteochondritis, partial or complete tears of the intercarpal ligaments and TFCC, and articular incongruity.

PITFALLS

OPEN: greater tissue damage could lead to pain, edema and a risk of recurrent stiffness. An extensive open

---

Panel 3—cont'd

capsular release can lead to joint instability requiring secondary stabilization.

ARTHROSCOPY: arthroscopy of both the RC joint and he DRUJ is very difficult in these cases and should only be done by experts in wrist arthroscopy. Conversion to open surgery is always an option.

CONCLUSION

The systematic review for this chapter demonstrates satisfactory results in both arthroscopic and open treatment for RC joint and DRUJ stiffness. The differences between the open and arthroscopic arthrolysis are, in our view, in the direction of the surgical procedure.

In open arthrolysis, the joint is opened from external capsular resection followed by internal resection of fibrosis ("out-in technique").

In arthroscopic arthrolysis we first release the internal fibrotic bands and fibrosis, then the external capsular resection if necessary ("in-out technique"). The last part of the technique is not always needed, if a sufficient wrist motion is obtained at the end of the first part. During the arthroscopic arthrolysis, the wrist motion is constantly evaluated and if the wrist motion gained is satisfactorily the capsular resection may not be done.

There are no major complications reported in the literature. One of the potential drawbacks for open surgery is a greater tissue damage that could lead to pain, edema and a risk of recurrent stiffness. An extensive open capsular release can lead to joint instability requiring secondary stabilization. The advantage with arthroscopy is that it may find associated lesions such as loose bodies, osteochondritis, partial or complete tears of the intercarpal ligaments and TFCC, and articular incongruity (step-off) that may not have been evident on preoperative investigations.[17, 18] The disadvantages with arthroscopy are that the extra-articular causes of wrist stiffness are not treated. They should be addressed at the same time with an associated open approach or alternatively as a separate secondary procedure.

The choice of surgical technique (open or arthroscopy) in cases with wrist contractures after DRF is not based by evidence as demonstrated in our chapter, but rather up to the experience of the surgeon. We suggest using the open volar approach when a palmar plate needs to be removed, leaving the arthroscopic technique to cases which was initially treated conservatively and to be done by expert arthroscopists.

REFERENCES

1. Yu YR, Makhni MC, Tabrizi S, Rozental TD, Mundanthanam G, Day CS. Complications of low-profile dorsal versus volar locking plates in the distal radius: a comparative study. *J Hand Surg Am.* 2011;36 (7):1135–1141.

2. Maloney MD, Sauser DD, Hanson EC, et al. Adhesive capsulitis of the wrist: arthrographic diagnosis. *Radiology.* 1988;167:187–190.

3. Hanson EC, Wood VE, Thiel AE, Maloney MD, Sauser DD. Adhesive capsulitis of the wrist. Diagnosis and treatment. *Clin Orthop Relat Res.* 1988;234:51–55.

4. Lee SK, Gargano F, Hausman MR. Wrist arthrofibrosis. *Hand Clin.* 2006;22:529–538 [abstract vii].

5. Sackett DL. Rules of evidence and clinical recommendation on the use of antithrombotic agent. *Chest.* 1989;95(Suppl. 2):3S.

6. Schünemann HJ, Bone L. Evidence-based orthopaedics: a primer. *Clin Orthop Relat Res.* 2003;413:117–132.

7. Guyatt G, Oxman AD, Akl EA, et al. GRADE guidelines: 1. Introduction-GRADE: evidence profiles and summary of findings tables. *J Clin Epidemiol.* 2011;64(4):383–394.

8. Kamal RN, Ruch DS. Volar capsular release after distal radius fractures. *J Hand Surg Am.* 2017;42:1034.e1–1034. e6.

9. Verhellen R, Bain GI. Arthroscopic capsular release for contracture of the wrist: a new technique. *Art Ther.* 2000;16:106–110.

10. Viegas SF, Patterson RM, Eng M, Ward K. Extrinsic wrist ligaments in the pathomechanics of ulnar translation instability. *J Hand Surg [Am].* 1995;20:312–318.

11. Hattori T, Tsunoda K, Watanabe K, et al. Arthroscopic mobilization for contracture of the wrist. *Art Ther.* 2006;22:850–854.

12. Luchetti R, Atzei A, Fairplay T. Arthroscopic wrist arthrolysis after wrist fracture. *Art Ther.* 2007;23(3): 255–260.

13. Bain GI, Munt J, Turner PC, Bergman J. Arthroscopic dorsal capsular release in the wrist: a new technique. *Tech Hand Up Extrem Surg.* 2008;12:191–194.

14. af Ekenstam FW. Capsulotomy of the distal radio-ulnar joint. *Scand J Plast Surg.* 1988;22:169–171.

15. Kleinman WB, Graham TJ. The distal radioulnar joint capsule: clinical anatomy and role in posttraumatic limitation of forearm rotation. *J Hand Surg Am.* 1998;23 (4):588–599.

16. Del Piñal F, Moraleda E, Rúas JS, et al. Effectiveness of an arthroscopic technique to correct supination losses of 90 degrees or more. *J Hand Surg Am.* 2018;43:676.e1–676.e6.

17. Luchetti R, Bain G, Morse L, McGuire D. Arthroscopic arthrolysis. In: Randelli P, et al., eds. *Arthroscopy.* Berlin, Heidelberg: Springer Verlag; 2016:935–951.

18. McGuire DT, Luchetti R, Atzei A, Bain GI. Arthroscopic arthrolysis. In: Geissler WB, ed. *Wrist and Elbow Arthroscopy.* New York: Springer Science Business Media; 2015:165–175.

Index

Note: Page numbers followed by *f* indicate figures, *t* indicate tables, and *b* indicate boxes.

Printed and bound by CPI Group (UK) Ltd, Croydon, CR0 4YY

12/05/2025

01867590-0001